The Impact of Vitamin D on Health and Disease

The Impact of Vitamin D on Health and Disease

Beyond the Bones

Edited by

Rehana Rehman

Department of Biological & Biomedical Sciences, Aga Khan University, Karachi, Pakistan

Faiza Alam

Pengiran-Anak-Puteri-Rashidah-Sa'adatul-Bolkiah Institute of Health Sciences, Universiti Brunei Darussalam, Bandar Seri Begawan, Brunei Darussalam

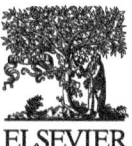

ELSEVIER

Elsevier
Radarweg 29, PO Box 211, 1000 AE Amsterdam, Netherlands
125 London Wall, London EC2Y 5AS, United Kingdom
50 Hampshire Street, 5th Floor, Cambridge, MA 02139, United States

Notices
Knowledge and best practice in this field are constantly changing. As new research and experience broaden our understanding, changes in research methods, professional practices, or medical treatment may become necessary.

Practitioners and researchers must always rely on their own experience and knowledge in evaluating and using any information, methods, compounds, or experiments described herein. In using such information or methods they should be mindful of their own safety and the safety of others, including parties for whom they have a professional responsibility.

To the fullest extent of the law, neither the Publisher nor the authors, contributors, or editors, assume any liability for any injury and/or damage to persons or property as a matter of products liability, negligence or otherwise, or from any use or operation of any methods, products, instructions, or ideas contained in the material herein.

ISBN: 978-0-443-34037-6

For Information on all Elsevier publications
visit our website at https://www.elsevier.com/books-and-journals

Publisher: Megan Ball
Acquisitions Editor: Patricia Osborn
Editorial Project Manager: Tracy Tugafa
Production Project Manager: Fahmida Sultana
Cover Designer: Mark Rogers

Typeset by MPS Limited, Chennai, India

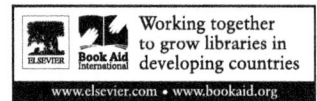

Working together
to grow libraries in
developing countries

www.elsevier.com • www.bookaid.org

Contents

Section 1   Unlocking the source code of vitamin D

Ambreen Surti, Haseeb Waheed and Rehana Rehman

Faiza Alam, Mussarat Ashraf and Maah Amir

Section 2   The power of D: health, performance, and global impact

Chapter 5: Vitamin D and sports performance 53

Mirza Mohammad Feisal Subhan

Chapter 14: Vitamin D: illuminating the shadows of pancreatic dysfunction.........203

Faiza Alam, Fasiha Fatima and Ihsan Nazurah Zulkipli

Chapter 15: Vitamin D and metabolic syndrome-associated diseases: interconnections and implications 227

Salaar Ahmed and Syeda Sadia Fatima

Chapter 16: Vitamin D and Reproductive health: a critical link of vitamin D deficiency with subfertility 245

Arfa Azhar, Rehana Rehman and Chaman Nasrullah

Chapter 21: Rare disorders of vitamin D metabolism

Aysha Habib Khan and Manju Chandran

Chapter 22: Vitamin D, pregnancy, and child health

Rehana Rehman and Shaheen Basheer

Chapter 23: Vitamin D and Mental Health: From Neurobiology to Clinical
Outcomes *337*

Aisha Noorullah, Nargis Asad and Shahina Pirani

Section 4   Optimising health with vitamin D: Clinical tools, public solutions, and future possibilities

Chapter 29: The Vitamin D supplementation protocols 431

Lena Jafri, Hafsa Majid and Nayab Afzal

Chapter 30: Vitamin D therapy: a promising appraoch for subfertility 445

Chaman Nasrullah, Fatima Syed and Rehana Rehman

List of contributors

Farzana Abubakar Department of Biological & Biomedical Sciences, Aga Khan University, Karachi, Pakistan

Nayab Afzal Pathology and Laboratory Medicine, Aga Khan University, Karachi, Sindh, Pakistan

Liyana Ahmad Pengiran-Anak-Puteri-Rashidah-Sa'adatul-Bolkiah Institute of Health Sciences, Universiti Brunei Darussalam, Bandar Seri Begawan, Brunei Darussalam

Siti Rohaiza Ahmad PAPRSB Institute of Health Sciences, Universiti Brunei Darussalam, Bandar Seri Begawan, Brunei-Muara, Brunei

Khalid Ahmed Department of Biological & Biomedical Sciences, Aga Khan University, Karachi, Pakistan

Salaar Ahmed Medical College, Aga Khan University, Karachi, Pakistan

Sibtain Ahmed Section of Chemical Pathology, Department of Pathology and Laboratory Medicine, Aga Khan University, Karachi, Sindh, Pakistan

Faiza Alam Pengiran-Anak-Puteri-Rashidah-Sa'adatul-Bolkiah Institute of Health Sciences, Universiti Brunei Darussalam, Bandar Seri Begawan, Brunei Darussalam

Rabiya Ali Karachi Institute of Medical Sciences, National University of Medical Sciences, Islamabad, Punjab, Pakistan

Bushra Madad Ali Malik Department of Health, Physical Education and Sport Sciences, University of Karachi, Karachi, Pakistan

Maah Amir Medical College, Aga Khan University, Karachi, Pakistan

Sofia Amjad Department of Physiology, Faculty of Medical Sciences, Azra Naheed Medical College, The Superior University, Lahore, Pakistan; Department of Physiology, Ziaudin University, Karachi, Pakistan

Amna Ansari Medical College, Aga Khan University, Karachi, Pakistan

Tarek Arabi College of Medicine, Alfaisal University, Riyadh, Saudi Arabia

Nargis Asad Department of Psychiatry, Aga Khan University, Karachi, Pakistan

Mussarat Ashraf Department of Biological & Biomedical Sciences, Aga Khan University, Karachi, Pakistan

Arfa Azhar University College of Medicine & Dentistry, The University of Lahore, Lahore, Pakistan

Shaheen Basheer Western Health and Social Care Trust, Obstetrics & Gynaecology, South West Acute Hospital, Enniskillen United Kingdom

Shiza Batool Instit fuer Didaktik und Ausbildungsforschung in der Medizin, Ludwig Maximilian University, Munich, Germany

Manju Chandran Osteoporosis and Bone Metabolism Unit, Department of Endocrinology, Singapore General Hospital, Singapore; DUKE NUS Medical School, Singapore

Fasiha Fatima Karachi Institute of Medical Sciences, National University of Medical Sciences, Punjab, Pakistan

Irum Fatima Department of Education, Sindh Madrasatul Islam University, Karachi, Pakistan

Kiran Fatima Department of Community Medicine, Sindh Medical College, Jinnah Sindh Medical University, Karachi, Pakistan

Syeda Sadia Fatima Department of Biological & Biomedical Sciences, Aga Khan University, Karachi, Pakistan

Kiren Habib Section of Adult Infectious Diseases, Department of Medicine, Aga Khan University, Karachi, Sindh, Pakistan

Mohammad Perwaiz Iqbal Biochemistry, Biological & Biomedical Sciences, Aga Khan University, Karachi, Pakistan; Life Sciences Department, School of Science, University of Management and Technology, Lahore, Pakistan

Nousheen Iqbal Department of Medicine, Aga Khan University, Karachi, Pakistan; Department of Medicine, Jinnah Medical and Dental College, Karachi, Pakistan

Saira Perwaiz Iqbal Infectious Diseases, Department of Medicine, Maimonides Medical Center, Brooklyn, NY, United States

Muhammad Irfan Department of Medicine, Aga Khan University, Karachi, Pakistan

Lena Jafri Section of Chemical Pathology, Department of Pathology and Laboratory Medicine, Aga Khan University, Karachi, Sindh, Pakistan

Aysha Habib Khan Department of Pathology & Laboratory Medicine, The Aga Khan University, Karachi, Pakistan

Nighat Nisar Khan Community Health Sciences, Dow Medical College, Dow University of Health Sciences, Karachi, Pakistan

Rabia Mahmood Khan Community Rehabilitation GP, Community Hospital, Oxford University Health and Care Trust, Oxford, United Kingdom; Bartlemas Surgery, Oxford, United Kingdom; Witney Community Hospital, Oxford University Health and Care Trust; Bartlemas Surgery, Manzil Way, Cowley, Oxfordshire, United Kingdom

Iffat Khanum Section of Adult Infectious Diseases, Department of Medicine, Aga Khan University, Karachi, Sindh, Pakistan

Ya Chee Lim PAPRSB Institute of Health Sciences, Universiti Brunei Darussalam, Bandar Seri Begawan, Brunei-Muara, Brunei

Hafsa Majid Pathology and Laboratory Medicine, Aga Khan University, Karachi, Sindh, Pakistan

Munazza Raza Mirza Dr. Panjwani Center for Molecular Medicine and Drug Research, International Center for Chemical and Biological Sciences, Karachi, Pakistan

Nosheen Nasir Section of Adult Infectious Diseases, Department of Medicine, Aga Khan University, Karachi, Sindh, Pakistan

Chaman Nasrullah University College of Medicine & Dentistry, The University of Lahore, Lahore, Pakistan

Mahwish Nida Geratology, Oxford University Hospital, Oxford, United Kingdom

Aisha Noorullah Department of Psychiatry, Aga Khan University, Karachi, Pakistan

Shahina Pirani Department of Psychiatry, Aga Khan University, Karachi, Pakistan

Rehana Rehman Department of Biological & Biomedical Sciences, Aga Khan University, Karachi, Pakistan

Nazra Remtulla Department of Biology, Western University, London, ON, Canada

Dileep Kumar Rohra Department of Pharmacology, College of Medicine, Alfaisal University, Riyadh, Saudi Arabia

Belal Nedal Sabbah College of Medicine, Alfaisal University, Riyadh, Saudi Arabia

Mirza Mohammad Feisal Subhan School of Biomedical Sciences, Faaculty of Health, University of Plymouth, Plymouth, Devon, United Kingdom

Rabia Sultan Dr. Panjwani Center for Molecular Medicine and Drug Research, International Center for Chemical and Biological Sciences, Karachi, Pakistan

Rashida Sultana Department of Obstetrics and Gynaecology, Azra Naheed Medical College, Faculty of Medical Sciences, The Superior University, Lahore, Punjab, Pakistan

Ambreen Surti Department of Biological & Biomedical Sciences, Aga Khan University, Karachi, Pakistan

Fatima Syed Department of Pathology, Fazaia Ruth Pfau Medical College, Karachi, Pakistan

Midrar Ullah Department of Medicine, Aga Khan University, Karachi, Pakistan

Soma Vankwani Dr. Panjwani Center for Molecular Medicine and Drug Research, International Center for Chemical and Biological Sciences, Karachi, Pakistan

Haseeb Waheed Aga Khan University Medical College, The Aga Khan University, Karachi, Pakistan

Samar Zaki Department of Family Medicine, Aga Khan University Hospital, Karachi, Sindh, Pakistan

Ihsan Nazurah Zulkipli Pengiran-Anak-Puteri-Rashidah-Sa'adatul-Bolkiah Institute of Health Sciences, Universiti Brunei Darussalam, Bandar Seri Begawan, Brunei Darussalam

Foreword

The understanding of the role of vitamin D in health and disease has advanced significantly in the last 10 years. From the well-recognized role in calcium homeostasis and musculoskeletal health to its role in immune function and mental health, interest in vitamin D has moved at pace. Vitamin D gained much attention during the COVID-19 pandemic as clinicians and researchers debated the role of vitamin D status and the severity of the disease. We have since continued deepening our understanding of the immune modulatory function of vitamin D—its role in innate immunity and defense from infectious diseases. This book brings together worldwide research, forming an up-to-date review of the dietary sources of vitamin D, its metabolism, and its influence on many physiological processes, including immunity. Crucially, it includes the latest advances in our understanding of genetic variability in vitamin D metabolism and the interplay of epigenetics.

Vitamin D is an interesting micronutrient as it can be obtained via dietary sources and synthesized in the body from the action of sunlight on 7-dehydrocholesterol, a cholesterol precursor. This makes it difficult to estimate a dietary requirement as people can synthesize significant amounts from sunlight exposure. However, vitamin D deficiency is all too common throughout the world, and this is explored in Chapter 12. Deficiency is common in higher latitudes due to insufficient UVB radiation at appropriate wavelengths in winter months, but it is also common in hotter climates as people avoid direct sunlight on the skin either for cultural and religious reasons or due to health and lifestyle choices. Chapters in this book highlight the detrimental effect of insufficient vitamin D status throughout the lifecycle on fertility, fetal and child development, aging, health outcomes, and sports performance. The detailed mechanisms by which vitamin D modulates disease risk, for example, in pancreatic dysfunction, cancer, and respiratory and cardiovascular diseases, are reviewed through its influence on inflammation, endothelial function, and oxidative stress.

There remains much work to be done to encourage sufficient consumption of vitamin D–rich foods, fortification of suitable products, and supplementation. Chapters 31 and 32 discuss tips for maintaining optimal vitamin D concentrations and supplementation protocols. Public health initiatives for promotion of awareness of the importance of vitamin D and supplementation programs are also covered in Chapter 34.

This book brings together authors of different specialist backgrounds to produce a comprehensive review of topics in vitamin D nutrition and metabolism, which will be of benefit to clinicians, researchers, educators, and students alike. It is vital for us all to stay informed, and this book advances our understanding of this important and fascinating nutrient. I hope you are enthused to learn more, collaborate, and work towards optimizing vitamin D status to advance the health of populations around the world.

Preface

Vitamin D is known to be the "sunshine vitamin," keeping our bony infrastructure strong and healthy. It also exerts a strong influence on various physiological functions, immune modulations, athletic abilities, and overall health status. However, millions of people around us are still falling short on the bare minimum knowledge of the benefits of vitamin D, hence improving the status and compromising a healthy life. This book is not just a dive into the deep seas of science, but it also establishes a pilot to make vitamin D drive our lives towards health, with a blend of cutting-edge research and multiple evidence.

We have systematized this book into four discrete segments to comprehensively understand the subject. The **first section** (Unlocking the Source Code of Vitamin D: Chapters 1–3) walks you through the sources, bioavailability, biochemistry, mechanism of action, target organs, and different research perspectives of vitamin D. The **second section** (The Power of D: Health, Performance, and Global Impact: Chapters 4–11) is dedicated to the vitamin D's association with bone integrity, epigenetic mechanisms, genetic predispositions, athletic abilities, and universal insinuations, contributing to regional disparities in evaluating vitamin D status. Chapters 12–26 in the **third section** (The Health Matrix: Vitamin D and the Many Systems It Touches) magnify its role across various physiological systems, incorporating the immune, cardiovascular, endocrine, and neurological systems. This section also emphasizes vitamin D's impact on exacerbations in diabetes mellitus, cardiovascular disorders, autoimmune diseases, and mental health, highlighting its broad-spectrum benefits and preventative potential. The **fourth section** (Optimizing Health with Vitamin D: Clinical Tools, Public Solutions, and Future Possibilities: Chapters 27–32) defines the "action plan," concentrating on the clinical guidelines and recommendations. This section accumulates lots of evidence-based policies for vitamin D supplementation, dietary consumption, and lifestyle alterations to boost health. Furthermore, it also offers recent endorsements from global health institutions, addressing dosage recommendations for different inhabitants of all age groups. While scientific novelties continue to untangle the intricacies of this indispensable nutrient, it is imperative to know and be practical in tackling vitamin D deficiency on individual and public health levels.

We hope this book brings transparency, sparks further inquiries, and supplements the ongoing dialogue on the grave character of vitamin D. We are gratified towards our readers and welcome their perspectives and opinions.

So, let us light our worlds, factually and metaphorically. "A big shout out to tougher bones, happier days, and a healthful world with one vitamin D molecule at a time."

Best Wishes,

Dr. Rehana Rehman, Professor

Department of Biological & Biomedical Sciences, Aga Khan University, Karachi, Pakistan

Dr. Faiza Alam, Assistant Professor Clinical Academia

PAPRSB Institute of Health Sciences, Universiti Brunei Darussalam, Bandar Seri Begawan, Brunei Darussalam

Fig. 1

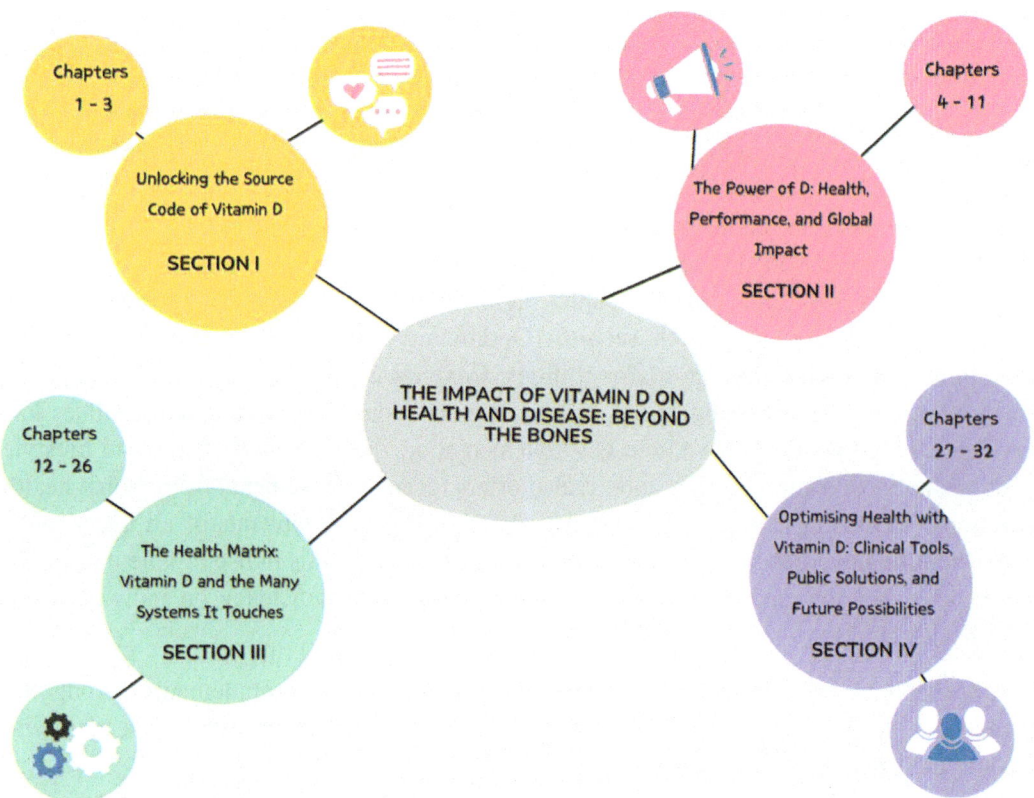

Figure 1
The book at a glance: a preface-inspired concept map.

Unlocking the source code of vitamin D

CHAPTER 1

Environmental factors and vitamin D

Ambreen Surti[1], Haseeb Waheed[2], and Rehana Rehman[1]

[1]*Department of Biological & Biomedical Sciences, Aga Khan University, Karachi, Pakistan* [2]*Aga Khan University Medical College, The Aga Khan University, Karachi, Pakistan*

1.1 Introduction

First species of Homonins developed receptors for vitamin D approximately 550 years ago. This receptor had the ability to bind to 1α,25-dihydroxyvitamin D3, a metabolite of vitamin D. Evolving from a subfamily of nuclear receptors, it can sense the derivatives of cholesterol and can control the genes taking part in immune responses. Vitamin D endocrinology started when some 550 million years ago first species developed a vitamin D receptor (VDR) that binds with the high-affinity vitamin D metabolite 1α,25-dihydroxyvitamin D3. The evolutionary development of the immune system and skeletal system exhibits a synchronous relationship. The close interaction between the osteogenic and immune systems is strongly regulated by vitamin D levels (DeLuca, 2004; Hanel & Carlberg, 2020).

Vitamin D is a crucial nutrient for the maintenance of bone health, support of the immune system, and regulation of calcium metabolism (Holick, 2008). In contrast to most nutrients, vitamin D is recognized not only as a vitamin but also as a prohormone due to its essential role in various biological processes (DeLuca, 2004). While diet plays a role in providing vitamin D, environmental factors that influence its synthesis and absorption are far more critical in ensuring the adequate maintenance of this essential nutrient (Vieth, 1999). Most significantly, sunlight exposure triggers the body's natural production of vitamin D, accounting for more than 85% of the regular intake in most individuals along (Holick, 2008). Several factors like pollution, aging, and geographic location play an impactful role in its synthesis and absorption (Rosen, 2011).

1.2 Sources of vitamin D
- Sunlight
- Dietary

The Impact of Vitamin D on Health and Disease. DOI: https://doi.org/10.1016/B978-0-443-34037-6.00027-3

1.2.1   Sunlight exposure

Sunlight is the primary source of vitamin D for the vast majority of individuals (MacLaughlin & Holick, 1985). The exposure of the skin to ultraviolet B (UVB) radiation initiates a multistep process that is finely regulated by the body. With an optimal wavelength of UVB between 290 and 315 nm, the process of vitamin D synthesis begins in the skin, making up nearly 90% of the body's requirement (Grant, 2010). The cholesterol-derived molecule, 7-dehydrocholesterol, present in the epidermis, undergoes a photochemical conversion to previtamin D3 upon UVB exposure (Sunyecz, 2008). This previtamin, being unstable, is subsequently isomerized within hours under the influence of body heat, transforming into vitamin D3 (cholecalciferol) (Holick & Slominski, 2024). However, it is essential to note that not all previtamin D3 is converted into its active forms (Holick & Chen, 2008). This thermal conversion signifies the end of the epidermal reactions, after which vitamin D3 is released into the bloodstream (Chakhtoura et al., 2020). Here, it binds to vitamin D-binding protein (DBP), and this complex is then transported to the liver and kidneys, where further metabolism occurs to produce the biologically active forms of vitamin D (Veldurthy et al., 2016).

1.2.1.1   Factors affecting sunlight exposure

Being the most important source of this nutrient, several factors influence the amount of UVB radiation an individual receives and, consequently, their ability to synthesize vitamin D.

1.2.1.1.1   Latitude

The radiations from the sun are concentrated most at the equator (Giannini et al., 2022). The greater availability of sun rays at the equator means a greater source of vitamin D for people living in equatorial regions (Holick, 1995). In contrast, those residing at higher latitudes (further north or south) experience reduced UVB exposure, particularly during winter months, which significantly impacts their vitamin D levels (Manisalidis et al., 2020).

1.2.1.1.2   Season

UVB radiation is more intense during the summer, leading to higher vitamin D synthesis (Hughes & Norton, 2009). In the winter, the sun's angle is lowest on the horizon, which leads to decreased UVB exposure and subsequently reduced vitamin D production (Yang et al., 2021).

1.2.1.1.3   Time of day

UVB radiation is most potent between 10 a.m. and 4 p.m., when the sun is at its highest point in the sky (Libon et al.,2013). Exposure during this time frame can significantly boost vitamin D production (Arshad & Zaidi, 2022). However, exposure outside these peak hours results in much lower synthesis (Neale et al., 2019).

1.2.1.1.4 Skin pigmentation

Melanin, the pigment responsible for skin color, acts as a natural sunscreen by absorbing UVB radiation (Gasparro, A Review of Sunscreen Safety and Efficacy, 1998). This means individuals with darker skin tones require more prolonged sunlight exposure to produce adequate amounts of vitamin D, as the higher melanin content reduces UVB penetration into the skin (Martin-Gorgojo et al., 2021).

1.2.1.1.5 Clothing

Clothing that covers the skin, such as long sleeves, hats, or veils, can block UVB rays and limit vitamin D synthesis (Yeum et al., 2016). The cultural and religious practice of wearing full-body clothing, prevalent in some regions, further exacerbates the risk of vitamin D deficiency in those populations (Wacker & Holick, 2013)

1.2.1.2 Recommendations for safe and effective sun exposure

While sunlight is essential for vitamin D production, it is equally important to balance this with the need for skin protection, particularly given the risks of skin cancer, such as melanoma, from excessive UV exposure (Raymond-Lezman & Riskin, 2023).Vitamin D synthesis and risk management can be achieved by following tested guidelines: 15–20 minutes of unprotected sun exposure during midday, exposing the face, arms, or legs, is optimal for most individuals (Jindal et al., 2020).

Sunscreen use with a sun protection factor (SPF) of 15 or higher when sun exposure exceeds the recommended duration is advisable (Neale et al., 2019). Sunscreen prevents skin damage but does not completely block vitamin D synthesis (Lergenmuller et al., 2022). Studies suggest that it can reduce UVB penetration by about 95%, so even with sunscreen, small amounts of vitamin D can still be synthesized (Neale et al., 2019). Intermittent sun exposure in short, frequent intervals, combined with protection during peak times, balances the risks and benefits of sun exposure effectively (Raymond-Lezman & Riskin, 2023).

1.2.2 Dietary vitamin D

Although sunlight is the primary source of vitamin D (80%), dietary intake becomes important, particularly for individuals with limited sun exposure or for those in high-latitude regions where UVB levels are insufficient (Wacker & Holick, 2013). The average daily intake ranges from 10 µgm/day (400iu/day) to 15 µgm (600IU/DAY) for infants (aged 7–11 months) and children (1–17 years) and adults (male, female, pregnant, and lactating women), respectively, as established by the European Food Safety Authority (Benedik, 2022). Certain foods naturally contain vitamin D, while others are fortified to help populations meet the daily intake recommendations.

1.2.2.1   Food sources of vitamin D

Fatty fish such as salmon, mackerel, and tuna are naturally rich in vitamin D, offering one of the best dietary sources (Lu et al., 2007). Egg yolks and liver also provide moderate amounts of vitamin D, though they are consumed less frequently in modern diets (Benedik, 2022). Fortified foods, including milk, orange juice, and breakfast cereals, are commonly enhanced with vitamin D, especially in regions where natural dietary sources may be scarce or cultural practices limit sun exposure (Nyakundi et al., 2023) (Table 1.1).

1.2.2.2   Factors affecting dietary vitamin D intake

Dietary preferences: Individuals following specific dietary patterns, such as vegans or vegetarians, may consume lower levels of vitamin D, as plant-based foods are limited in this nutrient. While certain mushrooms and fortified plant-based products provide some vitamin D, supplementation is often recommended for those on strict plant-based diets (Chan et al., 2009).

Food availability: Socioeconomic factors and geographic location also play a role in access to vitamin D-rich foods. In economically disadvantaged areas, fortified foods may not be readily available, and natural dietary sources may be too expensive for some populations.

1.2.2.2.1   Factors influencing vitamin deficiency
Environmental pollutants
Sunscreen
Geographic location and climate
Skin pigmentation
Aging

Environmental pollutants Environmental pollution can negatively affect vitamin D synthesis by limiting the amount of UVB radiation that reaches the Earth's surface (Manisalidis et al., 2020). Urban areas, in particular, suffer from air pollution, which acts as a barrier to sunlight (Holick, 1995). Pollution particles in the air scatter and absorb UVB radiation, thereby reducing the availability of these rays for vitamin D production (Yang et al., 2021). This is particularly evident in highly polluted regions like industrial areas or densely populated cities, where vitamin D deficiency is often more prevalent despite ample sunlight (Rahman & Elmi, 2021).

The role of sunscreen in blocking UV radiation Sunscreen plays a crucial role in protecting against harmful UV radiation and preventing skin cancer (Gasparro, A Review of Sunscreen Safety and Efficacy, 1998). However, it also blocks UVB rays to a significant extent, which can lead to reduced vitamin D synthesis if used excessively (Raymond-Lezman & Riskin, 2023). Individuals who use sunscreen regularly, particularly in regions where UVB exposure is already limited, should be mindful of their vitamin D intake, either through dietary sources or supplements.

Table 1.1 Cholecalciferol content per 100 g serving in dietary sources.

Dietary source	Serving	Cholecalciferol content	Reference
Salmon	100 g	6.0–33.48 µg	Polzonetti et al. (2020)
Herring	100 g	15–275 µg	
Cod liver oil	100 g of oil	85–1250 µg	
Tuna	100 g	1.0–10 µg	
Eggs	100 g	2.0–5.0 µg	
Wild mushrooms	100 g of fresh sample	–58 µg	
Milk	mL	0.0–8.0 µg	
Butter	100 g	0.18–1.0 µg	
50% Cheddar cheese	100 g	1.0 µg	

Balancing sun protection and vitamin D needs To strike a balance between protecting the skin from harmful UV rays and maintaining adequate vitamin D levels, individuals should: Use sunscreen when spending prolonged periods outdoors, especially during peak UV hours (Lergenmuller et al., 2022).

Consider supplements if regular sun exposure is limited due to geographic location, lifestyle factors, or medical reasons such as skin conditions that require UV protection (Raymond-Lezman & Riskin, 2023).

Geographic location and climate Geographic location is one of the most significant factors affecting vitamin D status (Yeum et al., 2016). Individuals living in regions with low sunlight exposure, especially those at higher latitudes or with frequent cloud cover, often report higher rates of vitamin D deficiency (Holick, 1995).

Vitamin D status in different regions Populations residing in northern Europe, Canada, and parts of the United States are at higher risk of vitamin D deficiency due to reduced UVB exposure, particularly during the winter months (Spiro & Buttriss, 2014). In contrast, individuals living closer to the equator generally maintain adequate vitamin D levels year-round, as they experience more consistent and intense UVB exposure (Yeum et al., 2016).

Implications for populations in high latitudes For populations living at higher latitudes, where sunlight exposure is limited, particularly in the winter, individuals may need to rely more heavily on dietary sources of vitamin D or take supplements to ensure sufficient intake (Wacker & Holick, 2013). In these regions, public health strategies often include food fortification programs and education on the importance of vitamin D supplementation, especially for children and older adults who are more vulnerable to deficiency (Wacker & Holick, 2013).

Skin pigmentation Melanin, the pigment responsible for skin color, has a significant influence on vitamin D synthesis. Darker skinned individuals possess higher melanin levels, which absorb UVB radiation and thus reduce the amount available for vitamin D production (Webb et al., 2018).

Risk of vitamin D deficiency in darker skinned individuals People with darker skin tones, particularly those living in areas with limited sunlight, are at a higher risk of vitamin D deficiency (Webb et al., 2018). These populations may need to pay extra attention to their vitamin D levels, focusing on consuming foods rich in nutrients or taking supplements. Studies have shown that darker skinned individuals living in northern climates are more likely to be deficient in vitamin D than their lighter skinned counterparts due to the dual challenge of low UVB exposure and higher melanin content.

Aging and vitamin D Aging affects the body's ability to both produce and metabolize vitamin D. The skin's capacity to synthesize vitamin D decreases with age, primarily due to reduced levels of 7-dehydrocholesterol (MacLaughlin & Holick, 1985). This reduction is compounded by the tendency for older adults to spend more time indoors, further limiting their sun exposure (Borecka et al., 2021).

Recommendations for older adults Older adults should monitor their vitamin D levels closely and consider dietary adjustments or supplementation to counteract the natural decline in vitamin D production. Healthcare providers often recommend regular screening for vitamin D deficiency in older populations, particularly those in residential care facilities or those with limited mobility (MacLaughlin & Holick, 1985). Encouraging safe outdoor activities can also help increase sunlight exposure for older individuals (Borecka et al., 2021).

1.3 Conclusion

Environmental factors play an essential and multifaceted role in determining vitamin D synthesis and absorption, directly influencing individual and population health outcomes. Among these factors, sunlight exposure stands out as the primary driver of vitamin D production, with UVB radiation triggering the conversion of 7-dehydrocholesterol in the skin to vitamin D3. However, this synthesis process is highly sensitive to variables such as latitude, season, time of day, and skin pigmentation. People living at higher latitudes or in regions with heavy pollution face particular challenges due to reduced UVB exposure, while individuals with darker skin tones, who naturally have higher melanin content, require more sun exposure to synthesize adequate vitamin D. Cultural practices, such as clothing choices that limit skin exposure, further complicate vitamin D production for certain populations.

Dietary intake becomes increasingly important in situations where sunlight exposure is insufficient, whether due to geographic, cultural, or personal health reasons. Natural sources of vitamin D, such as fatty fish, egg yolks, and liver, are vital, but fortification of foods like milk, orange juice, and cereals is critical in many regions to prevent widespread deficiency. Populations adhering to plant-based diets or living in economically disadvantaged areas face additional challenges in accessing vitamin D-rich or fortified foods, making supplementation a necessary intervention in many cases. Environmental pollutants, particularly in urban or industrialized areas, add another layer of complexity. Aging further complicates the vitamin D synthesis process, as older adults experience both a reduced capacity for skin production of vitamin D and diminished kidney function, which affects the activation of vitamin D into its biologically active form. Given these wide-ranging influences, it is crucial to strike a balance between obtaining adequate sunlight exposure and protecting against the harmful effects of excessive UV radiation.

References

Arshad, S., & Zaidi, S. J. A. (2022). Vitamin D levels among children, adolescents, adults, and elders in Pakistani population: A cross-sectional study. *BioMed Central Ltd, Pakistan BMC Public Health, 22*(1). https://doi.org/10.1186/s12889-022-14526-6, https://bmcpublichealth.biomedcentral.com/.

Benedik, E. (2022). Sources of vitamin D for humans. *International Journal for Vitamin and Nutrition Research, 92*(2), 118–125. https://doi.org/10.1024/0300-9831/a000733.

Borecka, O., Farrar, M. D., Osman, J. E., Rhodes, L. E., & Webb, A. R. (2021). Older adults who spend more time outdoors in summer and have higher dietary vitamin D than younger adults can present at least as high vitamin D status: A pilot study. *International Journal of Environmental Research and Public Health, 18*(7), 3364. https://doi.org/10.3390/ijerph18073364.

Chakhtoura, M., Chamoun, N., Rahme, M., & Fuleihan, G. E.-H. (2020). Impact of vitamin D supplementation on falls and fractures—A critical appraisal of the quality of the evidence and an overview of the available guidelines. *Bone, 131*, 115112. https://doi.org/10.1016/j.bone.2019.115112.

Chan, J., Jaceldo-Siegl, K., & Fraser, G. E. (2009). Serum 25-hydroxyvitamin D status of vegetarians, partial vegetarians, and nonvegetarians: The Adventist Health Study-2. *The American Journal of Clinical Nutrition, 89*(5), 1686S. https://doi.org/10.3945/ajcn.2009.26736x.

DeLuca, H. F. (2004). Overview of general physiologic features and functions of vitamin D. *The American Journal of Clinical Nutrition, 80*(6), 1689S. https://doi.org/10.1093/ajcn/80.6.1689s.

Gasparro (1998). A review of sunscreen safety and efficacy. Photochemistry and Photobiology.

Giannini, S., Giusti, A., Minisola, S., Napoli, N., Passeri, G., Rossini, M., & Sinigaglia, L. (2022). The immunologic profile of vitamin D and its role in different immune-mediated diseases: An expert opinion. *Nutrients, 14*(3), 473. https://doi.org/10.3390/nu14030473.

Grant, W. B. (2010). An ecological study of cancer mortality rates in the United States with respect to solar ultraviolet-B doses, smoking, alcohol consumption and urban/rural residence. *Dermato-Endocrinology, 2*(2), 68–76. https://doi.org/10.4161/derm.2.2.13812, http://www.landesbioscience.com/journals/dermatoendocrinology/Grant(2)DE2-2.pdf.

Hanel, A., & Carlberg, C. (2020). Vitamin D and evolution: Pharmacologic implications. *Biochemical Pharmacology, 173*, 113595. https://doi.org/10.1016/j.bcp.2019.07.024.

Holick, M. F. (1995). Environmental factors that influence the cutaneous production of vitamin D. *The American Journal of Clinical Nutrition, 61*(3), 638S. https://doi.org/10.1093/ajcn/61.3.638S.

Holick, M. F. (2008). Vitamin D: A D-lightful health perspective. *Nutrition Reviews, 66*(2), S182–S194. https://doi.org/10.1111/j.1753-4887.2008.00104.x.

Holick, M. F., & Chen, T. C. (2008). Vitamin D deficiency: A worldwide problem with health consequences. *The American Journal of Clinical Nutrition, 87*(4), 1080S. https://doi.org/10.1093/ajcn/87.4.1080s.

Holick, M. F., & Slominski, A. T. (2024). *Photobiology of vitamin D*. Elsevier BV, 27–45. https://doi.org/10.1016/b978-0-323-91386-7.00006-4.

Hughes, D. A., & Norton, R. (2009). Vitamin D and respiratory health. *Clinical and Experimental Immunology, 158*(1), 20–25. https://doi.org/10.1111/j.1365-2249.2009.04001.x.

Jindal, D., Kaur, H., Patil, R. K., & Patil, H. C. (2020). Validation – In pharmaceutical industry: Equipment validation: A brief review. *Adesh University Journal of Medical Sciences & Research, 2*(1), 94–98. https://doi.org/10.25259/aujmsr_15_2020.

Lergenmuller, S., Ghiasvand, R., Robsahm, T. E., Green, A. C., Lund, E., Rueegg, C. S., & Veierød, M. B. (2022). Sunscreens with high versus low sun protection factor and cutaneous squamous cell carcinoma risk: A population-based cohort study. *American Journal of Epidemiology, 191*(1), 75–84. https://doi.org/10.1093/aje/kwab216.

Libon, F., Cavalier, E., & Nikkels, A. F. (2013). Skin color is relevant to vitamin D synthesis. *Dermatology (Basel, Switzerland), 227*(3), 250–254. https://doi.org/10.1159/000354750.

Lu, Z., Chen, T. C., Zhang, A., Persons, K. S., Kohn, N., Berkowitz, R., Martinello, S., & Holick, M. F. (2007). An evaluation of the vitamin D3 content in fish: Is the vitamin D content adequate to satisfy the dietary requirement for vitamin D? *The Journal of Steroid Biochemistry and Molecular Biology, 103*(3-5), 642–644. https://doi.org/10.1016/j.jsbmb.2006.12.010.

MacLaughlin, J., & Holick, M. F. (1985). Aging decreases the capacity of human skin to produce vitamin D3. *Journal of Clinical Investigation, 76*(4), 1536–1538. https://doi.org/10.1172/JCI112134.

Manisalidis, I., Stavropoulou, E., Stavropoulos, A., & Bezirtzoglou, E. (2020). Environmental and health impacts of air pollution: A review. *Frontiers in Public Health, 8*. https://doi.org/10.3389/fpubh.2020.00014.

Martin-Gorgojo, A., Gilaberte, Y., & Nagore, E. (2021). Vitamin D and skin cancer: An epidemiological, patient-centered update and review. *Nutrients, 13*(12). https://doi.org/10.3390/nu13124292, https://www.mdpi.com/2072-6643/13/12/4292/pdf.

Neale, R. E., Khan, S. R., Lucas, R. M., Waterhouse, M., Whiteman, D. C., & Olsen, C. M. (2019). The effect of sunscreen on vitamin D: A review. *British Journal of Dermatology, 181*(5), 907–915. https://doi.org/10.1111/bjd.17980.

Nyakundi, P. N., Némethné Kontár, Z., Kovács, A., Járomi, L., Zand, A., & Lohner, S. (2023). Fortification of staple foods for household use with vitamin D: An overview of systematic reviews. *Nutrients, 15*(17). https://doi.org/10.3390/nu15173742, http://www.mdpi.com/journal/nutrients/.

Polzonetti, V., Pucciarelli, S., Vincenzetti, S., & Polidori, P. (2020). Dietary intake of vitamin d from dairy products reduces the risk of osteoporosis. *Nutrients, 12*(6), 1–15. https://doi.org/10.3390/nu12061743.

Rahman, A., & Elmi, A. (2021). Air pollutants are negatively associated with vitamin D-synthesizing UVB radiation intensity on the ground. *Scientific Reports, 11*(1). https://doi.org/10.1038/s41598-021-00980-6, www.nature.com/srep/index.html.

Raymond-Lezman, J. R., & Riskin, S. I. (2023). Benefits and risks of sun exposure to maintain adequate vitamin D levels. *Cureus, 15*(5). https://doi.org/10.7759/cureus.38578.

Rosen (2011). Clinical practice. Vitamin D insufficiency. *The New England Journal of Medicine, 364*(3), 248–254.

Spiro, A., & Buttriss, J. L. (2014). Vitamin D:An overview of vitamin D status and intake in E urope. *Nutrition Bulletin, 39*(4), 322–350. https://doi.org/10.1111/nbu.12108.

Sunyecz, J. A. (2008). The use of calcium and vitamin D in the management of osteoporosis. *Therapeutics and Clinical Risk Management, 4*(4), 827–836. https://doi.org/10.2147/tcrm.s3552, http://www.dovepress.com/therapeutics-and-clinical-risk-management-journal.

Veldurthy, V., Wei, R., Oz, L., Dhawan, P., Jeon, Y. H., & Christakos, S. (2016). Vitamin D, calcium homeostasis and aging. *Bone Research, 4*(1). https://doi.org/10.1038/boneres.2016.41.

Vieth, R. (1999). Vitamin D supplementation, 25-hydroxyvitamin D concentrations, and safety. *The American Journal of Clinical Nutrition, 69*(5), 842–856. https://doi.org/10.1093/ajcn/69.5.842.

Wacker, M., & Holick, M. F. (2013). Sunlight and vitamin D: A global perspective for health. *Landes Bioscience, United States Dermato-Endocrinology, 5*(1), 51–108. https://doi.org/10.4161/derm.24494, http://www.landesbioscience.com/journals/dermatoendocrinology/2013DE0239.pdf.

Webb, A. R., Kazantzidis, A., Kift, R. C., Farrar, M. D., Wilkinson, J., & Rhodes, L. E. (2018). Colour counts: Sunlight and skin type as drivers of vitamin D deficiency at UK latitudes. *Nutrients, 10*(4). https://doi.org/10.3390/nu10040457, http://www.mdpi.com/2072-6643/10/4/457/pdf.

Yang, C., Li, D., Tian, Y., & Wang, P. (2021). Ambient air pollutions are associated with vitamin D status. *International Journal of Environmental Research and Public Health, 18*(13), 6887. https://doi.org/10.3390/ijerph18136887.

Yeum, K. J., Song, B. C., & Joo, N. S. (2016). Impact of geographic location on vitamin D status and bone mineral density. *International Journal of Environmental Research and Public Health, 13*(2). https://doi.org/10.3390/ijerph13020184, http://www.mdpi.com/1660-4601/13/2/184/pdf.

CHAPTER 2

Sources of vitamin D

Faiza Alam[1], Mussarat Ashraf[2], and Maah Amir[3]

[1]*Pengiran-Anak-Puteri-Rashidah-Sa'adatul-Bolkiah Institute of Health Sciences, Universiti Brunei Darussalam, Bandar Seri Begawan, Brunei Darussalam* [2]*Department of Biological & Biomedical Sciences, Aga Khan University, Karachi, Pakistan* [3]*Medical College, Aga Khan University, Karachi, Pakistan*

2.1 Main sources of vitamin D: endogenous synthesis and dietary intake

Vitamin D, a fat-soluble vitamin essential for calcium homeostasis, immune function, and overall metabolic health, is obtained from two primary sources: endogenous synthesis in the skin and dietary intake.

2.1.1 Endogenous sources of vitamin D

2.1.1.1 Role of sunlight in vitamin D production

Vitamin D (VD), often known as the "sunshine vitamin," has been produced on Earth for over 500 million years. It has two existing forms, D2 and D3, both being essential to the human body for various physiological processes, including maintenance of bone health, calcium and phosphate metabolism, and other cellular processes. Vitamin D2 and D3 are metabolized in similar ways in the body and can be obtained exogenously from dietary sources and supplements. However, D3 is the only form that is primarily synthesized in the human body itself (Charoenngam et al., 2019; Nair & Maseeh, 2012). Sunlight plays a vital role in this endogenous synthesis of cholecalciferol (vitamin D3), specifically UVB rays which make up only 5% of the UV rays from sunlight (Humans, 2012).

The epidermis of the skin contains abundant quantities of the precursor for vitamin D3 synthesis, that is, 7-dehydrocholesterol, which, upon exposure to ultraviolet light, is converted to cholecalciferol, with maximal conversion occurring at wavelengths between 290 and 310 nm. UV irradiation cleaves the B ring in 7-dehydrocholesterol, leading to the formation of pre-vitamin D3, which subsequently undergoes isomerization to become vitamin D3 (Bikle, 2014).

Once formed, vitamin D enters the circulation where it weakly binds to vitamin D binding protein (DBP) and albumin and is transported to the liver and kidneys, respectively, to be converted into its active form, 1,25-dihydroxyvitamin D (Tuckey et al., 2019).

The Impact of Vitamin D on Health and Disease. DOI: https://doi.org/10.1016/B978-0-443-34037-6.00030-3

The cutaneous synthesis of vitamin D is influenced by several factors that affect the skin's exposure to UVB, these include geographical location, age, skin type, sunscreen use, as well as different clothing and cultural practices which may alter the skin's exposure.

2.1.1.2   Skin pigment

Melanin, being the skin's natural sunscreen, efficiently absorbs UV radiation but only allows some UVB rays to penetrate and produce vitamin D3. Early humans living near the equator developed darkly pigmented skin to shield against intense sunlight while still synthesizing sufficient vitamin D. However, as humans migrated to regions with lower UVB exposure, skin pigmentation lightened to enhance vitamin D production, which was vital for bone health and preventing conditions like rickets. These adaptations were critical for skeletal development, muscle function, and successful childbirth. This evolutionary shift underscores the intricate relationship between skin pigmentation, sunlight exposure, and the physiological demands of human health and reproduction (Wacker & Holick, 2013).

2.1.1.3   Clothing

Different fabrics also interfere with the transmission of UV rays, which may decrease the synthesis of cholecalciferol in the skin; light fabrics such as cotton and linen form a weaker barrier as compared to fabrics like wool or polyester, which are more effective in decreasing UV transmission to the skin. These effects may be attenuated by the use of sunscreen, thereby further decreasing UV transmission and effective VD synthesis (Tsiaras & Weinstock, 2011).

2.1.1.4   Geographical location

Geographical location also significantly influences the endogenous synthesis of vitamin D due to variations in the solar ultraviolet B (UVB) radiation exposure and the solar zenith angle (SZA). The SZA, which measures the angle of the sun relative to the observer's zenith, determines the intensity of UVB radiation reaching the Earth's surface. At higher latitudes, especially during winter, the SZA is large, leading to increased atmospheric scattering of UVB rays and reducing their penetration to the skin (Webb, 2006). Furthermore, research highlights that even a one- or two-degree latitude difference can significantly affect serum 25-hydroxyvitamin D concentrations, as demonstrated in a Korean population where individuals in southern regions had consistently higher vitamin D levels compared to those in northern regions (Yeum et al., 2016). These findings underscore the critical role of SZA and latitude in shaping vitamin D status, necessitating tailored interventions for populations in high-latitude regions to mitigate deficiency risks.

2.1.1.5 Season and time of day

Season and time of day further modulate the effects of geographical location on endogenous vitamin D synthesis by influencing the availability and intensity of ultraviolet B (UVB) radiation. During winter months, particularly at higher latitudes, the solar zenith angle (SZA) increases, causing UVB radiation to scatter more in the atmosphere, rendering it insufficient for cutaneous vitamin D production (Webb, 2006). Similarly, time of day plays a critical role, with peak synthesis occurring around solar noon when the SZA is smallest, and UVB penetration is highest. In contrast, mornings and late afternoons, characterized by larger SZAs, contribute little to vitamin D production (Harinarayan et al., 2013; Wacker & Holick, 2013). These variations across seasons and times of day underscore the complexity of vitamin D synthesis and highlight the need for supplementation or alternative sources during periods of low UVB availability.

2.1.1.6 Age

Age is a significant factor affecting the body's ability to synthesize vitamin D endogenously, primarily due to changes in skin physiology. As individuals age, the concentration of 7-dehydrocholesterol in the skin decreases, reducing the substrate available for ultraviolet B (UVB)-induced vitamin D production. Research shows that the capacity of elderly individuals to synthesize vitamin D can be up to three times lower than that of younger adults when exposed to the same amount of UVB radiation (Wacker & Holick, 2013). Additionally, aging is often associated with reduced outdoor activity and less direct sun exposure, further exacerbating the risk of vitamin D deficiency.

2.2 Balancing the risks: sunlight overexposure vs. vitamin D deficiency

Striking an appropriate balance in sunlight exposure is vital, as both excessive and insufficient exposure poses significant health risks.

Overexposure to sunlight is a well-established risk factor for various skin cancers, including melanoma, basal cell carcinoma, and squamous cell carcinoma. The DNA damage induced by UV radiation triggers mutations that can lead to malignancies, especially with prolonged and unprotected sun exposure. Squamous cell carcinoma of the skin is the most commonly reported type of skin cancer associated with sunlight as a significant risk factor (Mason & Reichrath, 2013).

On the other hand, VD deficiency poses significant risks to overall health, as it plays a vital role in calcium homeostasis and bone metabolism. Prolonged deficiency can lead to rickets in children, characterized by impaired mineralization of growth plates and osteomalacia in adults, resulting in weakened and soft bones. Additionally, vitamin D deficiency may contribute to osteoporosis by impairing calcium absorption and increasing bone turnover, thereby elevating the risk of fractures. Beyond its skeletal effects, emerging evidence suggests that vitamin D deficiency is associated with various nonskeletal disorders, including autoimmune diseases, infections, cardiovascular diseases, and metabolic syndromes. Populations at higher risk include those with limited sun exposure, darker skin pigmentation, obesity, or malabsorption syndromes, as well as the elderly, whose ability to synthesize vitamin D decreases with age (Sizar et al., 2025; Whyte & Thakker, 2013).

Public health strategies increasingly advocate for alternative solutions to address vitamin D deficiency without increasing skin cancer risk. These include fortifying foods with vitamin D, promoting dietary sources like fatty fish, and recommending vitamin D supplementation, particularly for high-risk groups such as the elderly. Such strategies can help mitigate vitamin D deficiency while minimizing reliance on sunlight exposure and reducing associated risks (Wacker & Holick, 2013).

2.2.1 Dietary sources of vitamin D

2.2.1.1 Natural food sources

Additionally, both vitamin D2 and D3 may be obtained via the diet, though foods that provide VD are limited; thus, the amount of VD obtained through diet varies largely in differing areas depending on the local dietary habits (Dominguez et al., 2021) Animal products are the main sources of vitamin D3, whereas vitamin D2 primarily comes from plants, though some dairy products may contain it as well (Janoušek et al., 2022) as shown in Fig. 2.1.

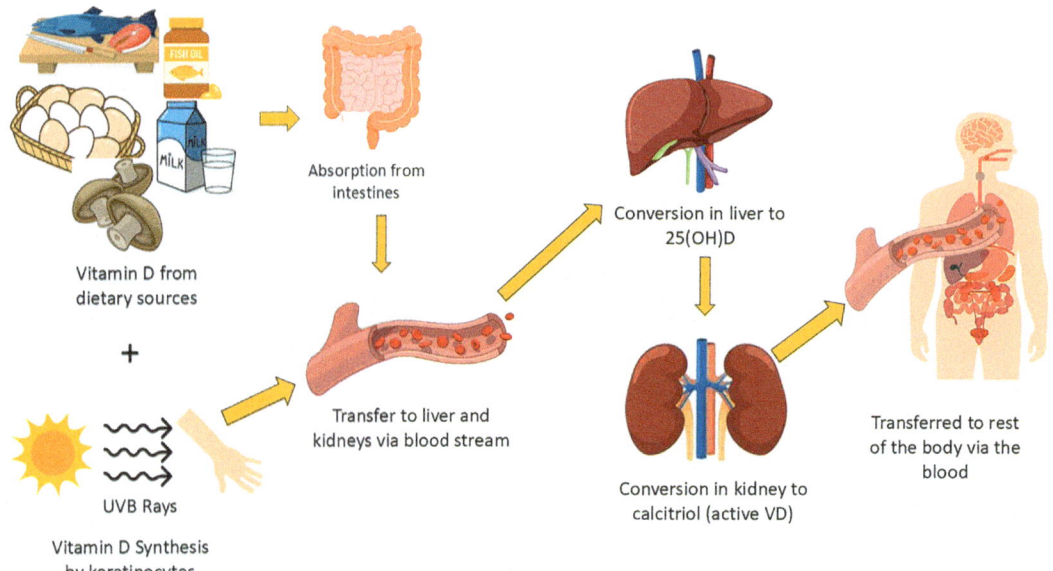

Figure 2.1
Sources of vitamin D.

2.2.1.2 Animal-based sources

2.2.1.2.1 Fatty fish and fish liver oil

The vast majority of VD comes from animal products, and of those products, fish and fish liver oil (particularly cod and tuna liver oils) contain the greatest amount per serving (Janoušek et al., 2022). Whole fish do not contain as much as the liver oil counterparts, with the greatest amounts of VD coming from rainbow trout and sockeye salmon (Dominguez et al., 2021); still, fish far outcompete other dietary sources for VD content. Other seafood products do not follow this trend; mussels, oysters, and shrimps all contain very small amounts of VD (Janoušek et al., 2022) and are not considered to be good dietary sources of VD.

2.2.1.2.2 Meat

Other sources of meat, such as chicken, beef, and pork, also contain small amounts of VD, but the amount varies with the animal's diet and exposure to sunlight; additionally, the VD is primarily stored in the fat (Janoušek et al., 2022).

2.2.1.2.3 Egg yolk

Following fish, eggs contain significant amounts of VD, particularly in the yolks. VD content appears to be the same in eggs across different animal species (Janoušek et al., 2022). Cooking eggs for consumption in the household causes some loss of VD content, but eggs remain a good source of VD due to comparable bioavailability compared to both supplements and other food sources, such as fish liver oil. Additionally, supplementing animal feed with vitamin D has a linear relationship with the amount of VD in eggs (Barnkob et al., 2020).

2.2.1.3 Natural plant-based sources

2.2.1.3.1 Mushrooms

VD from plants comes primarily from sun-exposed mushrooms and is in the form of vitamin D2. Other plants typically store VD in parts that are not edible to humans and are thus not counted as a dietary source. While most farmed mushrooms are grown in dark environments and thus contain little VD, exposure to sunlight for even 15 minutes following harvesting does increase VD content significantly. Wild mushrooms are exposed to sunlight before harvesting, but VD content is difficult to measure because growing conditions vary (Janoušek et al., 2022). Still, mushrooms appear to be the best unfortified plant-based source of VD.

2.3   Fortified plant-based foods

Other plant-based sources of VD are largely fortified products, such as fortified breakfast cereals, plant-based milks and yogurts, orange juice, baby foods, and supplemental or enteral nutrition and will be discussed further in the next section (Benedik, 2022).

2.3.1   Commonly fortified plant-based foods

2.3.1.1   Dairy products

Dairy products also contain small amounts of VD (both vitamins D2 and D3, depending on the product) (Janoušek et al., 2022); certain countries have adopted fortification policies or recommendations, leading to supplementation of VD in dairy products such as yogurts, milks, butters, and margarine to prevent deficiency in the population (Dominguez et al., 2021). Raw milk and yogurt contain very minor amounts of vitamin D; however, milk contains several small molecules that enable it to be a good carrier of fat-soluble molecules, including VD. Milk contains fat globules and large amounts of casein micelles, both of which are able to carry VD; additionally, cattle milk also contains VD-binding protein similar to that in human milk. Both the safety and effectiveness of VD supplementation in dairy have been shown in recent years in countries such as Finland, Sweden, and Canada; studies in Canada showed a marked increase in VD consumption and a decline in deficiency across all ages and sexes. Effects from other policies are still being studied (Pellegrino et al., 2021).

2.3.1.1.1   Plant-based milk

Plant-based milk beverages are a recent target of VD fortification, as there are very few natural sources of VD in a plant-based diet (Zhou, Zheng, et al., 2021). However, there have been very few studies assessing the bioavailability of VD in these milk alternatives. As VD is a lipid-soluble vitamin, it is important for emulsions to have smaller, oil-based emulsions for more effective intake (McClements, 2020). Additionally, as plant milks have a much less complete nutrition profile than cow's milk, they are commonly supplemented with other vitamins and minerals, which may change the bioavailability of VD. One in-vitro study found that increased levels of added calcium decreased the bioavailability of VD, likely due to the formation of calcium soaps, which prevented VD uptake (Zhou, Zheng, et al., 2021). Another in-vitro study had similar findings, showing only approximately 20% of VD added was bioavailable (Zhou, Liu, et al., 2021), suggesting a need to carefully consider the amounts of each nutrient added when creating these fortified milks.

2.3.1.1.2   Breakfast cereals

Aside from milk, many foods are commonly fortified with VD and play a large role in the dietary intake of vitamin D in some populations. Grains are an important target of fortification;

flour is commonly fortified with other nutrients such as iron and folate, and this may be especially impactful in countries in which bread is a dietary staple (Nikooyeh & Neyestani, 2022). In the United Kingdom, 13%–20% of dietary VD is consumed from fortified cereals, making them an important source in this demographic (Calame et al., 2020). These options for fortification make it easier for demographics similar to the United Kingdom, where sunlight exposure is limited and dietary sources are uncommon, to achieve healthy levels of V (Allen et al., 2015). Recent studies have begun to explore the efficacy of fortifying cooking oils with VD; one study in Iran found that using fortified sunflower oil was an effective way to increase VD intake and had better retention after cooking that fortified flat breads (Nikooyeh et al., 2020). Juices, such as orange juice, were also found to be an effective vehicle for VD supplementation but are not a recommended approach due to high levels of sugar and highly varied levels of consumption in the population (Nikooyeh & Neyestani, 2022).

2.3.2 Absorption and usage in the body

Dietary VD is VD is the absorbed from the GIT via emulsification and mixed micellar absorption; uptake by small intestine enterocytes is compromised in persons with certain gastrointestinal disorders affecting fat absorption, such as Crohn's disease (Janoušek et al., 2022). Regardless of dietary or cutaneous acquisition, VD is distributed through blood, where it is either the distributed to adipose tissue for storage or transferred to the liver, where it is metabolized into 25(OH)D (25-hydroxyvitamin D). It is then once again hydroxylated in the kidneys to 1,25(OH)D (1,25-hydroxyvitamin D, or calcitriol) (Dominguez et al., 2021). Calcitriol is the hormonally active form of VD, and it is this form that exerts its physiologic effects on the body (Janoušek et al., 2022).

2.3.2.1 Vitamin D supplements

2.3.2.1.1 Type of supplements

Both vitamin D2 and vitamin D3 are available orally in the form of tablets, capsules, and drops for pharmacologic supplementation, but due to a higher affinity for vitamin D binding protein (VDBP), some prefer vitamin D3 (Bilezikian et al., 2021). However, other studies report that clinically, neither is superior to the other (Vieth, 2020). Additionally, calcitriol and its synthetic analog, alfacalcidiol, are available to raise active VD levels whilst bypassing the kidney (Bilezikian et al., 2021). Other formulations, such as topical or transdermal delivery, are also being explored, though currently, topical delivery is mostly in use with psoriasis patients (Glowka et al., 2019).

Vitamin D supplementations can be given in various health conditions, including osteoarthritis, cardiovascular risks, preventing cancer, but it has shown variable effects (Michael et al., 2022). Although it does not seem to lower the risk of cardiovascular disease or cancer, new research indicates it might lessen the severity of COVID-19 and ease the symptoms of atopic dermatitis (Michael et al., 2022). Additionally, vitamin D may help with fibromyalgia pain, significant depression, and slowing the progression of prediabetic patients to type 2 diabetes by improving HbA1c (Abugoukh et al., 2022).

2.3.2.1.2 Indication for supplementation

There are several populations in which additional supplementation is required aside from general recommendations. Elderly patients are at higher risk for low bone density, as well as falls and fractures, and are thus recommended to have a minimum of 75 nmol/L (Pludowski et al., 2018). Patients with chronic kidney disease have similarly raised requirements, owing to the loss of the kidney's ability to convert VD into its active form as well as increased loss of proteins in the urine (Zhu et al., 2015). Patients with inflammatory bowel diseases (ulcerative colitis or Crohn's disease) and other gastrointestinal conditions (such as gluten enteropathy, short bowel syndrome, and bariatric surgery) also often suffer from VD deficiency due to impaired VD absorption from the small intestine but respond well to supplementation (Bilezikian et al., 2021). Pregnant patients are also recommended to supplement VD, as it plays a role in fetal bone development, has no associated adverse effects, and may reduce comorbidities related to gestation (Dobson et al., 2018).

2.3.3 Populations at risk of deficiency

Certain populations are also at risk for VD deficiency owing to a lack of sun exposure in their environment: several studies have found a possibility for increased risk of VD deficiency in urban areas as compared to rural areas, likely due to air pollution, tall buildings blocking sunlight, and the possibility of increased indoor work (Mendes et al., 2019).

Additionally, populations at high latitudes do not receive the correct UV wavelength for VD synthesis for several winter months, and levels of serum VD are inversely related with distance from the equator (Mendes et al., 2019). For these populations, VD supplementation may be indicated apart from simple food fortification.

2.3.4 Dosage recommendation

Adequate levels of VD are difficult to determine, and recommendations vary widely across populations due to differences in sun exposure, clothing, latitude, skin pigmentation, diet, and more (Pludowski et al., 2018). However, current guidelines recommend a concentration range of 25–75nmol/L of 25(OH)D in the serum, with levels under 25 or 30 nmol/L representing an increased risk of bone health conditions (Cashman, 2020). However, recommendations vary across ages. The Endocrine Society of USA recommends daily doses of 1500–2000 IU VD/day for adults for treatment and prevention of VD deficiency and 600–1000 IU VD/day for children older than one year (Pludowski et al., 2018).

2.3.5   Potential risks of over supplementation

There are some risks to VD supplementation at high doses. Symptoms associated with VD toxicity are due to raised levels of calcium in the blood and urine and include loss of appetite, vomiting, constipation, lethargy, polyuria, and renal stones (Ramasamy, 2020). However, VD toxicity is rare, and signs do not appear until a minimum serum concentration of 375 nmol/L (Pludowski et al., 2018).

2.4   Recent developments and research

2.4.1   Innovations in fortification

Food fortification is a cost-effective interventionwith significant economic returns, generating $27 for every dollar invested (Matthias, 2021). However, innovation in this field faces challenges due to unclear returns for private sector implementors and innovators. Recent advancements include fortifying bread with plant-based proteins to address malnutrition and meet the growing demand for plant-based options (Bashir et al., 2024).

2.4.2   New technologies and approaches in food fortification

The goal of recent developments in food fortification technology is to tackle issues, including stability, taste, and bioavailability. Food fortification, which involves adding different bioactive substances to food and consumer products, is necessary to address vitamin shortages globally (Piya et al., 2024).

2.4.3   Potential new dietary sources

Innovative food sources, including bioengineered foods, have the potential to address global nutritional difficulties and environmental concerns, according to recent studies. Insects, seaweed, and cultured meat are examples of future diets that provide vital micronutrients and have major environmental benefits (Parodi et al., 2018). There is potential for genetically modified crops to improve human nutrition by increasing the nutrient density of plant diets. As sustainable solutions to address protein deficit, alternative protein sources such as legumes, microalgae, and insects are becoming more and more well-liked (Dolganyuk et al., 2023).

2.4.4   Public health initiatives: current strategies to improve vitamin D intake globally

Currently, public education efforts, supplementation, and food fortification are used to increase vitamin D intake worldwide. Even in sunny areas, vitamin D insufficiency is common globally and poses a number of health problems. In certain nations, food fortification of staples like bread, milk, and eggs has proven effective and is regarded as a possible tactic to boost population intakes (Buttriss et al., 2022). Numerous fortification techniques have been investigated, such as the application of protein nanocapsules, liposomes, and nanoemulsions. Vitamin D stability and bioaccessibility are greatly influenced by the dietary matrix, with lipids, proteins, and antioxidants influencing absorption (Lavelli et al., 1989).

References

Abugoukh, T. M., Al Sharaby, A., Elshaikh, A. O., Joda, M., Madni, A., Ahmed, I., Abdalla, R. S., Ahmed, K., Elazrag, S. E., & Abdelrahman, N. (2022). Does vitamin D have a role in diabetes? *Cureus, 14*(10). https://doi.org/10.7759/cureus.30432.

Allen, R. E., Dangour, A. D., Tedstone, A. E., & Chalabi, Z. (2015). Does fortification of staple foods improve vitamin D intakes and status of groups at risk of deficiency? A United Kingdom modeling study. *American Journal of Clinical Nutrition, 102*(2), 338–344. https://doi.org/10.3945/ajcn.115.107409, http://ajcn.nutrition.org/content/102/2/338.full.pdf+html.

Barnkob, L. L., Argyraki, A., & Jakobsen, J. (2020). Naturally enhanced eggs as a source of vitamin D: A review. *Trends in Food Science and Technology, 102*, 62–70. https://doi.org/10.1016/j.tifs.2020.05.018, http://www.elsevier.com/wps/find/journaldescription.cws_home/601278/description#description.

Bashir, K., Jan, K., Maurya, V. K., & Shakya, A. (2024). *Food fortification: Trends and technologies food fortification: trends and technologies*. India: CRC Press, 1–405. https://www.routledge.com/Food-Fortification-Trends-and-Technologies/Bashir-Jan-Maurya-Shakya/p/book/9780367723927.

Benedik, E. (2022). Sources of vitamin D for humans. *International Journal for Vitamin and Nutrition Research, 92*(2), 118–125. https://doi.org/10.1024/0300-9831/a000733, https://econtent.hogrefe.com/loi/vit.

Bikle, D. D. (2014). Vitamin D metabolism, mechanism of action, and clinical applications. *Chemistry & Biology, 21*(3), 319–329. https://doi.org/10.1016/j.chembiol.2013.12.016.

Bilezikian, J. P., Formenti, A. M., Adler, R. A., Binkley, N., Bouillon, R., Lazaretti-Castro, M., Marcocci, C., Napoli, N., Rizzoli, R., & Giustina, A. (2021). Vitamin D: Dosing, levels, form, and route of administration: Does one approach fit all? *Reviews in Endocrine and Metabolic Disorders, 22*(4), 1201–1218. https://doi.org/10.1007/s11154-021-09693-7, https://link.springer.com/journal/11154.

Buttriss, J. L., Lanham-New, S. A., Steenson, S., Levy, L., Swan, G. E., Darling, A. L., Cashman, K. D., Allen, R. E., Durrant, L. R., Smith, C. P., Magee, P., Hill, T. R., Uday, S., Kiely, M., Delamare, G., Hoyland, A. E., Larsen, L., Street, L. N., Mathers, J. C., & Prentice, A. (2022). Implementation strategies for improving vitamin D status and increasing vitamin D intake in the UK: Current controversies and future perspectives: Proceedings of the 2nd Rank Prize Funds Forum on vitamin D. *British Journal of Nutrition, 127*(10), 1567–1587. https://doi.org/10.1017/S0007114521002555, http://journals.cambridge.org/BJN.

Calame, W., Street, L., & Hulshof, T. (2020). Vitamin d serum levels in the uk population, including a mathematical approach to evaluate the impact of vitamin d fortified ready-to-eat breakfast cereals: Application of the ndns database. *Nutrients, 12*(6), 1–14. https://doi.org/10.3390/nu12061868, https://www.mdpi.com/2072-6643/12/6/1868/pdf.

Cashman, K. D. (2020). Vitamin D deficiency: Defining, prevalence, causes, and strategies of addressing. *Calcified Tissue International, 106*(1), 14–29. https://doi.org/10.1007/s00223-019-00559-4, link.springer.de/link/service/journals/00223/index.htm.

Charoenngam, N., Shirvani, A., & Holick, M. F. (2019). Vitamin D for skeletal and non-skeletal health: What we should know. *Journal of Clinical Orthopaedics and Trauma, 10*(6), 1082–1093. https://doi.org/10.1016/j.jcot.2019.07.004, http://www.elsevier.com/wps/find/journaldescription.cws_home/724754/description#description.

Dobson, R., Cock, H. R., Brex, P., & Giovannoni, G. (2018). Vitamin D supplementation. *Practical Neurology, 18*(1), 35–42. https://doi.org/10.1136/practneurol-2017-001720, http://pn.bmj.com/content/by/year.

Dolganyuk, V., Sukhikh, S., Kalashnikova, O., Ivanova, S., Kashirskikh, E., Prosekov, A., Michaud, P., & Babich, O. (2023). Food proteins: Potential resources. *Sustainability, 15*(7), 5863. https://doi.org/10.3390/su15075863.

Dominguez, L. J., Farruggia, M., Veronese, N., & Barbagallo, M. (2021). Vitamin d sources, metabolism, and deficiency: Available compounds and guidelines for its treatment. *Metabolites, 11*(4). https://doi.org/10.3390/metabo11040255, https://www.mdpi.com/2218-1989/11/4/255/pdf.

Glowka, E., Stasiak, J., & Lulek, J. (2019). Drug delivery systems for vitamin D supplementation and therapy. *Pharmaceutics, 11*(7). https://doi.org/10.3390/pharmaceutics11070347, https://www.mdpi.com/1999-4923/11/7/347/pdf.

Harinarayan, C. V., Holick, M. F., Prasad, U. V., Vani, P. S., & Himabindu, G. (2013). Vitamin D status and sun exposure in India. *Dermato-Endocrinology, 5*(1), 130–141. https://doi.org/10.4161/derm.23873India, http://www.landesbioscience.com/journals/dermatoendocrinology/2012DE0213R.pdf.

Humans, I. W. GotEo. C. R. (2012). *Radiation*. International Agency for Research on Cancer.

Janoušek, J., Pilařová, V., Macáková, K., Nomura, A., Veiga-Matos, J., Silva, D. Dd, Remião, F., Saso, L., Malá-Ládová, K., Malý, J., Nováková, L., & Mladěnka, P. (2022). Vitamin D: sources, physiological role, biokinetics, deficiency, therapeutic use, toxicity, and overview of analytical methods for detection of vitamin D and its metabolites. *Republic Critical Reviews in Clinical Laboratory Sciences, 59*(8), 517–554. https://doi.org/10.1080/10408363.2022.2070595, http://www.tandfonline.com/loi/ilab20.

Lavelli, V., Incecco, P., & Pellegrino, L. (1989). Vitamin D incorporation in foods: Formulation strategies, stability, and bioaccessibility as affected by the food matrix. *Foods, 10*(9).

Mason, R. S., & Reichrath, J. (2013). Sunlight vitamin D and skin cancer. *Anti-cancer Agents in Medicinal Chemistry, 13*(1), 83–97. https://doi.org/10.2174/187152013804487272, http://www.eurekaselect.com/578/journal/anti-cancer-agents-medicinal-chemistry.

Matthias, D. (2021). *The continuing evolution of food fortification innovations*.

McClements, D. J. (2020). Development of next-generation nutritionally fortified plant-based milk substitutes: Structural design principles. *Foods, 9*(4). https://doi.org/10.3390/foods9040421, https://www.mdpi.com/2304-8158/9/4/421.

Mendes, M. M., Darling, A. L., Hart, K. H., Morse, S., Murphy, R. J., & Lanham-New, S. A. (2019). Impact of high latitude, urban living and ethnicity on 25-hydroxyvitamin D status: A need for multidisciplinary action? *Journal of Steroid Biochemistry and Molecular Biology, 188*, 95–102. https://doi.org/10.1016/j.jsbmb.2018.12.012, https://www.elsevier.com/locate/jsbmb.

Michael, W., Couture, A. D., Swedlund, M., Hampton, A., Eglash, A., & Schrager, S. (2022). An evidence-based review of vitamin D for common and high-mortality conditions. *Journal of the American Board of Family Medicine, 35*(6), 1217–1229. https://doi.org/10.3122/jabfm.2022.220115R1, https://www.jabfm.org/content/jabfp/35/6/1217.full.pdf.

Nair, R., & Maseeh, A. (2012). Vitamin D: The sunshine vitamin. *Journal of Pharmacology and Pharmacotherapeutics, 3*(2), 118–126. https://doi.org/10.4103/0976-500X.95506.

Nikooyeh, B., & Neyestani, T. R. (2022). The effects of vitamin D-fortified foods on circulating 25(OH)D concentrations in adults: a systematic review and meta-analysis. *British Journal of Nutrition, 127*(12), 1821–1838. https://doi.org/10.1017/S0007114521002816, http://journals.cambridge.org/BJN.

Nikooyeh, B., Zargaraan, A., Kalayi, A., Shariatzadeh, N., Zahedirad, M., Jamali, A., Khazraie, M., Hollis, B., & Neyestani, T. R. (2020). Vitamin D-fortified cooking oil is an effective way to improve vitamin D status: an institutional efficacy trial. *European Journal of Nutrition, 59*(6), 2547–2555. https://doi.org/10.1007/s00394-019-02103-4, http://www.springerlink.com/content/1436-6207.

Parodi, A., Leip, A., De Boer, I. J. M., Slegers, P. M., Ziegler, F., Temme, E. H. M., Herrero, M., Tuomisto, H., Valin, H., Van Middelaar, C. E., Van Loon, J. J. A., & Van Zanten, H. H. E. (2018). The potential of future foods for sustainable and healthy diets. *Nature Sustainability, 1*(12), 782–789. https://doi.org/10.1038/s41893-018-0189-7.

Pellegrino, L., Marangoni, F., Muscogiuri, G., D'incecco, P., Duval, G. T., Annweiler, C., & Colao, A. (2021). Vitamin d fortification of consumption cow's milk: Health, nutritional and technological aspects. A multidisciplinary lecture of the recent scientific evidence. *Molecules (Basel, Switzerland), 26*(17). https://doi.org/10.3390/molecules26175289, https://www.mdpi.com/1420-3049/26/17/5289/pdf.

Piya, N., Hussain, M., Uddin, I., Jahan, R. S., Bordoloi, T., Sharif, J., Das, A. M., Patowary, D., & Deka, A. (2024). *International Journal of Modern Pharmaceutical Research, 8*(12).

Pludowski, P., Holick, M. F., Grant, W. B., Konstantynowicz, J., Mascarenhas, M. R., Haq, A., Povoroznyuk, V., Balatska, N., Barbosa, A. P., Karonova, T., Rudenka, E., Misiorowski, W., Zakharova, I., Rudenka, A.,

Łukaszkiewicz, J., Marcinowska-Suchowierska, E., Łaszcz, N., Abramowicz, P., Bhattoa, H. P., & Wimalawansa, S. J. (2018). Vitamin D supplementation guidelines. *Journal of Steroid Biochemistry and Molecular Biology, 175*, 125–135. https://doi.org/10.1016/j.jsbmb.2017.01.021, https://www.elsevier.com/locate/jsbmb.

Ramasamy, I. (2020). Vitamin D metabolism and guidelines for vitamin D supplementation. *Clinical Biochemist Reviews, 41*(3), 103–126. https://doi.org/10.33176/aacb-20-00006.

Sizar, O., Khare, S., Goyal, A., & Givler, A. (2025). *Vitamin D Deficiency. StatPearls. Treasure Island (FL), StatPearls Publishing, Copyright © 2025*. StatPearls Publishing LLC.

Tsiaras, W., & Weinstock, M. (2011). Factors influencing vitamin D status. *Acta Dermato Venereologica, 91*(2), 115–124. https://doi.org/10.2340/00015555-0980.

Tuckey, R. C., Cheng, C. Y. S., & Slominski, A. T. (2019). The serum vitamin D metabolome: What we know and what is still to discover. *Journal of Steroid Biochemistry and Molecular Biology, 186*, 4–21. https://doi.org/10.1016/j.jsbmb.2018.09.003, https://www.elsevier.com/locate/jsbmb.

Vieth, R. (2020). Vitamin D supplementation: Cholecalciferol, calcifediol, and calcitriol. *European Journal of Clinical Nutrition, 74*(11), 1493–1497. https://doi.org/10.1038/s41430-020-0697-1.

Wacker, M., & Holick, M. F. (2013). Sunlight and vitamin D: A global perspective for health. *Dermato-Endocrinology, 5*(1), 51–108. https://doi.org/10.4161/derm.24494, http://www.landesbioscience.com/journals/dermatoendocrinology/2013DE0239.pdf.

Webb, A. R. (2006). Who, what, where and when-influences on cutaneous vitamin D synthesis. *Progress in Biophysics and Molecular Biology, 92*(1), 17–25. https://doi.org/10.1016/j.pbiomolbio.2006.02.004.

Whyte, M. P., & Thakker, R. V. (2013). Rickets and osteomalacia. *Medicine (United Kingdom), 41*(10), 594–599. https://doi.org/10.1016/j.mpmed.2013.07.012.

Yeum, K. J., Song, B. C., & Joo, N. S. (2016). Impact of geographic location on vitamin D status and bone mineral density. *International Journal of Environmental Research and Public Health, 13*(2). https://doi.org/10.3390/ijerph13020184, http://www.mdpi.com/1660-4601/13/2/184/pdf.

Zhou, H., Liu, J., Dai, T., Muriel Mundo, J. L., Tan, Y., Bai, L., & McClements, D. J. (2021). The gastrointestinal fate of inorganic and organic nanoparticles in vitamin D-fortified plant-based milks. *Food Hydrocolloids, 112*. https://doi.org/10.1016/j.foodhyd.2020.106310, https://www.sciencedirect.com/science/journal/0268005X.

Zhou, H., Zheng, B., Zhang, Z., Zhang, R., He, L., & McClements, D. J. (2021). Fortification of plant-based milk with calcium may reduce vitamin D bioaccessibility: An in vitro digestion study. *Journal of Agricultural and Food Chemistry, 69*(14), 4223–4233. https://doi.org/10.1021/acs.jafc.1c01525, http://pubs.acs.org/journal/jafcau.

Zhu, N., Wang, J., Gu, L., Wang, L., & Yuan, W. (2015). Vitamin D supplements in chronic kidney disease. *Renal Failure, 37*(6), 917–924. https://doi.org/10.3109/0886022X.2015.1043920.

CHAPTER 3

Biochemistry of vitamin D

Mohammad Perwaiz Iqbal[1,2]

[1]Biochemistry, Biological & Biomedical Sciences, Aga Khan University, Karachi, Pakistan [2]Life Sciences Department, School of Science, University of Management and Technology, Lahore, Pakistan

3.1 Background

Vitamin D is a fat-soluble vitamin that has a steroid nucleus in its structure. It is unique in several respects. It is endogenously produced in human skin upon exposure to sunlight (UV range 280–310 nm) (Michigami, 2017). It is also produced in plants from ergosterol under the influence of sunlight. It is one of the two vitamins that are also regarded as "hormones" (Reichrath et al., 2007). Its two major forms are ergocalciferol (vitamin D_2) and calciferol (vitamin D_3) as shown in Fig. 3.1 (Dusso et al., 2005; Malloy et al., 1999).

3.2 Discovery of vitamin D

Sir Edward Mellanby in the United Kingdom found that rickets was very common among Scottish people (Mellanby, 1919). He was keenly following the research work of McCollum who was working at the University of Wisconsin, USA, and had proposed that dietary factors could be responsible for the development of rickets. Sir Mellanby came to know that oatmeal was one of the major diets used in Scotland. Thus he carried out an experiment on dogs by feeding them only oatmeal for a number of weeks. Incidentally, dogs developed rickets similar to rickets in humans. He fed these dogs with cod liver oil, and to his surprise, the dogs were cured of the disease. Since vitamin A was considered to be a major component in cod liver oil, he concluded that vitamin A was the factor responsible for curing rickets. Later, McCollum tested the hypothesis of Sir Mellanby that vitamin A was the factor and that the deficiency of vitamin A could cause rickets (McCollum et al., 1922). In his experiment, he destroyed vitamin A in cod liver oil by bubbling oxygen through it, and then he fed the dogs with rickets with supplements of this cod liver oil and found that this new preparation of cod liver oil could not cure xerophthalmia (a disease which occurs due to deficiency of vitamin A) but still retained the ability to cure rickets. Based on these results, he inferred that there was a "new vitamin" present in cod liver which could cure rickets. This vitamin was named "vitamin D" (Deluca, 2014; Khalsa, 2009).

The Impact of Vitamin D on Health and Disease. DOI: https://doi.org/10.1016/B978-0-443-34037-6.00008-X

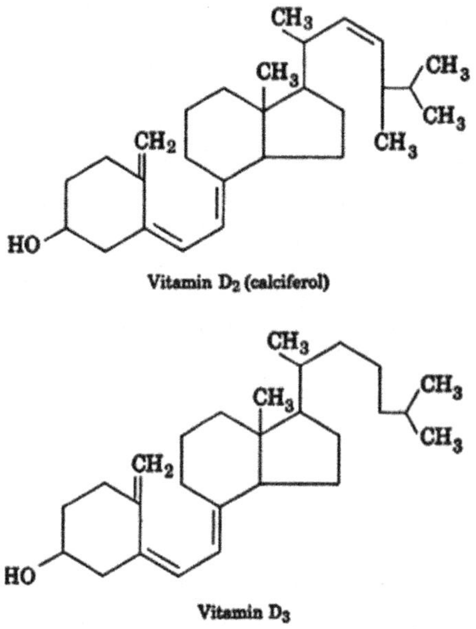

Figure 3.1
Structures of vitamin D_2 and vitamin D_3.
Source: Reproduced from Kalueff, A. L. (2005). Behavioural abnormalities in mice with partially deleted vitamin D receptor gene Academic dissertation. University of Tampere, Medical School, Finland.

3.2.1   Production of precursors of vitamin D

A number of clinicians in Europe observed that children suffering from rickets when exposed to sunlight during summer got cured alluding to the role of sunshine for the endogenous production of an antirachitic factor (Hess & Unger, 1921). Later experiments showed that it was the UV radiation from sun which led to the production of antirachitic factor in the plant-based animal feed (Hess & Weinstock, 1924; Steenbock & Black, 1924). This component in plants was later named "ergosterol," which had a molecular formula, $C_{28}H_{44}O$, and contained perhydrocyclopentanophenanthrene ring. Ergosterol, when exposed to sunlight or UV rays, would get converted into antirachitic factor (vitamin D2). This plant-based feed, when consumed by animals suffering from rickets, was able to cure them.

Dr. Steenbock in his experiment showed a link between this new antirachitic factor due to sunlight and calcium retention in animals (Steenbock & Black, 1924). This calcium retention as a result of the production of antirachitic factor was the biochemical phenomenon by which rickets was cured (Fitzpatrick et al., 2000).

3.2.2   Production of precursors of antirachitic factors in animals

Dr Steenbock in 1925 also showed that irradiating rats could result in the production of a fat-soluble factor which had antirachitic property (Steenbock & Black, 1924).

Later experiments revealed that the skin of animals contained a sterol-7 dehydrocholesterol which, when exposed to UV light, got converted into previtamins D3 and then to vitamin D3, also called "cholecalciferol" with molecular formula $C_{27}H_{44}O$ (Windaus et al., 1935).

In plants (through fungal pathogens):

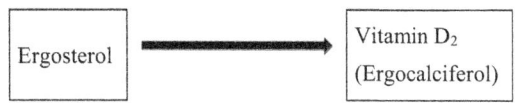

In animals:

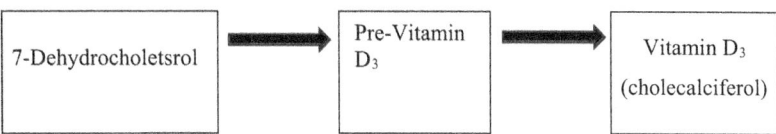

3.3 Sources

The richest dietary source of vitamin D is various types of fatty fish such as salmon, tuna, and sardine; however, small amounts are available in beef liver, egg, and cheese. Cod liver oil is the richest source of vitamin D and is being used as a major supplement (Cicek et al., 2023).

3.4 Conversion of dietary or endogenously synthesized vitamin D into active forms

Whether vitamin D is in the form of vitamin D_2 (ergocalciferol) or vitamin D_3 (colecalciferol), once in the blood steam, it is converted into 25-hydroxy cholecalciferol (calcidiol) in the liver through an enzyme 25-alpha hydroxylase (a mitochondrial or microsomal enzyme in liver). It is the major storage form of vitamin D (Cicek et al., 2023).

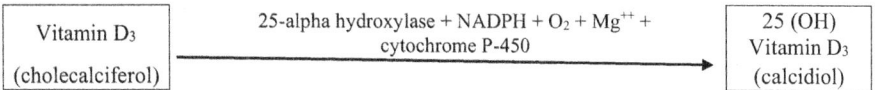

Being the main metabolite of vitamin D, its half-life has been determined to be 3 weeks (Zittermann, 2003). Calcidiol, found in the liver, goes to the circulation where it gets bound to vitamin D binding protein. Only about 1% calcidiol is in the unbound form. From the liver, 25-hydroxy vitamin D3 is taken to the kidney where it is converted into 1, 25-dihydroxy vitamin D3 by the action of another enzyme in the membranes of proximal tubules of the kidney, named 1-alpha hydroxylase. The resulting metabolite is now called "calcitriol" which is the most active form of vitamin D in humans. The 1-alpha hydroxylase is regulated by parathormone (parathyroid hormone) and 25 (OH) vitamin D_3 in circulation. Moreover, like

25-alpha hydroxylase, it also requires NADPH, cytochrome P-450, magnesium, and molecular oxygen.

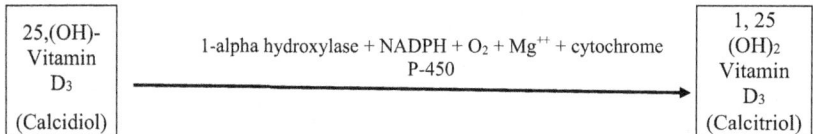

| 25,(OH)-Vitamin D$_3$ (Calcidiol) | 1-alpha hydroxylase + NADPH + O$_2$ + Mg^{++} + cytochrome P-450 $\longrightarrow$ | 1, 25 (OH)$_2$ Vitamin D$_3$ (Calcitriol) |

3.5   Action on target cells

Once calcitriol, the active form of vitamin D, is formed, it is transported to the target tissue where it exerts its function by binding to vitamin D receptor (VDR), which is a 50 KD protein comprising 427 amino acid residues (Cicek et al., 2023). These receptors could be located in the cytoplasm in certain target tissues or nucleus in certain other types of target cells. Calcitriol after binding to the vitamin D receptor forms a heterodimer with retinoic acid receptor (RXR) and translocates to cell nucleus and binds to the response elements on gene leading to its expression (Hossein-nezhad et al., 2013; Zella et al., 2010). It has been estimated that more than 900 genes are influenced by vitamin D (Battistini et al., 2020). Major functions include absorption of calcium through the expression of proteins such as calbindin. Another important function is its role in bone formation. Calcitriol in the presence of parathyroid hormone (PTH) increases the mobilization of calcium and phosphate from bones, thereby increasing their blood levels. Calcitriol then promotes the influx of calcium into osteoblasts and increases the expression of bone matrix proteins such as osteocalcin, osteopontin, alkaline phosphatase, and type I collagen (Jovicic et al., 2012).

3.6   Normal values of vitamin D in blood

Holick was the pioneer in developing the minimal optimal value of vitamin D in serum while keeping in view the threshold value of PTH (Holick, 2009). In adults, a value of 25 (OH) D less than 20 ng/ml was taken as deficiency of vitamin D, while a value between 21 and 29 ng/ml was marked as insufficiency of vitamin D. Bischoff-Ferrari et al. (2006) found a value of 25 (OH) D above 30 ng/ml to be an optimum concentration of vitamin D for a wide variety of functions in the human body.

3.7   Vitamin D deficiency in South Asia

Considering the normal value of 25(OH) D in serum to be above 30 ng/ml, a number of studies have been conducted on South Asian populations to determine the extent of vitamin D deficiency. A systematic review and metaanalysis of 65 studies comprising a total of 44,717 adults from 5 South Asian countries revealed that the average vitamin D levels in serum ranged from 4.7 to 32 ng/ml with a pooled prevalence of deficiency to be 68%. Pakistani adults had the highest prevalence of 73% followed by 67% among Bangladeshi and Indian adults, 57% among Nepalese, and 48% among Sri Lankans (Masood & Iqbal, 2008). Another study conducted on adult population in a peri-urban community in Karachi revealed vitamin D deficiency (< 20 ng/ml) to be 58.4% and vitamin D insufficiency (20 -29 ng/ml) 31.46% suggesting that nearly 90% of adult population in that community has been suffering from vitamin D deficiency or insufficiency (Mehboobali et al., 2015).

3.7.1　Vitamin D deficiency among pregnant women in South Asia

Prevalence of vitamin D deficiency or insufficiency among pregnant women is a serious public health problem because a deficiency during pregnancy has serious implications for a developing fetus. A metaanalysis and a systematic review on South Asian pregnant women revealed that 60% (95% CI: 38%–82%, $P<.001$) of women were suffering from vitamin D deficiency, while 25% (95% CI: 17%–32%, $P<.001$) suffered from vitamin D insufficiency (Nindrea & Hendriyani, 2024).

Unfortunately, this systematic review hardly included any studies from countries in South Asia where vitamin deficiency has reached epidemic proportions. However, a study on pregnant females in rural Bangladesh revealed vitamin D deficiency to be 17% but insufficiency of vitamin D up to 47.2% (Ahmed et al., 2021). Similarly, in South India, vitamin D deficiency among pregnant South Indian women was found to be 62% (Ravinder et al., 2022).

The situation was found to be even more grim in Pakistani urban and rural pregnant women. A study by Anwar and associates (Anwar et al., 2016) showed that 99.5% of pregnant women in urban Karachi and 89% of pregnant women in rural Jhelum were suffering from vitamin D deficiency. Later, it was reported that approximately 79.7% of pregnant women in general population failed to get sufficient quantities of vitamin D during pregnancy, thereby posing a serious risk to the neonates and the pregnant mothers (Final Key Findings Report 2019.pdf [Internet]. Available from: https://www.unicef.org/pakistan/media/1951/file/Final%20Key %20Findings%20Report%202019.pdf). A number of complications during pregnancy such as preeclampsia, diabetes, and miscarriages have been found to be associated with vitamin D deficiency (Salim et al., 2022).

3.8　Vitamin D and glycemic control in type 2 diabetes mellitus

Vitamin D, while influencing the expression of more than 300 genes, has been found to have some unique functions. Over the past few years, an association between vitamin D deficiency and poor glycemic control has been reported in some of the studies (Hutchinson et al., 2011; Kajbaf et al., 2014; Kositsawat et al., 2015; Kostoglou-Athanassiou et al., 2013; Minambres et al., 2015; Tahrani et al., 2010; Zoppini et al., 2013; Iqbal et al., 2016).

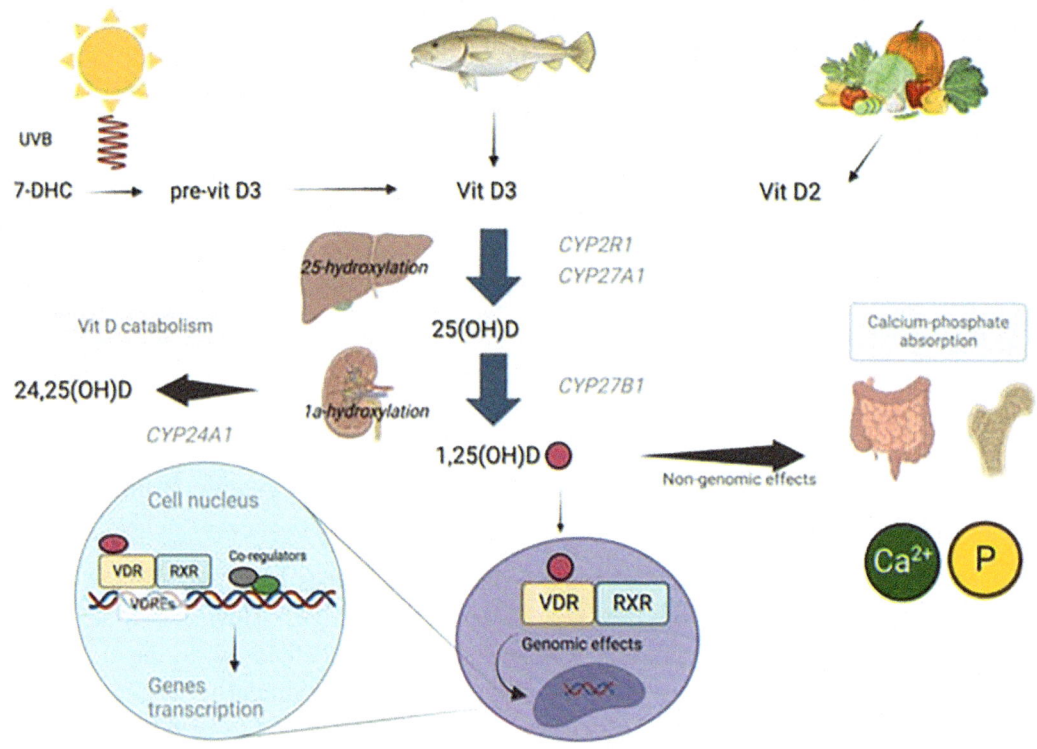

Figure 3.2

Synthesis of previtamin D3 by the action of UV rays from sun on 7-dehydrocholesterol (7 DHC); vegetables and fish are sources of vitamin D2 and vitamin D3, respectively. Vitamin D3 gets converted into 25 (OH) D in liver with the help of liver enzymes 25, hydroxylase (*CYP2R1*) and 24, hydroxylase (*CYP27A1*); conversion of 25 (OH) D into 1, 25 (OH)$_2$ D with the help of enzyme, 1, alpha hydroxylase (*CYP27B1*) in kidney tubules; entry of 1,25(OH)$_2$ into target cell and its binding to retinoid acid receptor (RXR) and translocation into nucleus to regulate the expression of gene (s); nongenomic action of 1, 25 (OH)$_2$ D by direct binding to cells of intestine and bone and increasing the absorption of both calcium and phosphate (Voltan et al., 2023).

Another study carried out in Iraq also reported similar results indicating poor vitamin D status in a diabetic population in Iraq. There was a direct relationship between hypovitaminosis D and poor glycemic control in these patients (Salih et al., 2021). These observations have led to the recommendation that type 2 diabetes mellitus patients should be supplemented with adequate amounts of vitamin D to maintain good glycemic control (Al-Daghri et al., 2012).

The biochemical basis for this action was ascribed to the association of deficiency of vitamin D with insulin resistance (Talaei et al., 2013). Another mechanism that has been put forward is through stimulation of the secretion of insulin from pancreatic beta cells by vitamin D, thereby playing a role in the regulation of insulin secretion (Bourlon et al., 1999). The notion that supplementation with vitamin D will improve glycemic control in diabetic patients has been questioned as there have been quite a few clinical trials showing no association of vitamin D status and glycemic control (Kampmann et al., 2014). Similar results have been reported by Sheth and his colleagues in a study from Western India (Sheth et al., 2015).

A recent systematic review and metaanalysis on this subject by Farahmand and associates (Farahmand et al., 2023) concluded that supplementation of a large dose of vitamin D in diabetic patients having low levels of vitamin D for a short period of time appeared to reduce fasting levels of plasma glucose, HbA1C levels, and HOMAIR in these type 2 diabetic patients.

It appears that the effects of vitamin D on glycemic control could be modulated by a number of factors. Therefore more in-depth studies are required to unravel the precise mechanism by which vitamin D could be influencing glycemic control in diabetes patients.

3.9 Nongenomic actions of vitamin D

In addition to the genomic actions of calcitriol (the active form of vitamin D), which are primarily through nuclear vitamin D receptor (nVDR), which, after forming a complex with retinoid acid receptor (RXR), regulates the expression of a number of genes, there are certain nongenomic actions performed by vitamin D (Hii & Ferrante, 2016).

These nongenomic actions include direct action on the cell membrane of certain target cells such as small intestine and bone and opening channels to facilitate calcium and phosphate absorption as shown in Fig. 3.2 (Voltan et al., 2023). In addition, calcitriol upon binding to target cells causes activation of signaling pathways resulting in phospholipase C, phospholipase A2, phosphatidylinositol-3-kinase (P13K), p21ras, cyclic AMP, and a number of protein kinases (Doroudi et al., 2015; Dwivedi et al., 2010; Fleet, 2004).

Acknowledgment

I thank Professor Filippo Ceccato, University of Padova, Italy, for permitting reproduction of a figure from one of his papers. The technical help provided by Ms. Tehreem Sajjad is also gratefully acknowledged.

References

Ahmed, F., Khosravi-Boroujeni, H., Khan, M. R., Roy, A. K., & Raqib, R. (2021). Prevalence and predictors of vitamin D deficiency and insufficiency among pregnant rural women in Bangladesh. *Nutrients, 13*(2), 449.

Al-Daghri, N. M., Alkharfy, K. M., Al-Othman, A., El-Kholie, E., Moharram, O., Alokail, M. S., & Chrousos, G. P. (2012). Vitamin D supplementation as an adjuvant therapy for patients with T2DM: an 18-month prospective interventional study. *Cardiovascular diabetology, 11*, 1–7.

Anwar, S., Iqbal, M. P., Azam, I., Habib, A., Bhutta, S., Soofi, S. B., & Bhutta, Z. A. (2016). Urban and rural comparison of vitamin D status in Pakistani pregnant women and neonates. *Journal of Obstetrics and Gynaecology, 36*(3), 318–323.

Battistini, C., Ballan, R., Herkenhoff, M. E., Saad, S. M. I., & Sun, J. (2020). Vitamin D modulates intestinal microbiota in inflammatory bowel diseases. *International Journal of Molecular Sciences, 22*(1), 362.

Bischoff-Ferrari, H. A., Giovannucci, E., Willett, W. C., Dietrich, T., & Dawson-Hughes, B. (2006). Estimation of optimal serum concentrations of 25-hydroxyvitamin D for multiple health outcomes. *The American Journal of Clinical Nutrition, 84*(1), 18–28.

Bourlon, P. M., Billaudel, B., & Faure-Dussert, A. (1999). Influence of vitamin D3 deficiency and 1, 25 dihydroxyvitamin D3 on de novo insulin biosynthesis in the islets of the rat endocrine pancreas. *Journal of Endocrinology, 160*(1), 87–96.

Cicek, H., Duyuran, R., Sri, R. M. M., & Ravichandran, S. (2023). Biochemistry and metabolism of vitamin D. *Int J Clin Biochem Res, 10*(1), 28–36.

Deluca, H. F. (2014). History of the discovery of vitamin D and its active metabolites. *BoneKEy Reports, 3*.

Doroudi, M., Schwartz, Z., & Boyan, B. D. (2015). Membrane-mediated actions of 1, 25-dihydroxy vitamin D3: A review of the roles of phospholipase A2 activating protein and Ca2+/calmodulin-dependent protein kinase II. *The Journal of Steroid Biochemistry and Molecular Biology, 147*, 81–84.

Dusso, A. S., Brown, A. J., & Slatofolsky, E. (2005). Vitamin D. *American Journal of Physiology-Renal Physiology, 289*, F8–28.

Dwivedi, P. P., Gao, X. H., Tan, J. C. T., Evdokiou, A., Ferrante, A., Morris, H. A., & Hii, C. S. (2010). A role for the phosphatidylinositol 3-kinase–protein kinase C zeta–Sp1 pathway in the 1, 25-dihydroxyvitamin D3 induction of the 25-hydroxyvitamin D3 24-hydroxylase gene in human kidney cells. *Cellular Signaling, 22*(3), 543–552.

Farahmand, M. A., Daneshzad, E., Fung, T. T., Zahidi, F., Muhammadi, M., Bellissimo, N., & Azadbakht, L. (2023). What is the impact of vitamin D supplementation on glycemic control in people with type-2 diabetes: a systematic review and meta-analysis of randomized controlled trails. *BMC Endocrine Disorders, 23*(1), 15.

Fitzpatrick, S., Sheard, N. F., Clark, N. G., & LeeRitter, M. (2000). Vitamin D-deficient rickets: a multifactorial disease. *Nutrition Reviews, 58*(7), 218–222.

Fleet, J. C. (2004). Rapid, membrane-initiated actions of 1, 25 dihydroxyvitamin D: what are they and what do they mean? *The Journal of Nutrition, 134*(12), 3215–3218.

Hess, A. F., & Unger, P. (1921). The cure of infantile rickets by sunlight as demonstrated by a chemical alteration of the blood. *Proceedings of the Society for Experimental Biology and Medicine, 19*(1), 31–34.

Hess, A. F., & Weinstock, M. (1924). Antirachitic properties imparted to lettuce and to growing wheat by ultraviolet irradiation. *Proceedings of the Society for Experimental Biology and Medicine, 22*(1), 5–6.

Hii, C. S., & Ferrante, A. (2016). The non-genomic actions of vitamin D. *Nutrients, 8*(3), 135.

Holick, M. F. (2009). Vitamin D status: Measurement, interpretation, and clinical application. *Annals of Epidemiology, 19*(2), 73–78.

Hossein-nezhad, A., Spira, A., & Holick, M. F. (2013). Influence of vitamin D status and vitamin D3 supplementation on genome wide expression of white blood cells: a randomized double-blind clinical trial. *PloS One, 8*(3), e58725.

Hutchinson, M. S., Figenschau, Y., Njolstad, I., Schirmer, H., & Jorde, R. (2011). Serum 25-hydroxyvitamin D levels are inversely associated with glycated haemoglobin (HbA1c). The Tromsø Study. *Scandinavian Journal of Clinical and Laboratory Investigation, 71*(5), 399–406.

Iqbal, K., Islam, N., Mehboobali, N., Asghar, A., & Iqbal, M. P. (2016). Association of vitamin D deficiency with poor glycaemic control in diabetic patients. *J Pak Med Assoc, 66*(12), 1562–1565.

Jovicic, S., Ignjatovic, S., & Majkic-Singh, N. (2012). Biochemistry and metabolism of vitamin D. *Journal of Medical Biochemistry, 31*(4), 309–315.

Kajbaf, F., Mentaverri, R., Diouf, M., Fournier, A., Kamel, S., & Lalau, J. D. (2014). The association between 25-hydroxyvitamin D and hemoglobin A1c levels in patients with type 2 diabetes and stage 1–5 chronic kidney disease. *International Journal of Endocrinology, 2014*(1), 142468.

Kalueff, A. L. (2005). Behavioural abnormalities in mice with partially deleted vitamin D receptor gene Academic dissertation. University of Tampere, Medical School, Finland. http://www.researchgate.net/publication/134442121.

Kampmann, U., Mosekilde, L., Juhl, C., Moller, N., Christensen, B., Rejnmark, L., & Orskov, L. (2014). Effects of 12 weeks high dose vitamin D3 treatment on insulin sensitivity, beta cell function, and metabolic markers in patients with type 2 diabetes and vitamin D insufficiency–a double-blind, randomized, placebo-controlled trial. *Metabolism, 63*(9), 1115–1124.

Khalsa, S. (2009). *Vitamin D Revolution: How the power of this amazing vitamin can change your life.* Hay House, Inc.

Kositsawat, J., Kuchel, G. A., Tooze, J. A., Houston, D. K., Cauley, J. A., & Kritchevsky, S. B. Health ABC. (2015). Vitamin D insufficiency and abnormal hemoglobin A1c in black and white older persons. *Journals of Gerontology Series A: Biomedical Sciences and Medical Sciences, 70*(4), 525–531.

Kostoglou-Athanassiou, I., Athanassiou, P., Gkountouvas, A., & Kaldrymides, P. (2013). Vitamin D and glycemic control in diabetes mellitus type 2. *Therapeutic Advances in Endocrinology and Metabolism, 4*(4), 122–128.

Malloy, P. J., Pike, J. W., & Feldman, D. (1999). The vitamin D receptor and the syndrome of hereditary 1,25-dihydrovitamin D resistant rickets. *Endocr Rev, 20*, 156–188.

Masood, S. H., & Iqbal, M. P. (2008). Prevalence of vitamin D deficiency in South Asia. *Angiogenesis, 1*(11), 12.

McCollum, E. V., Simmonds, N., Becker, J. E., & Shipley, P. G. (1922). Studies on experimental rickets: XXI. An experimental demonstration of the existence of a vitamin which promotes calcium deposition. *Journal of Biological Chemistry, 53*(2), 293–312.

Mehboobali, N., Iqbal, S. P., & Iqbal, M. P. (2015). High prevalence of vitamin D deficiency and insufficiency in a low-income peri-urban community in Karachi. *Journal of Pakistan Medical Association, 65*(9), 946.

Mellanby, E. (1919). An experimental investigation of rickets. *Lancet, 1*, 407–412.

Michigami, T. (2017). Update on recent progress in vitamin D research. Vitamin D Metabolism and Its Regulation. *Clinical Calcium, 27*(11), 1517–1523.

Minambres, I., Sánchez-Quesada, J. L., Vinagre, I., Sánchez-Hernández, J., Urgell, E., De Leiva, A., & Pérez, A. (2015). Hypovitaminosis D in type 2 diabetes: relation with features of the metabolic syndrome and glycemic control. *Endocrine research, 40*(3), 160–165.

Nindrea, R. D., & Hendriyani, H. (2024). Prevalence of vitamin D deficiency among pregnant women in Southeast Asia represents public health crisis: A systematic review and meta-analysis. *Clinical Epidemiology and Global Health* 101574.

Ravinder, S. S., Padmavathi, R., Maheshkumar, K., Mohankumar, M., Maruthy, K. N., Sankar, S., & Balakrishnan, K. (2022). Prevalence of vitamin D deficiency among South Indian pregnant women. *Journal of Family Medicine and Primary Care, 11*(6), 2884–2889.

Reichrath, J., Lehmann, B., Carlberg, C., Varani, J., & Zouboulis, C. C. (2007). Vitamins and hormones. *Horm Metab Res, 39*(2), 71–84.

Salih, Y. A., Rasool, M. T., Ahmed, I. H., & Mohammed, A. A. (2021). Impact of vitamin D level on glycemic control in diabetes mellitus type 2 in Duhok. *Annals of Medicine and Surgery, 64*, 102208.

Salim, N., Sattar, M. A., & Adnan, A. (2022). High prevalence of vitamin D deficiency in Pakistan and miscarriages: A hazard to pregnancies. *Annals of Medicine and Surgery, 82*.

Sheth, J. J., Shah, A., Sheth, F. J., Trivedi, S., Lele, M., Shah, N., & Vaidya, R. (2015). Does vitamin D play a significant role in type 2 diabetes? *BMC Endocrine Disorders, 15*(5), 1–7.

Steenbock, H., & Black, A. (1924). Fat-soluble vitamins: XVII. The induction of growth-promoting and calcifying properties in a ration by exposure to ultra-violet light. *Journal of Biological Chemistry, 61*(2), 405–422.

Tahrani, A. A., Ball, A., Shepherd, L., Rahim, A., Jones, A. F., & Bates, A. (2010). The prevalence of vitamin D abnormalities in South Asians with type 2 diabetes mellitus in the UK. *International Journal of Clinical Practice, 64*(3), 351–355.

Talaei, A., Mohamadi, M., & Adgi, Z. (2013). The effect of vitamin D on insulin resistance in patients with type 2 diabetes. *Diabetology & metabolic syndrome, 5*, 1–5.

Voltan, G., Cannito, M., Ferrarese, M., Ceccato, F., & Camozzi, V. (2023). Vitamin D: an overview of gene regulation, ranging from metabolism to genomic effects. *Genes, 14*(9), 1691.

Windaus, A., Lettre, H., & Schenck, F. (1935). 7-Dehydrocholesterol. *Annals of Chemistry, 520*, 98–107.

Zella, L. A., Meyer, M. B., Nerenz, R. D., Lee, S. M., Martowicz, M. L., & Pike, J. W. (2010). Multifunctional enhancers regulate mouse and human vitamin D receptor gene transcription. *Molecular Endocrinology, 24*(1), 128–147.

Zittermann, A. (2003). Vitamin D in preventive medicine: Are we ignoring the evidence? *British Journal of Nutrition, 89*(5), 552–572.

Zoppini, G., Galletti, A., Targher, G., Brangani, C., Pichiri, I., Negri, C., & Bonora, E. (2013). Glycated haemoglobin is inversely related to serum vitamin D levels in type 2 diabetic patients. *PLoS One, 8*(12), e82733.

The power of D: health, performance, and global impact

CHAPTER 4

Vitamin D and bone health

Saira Perwaiz Iqbal[1], and Mohammad Perwaiz Iqbal[2,3]

[1]*Infectious Diseases, Department of Medicine, Maimonides Medical Center, Brooklyn, NY, United States* [2]*Biochemistry, Biological & Biomedical Sciences, Aga Khan University, Karachi, Pakistan* [3]*Life Sciences Department, School of Science, University of Management and Technology, Lahore, Pakistan*

4.1 Introduction

Vitamin D is a fat-soluble vitamin that is derived from cholesterol. It is a secosteroid hormone with an incomplete ring that plays an essential role in bone growth and mineralization. Naturally, it exists in plants as ergocalciferol (vitamin D2) and in animals as cholecalciferol (vitamin D3). In humans, cholecalciferol can be obtained from diet or synthesized within deeper layers of the epidermis upon exposure to ultraviolet B rays in sunlight. However, this is an inactive metabolite that must undergo biological activation via two hydroxylation processes. The first hydroxylation takes place in the liver, resulting in the formation of 25-hydroxycholecalciferol or calcidiol. The second hydroxylation occurs in the kidney to form 1,25-dihydroxycholecalciferol or calcitriol, which is the active metabolite of vitamin D. The activated vitamin D then regulates the absorption of calcium, phosphate, and magnesium from the intestine and kidneys to maintain a balance between bone formation and bone resorption (Fig. 4.1).

4.2 History

Vitamin D deficiency has been around since the 15th century, but it was first described and documented in 1650 in Europe. A skeletal deformity was noted amongst affected children that significantly retarded their growth. It affected the long bones, joints, and even the ribcage. This affliction was initially called "the English disease" and later termed *Rickets* (Jones, 2022). Studies performed in the late 1700s in the United Kingdom showed marked improvement in disease after supplementation with cod liver oil, indicating some nutritional deficit (Percival, 1789). In contrast, another school of thought in the early 1800s from Poland suggested an environmental aspect to the disease, speculating fresh air or adequate sunlight exposure (Sniadecki & Sniadecki, 1840). Over the next 200 years, various experiments confirmed that vitamin D is not essential in diet and can be synthesized from UV exposure

The Impact of Vitamin D on Health and Disease. **DOI:** https://doi.org/10.1016/B978-0-443-34037-6.00031-5

(Raczynski, 1913; Rollier, 1923). However, deficiency can still ensue in different populations with inadequate exposure to sunlight, which can easily be overcome with diet and nutritional supplementation.

4.3   Vitamin D deficiency

Vitamin D is being extensively studied, and newer research has shown that its benefits are not only limited to bone metabolism but also has a significant role in cellular differentiation, cancer prevention, and immunity. Under this new light, there has been an exponential rise in vitamin D testing over the last few years. The most reliable marker for assessing vitamin D status is serum 25-hydroxyvitamin D because it is the main circulating form with a longer half-life of 3 weeks. According to the National Institute of Health (NIH), a range between 20 and 50 ng/mL (or 50–125 nmol/L) of 25(OH) D is considered adequate to sustain stable bone growth. A serum or plasma concentration of 25(OH) D less than 20 ng/mL (or 50 nmol/L) is considered vitamin D deficiency. Severe vitamin D deficiency is defined as 25(OH)D level of less than 12 ng/mL (or 30 nmol/L), and it significantly increases the risk of rickets and osteomalacia (Taylor et al., 2015).

The optimal level for vitamin D supplementation differs from country to country; however, there is a general consensus on recommending a daily allowance (RDA) of 400–1000 IU for children/adolescents under 18 years and 800–2000 IU for adults between 18 and 75 years. A higher RDA from 2000 to 4000 IU should be considered for pregnant females or older adults > 75 years of age (Bleizgys, 2021).

4.4   Prevalence

Deficiency of vitamin D has emerged as a global problem affecting almost one-third of the world's population. However, prevalence rates vary drastically among different populations. This can be attributed to numerous factors, such as the environment, climate, and industrialization.

According to a worldwide review, the prevalence of severe vitamin D deficiency has been found in 5.9% US population and 7.4% in the Canadian population. There is a slightly higher prevalence reported in Europe reaching around 13%. In South Asian countries, including Pakistan, India, Afghanistan, and Tunisia, low vitamin D status is reported to involve > 20% of the population (Amrein et al., 2020).

This indicates that population traits, such as age, education, ethnicity, type of skin, and traditions, also play a part in defining the vitamin status of a country.

4.5 Metabolism of vitamin D

Vitamin D3 is synthesized endogenously by the action of ultraviolet-B rays on 7-dehydrocholesterol present in keratinocytes and fibroblasts in the skin. Then, it binds to vitamin D binding protein (DBP) and is carried to the liver. Vitamin D, which is obtained from diet, is lipid soluble. Hence it gets absorbed by the villi in the small intestine and is packaged into chylomicrons and lipoproteins to be transported to the liver.

Once endogenous or dietary vitamin D reaches the liver, it is hydroxylated to form 25-hydroxycholecalciferol [25(OH)D]. This 25(OH)D binds to DBPs and circulates in the blood to be filtered through the glomerulus. It is then reabsorbed in the proximal tubules of kidneys and hydroxylated by 1-α hydroxylase to form active metabolite; 1,25-dihydroxycholecalciferol [1,25(OH)$_2$D] or Calcitriol. This active form 1,25(OH)$_2$D binds to the vitamin D receptor (VDR) and triggers gene transcription that results in calcium and phosphate absorption from the small intestine. Many factors stimulate the production of 1,25(OH)$_2$D, including low calcium and low phosphate states and hyperparathyroidism (Christakos et al., 2010; DeLuca, 1976; Horst et al., 2005).

When calcium levels drop in blood, parathyroid glands release parathyroid hormone (PTH), which increases the calcium level in blood by (1) stimulating kidneys to increase tubular reabsorption of calcium; (2) enhancing the activity of 1-α hydroxylase to produce 1,25 hydroxycholecalciferol and facilitate further calcium absorption from intestine; (3) acting on bone to increase osteoclastic activity and release bone calcium from stores.

Once the calcium level is adequate in the blood (normocalcemia), the active 1, 25(OH)$_2$D inactivates itself via negative feedback. High circulating levels of cholecalciferol stimulate fibroblast growth factor (FGF23) and the renal enzyme 24-α hydroxylase to create a negative feedback loop (Fig. 4.2). (1) 24-α hydroxylase inactivates 1, 25(OH)$_2$D by converting it into 24,25(OH)D, an inactive metabolite of vitamin D. (2) Fibroblast growth factor 23 (FGF23) is a phosphaturic hormone which is synthesized and released from osteocytes/osteoblasts. It inhibits 1-α hydroxylase and increases the expression of 24-α hydroxylase, hence reducing renal absorption of phosphate to maintain homeostasis (Fig. 4.2).

4.6 Causes of vitamin D deficiency

Vitamin D deficiency can occur due to multiple factors such as inadequate sun exposure, nutritional deficiency, coexisting liver, kidney, or gastrointestinal disease, or medications (Thomas & Demay, 2000). These factors have been summarized in Table 4.1.

4.6.1   *Reduced cutaneous synthesis*

Adequate sunlight exposure with high energy ultraviolet B rays (UV-B rays) is necessary to activate the vitamin D precursor in the skin. In certain parts of the world where the duration of sunshine is less, ultraviolet-B photons do not reach the earth's atmosphere; hence, an exceedingly small amount of vitamin D3 is produced. This is also seen in cold climate areas.

Among different ethnic groups, skin pigmentation also plays a key role. Light-skinned people need less UV-B exposure, while dark-skinned individuals require six times more exposure to UV-B to produce the same amount of vitamin.

Older adults are often deficient as their cutaneous vitamin D stores deplete with advancing age.

Whole-body clothing from head to toe in some religious cultures can minimize exposure to sunlight, especially seen in Muslim communities.

Similarly, the use of sunscreens in some populations can also reduce the effect of ultraviolet rays. A sunscreen with SPF 15 can decrease the skin penetration of UV-B up to 98%.

Patients with prolonged hospitalizations who are not exposed to outside sunshine will have deficiency unless provided with supplementation.

Extensive burn injury patients also have reduced synthesis of vitamin D despite adequate sun exposure because of reduced body surface area due to skin loss.

4.6.2   *Nutritional deficiency*

Despite adequate sun exposure, some people can still acquire vitamin D deficiency, especially in those who do not consume fortified food products. Fortification is the addition of essential minerals and micronutrients in different food groups to combat deficiency on a larger scale. Vitamin D fortification began in the 1930s with the addition of vitamin D in milk to prevent rickets. In the Western world, most foods are being fortified, such as yogurt, cheese, cereals, and orange juice. However, in many parts of the world, food fortification is still lacking.

Naturally occurring vitamin D is also found in abundance in meat products. The consumption of meat products should be encouraged; however, this may be unacceptable in some cultures that follow vegetarian diets.

Exclusively, breastfed infants can develop deficiency because breast milk is low in vitamin D. This deficiency should be overcome by exposing them to sunlight at least 30 minutes per week. Formula-fed infants do not require added vitamins because of the fortification of infant formula milk.

4.6.3 Renal diseases

In chronic kidney disease (CKD), structural renal damage results in the loss of enzyme 1-α hydroxylase, which is necessary for conversion to active vitamin D3 or 1,25 dihydroxycholecalciferol. This leads to hypocalcemia, secondary hyperparathyroidism, and bone disease, often referred to as renal osteodystrophy. Nutritional supplementation with vitamin D is recommended.

Proteinuria seen in nephrotic syndrome can also cause vitamin D deficiency by decreasing the amount of circulating vitamin D binding proteins (DBPs).

Distal renal tubular acidosis (RTA) triggers bone resorption; minerals are pulled from the bone in an attempt to buffer the acidosis, leading to hypocalcemia and hypophosphatemia. This is called hypophosphatemic rickets or vitamin D-resistant rickets. Calcium, phosphorus, and vitamin D replacement is necessary alongside correction of acidosis.

4.6.4 Gastrointestinal/liver disease

Malabsorption interferes with vitamin D metabolism. The disease of the hepatobiliary tree, pancreas, and small intestine can result in poor absorption and cause depletion of 25(OH) stores via interruption in the enterohepatic circulation. Commonest conditions include celiac disease, inflammatory bowel disease, cholestasis, and pancreatic insufficiency.

Obesity is known to cause deficiency because vitamin D, being lipid-soluble, gets sequestered into fat. Patients who have undergone bariatric surgeries such as bypass or gastrectomies (partial or total) lose gastric acidity, which again hinders vitamin D absorption from the proximal small bowel.

Parenchymal liver damage can cause loss of enzyme 25-α hydroxylase and reduce stores of 25 (OH)D.

4.6.5 Medications

Many medications can precipitate vitamin D deficiency by enhancing the catabolism of 25(OH)D (calcidiol) and 1,25 $(OH)_2D$ (calcitriol) by inducing the cytochrome P-450 enzyme. Certain anticonvulsants and antiretroviral drugs convert circulating calcidiol into inactive metabolites. Ketoconazole and some antifungals inhibit 1-hydroxylation to block the production of active vitamin D_3. Clinicians should be mindful when prescribing such drugs and ensure that the patient is on adequate supplementation. Another useful tactic would be to check vitamin D levels every 3 to 6 months while on medications. A detailed list of drugs causing vitamin D deficiency has been shown in Table 4.1.

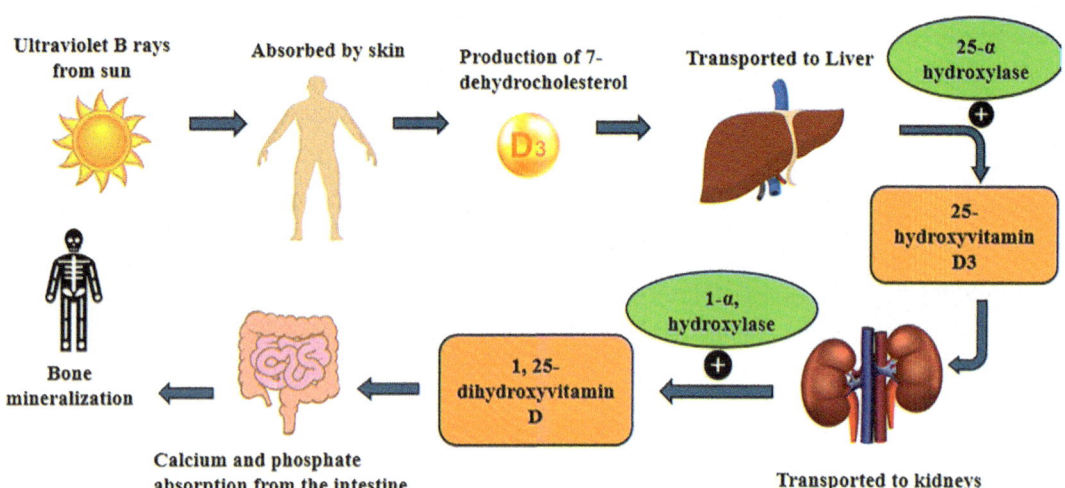

Figure 4.1
Overview of vitamin D and bone mineralization.
Production and activation of vitamin D and its role in increasing calcium deposition in bones.

4.7   Bone defects caused by vitamin D deficiency

There are two main types of cells found in bone: the bone-forming cells called osteoblasts and bone-remodeling cells called osteoclasts. Osteoblasts lay down the main framework or the osteoid, which undergoes subsequent mineralization by calcium salts. The process of mineralization gives the bone strength to withstand pressure and bear weight. Vitamin D is responsible for maintaining homeostasis between calcium and phosphorus to ensure proper bone growth and mineralization. Any deficiency in vitamin D or calcium will lead to a weaker bone matrix that will result in severe bone defects like rickets and osteomalacia.

Both rickets and osteomalacia belong to the same disease spectrum of unmineralized bone matrix. However, rickets is seen in young children and cause significant deformities such as frontal bossing and bowing of legs because the growth plates are still open, and long bones buckle under body weight. On the other hand, osteomalacia occurs in adults after fusion of the growth plates and may not cause obvious bone deformities (Whyte & Thakker, 2013).

4.8   Rickets

Rickets was first identified in children in the 16th century with severe skeletal deformities, but it took another two hundred years to establish its relation to sunlight exposure and vitamin D. With increased awareness and fortification of food products, the incidence of rickets has reduced globally. Multiple skeletal defects are pathognomonic of rickets, including bowing of legs, enlargement of the joint epiphyses of ribs, widening of wrists and ankles, and bossing of frontal and parietal skull bones. The severity and degree of deformity depend upon the age of acquiring the deficiency. For example, in infants, the defect is prominent in the forearms and skull bones. Toddlers will display an exaggeration of physiological tibial bowing, also called genu varum. Older children may have "knock knees" or genu valgum with kyphosis or scoliosis. Apart from skeletal deformities, these children also have a weak immune system and are prone to many infections, like pneumonia. This is consistent with recent research that has proven that vitamin D also plays a vital role in immunity. Children with rickets may be asymptomatic or have bone pains, irritability, paresthesia, delayed milestones, stunted growth, or waddling gait. Some patients may exhibit tetany resulting from severe hypocalcemia.

Rickets can be classified as nutritional or nonnutritional. Conditions that cause nutritional rickets include hypocalcemia, hypophosphatemia, and/or vitamin D deficiency (Chanchlani et al., 2020). Hypocalcemic rickets occurs if calcium intake is too low, even if vitamin D intake is adequate. Hypophosphatemic or nonnutritional rickets is caused by excess loss of phosphate from the kidneys. This is seen in renal tubular disorders like Fanconi's syndrome or certain genetic/hereditary conditions like X-linked hypophosphatemic rickets (XLHR), autosomal dominant (ADHR) or autosomal recessive hypophosphatemic rickets (ARHR).

4.9   Osteomalacia

Mineralization defect in adults is called osteomalacia which means "soft bone." The pathogenic mechanisms that can hinder bone mineralization and cause osteomalacia include:
1. Vitamin D deficiency or resistance to vitamin D.
2. Calcium deficiency (with or without vitamin D deficiency).
3. Renal wasting of phosphate salts.
4. Inhibitory effects of various drugs.
5. Oncogenic osteomalacia (increased FGF-23 release from neoplastic cells).

Osteomalacia can be identified with its characteristic radiological appearances, but there are many conditions that can mimic these findings, such as bone matrix disorders and high bone turnover states. Therefore, a definitive diagnosis can only be made by transiliac bone biopsy with histomorphometry.

4.10   Stages of hypovitaminosis D

Vitamin D deficiency or hypovitaminosis-related osteopathy can evolve into three stages based upon the biochemical profile and bone histomorphometry (Minisola et al., 2021). These stages have been elaborated in Table 4.2 (1) Initial stage of hypovitaminosis shows normal serum calcium and phosphate, elevated alkaline phosphatase, increased parathyroid hormone

(PTH), and consequently increased 1, 25-dihydroxyvitamin D. Bone histomorphometry reveals no mineralization defect. (2) The second stage of hypovitaminosis D reveals a decline in serum calcium and phosphate levels, alkaline phosphatase, and parathyroid hormone (PTH) increase further but because of lack of substrate 1,25-dihydroxyvitamin D returns to normal or low. Histomorphometry shows some degree of impaired mineralization. (3) In the third and final stage of severe deficiency there is hypocalcemia and hypophosphatemia with high alkaline phosphatase and remarkably high PTH levels (secondary hyperparathyroidism). Bone histomorphometry shows bone loss with porosity and thinning of the cortex.

4.11   Clinical manifestations

Most adults with early osteomalacia are asymptomatic. But as it progresses, they may develop generalized body pains that start from the weight-bearing areas, such as thighs, and lower back and gradually spread to involve arms and ribs. It is a nonradiating and symmetrical pain with associated tenderness in the affected bones. They eventually develop weakness of the proximal muscles, making it difficult to climb stairs, lift objects, and stand up from a squatting

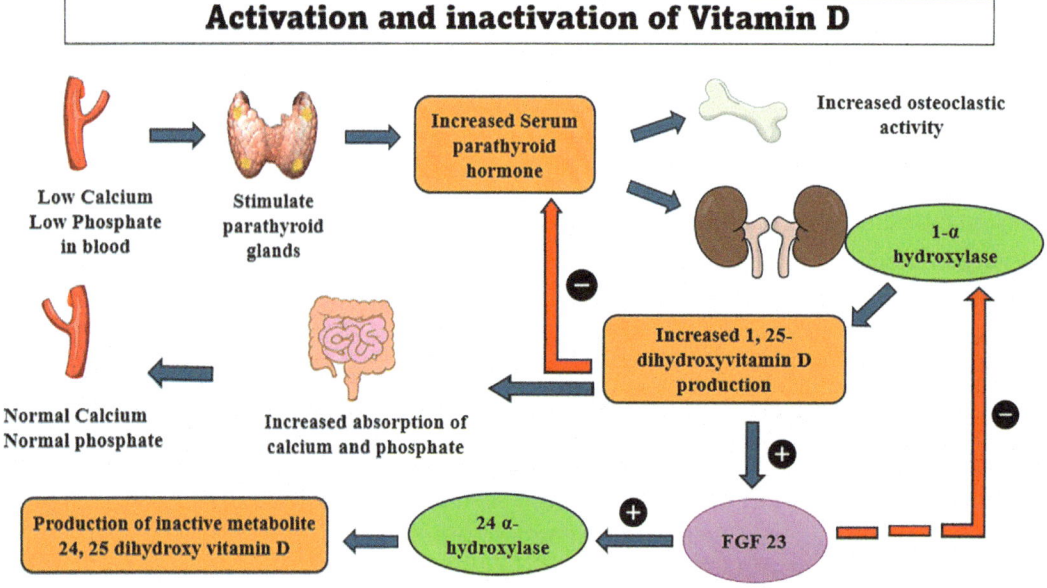

Figure 4.2
Activation and inactivation of vitamin D.
Positive and negative feedback mechanisms of vitamin D.

position. In severe disease, one may also develop pathological or fragility fractures from excess weight bearing on weak bones. Severe hypocalcemia may also cause tetany in adults.

Table 4.1 Causes of vitamin D deficiency.

Causes of vitamin D deficiency
Reduced sun exposure • Cold climate • Industrial pollution • Avoidance of sunlight/staying indoors • Use of sunscreens/sunblocks • Full body clothing
Skin conditions • Dark skin pigmentation • Advanced age • Extensive burns
Nutritional deficiency • Consumption of nonfortified foods • Vegetarians or "vegans"
Gastrointestinal abnormalities • Gastrectomy or bypass procedure • Intestinal resection • Gluten enteropathy (celiac disease) • Malabsorption syndromes • Pancreatic insufficiency
Hepatic conditions • Cirrhosis of liver • Primary biliary cholangitis • Neonatal hepatitis
Renal conditions • Chronic renal failure • Nephrotic syndrome • Distal renal tubular acidosis
Miscellaneous conditions • Obesity • Exclusive breastfeeding • Postmenopausal women
Medications • Anticonvulsants (phenytoin, phenobarbitone, carbamazepine) • Antiretrovirals (tenofovir, foscarnet, pentamidine) • Antimicrobials (rifampicin, isoniazid, ketoconazole) • Miscellaneous drugs (corticosteroids, theophylline, recombinant growth hormone)

4.12   Laboratory investigations and screening

Osteomalacia and rickets can be clinically diagnosed with a detailed history, including diet, medications, medical history of malabsorption, liver, or kidney disease. There are additional laboratory tests that can help in determining the etiology and diagnosis (Sahay & Sahay, 2012).

4.12.1   Blood tests

Serum alkaline phosphatase (ALP) represents osteoblastic activity and is a marker of active bone and cartilage growth and mineralization. Infants and children have higher levels due to rapid bone growth up to 350 IU/L, which gradually decreases after puberty. Normal levels of ALP in adults 18 years and above range between 30 IU/L to 130 IU/L. Serum alkaline phosphatase can be markedly elevated in rickets, osteomalacia, and osteoporosis.

Serum calcium and phosphorus concentrations are typically low in hypocalcemic rickets and osteomalacia. Calcium levels may be normal in hypophosphatemic rickets and in some stages of early disease due to the compensatory response of parathyroid hormone.

Serum parathyroid hormone (PTH) concentrations are elevated in osteomalacia and hypocalcemic rickets, but PTH may be normal in hypophosphatemic rickets.

High serum creatinine and low GFR levels may reflect bone disease related to kidney disease, also referred to as renal osteodystrophy. Other tests that will assist in diagnosis include urinary calcium and phosphorus levels, urine pH, urinary glucose, and liver enzymes.

4.12.2   Vitamin D assay

As discussed earlier, the main circulating form of vitamin D is 25-hydroxy vitamin D because of its longer half-life. It reflects the amount of vitamin stores and is the best indicator of vitamin D status. A serum 25(OH) D level of less than 20 ng/mL suggests deficiency. The lower the 25(OH)D concentration, the higher the risk of rickets and osteomalacia. Hence, this is the most reliable screening tool for the high-risk population. It can also be used as a prognostic marker by repeating levels every 3 months to ensure that supplementation is effective.

Screening is recommended only for symptomatic adults and high-risk populations, such as older adults > 65 years of age, children with high serum ALP levels, and pregnant females. According to the latest recommendations of the United States Preventive Services Task Force (USPSTF), universal screening of the general population has not been backed by research or evidence yet (Burnett-Bowie & Cappola, 2021).

4.12.3   Radiographs

Plain radiographs may help in determining the diagnosis of rickets and osteomalacia. Certain X-ray findings, such as cortical thinning and osteopenia, are nonspecific and may be present in a variety of bone defects, such as osteoporosis. Specific changes related to rickets are most prominent at the epiphyseal growth plates, which show widening, cupping, and splaying due to unmineralized osteoid (Adams, 2018). Hence, in children the diagnosis of rickets can be confirmed on radiographs of the distal ulna and knees.

Radiographs in adults with osteomalacia will show osteopenia and more pathognomonic "pseudo-fractures," which are 2–5 mm wide, transverse, radiolucent lines with sclerotic margins seen perpendicular to the long axis of the bone. These are also called Looser's zones or Milkman's lines, and they are commonly found at the femoral neck, shaft, scapula, ribs, ischial, and pubic rami. These are thought to be stress fractures that have healed improperly due to poorly mineralized osteoid, but the exact reason for these lines remains unclear. Fig. 4.3.

4.12.4   Bone densitometry

Another way to evaluate bone health and assess the risk of fractures is to measure bone mineral density (BMD). It is the measure of calcium and mineral contents of the bone using dual-energy X-ray absorptiometry (DXA) scan, also called bone density scan. Calcium salts and minerals make bone denser and stronger and less prone to fractures. It is a widely accepted screening tool for osteoporosis but reduced BMD can also occur because of osteomalacia (Cundy et al., 2020; Iqbal & Khan, 2010). This test does not differentiate between the two, but its clinical implication is similar (Chun, 2011).

The result of the DXA scan is based on T-scores:
- T- score equal to or greater than -1 indicates normal bone density.
- T- score between -1 and -2.5 suggests low bone density or osteopenia.
- T- score less than -2.5 indicates severe disease or osteoporosis.

DXA scans also give a Z-score which compares the individual's BMD with other people having the same age, gender, and body size.

4.12.5   Bone biopsy

The most accurate diagnostic test for osteomalacia/rickets is bone biopsy with tetracycline labeling. It is not routinely performed because it is invasive, and diagnosis can be made with clinical and radiological findings alone. Bone biopsy is taken from the iliac crest, and slides are prepared for histomorphometric analysis (Sahay & Sahay, 2012).

The following characteristics of osteomalacia will confirm the diagnosis: (1) widened osteoid with thickness > 15μm, (2) increased osteoid volume > 5%, and (3) prolonged mineralization lag time > 100 days.

All three features are necessary for the diagnosis of osteomalacia. Nonetheless, transiliac crest bone biopsy is now only used as an academic or research tool.

4.13   Prevention of vitamin D deficiency

According to the Institute of Medicine 2010 guidelines, the recommended daily allowance (RDA) for vitamin D in healthy children from ages 1 to 18 years is 600 IU/mL. This dose can be increased in children who are obese or on medications such as steroids, antiepileptics, and antiretroviral agents.

Similarly, adults aged 18–70 years require a recommended daily allowance of 600 IU/day. Adults older than 70 years of age should receive higher doses up to 800 IU/day.

Pregnant and lactating females require a minimum daily intake of at least 600 IU to maintain bone growth and this may be increased up to 4000 IU/ day.

According to the Endocrine Society practice guidelines (Ramasamy, 2020), higher doses of vitamin D, ranging from 1500 IU to 2000 IU/day, should be considered in high-risk populations such as pregnancy states, early diabetes, immunocompromised individuals, or children on medications.

4.14   Different formulations of vitamin D

Vitamin D is readily available in its generic forms, ergocalciferol (vitamin D2) and cholecalciferol (vitamin D3), which are effective and cost-effective at the same time.

Table 4.2 Stages of hypovitaminosis D.

Hypovitaminosis	Calcium	Phosphate	Parathyroid hormone	Alkaline Phosphatase	1,25 (OH) 2D level	Bone histomorphometry
Initial stage	Normal	Normal	High	High	Increased	No mineralization defect
Second stage	Low	Low	Normal or low	High	Low	Some degree of impaired mineralization
Final stage	Low	Low	Very high	High	Very low	Bone loss with porosity and cortical thinning

- Ergocalciferol is available in oral capsules, tablets, or liquid form. It is preferred for people who are strictly vegetarian or those who have cultural or religious restrictions that limit sun-exposure by full-body clothing.
- Cholecalciferol is available in capsules with multiple strengths, ranging from 400 to 60,000 international units (IU). It is also available as an intramuscular injection of 600,000 IU, which has long-lasting effects but is associated with injection site discomfort.

4.14.1   Vitamin D metabolites

Certain metabolites of vitamin D are available so that they can be used to treat deficiencies especially related to hepatic or renal abnormalities.

Calcidiol: This is also known as Calcifediol. It is three times more potent than cholecalciferol. It has good intestinal absorption and a high affinity to bind vitamin D-binding proteins. It is the preferred supplement for intestinal malabsorption, familial hypophosphatemia, and medication-induced osteoporosis.

Calcitriol: This is an expensive formulation with limited indications for use. It is useful for patients with hyperparathyroidism and metabolic bone disease secondary to renal disease who lack enzyme 1 alpha-hydroxylase. It has a short half-life of 6 hours, so it does not help in replenishing depleted stores of vitamin D.

4.14.2   Vitamin D analogs

Many analogs of vitamin D have been produced with variations in their chemical properties. These render them with selective attributes such as increased or reduced affinity for binding proteins and receptor sites. They were created to treat secondary hyperparathyroidism without the unwanted side effects such as hypercalcemia and hyperphosphatemia. However, comparative studies have not shown the superiority of these analogs over calcitriol in efficacy or safety. A few examples of these analogs include 22-oxacalcitriol, doxercalciferol, dihydrotachysterol, paricalcitol, and falecalcitriol (Steddon et al., 2001).

4.15   Treatment

There are various proposed regimens that can be used to treat vitamin D deficiency. However, the choice of regimen depends upon how rapid the correction is required.

Patients with 25-hydroxy vitamin D levels less than 20 ng/mL can be treated with high doses (50,000 IU) of vitamin D2 or D3 orally once a week for 6–8 weeks, followed by 800 IU of vitamin D daily.

Patients with 25-hydroxy vitamin D levels between 20 and 30 ng/mL can be treated with daily dosing of 600–800 IU of vitamin D daily.

Higher doses of 1500–2000 IU should be considered for high-risk populations such as diabetics, older adults, young children, pregnant females, and immunocompromised individuals.

4.16   Hypervitaminosis D

The normal concentration of vitamin D in blood ranges from 20 ng/mL to 50 ng/mL. Increasing awareness about vitamin D supplementation has triggered widespread fortification of foods and the use of unregulated vitamin D formulations, resulting in toxicity. Vitamin D intoxication is also called hypervitaminosis and is defined as a blood 25(OH)D concentration level of greater than 150 ng/mL (375 nmol/L). Excessive sun exposure does not cause toxicity because once the skin overcomes its vitamin D requirement, the excess vitamin D gets degraded. It is almost always caused by supplement overuse (Shodiqulovich, 2024). Other causes of hypervitaminosis D are granulomatous diseases such as sarcoidosis and lymphomas.

4.17   Diagnosis

Symptoms resulting from hypercalcemia and hypercalciuria may be vague, like weakness or fatigue, or more specific, such as confusion, irritability, dehydration, excessive thirst, polyuria, and nephrolithiasis. Some may develop mild gastrointestinal symptoms like abdominal pain and constipation or complications such as peptic ulcers and pancreatitis. Severe manifestations of hypercalcemia include metabolic encephalopathy and cardiac arrhythmias.

Diagnosis can be made using vitamin D assays, which will indicate the degree of hypervitaminosis. Supportive lab results will show hypercalcemia, hypercalciuria, and low or undetectable serum parathyroid hormone levels.

4.18   Treatment

It takes several months to reverse the effect of hypervitaminosis because vitamin D gets sequestered into fat cells. Some studies have shown that in some individuals, hypercalcemia may take up to 18 months to resolve. The following measures can effectively lower vitamin D levels:
• Discontinuation of vitamin D and calcium supplements.
• Normal saline infusion to correct dehydration and increase renal clearance of calcium.
• Use of calcitonin and bisphosphonates for severe hypercalcemia.
• Calcitonin 4 U/kg IM every 12 hours for 2 days OR IV pamidronate 90 mg over 2 hours or IV zoledronic acid 4 mg over 15 minutes.
• Steroids can be used for high vitamin D levels secondary to granulomatous disease.

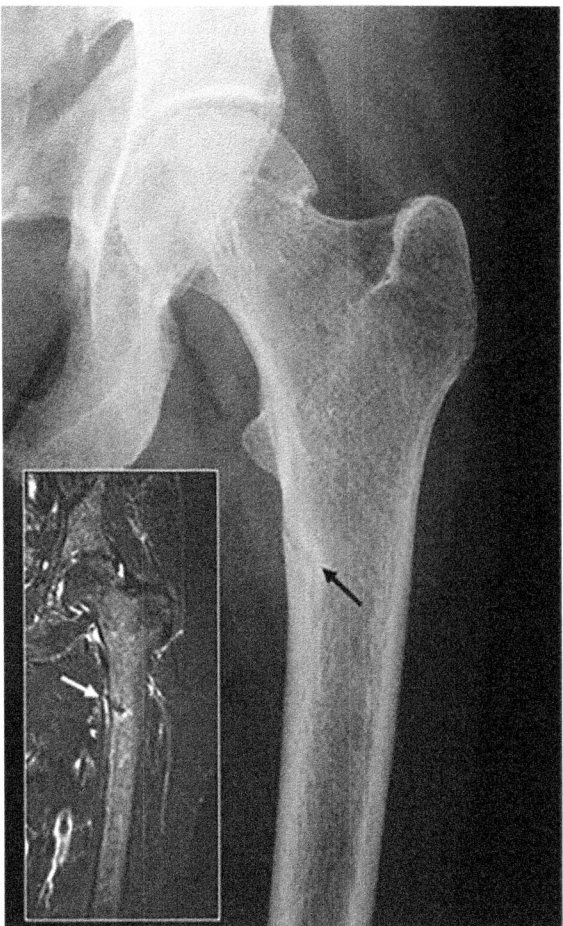

Figure 4.3
Looser's zones.
Looser's zones or Milkman's lines on the radiograph of the upper femur.
Source: *From Cundy, T., Que, L., Hassan, I. M., & Hughes, L. (2020). Bisphosphonate induced deterioration of osteomalacia in undiagnosed adult Fanconi syndrome.* Journal of Bone and Mineral Research Plus, *4(8).*

- Refractory hypercalcemia can be treated with hemodialysis.
- Monitoring vitamin D assays and serum calcium levels.
- Medication review and patient counseling.

4.19   Conclusion

Vitamin D is an essential element for bone health and many other processes that occur in the human body. Severe vitamin deficiency can have significant consequences on population health; therefore, screening should be employed for all individuals at risk. Current guidelines on vitamin D supplementation are vague but should be tailored according to patient needs. Physicians should be mindful of other predisposing medical conditions and treat them accordingly using various preparations of vitamin D compounds. Further studies and randomized control trials are underway to establish the safety and efficacy of newer analogs. Over the years, global awareness has led to the necessity of fortification of food groups with the addition of micronutrients for the benefit of public health.

Acknowledgments

We gratefully acknowledge the help provided by Professor Saima Iqbal, Shifa College of Medicine, Islamabad, in reviewing this chapter.

References

Adams, J. E. (2018). Radiology of rickets and osteomalacia. *Vitamin D: Fourth Edition, 1*, 975–1006. https://doi.org/10.1016/B978-0-12-809965-0.00054-9, http://www.sciencedirect.com/science/book/9780128099650.

Amrein, K., Scherkl, M., Hoffmann, M., Neuwersch-Sommeregger, S., Köstenberger, M., Tmava Berisha, A., Martucci, G., Pilz, S., & Malle, O. (2020). Vitamin D deficiency 2.0: An update on the current status worldwide. *European Journal of Clinical Nutrition, 74*(11), 1498–1513. https://doi.org/10.1038/s41430-020-0558-y.

Bleizgys, A. (2021). Vitamin D dosing: Basic principles and a brief algorithm (2021 Update). *Nutrients, 13*(12), 4415. https://doi.org/10.3390/nu13124415.

Burnett-Bowie, S. A. M., & Cappola, A. R. (2021). The USPSTF 2021 Recommendations on screening for asymptomatic vitamin D deficiency in adults: The challenge for clinicians continues. *JAMA - Journal of the American Medical Association, 325*(14), 1401–1402. https://doi.org/10.1001/jama.2021.2227, http://jama.jamanetwork.com/journal.aspx.

Chanchlani, R., Nemer, P., Sinha, R., Nemer, L., Krishnappa, V., Sochett, E., Safadi, F., & Raina, R. (2020). An overview of rickets in children. *Kidney International Reports, 5*(7), 980–990. https://doi.org/10.1016/j.ekir.2020.03.025.

Christakos, S., Ajibade, D. V., Dhawan, P., Fechner, A. J., & Mady, L. J. (2010). Vitamin D: Metabolism. *Endocrinology and Metabolism Clinics of North America, 39*(2), 243–253. https://doi.org/10.1016/j.ecl.2010.02.002.

Chun, K. J. (2011). Bone densitometry. *Seminars in Nuclear Medicine, 41*(3), 220–228. https://doi.org/10.1053/j.semnuclmed.2010.12.002, http://www.elsevier.com/inca/publications/store/6/2/3/1/8/4/index.htt.

Cundy, T., Que, L., Hassan, I. M., & Hughes, L. (2020). Bisphosphonate induced deterioration of osteomalacia in undiagnosed adult Fanconi syndrome. *Journal of Bone and Mineral Research Plus, 4*(8).

DeLuca, H. F. (1976). Metabolism of vitamin D: current status. *The American Journal of Clinical Nutrition, 29*(11), 1258–1270. https://doi.org/10.1093/ajcn/29.11.1258.

Horst, R. L., Reinhardt, T. A., & Reddy, G. S. (2005). Vitamin D metabolism. *Vitamin D, 1*, 15–36. https://doi.org/10.1016/B978-012252687-9/50005-X, http://www.sciencedirect.com/science/book/9780122526879.

Iqbal, R., & Khan, A. H. (2010). Possible causes of vitamin D deficiency (VDD) in Pakistani population residing in Pakistan. *Journal of the Pakistan Medical Association, 60*(1), 1–2. http://jpma.org.pk//PdfDownload/1888.pdf.

Jones, G. (2022). 100 YEARS OF VITAMIN D: Historical aspects of vitamin D. *Endocrine Connections, 11*(4). https://doi.org/10.1530/ec-21-0594.

Minisola, S., Colangelo, L., Pepe, J., Diacinti, D., Cipriani, C., & Rao, S. D. (2021). Osteomalacia and vitamin D status: A clinical update 2020. *JBMR Plus, 5*(1). https://doi.org/10.1002/jbm4.10447, https://asbmr.onlinelibrary.wiley.com/journal/24734039.

Percival, T. (1789). *Essays medical, philosophical, and experimental.* 1740–1804.

Raczynski, W. E. (1913). Recherches Experimentales sur le Manque D'action au Soleil Comme Cause du Rachitisme. *C. R. de l'Association Internationale de Pédiatrie,* 308–309.

Ramasamy, I. (2020). Vitamin D metabolism and guidelines for vitamin D supplementation. *Clinical Biochemist Reviews, 41*(3), 103–126. https://doi.org/10.33176/aacb-20-00006.

Rollier, A. (1923).

Sahay, M., & Sahay, R. (2012). Rickets-vitamin D deficiency and dependency. *Indian Journal of Endocrinology and Metabolism, 16*(2), 164. https://doi.org/10.4103/2230-8210.93732.

Shodiqulovich, B. K. (2024). Hypervitaminosis D or vitamin D toxicity. *Web of Medicine: Journal of Medicine, Practice and Nursing, 2*(5), 17–25.

Sniadecki, S. J., & Sniadecki, J. (1840). On the cure of rickets. *Nature, 143.*

Steddon, S. J., Schroeder, N. J., & Cunningham, J. (2001). Vitamin D analogues: How do they differ and what is their clinical role? *Nephrology Dialysis Transplantation, 16*(10), 1965–1967. https://doi.org/10.1093/ndt/16.10.1965, http://ndt.oxfordjournals.org/.

Taylor, C. L., Thomas, P. R., Aloia, J. F., Millard, P. S., & Rosen, C. J. (2015). Questions about vitamin D for primary care practice: Input from an NIH conference. *American Journal of Medicine, 128*(11), 1167–1170. https://doi.org/10.1016/j.amjmed.2015.05.025, https://www.elsevier.com/locate/amjmed.

Thomas, M. K., & Demay, M. B. (2000). Vitamin D deficiency and disorders of vitamin D metabolism. *Endocrinology and Metabolism Clinics of North America, 29*(3), 611–627. https://doi.org/10.1016/S0889-8529(05)70153-5, http://www.endo.theclinics.com/.

Whyte, M. P., & Thakker, R. V. (2013). Rickets and osteomalacia. *Medicine (United Kingdom), 41*(10), 594–599. https://doi.org/10.1016/j.mpmed.2013.07.012.

CHAPTER 5

Vitamin D and sports performance

Mirza Mohammad Feisal Subhan

School of Biomedical Sciences, Faaculty of Health, University of Plymouth, Plymouth, Devon, United Kingdom

5.1 Introduction

It has been approximately two decades since (Lovell, 2008) research has highlighted the link between levels of vitamin D and physical performance (Bischoff-Ferrari et al., 2004; Houston et al., 2007). Research has clearly shown a strong link between higher vitamin D concentrations and lower extremity function in active and inactive women and men over 60 years of age in the US population (Bischoff-Ferrari et al., 2004). Similarly, a study in Italian women and men > 65 years old showed a dose effect, where persons with higher vitamin D levels had greater handgrip strength and lower extremity performance (Houston et al., 2007). At roughly the same time, evidence was building up that large numbers of children and adults had vitamin D deficiency (Holick, 2006). This leads to an obvious question, whether athletes also had inadequate levels of vitamin D, and if this was negatively affecting them (Willis et al., 2008). Several randomized controlled trials have shown that a significant percentage of athletes had inadequate vitamin D levels, irrespective of whether this was in elite female gymnasts in Australia (Lovell, 2008), male athletes in Qatar (Hamilton et al., 2010), or athletes in Germany (Hacker et al., 2025).

This chapter will first investigate the prevalence of Vitamin D deficiency in athletes and the possible causes behind this. Before the discussion of the effects of vitamin D on athletic performance, it is imperative to cover the prevalence of inadequate vitamin D levels in athletes and then explain what the reasons for this in this population can be. It is important to understand what the causes of Vitamin D deficiency in athletes can be, as reports indicate their deficiency rates can be higher than that found in the general population. With regard to the question on how lower levels of vitamin D affect athletes' performance, there is a growing body of evidence to show that their performance is negatively affected, and additionally, this can also result in more musculoskeletal injuries too (Yoon, Kwon, & Kim, 2021), which will be covered in this chapter. The complex relationship between vitamin D and muscle performance will also be looked at. Lastly, current guidelines for athletes for an adequate status of this vitamin and the safety of supplements will be covered.

The Impact of Vitamin D on Health and Disease. DOI: https://doi.org/10.1016/B978-0-443-34037-6.00025-X

5.2   Vitamin D deficiency in athletes: prevalence, risk factors, and causes

In the United Kingdom, adequate vitamin D levels in the general adult population are suggested to be above 50 nmol/L (Nhs, 2018; National Institute for Health and Care Excellence NICE, 2022). In North America, the Institute of Medicine similarly suggests that a concentration of 50 nmol/L (20 ng/ml) meets the needs of 97.5% of the population (Ross et al., 2011). As found in the general population, vitamin D status is affected by several factors, including age, skin color, season, latitude, sport type (indoor/outdoor), and diet. Before discussing issues with vitamin D levels in athletes, it is imperative that we decide what definition of deficient, insufficient, and sufficient we will use. We have decided to define serum 25-hydroxyvitamin D (vitamin D) below 50 nmol/L as deficient, between 50 and 75 nmol/L as insufficient, and above 75 nmol/L as sufficient, as used by several authors (Hacker et al., 2025; Hamilton et al., 2010), although previous work has had slight variations (Houston et al., 2007). Fig. 5.1 clearly shows how different athletic and other organizations define a normal vitamin D value (Ribbans et al., 2021).

A recent metaanalysis looked at 5456 athletes and found that 30% of adult athletes and 39% of adolescent athletes had vitamin D insufficiency (Harju et al., 2022). These authors defined vitamin D insufficiency as values below the cut-off value of 50 nmol/L. No female versus male differences were found, although only 21% of participants were female. Interestingly, a

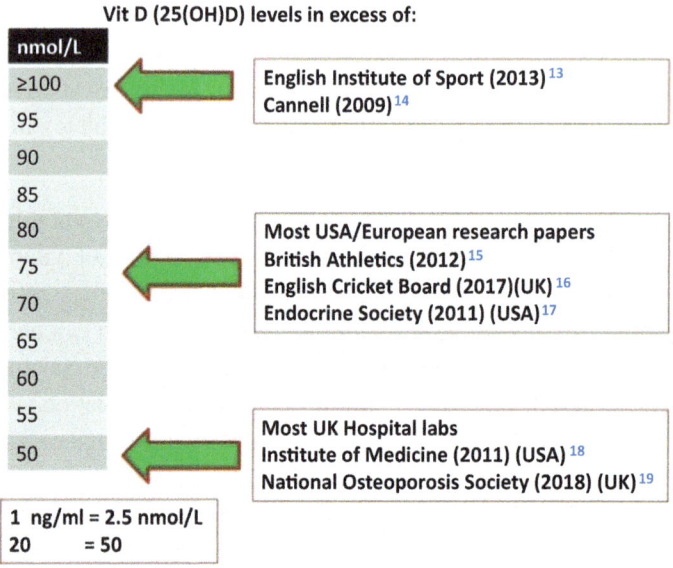

Figure 5.1
Various definitions of normal serum vitamin D levels.
Source: *Reproduced with permission from Ribbans, W. J., Aujla, R., Dalton, S., & Nunley, J. A. (2021). Vitamin D and the athlete-patient: State of the art.* Journal of ISAKOS, 6(1), 46–60.

metaanalysis from 2015, which used a higher cut-off value of 80 nmol/L, found a higher prevalence of vitamin D inadequacy (Farrokhyar et al., 2015). These authors found that 56% of their athletes were inadequate in this vitamin, using a sample of 2313. The more recent metaanalysis used 51 studies compared to the latter one, which had 23.

As para-athletics gets more popular, it would be good to include these data too. A metaanalysis in female and male para-athletes was conducted in 2025, looking at 355 para-athletes from 10 studies. Rather than use a standard cut-off value for vitamin D insufficiency, the authors followed levels set by each individual study. Of all the samples, 43.2% were insufficient, while 28.1% were deficient (Langley et al., 2024). The 10 studies used different definitions of vitamin D deficiency and insufficiency, which does complicate matters, however, both of these could be referred as low vitamin D. Most of these studies used a cut-off value of > 80 nmol/L as a sufficiency threshold, with insufficiency defined as being between 75 and 50 nmol/L, and deficiency being below 50 nmol/L. In spite of these differences, this metaanalysis did show large numbers of para-athletes with low vitamin, and more so in winter than summer. Wheelchair para-athletes, who participate in indoor events, had lower levels than other para-athletes.

When contrasting low vitamin D prevalence rates in athletes and para-athletes to that of the general population, we find that prevalence rates are comparable. A systematic review has investigated the vitamin D levels in approximately 8 million participants from 308 studies (Cui et al., 2023). These studies collected data from 81 countries and found that 47.9% had vitamin D levels below 50 nmol/L. It is surprising that athletic and nonathletic populations vitamin D levels show such similarity, while some authors have suggested that low vitamin D prevalence may even be higher in athletes (Ip et al., 2022). With athletes being more health conscious and often exercising outdoors, it would be assumed that they have a greater bioavailability of vitamin D from their diet and sunlight. Ip and coworkers imply that other factors such as how athletes utilize and store vitamin D could be important (Ip et al., 2022). More research is needed to investigate the prevalence of vitamin D levels in athletes, especially in female athletes.

In terms of risk factors, research has shown that seasons are a factor, with vitamin D levels higher in summer compared to winter (Abulafia et al., 2024; Farrokhyar et al., 2015; Langley et al., 2024; Perrone et al., 2024). Indoor sports are also a factor (Farrokhyar et al., 2015; Langley et al., 2024). Geographical location and vitamin D inadequacy have been shown in the United Kingdom and the Middle East (Harju et al., 2022). Data from the Middle East have shown opposing results, with 91% of football players in Qatar showing levels below 50 nmol/L (Hamilton et al., 2010), while Israeli Olympic athletes only have a prevalence of 7.5% (Abulafia et al., 2024). As the Israeli study was conducted recently, it is possible that they were more aware of the risks of vitamin D deficiency and were taking supplements. Using the same vitamin D cutoff, Australian elite female gymnasts (Lovell, 2008) had a 33% deficiency, while for German Olympic athletes (Hacker et al., 2025), it was 16%. Latitude was not a major factor in one study (Langley et al., 2024), yet an Italian study of professional football players has clearly shown players in a higher latitude (more North) had lower vitamin D levels than similar players based at a lower latitude, during winter and spring (Perrone et al., 2024). However, during summer, both teams showed no difference in vitamin D levels. The type of sport may also be a factor, with power sports (wrestling, track, and field) having lower vitamin levels than endurance sports (cycling and rowing), along with darker skin also being a risk factor (Ip et al., 2022).

From Fig. 5.2, we can see that one cause of vitamin D deficiency can be insufficient sunlight and low levels of vitamin D in the diet. Another is the failure of liver and kidney conversion of vitamin D metabolites. Lastly, increased use or decreased release of vitamin D from storage in fat and muscle tissue is a recent and underresearched phenomenon (Ip et al., 2022).

5.3   Impact on muscle strength, power, and endurance

Physiological, psychological, anthropometric, health, genetic, training, and environmental factors all contribute to athletic performance. In the 1930s, 1940s, and 1950s, many studies in Russia and Germany on adults and children clearly showed that subjects exposed to

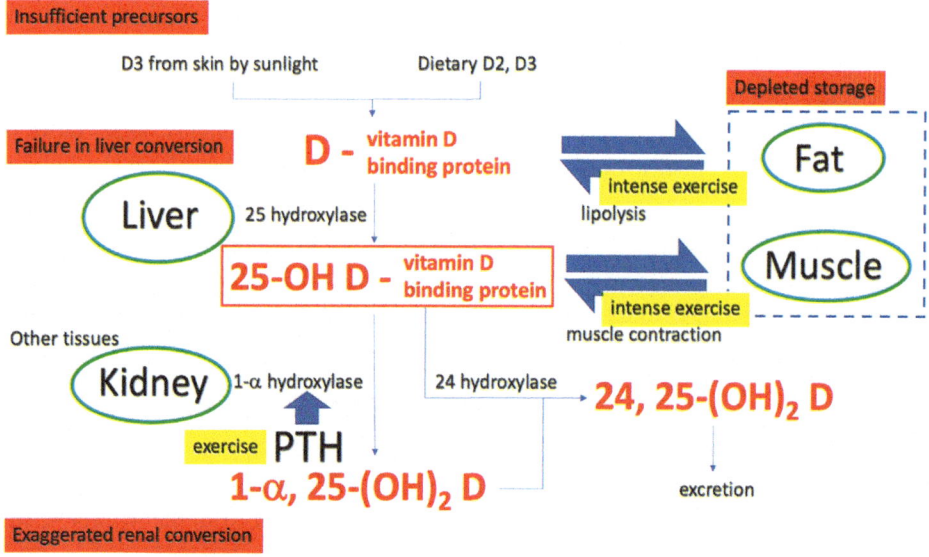

Figure 5.2

The potential reasons of low vitamin D in athletes.

Source: *Reproduced with permission from Ip, T. S. T., Fu, S. C., Ong, M. T. Y., & Yung, P. S. H. (2022). Vitamin D deficiency in athletes: Laboratory, clinical and field integration.* Asia-Pacific Journal of Sports Medicine, Arthroscopy, Rehabilitation and Technology, 29, 22–29.

ultraviolet light improved speed, performance, cardiovascular fitness, and reaction times (Cannell et al., 2009). Several of these studies also showed performance was best during or just after summer, clearly showing a seasonal relationship. In the previous section, the timing of training and the effect of season were mentioned, and data to support this are shown in Fig. 5.3. This image shows a significant peak increase in forearm wrist strength after the summer months in German subjects, indicative of the increased vitamin D production due to the longest summer months and greater exposure to ultraviolet light (Cannell et al., 2009).

In terms of muscle strength, there is mounting evidence to show that vitamin D supplementation has no significant effect on muscle strength (Cannell et al., 2009; Farrokhyar et al., 2015; Ip et al., 2022; Książek et al., 2019), after sufficient levels are found in athletes. Fig. 5.4 shows how an increase in vitamin D is related to an increase in musculoskeletal performance, but this reaches a plateau after 125 nmol/L (50 ng/mL), and athletes with low vitamin D levels (< 75 nmol/L) would benefit the most with increasing vitamin D levels (Shuler et al., 2012).

Studies on rodents and vitamin D-deficient patients have shown muscle protein synthesis after vitamin D administration, specifically type 2 muscle fibers (Cannell et al., 2009). Patient groups did show an increase in muscle strength after treatment. This is in contrast to several

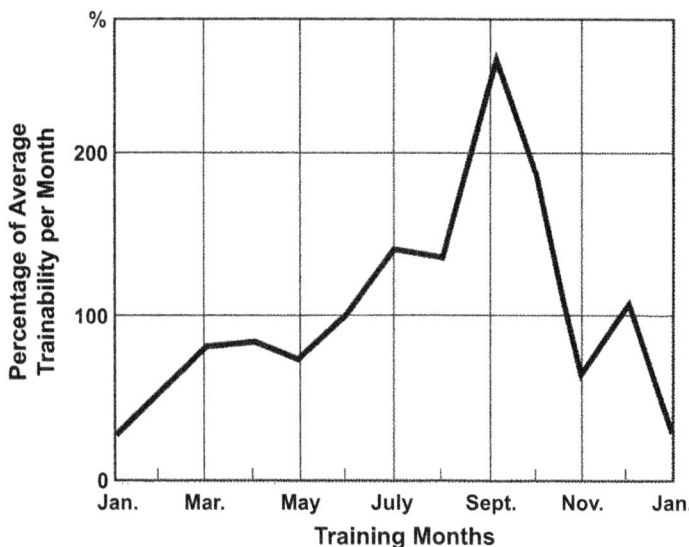

Figure 5.3

Image showing the trainability of muscle (% increase in strength/mean strength increase) in seven subjects after daily exercise over a complete year.

Source: *Reproduced with permissionfrom Cannell, J.J., Hollis, B.W., Sorenson, M.B., Taft, T.N., & Anderson, J.J.B. (2009). Athletic performance and vitamin D. Medicine and Science in Sports and Exercise, 41(5), 1102–1110.*

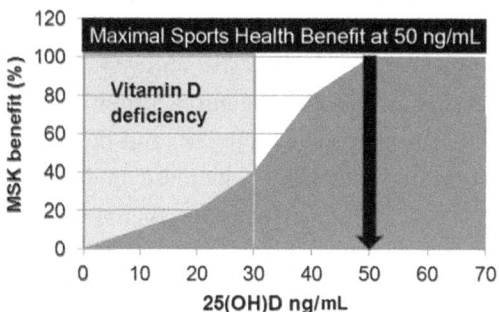

Figure 5.4
Relationship of vitamin D and musculoskeletal (MSK) performance in athletes. *MSK,*
Musculoskeletal.
Source: *Reproduced with permission from Shuler, F. D., Wingate, M. K., Moore, G. H., & Giangarra, C.*
(2012). Sports health benefits of vitamin D. Sports Health, 4(6), 496–501.

physiological and pathological conditions, such as space travel, long term best rest, Type 2 diabetes mellitus, chronic heart failure and chronic obstructive pulmonary disease whereby there is a gradual change in type of muscle fiber from slow oxidative type 1 to fast glycolytic type 2b, with some of these conditions also showing atrophy of type 1 fibers. Type 2 muscle fibers are known for their higher force production and also fall prevention, and patient studies have shown supplementation of vitamin D can lower the risk of falls (Shuler et al., 2012).

At the cellular and molecular level, vitamin D binds to cellular and nuclear vitamin D receptors (VDR) in muscle cells and then binds to retinoid X receptors, before acting on DNA in the nucleus for gene and protein transcription (Książek et al., 2019). This directly can improve muscle growth, but indirectly, second messenger molecules increase the amount of intracellular calcium ions, which are also thought to increase muscle strength. A case study in a severely vitamin D-deficient patient does clearly show a benefit with vitamin D supplementation, with the patient improving their physical performance after therapy, and also their muscle pain going away (Gunton & Girgis, 2018). However, this report does show the complexity of research in this area, as several studies show inconclusive results with regard to muscle strength and function with improved vitamin D status. It is possible that this could be due to variations in doses of vitamin D supplements, baseline levels of vitamin D (see Fig. 5.2), the population type (patients vs athletes), and how performance is measured (Gunton & Girgis, 2018).

From the data above, it is apparent that a large portion of research on vitamin D and muscle strength has been performed on animal and patient models. Recently, a metaanalysis has looked at these effects in athletes per se and has collated 11 randomized controlled trials which had a total of 436 athletes (Sist et al., 2023) who were given supplemental vitamin D. The results showed no significant difference in therapy in upper or lower body muscle strength. It was noted that some studies had a baseline of vitamin D status of > 75 nmol/L, while some had a status below this. One clear conclusion from this metaanalysis is that more randomized controlled trials need to be performed in athletes. One aspect that is apparent is the important role vitamin D has in muscle function and regeneration, and Fig. 5.5 shows how this nutrient affects mitochondrial function, reactive oxygen species (ROS), and VDRs (Fig. 5.5).

Muscle tissue can be damaged by several factors, including a lack of vitamin D and muscle overuse. In murine models, greater levels of vitamin D increase VDR expression. While in equine data, muscle damage caused by high-intensity exercise also resulted in greater protein expression of VDR, although serum vitamin D levels were lower postexercise (Latham et al., 2021). Both

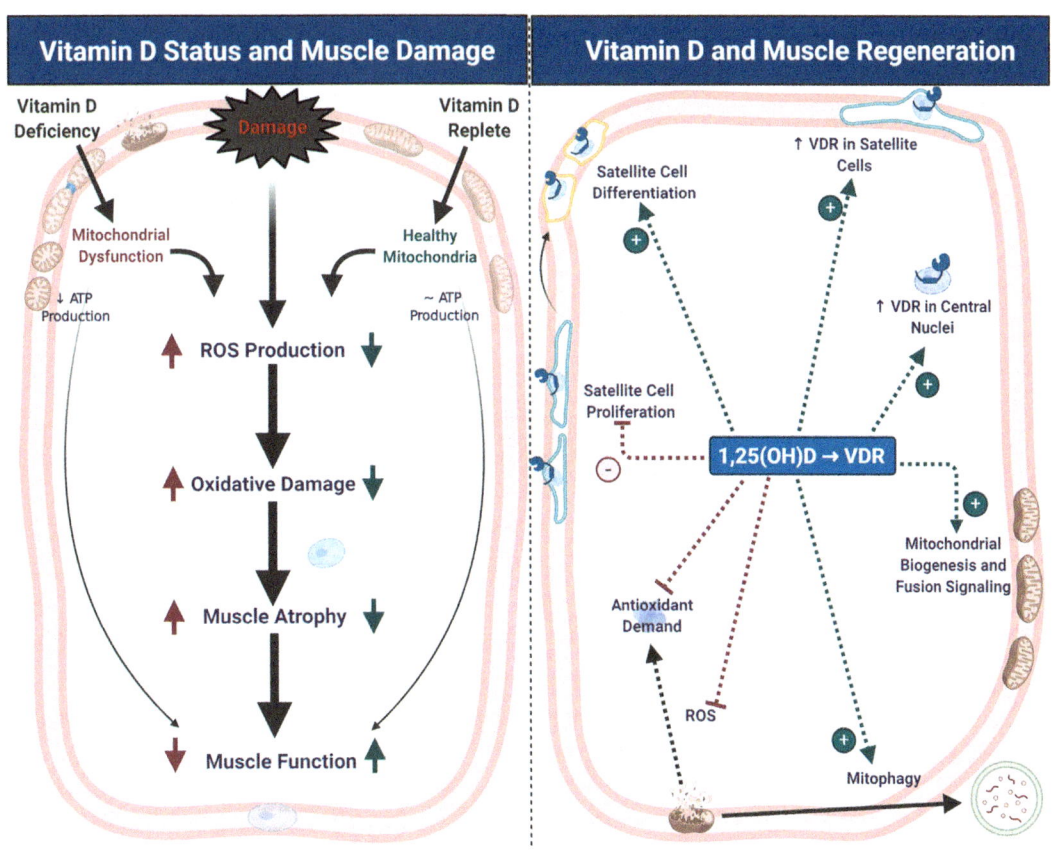

Figure 5.5

Effect of vitamin D on muscle regeneration. Image showing how vitamin D deficiency can damage muscle, and with sufficiency, muscle can regenerate.

Source: Reproduced with permission from Latham, C. M., Brightwell, C. R., Keeble, A. R., Munson, B. D., Thomas, N. T., Zagzoog, A. M., Fry, C. S., & Fry, J. L. (2021). Vitamin D promotes skeletal muscle regeneration and mitochondrial health. Frontiers in Physiology, 12.

results show a close relationship between the muscle repair and vitamin D systems, which occur together after muscle damage. In a human study, elderly females in the United States were given vitamin D supplements over four months, and they showed greater muscle VDR concentrations and type 2 muscle fiber size compared to placebo (Ceglia et al., 2013). Regression analysis of data from this study showed a strong correlation with serum vitamin D levels and muscle VDR concentrations in the placebo and supplemented groups, though further work is needed to show if higher levels of vitamin D increase muscle fibre cross-sectional area (FCSA) due to VDR activation.

More evidence is also showing a link between vitamin D and mitochondrial health, which is important for energy production. Most studies have been conducted on adults with vitamin D deficiency, and they clearly show an increase in mitochondrial function improving oxidative phosphorylation therefore muscle energy (Latham et al., 2021), and work in rodents has also confirmed similar results.

From Fig. 5.5, we can see that vitamin D deficiency can cause increased mitochondrial ROS, which can negatively affect mitochondria and lead to muscle atrophy. It can also cause changes in antioxidant enzyme activity. Supplementation can reverse these changes; yet more work in this field needs to be done looking specially at athletic populations.

Vitamin D possibly has an effect on satellite cells too. Satellite cells are resident stem cells found in muscle, responsible for muscle repair and maintenance. It is thought that the role of vitamin D is to regulate the activity of these cells (Książek et al., 2019; Latham et al., 2021).

Maximal oxygen consumption (VO_2max) is often used as a marker of aerobic fitness, and it correlates closely with muscle mass and aerobic endurance. Data have not shown a clear link between vitamin D levels and VO_2max in athletes, though a correlation has been seen in physically inactive subjects (Książek et al., 2019). Similarly, there is inconclusive evidence of a link between vitamin D supplementation and VO_2max and athletic performance. There is evidence showing that supplementation in athletes improves vitamin D levels and lower limb quadricep muscle strength, giving rise to the possibility that vitamin D might act on varied muscle groups and muscle capacity (Han et al., 2024; Książek et al., 2019). A recent cross-sectional study in German Olympic athletes has shown that serum vitamin D levels had a positive linear correlation with handgrip strength (Hacker et al., 2025).

Cardiorespiratory function is also important for athletic performance, especially as it is an important factor in determining VO_2max. Vitamin D deficiency has been seen to show a negative effect on lung function in athletes, and it increases lung infections too, yet whether this reduces VO_2max in athletes is unclear (de la Puente Yagüe et al., 2020).

In terms of cardiac function, low levels of vitamin D in the general population have been shown to relate to decreased cardiac function and increased levels of cardiac morbidity and mortality (Owens et al., 2018). Due to regular intensive exercise, athletes' hearts are well known to adapt to have lower resting heart rates and allow a greater cardiac output. Vitamin D deficient athletes have showed smaller hearts, decreased cardiac function and greater prevalence of sudden cardiac death, compared to athletes who were sufficient or insufficient in vitamin D. Although the physiological mechanisms still need to be determined, an increase in parathyroid hormone due to vitamin D deficiency can be a direct cause of cardiac muscle hypertrophy. Loss of cardiorespiratory function due to low vitamin D levels can be a major issue in athletes, as both of these organs are responsible to supply nutrients and oxygen to muscle tissue.

An aspect not directly related to athletic performance is the effect vitamin D has on the innate and acquired immune system, which can keep athletes healthy, and keep them training thereby increasing endurance and VO$_2$max. Most immune cells, including macrophages, neutrophils, and lymphocytes, have VDR in them. In terms of the innate system, vitamin D is known to upregulate antimicrobial peptides, and for the acquired system, it has a positive effect on B and T lymphocytes (Owens et al., 2018). Looking specifically at athletes, evidence does show an inverse relationship between vitamin D and upper respiratory tract infections. A cutoff of 95 nmol/L seems to differentiate athletes who have one or more illnesses to ones above this cutoff who have one or less illness.

In future, organizations and athletic bodies should have standard cutoff points for levels of vitamins to determine deficiency, insufficiency, and sufficiency. Also, there needs to be a clear agreement over the measurement of vitamin D as the active calcitriol (1,25-dihydroxyvitamin D), measured in pmol/L, or the inactive 25-hydroxyvitamin D, measured in nmol/L. The relationship between these two chemicals is not clear cut. This will greatly improve the ability to make interstudy comparisons, such as systematic reviews and/or metaanalyses. One aspect of athletic performance and vitamin D is injuries and their recovery, which is covered in the next section, and bone health, as both of these also affect athletic performance and training schedules (Harju et al., 2022).

5.3.1 Injury prevention and recovery

The previous section has covered the effects of vitamin D on muscle repair, and now we will discuss the effects of vitamin D on injury prevention and recovery from injury.

Before we discuss injury and injury prevention, it is imperative to discuss bone health. Vitamin D has been long been known to improve calcium absorption, bone mineralization, and osteoclast activity, all resulting in athletes having greater bone mineral density (Cannell et al., 2009), yet conversely, evidence in a study of 950 ethnically diverse male athletes has shown no association between vitamin D levels and bone density, when taking age, ethnicity and type of sport into account (Allison et al., 2015). The same study did, however, show greater bone mineral density in some bones (hip, spine, and neck) for African and Caucasian athletes compared to athletes from other ethnic backgrounds. Bone density is also likely to be higher in athletes due to mechanical stress on bone during training resulting in bone remodeling. Evidence points to the fact that even with vitamin D deficiency, bone health is maintained in high-intensity athletic activities, but this is not the case with deficiency in nonweight-bearing activities, where lower bone mineral density can be seen (Allison et al., 2015; Owens et al., 2018). Although stress fractures or bone injuries can account for up to a fifth of all injuries in sports medicine, the total prevalence of athletic injuries can be up to 43%, and of this, about two-fifths are soft tissue or muscle injuries (Farrokhyar et al., 2015). The relationship between injury prevalence and levels of vitamin D in this population is uncertain. Current evidence for any benefits of vitamin D in athletes in fracture healing is inconclusive (de la Puente Yagüe et al., 2020). Several patient studies have clearly shown that the majority of those with musculoskeletal injuries had low levels of vitamin D (Yoon, Kwon, & Kim, 2021). Fig. 5.6 links a dose effect of vitamin D with musculoskeletal conditions, where low levels can result in rickets and adequate levels can enhance performance.

Ethnic differences in bone density in athletes was previously mentioned. Evidence also shows that Black and Hispanic men have a great risk of having vitamin D deficiency, yet they have a lower risk of fracture, bone loss, and osteoporosis (Owens et al., 2018). Blacks do not show bone loss if they have lower vitamin D levels, unlike Caucasians (Owens et al., 2018). Data from Arab athletes showed 91% were deficient in vitamin D, and a subset had low bone density, yet none reported a stress fracture (Hamilton et al., 2010). Additionally, their skin color did not correlate with vitamin D levels.

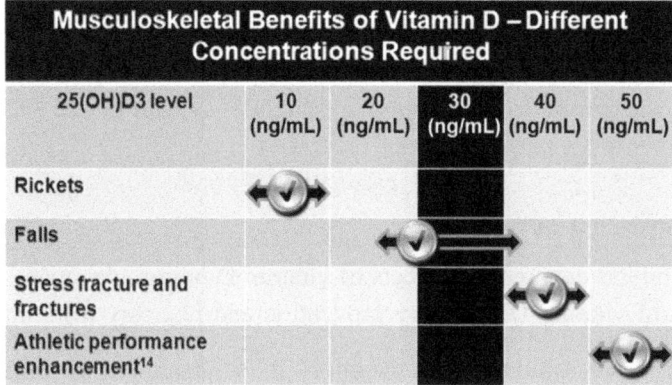

Musculoskeletal Benefits of Vitamin D – Different Concentrations Required					
25(OH)D3 level	10 (ng/mL)	20 (ng/mL)	30 (ng/mL)	40 (ng/mL)	50 (ng/mL)
Rickets	✓				
Falls			✓		
Stress fracture and fractures				✓	
Athletic performance enhancement[14]					✓

Figure 5.6
Levels of vitamin D affecting musculoskeletal status. This image shows how differing levels of vitamin D can result in various musculoskeletal effects, with the shaded column of 30 ng/mL (75 nmol/L) being a sufficient level of vitamin D.
Source: *Reproduced with permission from Shuler, F. D., Wingate, M. K., Moore, G. H., & Giangarra, C. (2012). Sports health benefits of vitamin D. Sports Health, 4(6), 496–501.*

One potential explanation for these differences could be vitamin D binding protein. This protein transports vitamin D and its metabolites in blood. Different ethnicities have genetic variations in this protein, and this could account for differences in vitamin D binding and serum concentrations, though more studies need to be conducted.

The relationship between stress fractures and vitamin D in athletes is well known, as low vitamin D levels result in less calcium gut absorption, which in turn triggers the release of parathyroid hormone to homeostatically raise calcium levels. The function of this latter hormone is increasing osteoclastic bone activity, which increases bone resorption and results in demineralization of bone, weakening it (Yoon, Kwon, & Kim, 2021). One of the main preventative measures that athletes, trainers, coaches, and healthcare professionals can do is to make sure vitamin D levels are adequate in athletes. A section below will discuss doses of vitamin D for supplementation, but we will discuss the benefits in this section. Evidence shows that vitamin D supplementation in deficient or insufficient athletes reduces stress fractures. A study in US college athletes showed supplementation helped significantly reduce the stress fracture incidence from 8% to 2% (Williams et al., 2020). In a previous section, we have discussed the molecular and cellular aspects of muscle repair in relation to vitamin D, though when discussing skeletal injuries, we should also include muscle injury too. Studies in healthy men show supplementation with vitamin D can protect against muscle injury, yet in contrast, studies in athletes also being supplemented showed no effect on exercise-related muscle injury, so more research needs to be undertaken in this area (Yoon, Kwon, & Kim, 2021). From Fig. 5.6 and other literature (Cannell et al., 2009), it is clear that there are skeletal and muscular risks in athletes if they are deficient in vitamin D, and serum target values should be more than 75 nmol/L for optimum muscle health and function and > 100 nmol/L for prevention of fractures, while being above 125 nmol/L has no known benefit (Cannell et al., 2009).

5.3.2 Vitamin D and cognitive function in athletes

All sports require athletes to have good cognitive skills, so they can support and communicate with other team members, make reasonably quick judgments, and follow through with complex movements. Studies of vitamin D in athletes and its effects on cognition are very limited, so comparable work in healthy humans will often be discussed.

A recent cross-sectional study in 350 elite German athletes has shown that higher levels of vitamin D were correlated with better cognitive flexibility (Wiedenbrüg et al., 2024). This was assessed using a validated puzzle and tested whether the athlete would abandon one cognitive approach in place of another when a demand arose. The authors believe that the results could relate to Vitamin D affecting neurotransmitter production. Limitations of the study were that two-thirds of this cohort had deficient or insufficient vitamin D levels, and that vitamin D had no correlations with other cognitive tests, such as processing speed, attention, or visuo-spatial memory (Silva et al., 2022). Vitamin D has also been shown to be linked to better reaction times in older adults (Cannell et al., 2009). A systematic review of the effects of vitamin D on cognitive function in healthy persons showed that vitamin D improved the following three out of five cognitive domains: verbal learning/memory, executive function, and general cognitive functions. Nine studies were included with 5588 participants, although only 4 studies showed cognitive improvements. The authors mention that confounding factors in these studies included variations in age, ethnicity, diet, geographic location, levels of vitamin D supplementation, and types of cognitive testing (Silva et al., 2022). A metaanalysis in mid to older adults showed no cognitive effect of vitamin D (Lehert et al., 2015). From these limited numbers of studies, it is apparent that very little published data are available on athletes, and although more data are available on healthy or aged adults, the results are not conclusive.

5.3.2.1 *Supplementation guidelines for athletes*

Athletes can obtain vitamin D from several sources, including natural sunlight, artificial ultraviolet B light, supplementation, and small amounts in their diet. Public Health England recommends that in the autumn and winter months (October–March), persons take $10 \, \mu g$ (400 IU) of vitamin D daily (Public Health, England, 2016), although other organizations suggest higher amounts (Ip et al., 2022). Studies have shown an increase in serum vitamin D in athletes after supplementation (Williams et al., 2020), although athletes in this study were given 50,000 IU per week.

In previous sections, we have stated that athletes with deficient or insufficient vitamin D levels would benefit from supplemental vitamin D, with regard to muscle strength and stress fractures. Fig. 5.6 shows the relationship between serum vitamin D levels and effects on the musculoskeletal system. Fig. 5.3 shows no reported sports benefits after 125 nmol/L (50 ng/mL). Yet, there is no standard regimen for vitamin D supplementation in athletes for maintenance of serum levels or supplementation in general (Ip et al., 2022). An important aspect for all involved is that supplements should improve serum vitamin D levels in a particular athlete to recommended sufficient levels, but not be excessive. Some authors suggest that a preferable serum for athletes should be more than 100 nmol/L (Yoon, Kwon, & Kim, 2021).

In terms of which type of supplement to take, it is generally recommended that vitamin D_3 (cholecalciferol), the form made in humans by sunlight, is better than D_2 (ergocalciferol), mostly found in plants or fungi, or a combination of both (Ip et al., 2022). D_3 binds to vitamin D binding protein better than D_2, therefore having a better bioavailability and stability. Some evidence shows that D_3 may be better at improving muscle strength than D_2 (Yoon, Kwon, & Kim, 2021).

Although there is no consensus on a recommended dose for athletes, literature does mention a daily vitamin D dose of 2000–6000 IU, with some athletes possibly requiring more than this in specific conditions (Yoon, Kwon, & Kim, 2021). Fig. 5.7 shows an algorithm to use for athletes with regard to vitamin D supplementation, and this image suggests that athletes take 2000–6000 IU/day if they are insufficient in vitamin D levels (Owens et al., 2018).

It has also been suggested that a dose of < 2000 IU would be enough for athletes throughout the year (Ip et al., 2022). Other guidance suggests that after diagnostic testing, athletes not deficient should have a dose of 600 IU/day, and if this is not enough to maintain a serum level of > 75 nmol/L, the daily supplemental dose should be increased (Abushamma, 2022). Athletes most likely utilize more vitamin D than nonathletes, and this greater usage adds another complication when correcting deficient or insufficient vitamin D in this population.

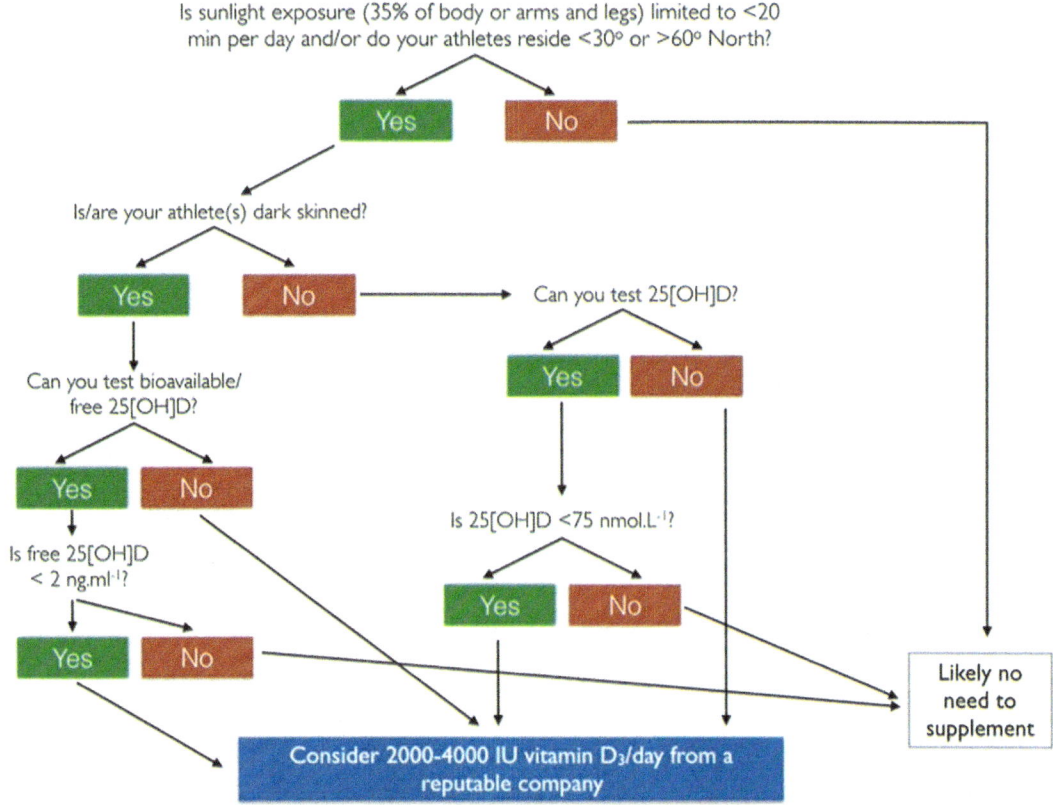

Figure 5.7

An algorithm for athletes to assess need of vitamin D supplementation. An algorithm for athletes to assess if they need vitamin D supplementation or not.

Source: *Reproduced with permission from Owens, D. J., Allison, R., & Close, G. L. (2018). Vitamin D and the athlete: Current perspectives and new challenges.* Sports Medicine, *48, 3–16.*

This complication along with type of sport, season, form of training, and diet could be the reason there is no clear consensus on recommended doses in athletes (de la Puente Yagüe et al., 2020). Additionally, data from the United States suggest that most structured athletic teams neither diagnostically test for vitamin D levels nor offer supplementation (Abushamma, 2022).

5.3.3   Factors influencing vitamin D requirements in athletes

Several factors such as season, latitude, type of sport (indoor/outdoor), diet, and supplementation can all affect vitamin D levels in athletes. Healthcare practitioners and coaches should be aware of these factors and a detailed dietary history before deciding if their athletes need supplementation. Analysis of serum levels of vitamin D should be assessed. Recently, in-office finger-prick blood tests have become available, and studies show they are reliable. A small study on 20 dental patients showed no statistical difference between gold standard lab testing and two finger-prick testing devices (Paz et al., 2021); however, both finger-prick tests showed that their mean vitamin D concentrations were approximately 30% higher than lab values.

Along with vitamin D levels, it is important to be aware of serum calcium levels in athletes, too. If these are low in the diet, parathyroid hormone can cause low bone mineral density, as we have discussed above. Although the type of diet has not been mentioned in detail in this chapter, healthcare practitioners and coaches should be aware that a greater number of vegan and vegetarian athletes need extra considerations with regard to vitamin D requirements (West et al., 2023). The prevalence of vegan athletes is unknown; however, it would be sensible to assume that as numbers in the general population increase, so would the prevalence in the athletic population. There is no data on vitamin D levels in vegan athletes. However, from the general population, it can be seen that vegan persons have lower vitamin D intake and lower serum levels compared to persons following an omnivorous diet. For this reason, it has been suggested that vegan athletes regularly take vitamin D supplements (West et al., 2023).

5.3.4   Safety, side effects, and toxicity of vitamin D supplementation

From our previous discussion on the role of vitamin D in exercise and the supplementation of D in athletes, it should be clear that supplementation is common in many athletes. Several studies on vitamin D supplementation have been published, including randomized trials, systematic reviews, and metaanalyses (Abushamma, 2022; Ceglia et al., 2013; Han et al., 2024; Sist et al., 2023; Williams et al., 2020). Ironically, there is little evidence on the prevalence of vitamin D supplementation in athletes. Due to the fact athletes are taking exogenous doses of vitamin D, there is the danger of an effect of high doses on safety, side effects, and also toxicity, though there is limited evidence of the effect of mega-doses in athletes, and further research is needed (Yoon, Kwon, & Kim, 2021). An interesting case study is of two elderly nursing home patients who were accidentally given mega-doses of 2,000,000 IU each via oral solution (van den Ouweland et al., 2014). Neither showed any signs nor symptoms of vitamin D toxicity, and serum vitamin D did increase sharply, and serum calcium only slightly increased. Although this is an extreme example, it does show the body adapting well to such high levels. It might not be comparable to athletes regularly taking high doses. Most researchers agree that toxic concentrations of vitamin D are > 180 nmol/L (Owens et al., 2018), though some others suggest that it could be > 150 nmol/L (de la Puente Yagüe et al., 2020), or as high as 375 nmol/L (Marcinowska-Suchowierska et al., 2018).

Dangers of vitamin D toxicity include increased serum calcium and phosphate, as vitamin D increases bone resorption and greater calcium gut absorption, and this can occur when serum vitamin D goes above 250 nmol/L. This can lead to weakness, nausea, vomiting, greater urination, and with greater hypercalcemia, heart dysfunction and kidney failure (de la Puente Yagüe et al., 2020; Ribbans et al., 2021). Such mishaps can be prevented by qualified healthcare professionals guiding athletes on the correct or recommended amount of supplementation required. Ip et al. (2022) suggest that as vitamin D toxicity is rare, and that most adults can tolerate high dosages that can advocate giving higher supplemental doses of vitamin D to athletes, although others disagree, on the basis that there are limited benefits for athletes at higher dosages of vitamin D (Owens et al., 2018). Data on athletes given 5000 versus 10,000 IU for 12 weeks have shown a potential negative effect on the conversion of the inactive 25-hydroxyvitamin D to the active 1,25-dihydroxyvitamin D, and these effects could occur even after the period of supplementation was over (Owens et al., 2017).

5.4 Future research and conclusion

In conclusion, vitamin D is an important hormone that can be more significant in athletes if serum levels are low, and once at sufficient levels, increasing the dose will have a minimal effect. Vitamin D has important biochemical and physiological functions affecting cardiac, muscle, bone, and metabolic tissues. As with the general population, there is a high prevalence of vitamin D deficiency and insufficiency in athletes. These low levels can be combatted with supplementation, and if taken in safe doses, under the supervision of healthcare professionals, they can be very effective.

Several areas mentioned in the sections above could do with more primary data through randomized controlled trials and then eventually with systematic reviews and metaanalyses. Such areas include as follows:

1. the use of generation artificial intelligence and large language models to help find patterns of where vitamin deficiency occurs globally and how supplementation can be best effective,
2. determine the exact relationship between active and nonactive forms of vitamin D and which is better for athletic performance and as a diagnostic biomarker in athletes,

3. why low levels of vitamin result in low stress fractures in specific ethnic groups,
4. the effects of vitamin D on cognitive function in athletes.

References

Abulafia, O., Ashkenazi, E., Epstein, Y., Eliakim, A., & Nemet, D. (2024). Characteristics of vitamin D concentration in elite Israeli olympic athletes. *Nutrients, 16*(16), 2627. https://doi.org/10.3390/nu16162627.

Abushamma, A. (2022). The effects of vitamin D supplementation on athletic performance and injury prevention. *Journal of Sports Medicine and Allied Health Sciences: Official Journal of the Ohio Athletic Trainers' Association, 8*(2). https://doi.org/10.25035/jsmahs.08.02.03.

Allison, R. J., Farooq, A., Hamilton, B., Close, G. L., & Wilson, M. G. (2015). No association between vitamin D deficiency and markers of bone health in athletes. *Medicine and Science in Sports and Exercise, 47*(4), 782–788. https://doi.org/10.1249/MSS.0000000000000457, http://www.lww.com/product/?0195-9131.

Bischoff-Ferrari, H. A., Dietrich, T., Orav, E. J., Hu, F. B., Zhang, Y., Karlson, E. W., & Dawson-Hughes, B. (2004). Higher 25-hydroxyvitamin D concentrations are associated with better lower-extremity function in both active and inactive persons aged ≥60 y. *American Journal of Clinical Nutrition, 80*(3), 752–758. https://doi.org/10.1093/ajcn/80.3.752, http://www.ajcn.org/contents-by-date.2005.shtml.

Cannell, J. J., Hollis, B. W., Sorenson, M. B., Taft, T. N., & Anderson, J. J. B. (2009). Athletic performance and vitamin D. *Medicine and Science in Sports and Exercise, 41*(5), 1102–1110. https://doi.org/10.1249/MSS.0b013e3181930c2b.

Ceglia, L., Niramitmahapanya, S., Da Silva Morais, M., Rivas, D. A., Harris, S. S., Bischoff-Ferrari, H., Fielding, R. A., & Dawson-Hughes, B. (2013). A Randomized study on the effect of vitamin D3 supplementation on skeletal muscle morphology and vitamin d receptor concentration in older women. *Journal of Clinical Endocrinology and Metabolism, 98*(12), E1927. https://doi.org/10.1210/jc.2013-2820United, http://jcem.endojournals.org/content/98/12/E1927.full.pdf+html.

Cui, A., Zhang, T., Xiao, P., Fan, Z., Wang, H., & Zhuang, Y. (2023). Global and regional prevalence of vitamin D deficiency in population-based studies from 2000 to 2022: A pooled analysis of 7.9 million participants. *Frontiers in Nutrition, 10*. https://doi.org/10.3389/fnut.2023.1070808.

de la Puente Yagüe, M., Collado Yurrita, L., Ciudad Cabañas, M., & Cuadrado Cenzual, M. (2020). Role of vitamin D in athletes and their performance: Current concepts and new trends. *Nutrients, 12*(2), 579. https://doi.org/10.3390/nu12020579.

Farrokhyar, F., Tabasinejad, R., Dao, D., Peterson, D., Ayeni, O. R., Hadioonzadeh, R., & Bhandari, M. (2015). Prevalence of vitamin D inadequacy in athletes: A systematic-review and meta-analysis. *Sports Medicine, 45*(3), 365–378. https://doi.org/10.1007/s40279-014-0267-6, http://rd.springer.com/journal/40279.

Gunton, J. E., & Girgis, C. M. (2018). Vitamin D and muscle. *Bone Reports, 8*, 163–167. https://doi.org/10.1016/j.bonr.2018.04.004, http://www.journals.elsevier.com/bone-reports/.

Hacker, S., Lenz, C., Reichert, L., Ringseis, R., Zentgraf, K., & Krüger, K. (2025). Vitamin D status and its determinants in German elite athletes. *European Journal of Applied Physiology*. https://doi.org/10.1007/s00421-024-05699-6.

Hamilton, B., Grantham, J., Racinais, S., & Chalabi, H. (2010). Vitamin D deficiency is endemic in Middle Eastern sportsmen. *Public Health Nutrition, 13*(10), 1528–1534. https://doi.org/10.1017/s136898000999320x.

Han, Q., Xiang, M., An, N., Tan, Q., Shao, J., & Wang, Q. (2024). Effects of vitamin D3 supplementation on strength of lower and upper extremities in athletes: An updated systematic review and meta-analysis of randomized controlled trials. *Frontiers in Nutrition, 11*. https://doi.org/10.3389/fnut.2024.1381301.

Harju, T., Gray, B., Mavroedi, A., Farooq, A., & Reilly, J. J. (2022). Prevalence and novel risk factors for vitamin D insufficiency in elite athletes: Systematic review and meta-analysis. *European Journal of Nutrition, 61*(8), 3857–3871. https://doi.org/10.1007/s00394-022-02967-z, https://www.springer.com/journal/394.

Holick, M. F. (2006). High prevalence of vitamin D inadequacy and implications for health. *Mayo Clinic Proceedings, 81*(3), 353–373. https://doi.org/10.4065/81.3.353, http://www.journals.elsevier.com/mayo-clinic-proceedings.

Houston, D. K., Cesari, M., Ferrucci, L., Cherubini, A., Maggio, D., Bartali, B., Johnson, M. A., Schwartz, G. G., & Kritchevsky, S. B. (2007). Association between vitamin D status and physical performance: The InCHIANTI study. *The Journals of Gerontology Series A: Biological Sciences and Medical Sciences, 62*(4), 440–446. https://doi.org/10.1093/gerona/62.4.440.

Ip, T. S. T., Fu, S. C., Ong, M. T. Y., & Yung, P. S. H. (2022). Vitamin D deficiency in athletes: Laboratory, clinical and field integration. *Asia-Pacific Journal of Sports Medicine, Arthroscopy, Rehabilitation and Technology, 29*, 22–29. https://doi.org/10.1016/j.asmart.2022.06.001, http://www.elsevier.com/journals/asia-pacific-journal-of-sports-medicine-arthroscopy-rehabilitation-and-technology/2214-6873.

Książek, A., Zagrodna, A., & Słowińska-Lisowska, M. (2019). Vitamin D, skeletal muscle function and athletic performance in athletes—A narrative review. *Nutrients, 11*(8), 1800. https://doi.org/10.3390/nu11081800.

Langley, C. K., Morse, C. I., & Buffey, A. J. (2024). The prevalence of low vitamin D in elite para-athletes: A systematic review. *Sports Medicine - Open, 10*(1). https://doi.org/10.1186/s40798-024-00756-y, https://sportsmedicine-open.springeropen.com/.

Latham, C. M., Brightwell, C. R., Keeble, A. R., Munson, B. D., Thomas, N. T., Zagzoog, A. M., Fry, C. S., & Fry, J. L. (2021). Vitamin D promotes skeletal muscle regeneration and mitochondrial health. *Frontiers in Physiology, 12*. https://doi.org/10.3389/fphys.2021.660498, http://www.frontiersin.org/Physiology/archive/.

Lehert, P., Villaseca, P., Hogervorst, E., Maki, P. M., & Henderson, V. W. (2015). Individually modifiable risk factors to ameliorate cognitive aging: A systematic review and meta-analysis. *Climacteric the Journal of the International Menopause Society, 18*(5), 678–689. https://doi.org/10.3109/13697137.2015.1078106.

Lovell, G. (2008). Vitamin D status of females in an elite gymnastics program. *Clinical Journal of Sport Medicine, 18*(2), 159–161. https://doi.org/10.1097/jsm.0b013e3181650eee.

Marcinowska-Suchowierska, E., Kupisz-Urbańska, M., Łukaszkiewicz, J., Płudowski, P., & Jones, G. (2018). Vitamin D toxicity–A clinical perspective. *Frontiers in Endocrinology, 9*. https://doi.org/10.3389/fendo.2018.00550.

National Institute for Health and Care Excellence (NICE). 2022. https://cks.nice.org.uk/topics/vitamin-d-deficiency-in-adults/#:~:text=An%20increased%20risk%20of%20vitamin,greater%20than%2050%20nmol%2FL (Accessed 22 Jan 2025).

Nhs, Guidance on Vitamin D Deficiency/Insufficiency. (2018).

Owens, D. J., Tang, J. C. Y., Bradley, W. J., Sparks, A. S., Fraser, W. D., Morton, J. P., & Close, G. L. (2017). Efficacy of high-dose vitamin D supplements for elite athletes. *Medicine and Science in Sports and Exercise, 49*(2), 349–356. https://doi.org/10.1249/MSS.0000000000001105, http://www.lww.com/product/?0195-9131.

Owens, D. J., Allison, R., & Close, G. L. (2018). Vitamin D and the athlete: Current perspectives and new challenges. *Sports Medicine, 48*, 3–16. https://doi.org/10.1007/s40279-017-0841-9, http://rd.springer.com/journal/40279.

Paz, A., Stanley, M., Mangano, F. G., & Miron, R. J. (2021). Vitamin D deficiency and early implant failure: Outcomes from a pre-surgical supplementation program on vitamin D levels and antioxidant scores. *Oral Health & Preventive Dentistry, 19*(1), 495–502. https://doi.org/10.3290/j.ohpd.b2082063.

Perrone, M. A., Pieri, M., Caminiti, G., Ali, W., Bernardini, S., Parisi, A., Iellamo, F., Barone, R., & Farsetti, P. (2024). Vitamin D deficiency in professional football players during competitive season of Italian First Division (Serie A). *Sports, 12*(6), 153. https://doi.org/10.3390/sports12060153.

Public Health, England, PHE publishes new advice on vitamin D. Retrieved. (2016).

Ribbans, W. J., Aujla, R., Dalton, S., & Nunley, J. A. (2021). Vitamin D and the athlete-patient: State of the art. *Journal of ISAKOS, 6*(1), 46–60. https://doi.org/10.1136/jisakos-2020-000435, http://jisakos.bmj.com/.

Ross, A. C., Manson, J. A. E., Abrams, S. A., Aloia, J. F., Brannon, P. M., Clinton, S. K., Durazo-Arvizu, R. A., Gallagher, J. C., Gallo, R. L., Jones, G., Kovacs, C. S., Mayne, S. T., Rosen, C. J., & Shapses, S. A. (2011). The 2011 report on dietary reference intakes for calcium and vitamin D from the Institute of Medicine: What clinicians need to know. *Journal of Clinical Endocrinology and Metabolism, 96*(1), 53–58. https://doi.org/10.1210/jc.2010-2704, http://jcem.endojournals.org/cgi/reprint/96/1/53.

Shuler, F. D., Wingate, M. K., Moore, G. H., & Giangarra, C. (2012). Sports health benefits of vitamin D. *Sports Health, 4*(6), 496–501. https://doi.org/10.1177/1941738112461621.

Silva, A. B. Jd, Barros, W. M. A., Silva, M. Ld, Silva, J. M. L., Souza, A. Pd. S., Silva, K. Gd, de Sousa Fernandes, M. S., Carneiro, A. C. Bd. F., Souza, Vd. O. N., & Lagranha, C. J. (2022). Impact of vitamin D on cognitive functions in healthy individuals: A systematic review in randomized controlled clinical trials. *Frontiers in Psychology, 13*. https://doi.org/10.3389/fpsyg.2022.987203, http://www.frontiersin.org/Psychology.

Sist, M., Zou, L., Galloway, S. D. R., & Rodriguez-Sanchez, N. (2023). Effects of vitamin D supplementation on maximal strength and power in athletes: A systematic review and meta-analysis of randomized controlled trials. *Frontiers in Nutrition, 10*. https://doi.org/10.3389/fnut.2023.1163313 http://journal.frontiersin.org/journal/nutrition.

van den Ouweland, J., Fleuren, H., Drabbe, M., & Vollaard, H. (2014). Pharmacokinetics and safety issues of an accidental overdose of 2,000,000 IU of vitamin D3 in two nursing home patients: A case report. *BMC Pharmacology and Toxicology, 15*(1). https://doi.org/10.1186/2050-6511-15-57.

West, S., Monteyne, A. J., van der Heijden, I., Stephens, F. B., & Wall, B. T. (2023). Nutritional considerations for the vegan athlete. *Advances in Nutrition, 14*(4), 774–795. https://doi.org/10.1016/j.advnut.2023.04.012, https://www.sciencedirect.com/journal/advances-in-nutrition.

Wiedenbrüg, K., Will, L., Reichert, L., Hacker, S., Lenz, C., Zentgraf, K., Raab, M., & Krüger, K. (2024). Inflammation and cognitive performance in elite athletes: A cross-sectional study. *Brain, Behavior, & Immunity - Health, 42*, 100872. https://doi.org/10.1016/j.bbih.2024.100872.

Williams, K., Askew, C., Mazoue, C., Guy, J., Torres-McGehee, T. M., & Jackson III, J. B. (2020). Vitamin D3 supplementation and stress fractures in high-risk collegiate athletes – A pilot study. *Orthopedic Research and Reviews, Volume 12*, 9–17. https://doi.org/10.2147/orr.s233387.

Willis, K. S., Peterson, N. J., & Larson-Meyer, D. E. (2008). Should we be concerned about the vitamin D status of athletes? *International Journal of Sport Nutrition and Exercise Metabolism, 18*(2), 204–224. https://doi.org/10.1123/ijsnem.18.2.204, http://www.humankinetics.com/eJournalMedia/pdfs/15665.pdf.

Yoon, S., Kwon, O., & Kim, J. (2021). Vitamin D in athletes: Focus on physical performance and musculoskeletal injuries. *Physical Activity and Nutrition, 25*(2), 20–25. https://doi.org/10.20463/pan.2021.0011.

CHAPTER 6

Vitamin D and the immune system

Ihsan Nazurah Zulkipli, and Liyana Ahmad

Pengiran-Anak-Puteri-Rashidah-Sa'adatul-Bolkiah Institute of Health Sciences, Universiti Brunei Darussalam, Bandar Seri Begawan, Brunei Darussalam

6.1 Introduction to vitamin D and immune health

6.1.1 Overview of vitamin D

Vitamin D is a fat-soluble vitamin that facilitates various bodily functions, including maintaining healthy bones and supporting the immune system. The body synthesizes vitamin D in the skin upon exposure to ultraviolet B (UVB) radiation from sunlight. It can also be obtained through dietary sources such as fatty fish, egg yolks, and cheese. It may also be ingested as a supplement in the form of Vitamin D2 (ergocalciferol) and D3 (cholecalciferol), which are commonly derived from plants and animals, respectively.

6.1.2 Synthesis and activation of vitamin D

The synthesis of vitamin D begins when UVB rays convert 7-dehydrocholesterol, a compound found in the skin, into previtamin D3 and ultimately into vitamin D3 (cholecalciferol). Following synthesis, vitamin D3 enters the bloodstream and is transported to the liver, where it undergoes its first metabolic conversion. In the liver, vitamin D3 is hydroxylated by the enzyme vitamin D 25-hydroxylase to form 25-hydroxyvitamin D (25(OH)D), also known as calcidiol. This form of vitamin D is the primary circulating metabolite and is often measured (Young et al., 2022) to assess an individual's vitamin D status. The next step in vitamin D metabolism occurs in the kidneys, where calcidiol is further hydroxylated by the enzyme 1α-hydroxylase to produce the biologically active form, 1,25-dihydroxyvitamin D (1,25(OH)₂D), also referred to as calcitriol (Engelsen, 2010).

Vitamin D metabolism is tightly regulated by various factors, including parathyroid hormone (PTH), serum calcium levels, and phosphate levels. For instance, low serum calcium levels stimulate PTH secretion, which in turn enhances the activity of 1α-hydroxylase in the kidneys, leading to increased production of calcitriol. Conversely, high levels of 1,25(OH)₂D can exert negative feedback on its own synthesis by inhibiting the expression of 1α-hydroxylase (Anderson et al., 2003; Young et al., 2022).

The Impact of Vitamin D on Health and Disease. **DOI:** https://doi.org/10.1016/B978-0-443-34037-6.00033-9

6.2 Immune modulation by vitamin D

6.2.1 Overview of the immune system

Innate immunity is a forefront defense system that immediately protects the body against pathogens and injury. Its responses are fast and broad, owing to the pattern-recognition receptors (PRRs) on cells that recognize molecular signatures of pathogens. Intracellular PRRs, such as Toll-like receptors (TLRs), can detect pathogens in the cells, which trigger the activation of inflammatory signaling pathways that lead to the production of an array of host defenses such as antimicrobial peptides (AMPs), chemokines, and pro-inflammatory cytokines, and the initiation of adaptive immune responses. Additionally, the detection of pathogens by phagocytes such as macrophages will stimulate the internalization of the pathogen in phagosome vesicles, which are enriched with AMPs such as cathelicidin and defensin, as well as nitric oxide (Pieters, 2008). These molecules are cytotoxic, which can potentiate the killing of the pathogen contained within through the process of phagocytosis. Alternatively, the pathogen may also be engulfed by autophagosomal vesicles, which direct the pathogen toward degradation via the autophagy pathway (Wu & Sun, 2011).

Although delayed, adaptive immunity works in concert with innate immunity in eliminating pathogens, via its specific targeting of the pathogens with the help of T and B lymphocytes. CD4$^+$ T cells can proliferate and differentiate into specific subtypes, such as T helper (Th)-1 and Th17, which actively promote inflammation and perform direct killing of the infected cells and pathogens. On the other hand, B cells produce antibodies that can effectively neutralize and eradicate the offending pathogens. Following a successful elimination, inflammation shall resolve with the help of immunomodulators such as regulatory T (Treg) cells and antiinflammatory cytokines, returning the body to homeostasis.

6.2.2 Role of vitamin D in innate immunity

Vitamin D exerts its effect in its active form calcitriol (1,25-dihydroxyvitamin D3) which interacts with nuclear vitamin D receptor (VDR). VDR is ubiquitously expressed in various immune cells of both innate and adaptive immunity, including monocytes, macrophages, dendritic cells, T cells, and B cells (Baeke et al., 2010; White, 2012). As such, vitamin D has a great influence on both innate and adaptive immune responses (Baeke et al., 2010; Kamen & Tangpricha, 2010; White, 2012). Upon binding to its receptor, vitamin D influences gene expression related to immune function and inflammation, thereby promoting the body's ability to respond to pathogens. In parallel, it plays a regulatory role in the immune system by preventing excessive inflammation, which evidently underlies multiple autoimmune diseases and chronic inflammatory conditions (Ao et al., 2021).

The role of vitamin D in innate immunity is best exemplified in tuberculosis, a disease caused by *Mycobacterium tuberculosis* (Fabri et al., 2011; Verway et al., 2013). It participates by enhancing the production of antimicrobial peptides (AMPs) (Al-Jaberi et al., 2022; Svensson et al., 2016), elimination of intracellular pathogens via autophagy (Yuk et al., 2009), and modulating the expression of pathogen recognition receptors (Ao et al., 2021). Upon binding to VDR on macrophages and monocytes, vitamin D activates the transcription of the cathelicidin gene (CAMP) resulting in an enhanced production of LL-37, the mature form of cathelicidin, which is known to disrupt mycobacterial cell walls and thus kill the pathogen (Martineau et al., 2007). Additionally, vitamin D activates the autophagic process in macrophages, which is crucial for the elimination of intracellular pathogens, including *M. tuberculosis*. Autophagy facilitates the delivery of AMPs to autophagosome vesicles containing the bacteria, thereby enhancing the macrophage's ability to kill the pathogen (Klug-Micu et al., 2013; Yuk et al., 2009).

Moreover, vitamin D has been shown to modulate the expression of toll-like receptors (TLRs) on immune cells, thereby influencing their responsiveness to pathogens. For instance, vitamin D can enhance TLR2-mediated signaling in macrophages, which is vital for the activation of innate immune responses against bacterial infections (Larcombe et al., 2012). By modulating the responsivity of the innate recognition, vitamin D can thus influence the secretion of downstream pro-inflammatory cytokines, such as interleukin-1β (IL-1β), which plays a role in the inflammatory response to mycobacterial infections (Verway et al., 2013). This interplay between vitamin D and cytokine signaling highlights its role in shaping both innate and adaptive immune responses (Baeke et al., 2010; Wei & Christakos, 2015; White, 2012).

6.2.3   Role of vitamin D in adaptive immunity

On the other hand, vitamin D can also impact on cytokine production, inflammation regulation, and immune cell differentiation. Vitamin D can downregulate inflammation in macrophages by inhibiting TLR4 receptor signaling, consequently dampening down the production of pro-inflammatory cytokines (Chen et al., 2013). Furthermore, vitamin D plays a significant role in the adaptive immune system by influencing T cell differentiation and function. Vitamin D can promote the differentiation of T cells into IL-22-producing cells, which are important for maintaining mucosal immunity (Sommer & Fabri, 2015). It also promotes the development of regulatory T (Treg) cells while inhibiting the proliferation of pro-inflammatory Th1 and Th17 cells and production of autoantibodies, thereby reducing the risk of autoimmune conditions (Chang et al., 2010; Lemire et al., 1992; Liu et al., 2019; Mattner et al., 2000; Sassi, 2018; Unal et al., 2014).

6.2.4   Implications for immune function

Studies have demonstrated that vitamin D deficiency or insufficiency is associated with increased susceptibility to infections and inflammatory diseases, suggesting that adequate vitamin D levels are essential for optimal immune function (Ao et al., 2021). For instance, vitamin D insufficiency has been linked to severe malaria in children, indicating its protective role in infectious diseases (Cusick et al., 2014). Experimental mice models have illustrated the benefits of vitamin D in malarial infection whereby its coadministration with antimalarial drug arteether improved the outcome (Dwivedi et al., 2016).

Similarly, vitamin D supplementation has been shown to improve immune responses in both acute and chronic respiratory infections. A low dose daily supplementation of vitamin D has been shown to be beneficial for acute respiratory infections (Jolliffe et al., 2021; Martineau et al., 2017). Although the link between COVID-19 and vitamin D is yet to be established, it is speculated that vitamin D may pose a therapeutic potential for COVID-19. COVID-19 is a respiratory disease caused by the coronavirus SARS-CoV-2, and severe cases may present with acute respiratory distress syndrome (ARDS) and cytokine storm, which may benefit from the immunomodulatory effects of vitamin D (Quesada-Gomez et al., 2020).

Vitamin D deficiency is associated with susceptibility to tuberculosis (TB) and disease progression, highlighting the role of vitamin D in host defense against mycobacterial infection (Nnoaham & Clarke, 2008; Talat et al., 2010). A clinical trial on active TB patients who were given daily doses of vitamin D also observed similar protective effects. Macrophages from TB patients who consumed vitamin D produced more antibacterial cathelicidin and showed greater reduction in bacterial growth than those who did not (Mily et al., 2015).

The protective role of vitamin D in TB also extends to immunomodulation, where it helps minimize excessive inflammation and tissue damage that can worsen disease outcome. It exerts this role via two ways: (1) reducing inflammation by downregulating nuclear factor kappa B (NF-κB) inflammatory signaling pathway and matrix metalloproteinases (Coussens et al., 2009; Deng et al., 2021) and (2) inhibiting the expression of major histocompatibility complex (MHC)-II thus antigen presentation, which consequently dampens the activation of T helper (Th) cell activation and promotes the proliferation of regulatory T (Treg) cells (Harishankar et al., 2016). This immunoregulatory capacity of vitamin D is particularly relevant in the context of autoimmune diseases where it evidently helps reduce the expansion of pro-inflammatory Th1 and Th17 and stimulates the production of Treg cells (Chang et al., 2010; Dankers et al., 2017; Treiber et al., 2015).

6.3   Vitamin D deficiency: prevalence, risk factors, and immune implications

6.3.1   Global and regional prevalence

Vitamin D deficiency, or hypovitaminosis D, is defined as plasma 25-hydroxyvitamin D [25(OH)D] < 50 nmol/L. Globally, it is alarmingly common in both genders and is affecting an estimated 1 billion people, with varying prevalence across different populations and regions. It is influenced by factors such as geographical location, lifestyle, dietary habits, and socioeconomic status. For instance, studies have shown that vitamin D deficiency is particularly prevalent in regions with limited sunlight exposure, such as northern Europe and parts of Asia (Cashman, 2018; Holick, 2006, 2007). In the United States, approximately 41.6% of adults are estimated to be vitamin D deficient, with higher rates observed among African Americans and Hispanics (Forrest & Stuhldreher, 2011). In specific regions, such as the Middle East and South Asia, vitamin D deficiency is widespread due to cultural practices that limit sun exposure and dietary insufficiencies (AlFaris et al., 2019; Siddiqee et al., 2021). A study in northwestern Chinese population reported a high prevalence of vitamin D deficiency, particularly among the middle-aged and elderly, highlighting the need for targeted public health interventions (Chen et al., 2017; Zhen et al., 2015). Similarly, research in Georgia indicated that a significant proportion of pulmonary tuberculosis patients exhibited vitamin D deficiency, suggesting a correlation between vitamin D status and health outcomes in specific populations (Desai et al., 2012).

Vitamin D deficiency has significant implications for immune function and the prevalence of immune-related diseases. As previously discussed, vitamin D plays a critical role in modulating the immune system, influencing both innate and adaptive immune responses. Hence, deficiency in vitamin D is linked to an increased risk of various autoimmune diseases, including type 1 diabetes (T1D), multiple sclerosis (MS), and rheumatoid arthritis (RA) (Balasooriya et al., 2024; Harrison et al., 2019; Infante et al., 2019).

In the context of infectious diseases, vitamin D deficiency has been shown to impair the immune response to pathogens, increasing the risk of respiratory infections (Ginde et al., 2009; Nnoaham & Clarke, 2008; Raju et al., 2022; Wayse et al., 2004) and exacerbating conditions such as asthma and chronic obstructive pulmonary disease (COPD) (Brehm et al., 2010; Ferrari et al., 2011; Janssens et al., 2010). A metaanalysis indicated that vitamin D supplementation could reduce the risk of acute respiratory tract infections, highlighting its potential protective role (Martineau et al., 2017). Furthermore, vitamin D deficiency has been implicated in the pathogenesis of tuberculosis, with studies showing that adequate vitamin D levels may enhance the immune response against *M. tuberculosis* (Larcombe et al., 2012; Martineau et al., 2012; Morcos et al., 1998). Certain VDR gene polymorphisms have also been implicated in the genetic susceptibility to *M. tuberculosis*, highlighting the importance of vitamin D in combating mycobacterial infections (Al-Jaberi et al., 2022; Joshi et al., 2014; Tiosano et al., 2013). Additionally, vitamin D deficiency during pregnancy has been associated with impaired fetal immune responses, potentially leading to increased susceptibility to infections and autoimmune diseases later in life (Dragomir et al., 2024).

6.3.2 Risk factors

Vitamin D deficiency is a significant public health concern globally as it has been associated with various health issues, including osteoporosis, autoimmune diseases, and increased susceptibility to infections (Holick & Chen, 2008; Holick, 2007). There are various risk factors contributing to its prevalence, and therefore understanding these risk factors is crucial for developing effective prevention strategies.

1. *Geographical location and sun exposure*: Deficiencies in vitamin D can arise from inadequate synthesis due to factors such as limited sun exposure, skin pigmentation, and the use of sunscreen. Individuals living in regions with limited sunlight, particularly during winter months, are at a higher risk of vitamin D deficiency (Reichrath, 2006). This is especially true for populations residing at higher latitudes where UVB radiation is insufficient for vitamin D synthesis in the skin (Mendes et al., 2019). Additionally, cultural practices that limit sun exposure, such as wearing clothing that covers most of the skin or spending excessive time indoors, further exacerbate the risk (AlFaris et al., 2019; Al-Taiar et al., 2018).

2. *Skin pigmentation*: Darker skin contains more melanin, which reduces the skin's ability to produce vitamin D in response to sunlight. Consequently, individuals with darker skin tones are at a higher risk of deficiency, particularly in areas with low UV exposure (Nesby-O'Dell et al., 2002). This is particularly relevant in populations such as African Americans and certain ethnic groups in Europe and Asia (Nessvi et al., 2011; Powe et al., 2013).

3. *Age*: Older adults are at increased risk of vitamin D deficiency due to several factors, including reduced skin synthesis of vitamin D, decreased dietary intake, and potential malabsorption issues. Aging also affects the kidneys' ability to convert vitamin D to its active form (Gallagher, 2013; Kweder & Eidi, 2018; Lips, 2001).

4. *Obesity*: There is a well-established link between obesity and vitamin D deficiency. Vitamin D is a lipid-soluble vitamin, and higher body fat percentages can sequester vitamin D, making it less biologically available in the bloodstream (Wortsman et al., 2000). Studies have shown that individuals with obesity often have lower serum levels of vitamin D compared to those with normal weight (Carrelli et al., 2016).

5. *Dietary factors*: Insufficient dietary intake of vitamin D-rich foods, such as fatty fish, fortified dairy products, and egg yolks, can lead to deficiency. This is particularly concerning in populations with limited access to these foods or those following strict vegetarian or vegan diets (Crowe et al., 2011).

6. *Medical conditions*: Certain medical conditions can impair the metabolism of vitamin D, leading to insufficient levels of its active form. Gastrointestinal diseases such as celiac disease, Crohn's disease, and cystic fibrosis can hinder the absorption of vitamin D from the diet causing a reduction in bioavailability (Aris et al., 2005; Lo et al., 1985). Additionally, chronic kidney disease can affect the conversion of vitamin D to its active form leading to vitamin D deficiency (Holick, 2005).

7. *Pregnancy and lactation*: Pregnant and breastfeeding women are at increased risk of vitamin D deficiency due to the higher demands for vitamin D during these periods (Hollis

& Wagner, 2004a). Insufficient maternal vitamin D levels can also affect the vitamin D status of the infant (Hollis & Wagner, 2004b).

8. *Gender*: Studies have shown that females are more likely to be vitamin D deficient compared to males. This may be attributed to factors such as hormonal differences, dietary habits, and lifestyle choices that limit sun exposure (Ning et al., 2016; Wallace et al., 2013).

9. *Socioeconomic status*: Individuals from lower socioeconomic backgrounds may have limited access to vitamin D-rich foods, healthcare, and opportunities for outdoor activities, increasing their risk of deficiency (Santana et al., 2022; Scully et al., 2022).

In conclusion, vitamin D deficiency is influenced by a complex interplay of environmental, biological, and lifestyle factors. Addressing these risk factors through public health initiatives, dietary recommendations, and lifestyle modifications is essential for improving vitamin D status in at-risk populations.

6.4 Vitamin D deficiency and autoimmune diseases

6.4.1 Multiple sclerosis

MS is a chronic autoimmune disease where the immune system which is mediated by Th1 and Th17 cells attacks the protective covering of nerve fibers in the central nervous system (CNS). This causes the demyelination of nerve fibers, leading to a range of neurological symptoms. The relationship between vitamin D and MS has been a topic of considerable interest in recent years, with growing evidence suggesting that vitamin D may play a protective role in the development and progression of this autoimmune disease. Vitamin D deficiency is prevalent among MS patients, suggesting that adequate vitamin D levels might be protective against the development of this disease (Balasooriya et al., 2024).

Vitamin D deficiency has been linked to an increased risk for developing MS. Mendelian randomization studies performed on different populations demonstrated a strong causal effect of low vitamin D on MS risk, reinforcing the hypothesis that vitamin D deficiency may contribute to the pathogenesis of the disease (Mokry et al., 2015; Rhead et al., 2016). Similarly, Simpson et al. (2010) reported that higher serum levels of vitamin D are associated with a lower risk of MS relapses, suggesting that maintaining adequate vitamin D levels may be beneficial for individuals with MS. Geographic studies also indicate that MS is more common in areas with lower sunlight exposure, supporting the role of vitamin D (Hedström et al., 2019; Sintzel et al., 2017).

Vitamin D is known to modulate immune responses by shifting the balance from pro-inflammatory to antiinflammatory pathways by influencing lymphocyte activation and differentiation, which are critical processes in the context of autoimmune diseases like MS (Mora et al., 2008). For example, vitamin D has been shown to reduce the proliferation of Th1 and Th17 cells, which are implicated in the inflammatory processes of MS (Chang et al., 2010). Additionally, Wang et al. (2012) demonstrated that the development of experimental autoimmune encephalomyelitis (EAE), a mouse model of MS, requires vitamin D and the vitamin D receptor (VDR), indicating that vitamin D signaling is crucial for the regulation of immune responses in the context of MS. This suggests that vitamin D may help to mitigate the autoimmune attack on myelin sheaths in the CNS.

6.4.2   Rheumatoid arthritis

RA is an autoimmune disease in which the immune system attacks the joints, causing chronic inflammation, pain, swelling, and eventual joint destruction. Emerging evidence suggests that vitamin D may play a crucial role in the pathogenesis and management of this autoimmune disease.

Studies showed that there is a high prevalence of vitamin D deficiency among individuals with RA, and that low levels of vitamin D can exacerbate the disease and increase the severity of joint inflammation. Studies in various RA cohorts demonstrated a prevalence of low vitamin D levels in patients which are associated with disease severity (Cutolo et al., 2006; Haque & Bartlett, 2010; Kerr et al., 2011; Rossini et al., 2010; Welsh et al., 2011). Similarly, a metaanalysis by Lin et al. (2016) demonstrated that RA patients have lower serum vitamin D levels compared to healthy controls, and there is an inverse relationship between vitamin D levels and disease activity scores. These findings suggest that vitamin D deficiency may be common in RA patients and could potentially influence disease severity.

The pathophysiological role of vitamin D in RA involves promoting antiinflammatory pathways while inhibiting pro-inflammatory cytokines. For example, in RA mouse model, the absence of VDR leads to an increase in inflammation, bone erosion, and disease severity, suggesting a suppressive role of vitamin D on arthritis (Zwerina et al., 2011). In synergy with conventional RA therapy, vitamin D can also limit the production of pro-inflammatory cytokines such as IL-6 and IL-17 and restrict the proliferation of bone-eroding osteoclasts, further contributing to its potential therapeutic effects in RA (Huhtakangas et al., 2017; Kim et al., 2020).

The relationship between vitamin D and RA may also be influenced by environmental factors, such as geographic location and sun exposure. Individuals living in regions with limited sunlight exposure are at a higher risk of vitamin D deficiency, which may contribute to the higher incidence of RA observed in these populations (Arkema et al., 2013; Staples et al., 2003; Vieira et al., 2010). Furthermore, seasonal variations in vitamin D levels have been associated with fluctuations in RA disease activity, suggesting that maintaining adequate vitamin D levels throughout the year may be beneficial for managing the disease (Mori et al., 2019).

6.4.3 Type 1 diabetes

T1D is an autoimmune condition where the body's immune system attacks insulin-producing β-cells in the pancreas, leading to hyperglycemia and a lifelong dependence on exogenous insulin. The relationship between vitamin D levels and T1D is complex, with various studies suggesting that vitamin D deficiency may be associated with an increased risk of developing the disease, as well as influencing glycemic control in affected individuals. A metaanalysis study by Dong et al. (2013) found that higher vitamin D intake in early life is associated with a reduced risk of T1D. Similarly, another study found that maternal serum levels of vitamin D during pregnancy were inversely related to the risk of T1D in offspring, highlighting the importance of maternal vitamin D status during critical developmental periods (Sørensen et al., 2012).

In terms of glycemic control, vitamin D supplementation has shown mixed results in individuals with T1D. A case report showed that supplementing T1D patients with vitamin D improved insulin sensitivity (Schwalfenberg, 2008). While other studies indicated that vitamin D3 supplementation at doses up to 4000 IU or ≥30 µg was safe and could potentially improve glycemic control (Ahola et al., 2024; Aljabri et al., 2010), a study in Sudanese children with T1D reported no significant improvements in HbA1c levels following vitamin D supplementation, suggesting that while vitamin D may have a role in metabolic processes, its direct impact on glycemic control in T1D may be limited (Suliman et al., 2024).

The potential mechanisms by which vitamin D may influence T1D include its role in immune regulation, insulin secretion and sensitivity, and β-cell function. Vitamin D may help prevent the autoimmune destruction of pancreatic β-cells by promoting immune tolerance and reducing inflammation. It exerts its effects primarily through the vitamin D receptor (VDR), which is expressed in various immune cells, including T cells and B cells. Activation of VDR on T cells has been shown to inhibit the production of pro-inflammatory cytokines, such as interleukin-1β (IL-1β) and interferon-gamma (IFN-γ), which are implicated in the pathogenesis of T1D (Wolden-Kirk et al., 2011). Numerous studies that used T1D mouse model demonstrated that vitamin D supplementation can reduce the activation of autoreactive T cells and thus prevent pancreatic destruction (Driver et al., 2007; Gregori et al., 2002; Lai et al., 2022). Additionally, vitamin D may enhance the function of regulatory T cells, which are essential for maintaining immune tolerance and preventing autoimmunity (Gregori et al., 2002). In randomized controlled trials (RCTs), patients given long-term vitamin D supplementation showed an improvement in Treg cell proliferation with enhanced regulatory capacity (Gabbay et al., 2012; Treiber et al., 2015). In terms of glycemic control, vitamin D interacts with VDRs that are present in pancreatic β-cells to modulate insulin secretion and sensitivity (Wolden-Kirk et al., 2011).

The relationship between vitamin D and T1D may also be influenced by genetic factors. Cooper et al. (2011) highlighted that inherited variations in vitamin D metabolism genes are associated with an increased risk of autoimmune diseases, including T1D. This suggests that genetic predisposition may interact with environmental factors, such as vitamin D status, to influence the development of T1D. In conclusion, vitamin D appears to play a significant role in the pathogenesis and management of T1D.

6.5   Therapeutic potential of vitamin D in immune disorders

6.5.1   Benefits of supplementation for disease management and evidence from human trials

Numerous studies have established a link between vitamin D deficiency and various autoimmune and infectious diseases, highlighting the potential of vitamin D supplementation as a therapeutic strategy to mitigate disease activity. Many case studies and RCTs have shown promising results from using vitamin D supplementation with general improvements in disease markers and clinical outcomes.

Exaggerated inflammation is a hallmark in severe and complicated autoimmune disorders and infectious diseases where vitamin D's immunomodulatory potential appears to have the most impact. It evidently can slow down tuberculosis (TB) progression into an active course and provides an additive power to current treatments against malaria and COVID-19 infections. Moreover, its antiinflammatory effects are beneficial in many autoimmune conditions such as MS and RA. By preserving insulin sensitivity and promoting immune tolerance, vitamin D also helps retain metabolic control over glucose in type 1 diabetes.

A RCT on TB patients who received vitamin D supplementation demonstrated an improvement in clinical and radiographic outcomes compared to those receiving a placebo (Salahuddin et al., 2013). Many believed that vitamin D can arrest disease progression from active to latent TB and improve overall survival (Nnoaham & Clarke, 2008; Talat et al., 2010). Vitamin D is also shown to inhibit the growth of *M. tuberculosis* in vitro, which may be mediated by enhanced autophagy response and nitric oxide that promotes intracellular elimination of the bacteria by infected macrophages (Rockett et al., 1998; Yuk et al., 2009). By promoting the antimicrobial peptide cathelicidin, Vitamin D also reduces the production of pro-inflammatory TNF-α and IL-17 cytokines and increases the production of antiinflammatory IL-10 and TGF-β cytokines by macrophages, which is crucial in controlling the severity of TB (Torres-Juarez et al., 2015).

Clinical trials investigating the efficacy of vitamin D supplementation in reducing malaria incidence or improving treatment outcomes are relatively limited. The potency of vitamin D emerged as an adjunctive, whereby its antiplasmodial protective effect in the cerebral malaria mouse model was only seen in combination with an antimalarial drug as opposed to on its own (Dwivedi et al., 2016). Furthermore, while some animal studies have shown that high doses of vitamin D can decrease parasite growth, the effects observed at lower doses have been inconsistent (Bivona et al., 2019; Waisberg et al., 2012). Nevertheless, the clinical significance of this association remains debated, and further research is needed to clarify the immunological mechanisms involved and the potential benefits of vitamin D supplementation in malaria management.

The role of vitamin D in reducing the severity of COVID-19 has garnered significant attention. Evidence suggests that adequate levels of vitamin D may mitigate the inflammatory cytokine storm and acute respiratory distress syndrome (ARDS) associated with severe COVID-19 cases, thereby improving clinical outcomes (Zelini et al., 2022). Moreover, vitamin D's ability to modulate the immune response means that it may act as an adjuvant, enhancing COVID-19 vaccine efficacy and promoting the production of neutralizing antibodies against SARS-CoV-2 virus, particularly in populations with high rates of vitamin D deficiency (Zelini et al., 2022). An observational study conducted in the United Kingdom in 2020 showed the benefit of high-dose (40,000 IU) vitamin D daily supplementation in reducing COVID-19 mortality in a cohort of 986 patients regardless of their baseline vitamin D levels (Ling et al., 2020). Lower daily dose of 10,000–25,000 IU seemed to confer similar benefits in reducing length of COVID-19 hospitalization and oxygen ventilation in two separate trials (Cervero et al., 2022; De Niet et al., 2022). The COvid-19 and VITamin d TRIAL (COVIT-TRIAL) is a multicenter RCT conducted in 2021 across nine medical centers in France on 254 older COVID-19 patients. It was set out to test the therapeutic effect of high (400,000 IU) versus low (50,000 IU) single doses of vitamin D on COVID-19. In line with others, this RCT found that either dose given once at the beginning of infection was able to reduce overall mortality in high-risk COVID-19 patients within 14 days, albeit this protective effect waned at day 28 of the disease (Annweiler et al., 2022).

In other respiratory infections, vitamin D was also observed to be preventative by reducing the risk of infection. In 2017 a metaanalysis of 11,321 participants across 25 RCTs observed a strong reduction in risk of acute respiratory infections following vitamin D supplementation, although this protection was more significant in individuals with severe vitamin D deficiency at baseline (Martineau et al., 2017). However, some studies have reported inconsistent results, indicating that individual responses may vary based on factors such as baseline vitamin D status, age, and underlying health conditions (Marusca et al., 2023). For example, an RCT on 703 healthy children found no significant protective effect of high-dose 2000 IU per day of vitamin D supplementation on the incidence of upper respiratory infections, suggesting that further research is needed to clarify the optimal dosing and timing of supplementation (Aglipay et al., 2017).

The evidence on the therapeutic effects of vitamin D on the progression of MS patients is rather conflicting. Some studies demonstrated a protective effect, while others did not. For example, a prospective cohort study on 170 relapsing-remitting MS (RRMS) patients who were vitamin D deficient revealed an improvement in disability score and disease relapses after taking up to 4000 IU of vitamin D daily (Laursen et al., 2016). Similarly, an RCT administering a weekly vitamin D supplementation to 15 MS patients who were pregnant and had low baseline vitamin D levels also demonstrated protective effects, where patients showed a reduced disability progression and relapse rates during pregnancy and within 6 months after delivery (Janghorbani et al., 2015). In contrast, an RCT that compared high (5000 IU) and low (600 IU) doses of vitamin D on RRMS patients did not observe any significant protective effects on the disease relapse rates (Cassard et al., 2023).

The effects of vitamin D supplementation on the recurrence and severity of RA are also an active area of debate. An RCT in 2017 by Buondonno et al. (2017) demonstrated that supplementation with a single dose of vitamin D (300,000 IU) in early RA patients receiving methotrexate led to improvements in disease activity score. Conversely, other studies have found no significant effects of vitamin D supplementation on disease activity scores, indicating that individual responses may vary based on factors such as baseline vitamin D status and genetic predispositions (Hansen et al., 2014; Singh et al., 2023). These conflicting findings therefore highlight the need for further research to clarify the therapeutic potential of vitamin D in RA management.

Type 1 diabetes (T1D) is another chronic inflammatory disease that appears to benefit from supplemental vitamin D intake, as demonstrated by some studies that reported improvements in glycemic control. For example, two studies demonstrated that vitamin D supplementation of 50,000 and 300,000 IU in children with T1D and vitamin D deficiency resulted in improved HbA1c levels, indicating better glycemic control (Dehkordi et al., 2018; Mohammadian et al., 2015). Another study on 80 diabetic patients with vitamin D deficiency also showed an improvement in HbA1c levels after 12 weeks of taking 4000 IU of vitamin D supplement (Aljabri et al., 2010). Conversely, other studies have found no significant effects of vitamin D supplementation on disease progression or metabolic control. For example, a study on pediatric T1D patients who were vitamin D deficient at baseline and given daily doses of vitamin D did not report an improvement in HbA1c levels after 3 months (Suliman et al., 2024).

In summary, vitamin D levels are influenced by factors like geography, diet, and socio-economic status, impacting risk for these diseases. While supplementation offers therapeutic potential, further research is needed to establish guidelines and determine optimal dosing, timing, and individual responses, particularly for high-risk groups. Robust RCTs are essential to clarify vitamin D's role across these conditions and refine treatment approaches.

6.5.2 Limitations and risks

Vitamin D supplementation has gained considerable attention due to its essential roles in bone health, immune function, and potential protective effects against various diseases. However, the practice of supplementation is not without its challenges, particularly concerning the risks of oversupplementation, variability in individual responses, and the complexities surrounding optimal dosing.

Excessive intake of vitamin D can lead to hypervitaminosis D, characterized by hypercalcemia, which manifests through symptoms such as nausea, vomiting, weakness, and frequent urination. In severe cases, it can result in kidney damage and calcification of soft tissues (Janoušek et al., 2022). The fat-soluble nature of vitamin D allows it to accumulate in the body, raising concerns about toxicity, especially when high doses are consumed over extended periods (Bell et al., 2013). The risk of oversupplementation is exacerbated by the widespread availability of high-dose vitamin D supplements and a general lack of awareness regarding safe upper limits, which leads to overdosing and potential adverse effects (Taylor & Davies, 2018).

Individual responses to vitamin D supplementation vary significantly due to several factors, including genetics, baseline vitamin D status, age, body weight, sun exposure, and dietary habits. Genetic polymorphisms in vitamin D receptor (VDR) genes can influence how effectively the body metabolizes and utilizes vitamin D (Ahn et al., 2010; Tomei et al., 2020). For instance, variations in the CYP2R1 gene, which is crucial for converting vitamin D to its active form, can lead to differences in serum vitamin D levels among individuals (Ahn et al., 2010). Additionally, conditions such as obesity and malabsorption disorders can further complicate vitamin D bioavailability and efficacy (Earthman et al., 2011). This variability underscores the necessity for personalized supplementation approaches rather than a one-size-fits-all regimen.

Despite extensive research, there remains no universally accepted optimal dose of vitamin D for different populations. Recommendations from health organizations vary widely, with suggested daily allowances ranging from 400 to 4000 IU, depending on factors such as age, health status, and risk factors (Cashman, 2018; Pilz et al., 2018). The lack of consensus is largely due to inconsistent findings in clinical trials and the challenges in establishing clear thresholds for vitamin D sufficiency and deficiency (Cashman, 2018). Seasonal variations, geographical differences, and lifestyle factors further complicate dosing guidelines, as individuals in different regions may have varying sun exposure levels that affect their vitamin D synthesis. Moreover, the absence of standardized testing methods for vitamin D levels adds another layer of complexity to establishing appropriate supplementation protocols (Lai et al., 2012).

In conclusion, while vitamin D supplementation offers significant benefits for bone health and immune function, it must be approached with caution. The potential for oversupplementation, the considerable variability in individual responses, and the ongoing debate regarding optimal dosing highlight the need for careful monitoring and tailored supplementation strategies.

Healthcare providers should prioritize individualized assessments and foster awareness about the risks associated with excessive vitamin D intake.

6.5.3   Innovative therapeutics

Vitamin D analogs are structurally modified compounds designed to enhance the beneficial effects of vitamin D while minimizing hypercalcemic side effects. Several analogs have demonstrated efficacy in preclinical and clinical trials for various conditions. Paricalcitol and calcipotriol analogs are used to manage secondary hyperparathyroidism and psoriasis, respectively. Moreover, paricalcitol has shown promise in reducing inflammation and fibrosis in chronic kidney disease, while calcipotriol effectively modulates keratinocyte proliferation. Eldecalcitol and maxacalcitol are developed for osteoporosis to promote bone mineral density with a reduced risk of hypercalcemia. Preclinical studies indicate that certain vitamin D analogs, such as inecalcitol, may inhibit tumor growth in prostate and breast cancers by modulating cell cycle and apoptosis pathways (Chen et al., 2020; Leyssens et al., 2014).

Targeted immunotherapies aim to harness the immune system to combat cancers precisely. Vitamin D's role in immune regulation complements these cancer therapies by enhancing the efficacy of immune checkpoint inhibitors and CAR-T cell therapies. Research suggests that adequate vitamin D levels may improve responses to PD-1/PD-L1 inhibitors by reducing tumor-associated inflammation and promoting T cell infiltration (Dimitrov et al., 2017). Additionally, vitamin D can enhance persistence and reduce exhaustion of antitumor $CD8^+$ T cells, potentially improving outcomes in malignancies (Li et al., 2022).

While the therapeutic potential of vitamin D and its analogs is promising, challenges remain in optimizing dosing, minimizing side effects, and understanding individual variability in response. Personalized medicine approaches, leveraging genetic and microbiome data, could refine vitamin D-based therapies for enhanced efficacy. As research progresses, integrating vitamin D into targeted immunotherapies holds the potential to revolutionize treatment paradigms.

6.6   Emerging areas in vitamin D and immune health

6.6.1   Vitamin D and the gut microbiota

There is growing evidence on the strong association between vitamin D levels and gut microbiota composition, which in turn plays a crucial role in shaping the immune system. For instance, a study by Kassem et al. (2020) demonstrated that maternal vitamin D levels during pregnancy are linked to the gut microbiota of infants, suggesting that adequate vitamin D may promote a healthy microbial community in early life. Similarly, Boughanem et al. (2023) found that optimal vitamin D levels were associated with increased gut microbiota diversity, which is often correlated with better health outcomes. A diverse gut microbiome is critical for immune resilience, as it helps regulate inflammatory responses, supports immune tolerance, and enhances pathogen defense through microbial-derived metabolites. These findings underscore the potential role of vitamin D in shaping the gut microbiome, particularly during critical developmental periods.

Mechanistically, vitamin D influences gut microbiota through the VDR receptor, which is also expressed in various cells within the gastrointestinal tract. VDR activation has been shown to regulate the expression of genes involved in maintaining intestinal homeostasis, inflammation, and microbial colonization (Singh et al., 2020). The VDR pathway is also central to immune function, as it regulates antimicrobial peptides such as cathelicidins and defensins, which not only help maintain gut barrier integrity but also play a direct role in host immune defense against pathogens. For example, Wang et al. (2020) reported that vitamin D decreases plasma trimethylamine-N-oxide levels in mice by modulating gut microbiota, thereby potentially reducing inflammation and metabolic disorders (Wang et al., 2020). Furthermore, vitamin D signaling has been linked to the production of antimicrobial peptides such as defensins, which play a crucial role in maintaining gut barrier integrity and preventing dysbiosis (Su et al., 2016). By strengthening gut barrier function, vitamin D helps prevent microbial translocation, which can otherwise trigger systemic inflammation and contribute to immune dysregulation.

Research has also highlighted the impact of vitamin D deficiency on gut microbiota composition. Robles-Vera et al. (2019) found that vitamin D deficiency increases the abundance of opportunistic pathogens, which can compromise intestinal barrier function and lead to systemic inflammation. This is particularly relevant for immune health, as dysbiosis-induced inflammation has been linked to immune-mediated diseases such as inflammatory bowel disease, MS, and RA. Vitamin D deficiency will not only alter the composition of the gut microbiome but may also impair immune tolerance, leading to increased susceptibility to chronic inflammation and autoimmunity. This suggests that maintaining adequate vitamin D levels is essential for preserving a healthy gut microbiome and preventing dysbiosis, which is associated with various health conditions, including obesity and inflammatory bowel diseases (Akimbekov et al., 2020).

The bidirectional relationship between vitamin D and gut microbiota is becoming increasingly evident. Studies have shown that gut microbiota can influence vitamin D metabolism and bioavailability. For instance, certain gut bacteria are involved in the metabolism of vitamin D, potentially affecting its systemic levels (Jones et al., 2013). Additionally, the gut microbiome can modulate the immune response, which may further impact vitamin D metabolism and its effects on health (Clark & Mach, 2016). Gut microbiota influences the differentiation and function of key immune cells, including regulatory T cells (Tregs) and antigen-presenting cells, both of which are crucial for maintaining immune balance. Microbial-derived short-chain fatty acids (SCFAs), such as butyrate, play a crucial role in immune regulation. As both butyrate and vitamin D independently contribute to immune homeostasis, their potential synergistic effects on immune function remain an area for further investigation. This interplay highlights the complexity of the relationship and the need for more studies into how gut microbiota can influence vitamin D status and vice versa.

Clinical trials exploring the effects of vitamin D supplementation on gut microbiota have yielded promising results, although findings remain inconsistent. Naderpoor et al. (2019) conducted a randomized clinical trial that demonstrated changes in fecal microbiota composition in overweight adults following vitamin D supplementation, suggesting a potential role for vitamin D in modulating gut health. However, other studies have reported mixed outcomes regarding the efficacy of vitamin D supplementation in altering gut microbiota profiles, indicating that individual responses may vary based on factors such as baseline vitamin D status and dietary habits. For example, in investigating the effect of vitamin D (5000 IU/daily) on dysbiosis in HIV patients, a RCT found no significant changes to gut microbiota following supplementation (Missailidis et al., 2019). Similarly, in an older Australian cohort, monthly supplementation of vitamin D at 60,000 IU did not influence the composition of the gut microbiota (Pham et al., 2023). Another observational study also did not find a link between habitual vitamin D intake among healthy Japanese women and their fecal microbiota composition (Seura & Fukuwatari, 2017).

In conclusion, the association between vitamin D and gut microbiota represents an emerging field of research with significant implications for health. Evidence suggests that vitamin D plays a crucial role in shaping gut microbiota composition and function while also being influenced by the gut microbiome. Given the central role of the gut microbiome in regulating immune responses, understanding how vitamin D-mediated microbiota modulation affects immune function is crucial. A well-balanced microbiota supports immune surveillance, mitigates excessive inflammation, and protects against autoimmune diseases, all of which may be influenced by vitamin D status. Understanding the mechanisms underlying this relationship may provide insights into novel therapeutic strategies for managing conditions associated with dysbiosis and vitamin D deficiency. Future research should focus on elucidating the specific pathways through which vitamin D affects gut microbiota and exploring the potential benefits of vitamin D supplementation in promoting gut health. Further, interdisciplinary studies should investigate the integration of microbiome-targeted interventions, such as probiotics or dietary modifications, with vitamin D supplementation to optimize immune function and disease prevention.

6.6.2   Cancer immunotherapy

The potential of vitamin D as an immunotherapeutic agent in cancer treatment has gained increasing attention in recent years. The immunomodulatory effect of vitamin D is particularly relevant in the context of cancer, where inflammation plays a crucial role in tumor progression and metastasis (El-Sharkawy & Malki, 2020). Vitamin D helps regulate nuclear factor kappa B (NF-κB) signaling in T cells in vitro (Yu et al., 1995). By mitigating this inflammation pathway, vitamin D may contribute to a less favorable environment for tumor growth and spread.

Several studies have suggested that vitamin D may have chemopreventive and therapeutic roles in various cancers. Grimm et al. (2015) reported that precancerous lesions of oral squamous cell carcinoma (OSCC) express VDR, indicating that vitamin D signaling could be leveraged for chemopreventative purposes. Additionally, Udeabor et al. (2020) found that low serum vitamin D levels were associated with an increased risk of OSCC, suggesting that vitamin D supplementation could be beneficial in this context (Udeabor et al., 2020). Interestingly, vitamin D has been shown to induce apoptosis and inhibit cancer proliferation in oral cancer, enhancing the efficacy of conventional therapies (Grimm et al., 2015; Hung et al., 2023; Jin et al., 2020).

In colorectal cancer, vitamin D has been linked to improved outcomes. In a RCT, Haidari et al. (2020) reported that vitamin D (dosage of 50,000 IU) and omega-3 fatty acids cosupplementation significantly reduced pro-inflammatory biomarkers (NF-κB, TNF-α, IL-1β, IL-6, and IL-8) and tumor marker CEA (carcinoembryonic antigen) in colorectal cancer patients. This suggests that vitamin D may enhance the effectiveness of existing treatments by modulating the immune response and reducing inflammation. Additionally, a systematic review by Deuster et al. emphasized the potential of vitamin D in various gynecological cancers, noting that adequate vitamin D levels may reduce cancer risk (Deuster et al., 2017).

The relationship between vitamin D and breast cancer has also been extensively studied. Thabet et al. (2022) discussed the antiinflammatory and immunomodulatory effects of vitamin D in breast cancer, particularly in triple-negative tumors, which are often more aggressive and harder to treat. Vitamin D may induce the expression of estrogen receptor (ER)-α in ER-negative breast cancer cells. This helps increase the sensitivity of the cancer cells to tamoxifen, a common therapeutic agent, thereby improving treatment outcomes. Moreover, a metaanalysis on 30 prospective studies found that higher serum levels of vitamin D were associated with better survival rates among breast cancer patients, reinforcing the notion that vitamin D status may influence cancer prognosis (Kim & Je, 2014).

Despite the promising findings, the clinical application of vitamin D in cancer immunotherapy remains complex. While observational studies suggest a beneficial association between vitamin D levels and cancer outcomes, RCTs are necessary to establish causality and determine optimal dosing strategies. For instance, while some studies indicate that vitamin D supplementation may reduce cancer mortality, others have reported mixed results regarding its efficacy in reducing cancer incidence (Kuznia et al., 2023; Manson et al., 2019; Rita et al., 2018). For example, supplementing colorectal cancer patients with vitamin D at 1000 IU daily did not significantly reduce the risk of cancer recurrence (Baron et al., 2015). Similarly, daily supplementation of 2000 IU of vitamin D did not result in a significantly lower risk of all-type cancer in older women (Lappe et al., 2017).

Furthermore, the mechanisms through which vitamin D influences cancer biology are still being elucidated. Vitamin D's role in modulating the tumor microenvironment, enhancing immune cell infiltration, and regulating angiogenesis is area of active research (El-Sharkawy & Malki, 2020). Understanding these mechanisms will be crucial for developing targeted therapies that harness the potential of vitamin D in cancer treatment.

In conclusion, vitamin D shows promise as an immunotherapeutic agent in cancer treatment, with evidence supporting its role in modulating immune responses, inducing apoptosis, and enhancing the efficacy of conventional therapies. However, further research is needed to clarify its mechanisms of action, establish optimal dosing regimens, and conduct well-designed clinical trials to validate its therapeutic potential. As our understanding of vitamin D's role in cancer biology continues to evolve, it may become an integral component of cancer immunotherapy strategies.

6.6.3   Synergistic interplay with other nutrients

The interplay between vitamin D and other essential nutrients, particularly vitamins A, C, and E, has garnered increasing attention in recent years, particularly in the context of immune modulation. These vitamins are known to play critical roles in supporting immune function, and their synergistic effects with vitamin D may enhance its immune-modulating effects, thereby improving overall immune function (Mora et al., 2008).

Vitamin A, particularly in its active form retinoic acid, is crucial for maintaining the integrity of mucosal barriers and regulating immune responses. It has been shown to enhance the differentiation and function of T cells and B cells, which are vital for adaptive immunity (Mora et al., 2008). The combination of vitamin D and vitamin A has been suggested to have a synergistic effect on immune modulation. For instance, both vitamins promote the expression of the antimicrobial peptide cathelicidin in an additive manner, which is essential for the innate immune response to pathogens (Jacobo-Delgado et al., 2021; Liggins et al., 2019).

Vitamin C is another critical nutrient that plays a significant role in immune function. It is known for its antiinflammatory and antioxidant properties (Gombart et al., 2020). The interplay between vitamin D and vitamin C has been highlighted in multiple studies, suggesting that adequate levels of both vitamins may reduce complications during chemotherapy, strengthen the epithelial barrier in the intestinal mucosa, and enhance bone mineralization. For example, supplementing acute myeloid leukemia patients with both vitamin C and D lessened the number of adverse events during chemotherapy (Mouchel et al., 2023). Furthermore, the combined supplementation of vitamins C and D upregulated the expression of the tight junction protein claudin-2, promoting the integrity of the intestinal barrier in colitis (Qiu et al., 2021). Additionally, combined vitamin C and D deficiency was found to be associated with osteoporosis, and cosupplementation with both vitamins may be a potential strategy to prevent further bone loss by reducing inflammation and promoting bone growth (He et al., 2024; Stevens et al., 2023).

Vitamin E, known for its antioxidant properties, also plays a vital role in immune modulation. It helps to protect cell membranes from oxidative damage and enhances the proliferation of immune cells (Lewis et al., 2018). The interaction between vitamin D and vitamin E has been explored in various contexts, with evidence suggesting that these vitamins may work synergistically to combat oxidative stress and excessive inflammation. For instance, combined vitamin E and D supplementation promoted lipid peroxidation by modulating superoxide dismutase, demonstrating the potential of these vitamins as an antioxidant therapy (Ismiyati et al., 2016). Moreover, the combination of vitamins E and D has been reported to decrease pro-inflammatory IL-6 cytokine levels in adipose tissue, highlighting their benefit in downregulating inflammation seen in obesity (Lira et al., 2011).

The implications of these synergistic interactions extend to various health conditions, including respiratory infections and chronic diseases. Nutrient deficiencies, particularly in vitamins A, C, D, and E, have been associated with impaired immune function and increased susceptibility to infections (Gombart et al., 2020). The prevalence of inadequate intakes of these vitamins in the general population underscores the need for public health measures to promote adequate nutrition and supplementation where necessary (Reider et al., 2020). For instance, during the COVID-19 pandemic, the potential role of vitamins A, C, D, and E in supporting immune health has been emphasized, with recommendations for maintaining optimal levels to enhance resilience against infections (Carr & Gombart, 2022; Gasmi et al., 2020).

Despite the promising evidence regarding the synergistic effects of these vitamins on immune modulation, further research is needed to elucidate the specific mechanisms underlying these interactions and their clinical implications. RCTs are essential to determine the optimal dosages and combinations of these vitamins for enhancing immune function and preventing infections. Additionally, understanding the role of dietary sources of these vitamins and their bioavailability in different populations will be crucial for developing effective nutritional strategies.

6.7 Current research, methodologies, and future directions

6.7.1 Advances in research: recent discoveries in molecular and clinical studies

Recent discoveries have significantly advanced our understanding of vitamin D's role in immune health. Vitamin D's influence extends far beyond its well-established role in calcium and bone metabolism, with a wide array of nonclassical actions that are increasingly recognized for their impact on human health. Molecular studies have elucidated pathways through which vitamin D modulates immune cell function, including its regulation of cytokine production and its role in antimicrobial peptide synthesis. Recent research has continued to explore the multifaceted role of vitamin D and immune health, with a focus on potential therapeutic applications as well as underlying mechanisms. A recent systematic review suggested that maintaining serum 25(OH)D concentrations of more than 50 ng/mL reduces the risk of microbial infections and autoimmunity (Wimalawansa, 2023). The role of salivary vitamin D and its associated antimicrobial peptide LL-37 was studied in association with the severity of dental caries, where increasing salivary vitamin D and LL-37 levels were negatively associated with the severity of dental caries (Nireeksha et al., 2024). This further expands the role of vitamin D antimicrobial peptides in immune function. Vitamin D has demonstrated the ability to modulate the composition and function of the intestinal microbiota, which may contribute to protective effects against pneumonia. In animal studies, vitamin D supplementation has been shown to support the immune response against respiratory infections like pneumonia (Hu et al., 2024). However, these findings are based on preclinical models, and the underlying mechanisms and clinical relevance remain to be fully elucidated. Rigorous human studies are essential to validate these findings, determine optimal dosing, and explore potential therapeutic applications for vitamin D in respiratory health.

Clinically, RCTs have tried to demonstrate vitamin D's potential to mitigate the severity of respiratory infections and autoimmune diseases. In MS, while vitamin D deficiency increases the risk and progression of the disease, multiple studies have shown that vitamin D supplementation appears to have no therapeutic benefit (Cassard et al., 2023; Feige et al., 2020; Mahler et al., 2024). These findings underscore the complexity of vitamin D's role in health and disease, highlighting the need for a nuanced approach to supplementation. Risks and benefits of vitamin D supplementation should be carefully evaluated for each condition, as its efficacy may vary significantly depending on the disease, patient demographics, baseline vitamin D levels, and the dosage administered. Future research should focus on identifying specific populations that might benefit most from supplementation, determining optimal dosing strategies, and exploring potential adverse effects, particularly in individuals with adequate or high baseline levels of vitamin D. Personalized treatment plans and further large-scale clinical trials are crucial to fully understand the implications of vitamin D supplementation across various diseases and conditions.

The impact of vitamin D on immune-related conditions like COVID-19 has also emerged as a prominent area of research, with studies highlighting its role in improving patient outcomes. Emerging findings also suggest potential applications of vitamin D in enhancing cancer immunotherapy and modulating gut microbiota, providing a broader scope for future exploration.

6.7.2   Methodological challenges: addressing confounders, standardizing measurement of vitamin D levels, and improving study design

The literature on vitamin D is not without limitations. A significant challenge lies in the variability of vitamin D status assessments, as serum 25(OH)D levels remain the standard measure, yet lack global consensus on deficiency thresholds. Variability in measurement techniques across different laboratories can result in inconsistent data. Additionally, serum 25(OH)D may not reflect the bioavailability or functional activity of vitamin D in tissues (Chun et al., 2019). Confounding factors complicate data interpretation. For example, genetic polymorphisms in VDR and CYP enzymes can significantly affect vitamin D metabolism, absorption, and activation, which will complicate the interpretation of results in diverse populations. Genetic profiling to stratify participants in future studies may help us better understand these interactions. Additionally, geographic and seasonal differences in sunlight exposure will also significantly affect vitamin D synthesis. Finally, the heterogeneity in dosing regimens and endpoints across studies hinders the ability to draw definitive conclusions regarding optimal supplementation strategies. Wimalawansa noted in their systematic review that the studies that failed to conclude that vitamin D supplementation had beneficial effects in improving infection outcomes often had major study design issues (Wimalawansa, 2023). Therefore addressing these methodological issues is crucial and requires standardization in study design, robust control of confounding variables, and larger, well-powered clinical trials. Global consensus on these issues and establishing optimal dosing regimens will enhance the comparability of studies and the reliability of their findings. By integrating genetic, geographic, and lifestyle factors into research, the field may be able to move closer to personalized recommendations that maximize the health benefits of vitamin D.

6.7.3   Future perspectives: personalized medicine approaches, integration of genomics and proteomics, and technological innovations in monitoring vitamin D status

Indeed, the future of vitamin D research lies in personalized medicine, integrating genomic, proteomic, and metabolomic data to tailor supplementation and therapeutic approaches. Innovations in wearable technology and digital health tools may facilitate real-time monitoring of vitamin D levels and sun exposure, enabling dynamic adjustments in supplementation. Educational tools, such as the vitamin D toolkit demonstrated by Sanford et al. (2023), which improved knowledge of vitamin D best practices among nurses and dietitians, highlight the importance of disseminating evidence-based guidelines to healthcare professionals. Research should focus on novel delivery mechanisms, such as vitamin D analogs, to maximize efficacy while minimizing risks of hypercalcemia. Interdisciplinary studies exploring the interplay between vitamin D, microbiota, and other nutrients will further elucidate its role in immune health. Such studies can provide a comprehensive understanding of how vitamin D influences the gut–lung axis, a critical pathway linking intestinal microbiota and respiratory immunity. For instance, vitamin D's ability to modulate microbial composition may not only enhance gut barrier integrity but also reduce systemic inflammation, thereby supporting a robust immune response to pathogens. Additionally, investigating synergistic effects between vitamin D and other nutrients, such as omega-3 fatty acids, zinc, or fiber, could uncover combinatory strategies that optimize immune function.

Future studies could also explore how these interactions vary across life stages, genetic profiles, and health conditions, potentially identifying tailored dietary and supplementation approaches. Moreover, advancing methodologies, such as high-throughput sequencing and metabolomic profiling, will enable researchers to map intricate molecular pathways and pinpoint biomarkers indicative of vitamin D's immunomodulatory effects. Additionally, expanding research into underrepresented populations and geographic regions is crucial for addressing global health disparities associated with vitamin D deficiency. Expanding these investigations to include the impact of environmental factors, such as diet, antibiotics, and geographic location, will help unravel the complex dynamics between vitamin D, the microbiome, and overall immune health.

6.8   Conclusion

6.8.1   Summary of key findings

Vitamin D plays a critical role in immune health by modulating both innate and adaptive immune responses. The active form, $1,25(OH)_2D$, is essential for maintaining mineral homeostasis and regulating immune function. Adequate vitamin D levels are necessary to reduce the risk of immune-related diseases and infections. A deficiency in vitamin D is a widespread global health issue, with correlations observed between low vitamin D levels and an increased prevalence of infectious diseases and autoimmune conditions. This highlights the necessity of maintaining sufficient vitamin D status to ensure optimal immune health and overall well-being.

6.8.2   Clinical implications and public health relevance

Addressing vitamin D deficiency requires a multifaceted approach involving public health initiatives and clinical recommendations. Strategies such as increasing awareness about the benefits of vitamin D, promoting safe sun exposure, and encouraging the consumption of vitamin D-rich foods are crucial in mitigating deficiency risks. Supplementation guidelines should be tailored to individual needs, accounting for genetic variations (such as VDR gene polymorphisms) and lifestyle factors that influence vitamin D metabolism. Special attention should be directed toward populations at higher risk for deficiency, including those with limited sun exposure, darker skin tones, or underlying health conditions that affect nutrient absorption.

6.8.3   Final thoughts

Vitamin D's potential to shape the future of immune-related therapies and public health policy is significant. Its role in enhancing antimicrobial defenses, reducing inflammation, and modulating immune cell activity positions vitamin D as a valuable asset in preventing and managing infections and autoimmune diseases. As research continues to uncover the complexities of vitamin D's interactions with the immune system, personalized supplementation and population-level interventions will be vital. Optimizing vitamin D levels across diverse populations could play a transformative role in improving immune health and reducing the burden of chronic and emerging diseases globally.

AI disclosure

During the preparation of this work, the author(s) used ChatGPT to improve readability and clarity of written work. After using this tool/service, the author(s) reviewed and edited the content as needed and take(s) full responsibility for the content of the publication.

References

Aglipay, M., Birken, C. S., Parkin, P. C., Loeb, M. B., Thorpe, K., Chen, Y., Laupacis, A., Mamdani, M., Macarthur, C., Hoch, J. S., Mazzulli, T., & Maguire, J. L. (2017). Effect of high-dose vs standard-dose wintertime vitamin D supplementation on viral upper respiratory tract infections in young healthy children. *JAMA, 318*(3), 245–254. https://doi.org/10.1001/JAMA.2017.8708, https://jamanetwork.com/journals/jama/fullarticle/2643763.

Ahn, J., Yu, K., Stolzenberg-Solomon, R., Simon, K. C., McCullough, M. L., Gallicchio, L., Jacobs, E. J., Ascherio, A., Helzlsouer, K., Jacobs, K. B., Li, Q., Weinstein, S. J., Purdue, M., Virtamo, J., Horst, R., Wheeler, W., Chanock, S., Hunter, D. J., Hayes, R. B., ... Albanes, D. (2010). Genome-wide association study of circulating vitamin D levels. *Human Molecular Genetics, 19*(13), 2739–2745. https://doi.org/10.1093/HMG/DDQ155, https://doi.org/10.1093/hmg/ddq155.

Ahola, A. J., Harjutsalo, V., & Groop, P. H. (2024). The use of dietary supplements, and the association between supplemental vitamin D and glycaemic control in adult individuals with type 1 diabetes. *Diabetic Medicine, 41*(5), e15308. https://onlinelibrary.wiley.com/doi/full/10.1111/dme.15308.

Akimbekov, N. S., Digel, I., Sherelkhan, D. K., Lutfor, A. B., & Razzaque, M. S. (2020). Vitamin D and the host-gut microbiome: A brief overview. *Acta Histochemica et Cytochemica, 53*(3), 33. https://doi.org/10.1267/AHC.20011, https://pmc.ncbi.nlm.nih.gov/articles/PMC7322162/.

AlFaris, N. A., AlKehayez, N. M., AlMushawah, F. I., Abdul, AlNaeem, R. N., AlAmri, N. D., & AlMudawah, E. S. (2019). Vitamin D deficiency and associated risk factors in women from Riyadh, Saudi Arabia. *Scientific Reports, 9*(1), 1–8. https://doi.org/10.1038/s41598-019-56830-z, https://www.nature.com/articles/s41598-019-56830-z.

Al-Jaberi, F. A. H., Geisler Crone, C., Lindenstrøm, T., Arildsen, N. S., Lindeløv, E. S., Aagaard, L., Gravesen, E., Mortensen, R., Andersen, A. B., Olgaard, K., Hjaltelin, J. X., Brunak, S., Bonefeld, C. M., Kongsbak-Wismann, M., & Geisler, C. (2022). Reduced vitamin D-induced cathelicidin production and killing of Mycobacterium tuberculosis in macrophages from a patient with a non-functional vitamin D receptor: A case report. *Frontiers in Immunology.* https://doi.org/10.3389/fimmu.2022.1038960.

Aljabri, K. S., Bokhari, S. A., & Khan, M. J. (2010). Glycemic changes after vitamin D supplementation in patients with type 1 diabetes mellitus and vitamin D deficiency. *Annals of Saudi Medicine, 30*(6), 454. https://doi.org/10.4103/0256-4947.72265, https://www.annsaudimed.net/doi/10.4103/0256-4947.72265.

Al-Taiar, A., Rahman, A., Al-Sabah, R., Shaban, L., & Al-Harbi, A. (2018). Vitamin D status among adolescents in Kuwait: A cross-sectional study. *BMJ Open, 8*(7), e021401. https://doi.org/10.1136/bmjopen-2017-021401.

Anderson, P. H., May, B. K., & Morris, H. A. (2003). Vitamin D metabolism: New concepts and clinical implications. *The Clinical biochemist. Reviews.*

Annweiler, C., Beaudenon, M., Gautier, J., Gonsard, J., Boucher, S., Chapelet, G., Darsonval, A., Fougère, B., Guérin, O., Houvet, M., Ménager, P., Roubaud-Baudron, C., Tchalla, A., Souberbielle, J. C., Riou, J., Parot-Schinkel, E., & Célarier, T. (2022). High-dose versus standard-dose vitamin D supplementation in older adults with COVID-19 (COVIT-TRIAL): A multicenter, open-label, randomized controlled superiority trial. *PLoS Medicine, 19*(5), e1003999. https://doi.org/10.1371/JOURNAL.PMED.1003999, https://pmc.ncbi.nlm.nih.gov/articles/PMC9154122/.

Ao, T., Kikuta, J., & Ishii, M. (2021). *The effects of vitamin D on immune system and inflammatory diseases.*

Aris, R. M., Merkel, P. A., Bachrach, L. K., Borowitz, D. S., Boyle, M. P., Elkin, S. L., Guise, T. A., Hardin, D. S., Haworth, C. S., Holick, M. F., Joseph, P. M., O'Brien, K., Tullis, E., Watts, N. B., & White, T. B. (2005). Guide to bone health and disease in cystic fibrosis. *The Journal of Clinical Endocrinology and Metabolism, 90*(3), 1888–1896. https://doi.org/10.1210/JC.2004-1629, https://pubmed.ncbi.nlm.nih.gov/15613415/.

Arkema, E. V., Hart, J. E., Bertrand, K. A., Laden, F., Grodstein, F., Rosner, B. A., Karlson, E. W., & Costenbader, K. H. (2013). Exposure to ultraviolet-B and risk of developing rheumatoid arthritis among women in the Nurses' Health Study. *Annals of the rheumatic diseases, 72*(4), 506–511. https://doi.org/10.1136/ANNRHEUMDIS-2012-202302, https://pubmed.ncbi.nlm.nih.gov/23380431/.

Baeke, F., Takiishi, T., Korf, H., Gysemans, C., & Mathieu, C. (2010). *Vitamin D: Modulator of the immune system.*

Balasooriya, N. N., Elliott, T. M., Neale, R. E., Vasquez, P., Comans, T., & Gordon, L. G. (2024). The association between vitamin D deficiency and multiple sclerosis: An updated systematic review and meta-analysis. *Multiple Sclerosis and Related Disorders, 90*, 105804. https://doi.org/10.1016/J.MSARD.2024.105804.

Baron, J. A., Barry, E. L., Mott, L. A., Rees, J. R., Sandler, R. S., Snover, D. C., Bostick, R. M., Ivanova, A., Cole, B. F., Ahnen, D. J., Beck, G. J., Bresalier, R. S., Burke, C. A., Church, T. R., Cruz-Correa, M., Figueiredo, J. C., Goodman, M., Kim, A. S., Robertson, D. J., ... Summers, R. W. (2015). A trial of calcium and vitamin D for the prevention of colorectal adenomas. *The New England journal of medicine, 373*(16), 1519–1530. https://doi.org/10.1056/NEJMOA1500409, https://pubmed.ncbi.nlm.nih.gov/26465985/.

Bell, D. A., Crooke, M. J., Hay, N., & Glendenning, P. (2013). Prolonged vitamin D intoxication: Presentation, pathogenesis and progress. *Internal Medicine Journal, 43*(10), 1148–1150. https://doi.org/10.1111/IMJ.12269, https://pubmed.ncbi.nlm.nih.gov/24134173/.

Bivona, G., Agnello, L., Sasso, B. L., Scazzone, C., Butera, D., Gambino, C. M., Iacolino, G., Bellia, C., & Ciaccio, M. (2019). Vitamin D in malaria: More hypotheses than clues. *Heliyon, 5*(2), e01183. http://www.cell.com/article/S240584401838441X/fulltext.

Boughanem, H., Ruiz-Limón, P., Pilo, J., Lisbona-Montañez, J. M., Tinahones, F. J., Moreno Indias, I., & Macías-González, M. (2023). Linking serum vitamin D levels with gut microbiota after 1-year lifestyle intervention with Mediterranean diet in patients with obesity and metabolic syndrome: A nested cross-sectional and prospective study. *Gut Microbes, 15*(2). https://doi.org/10.1080/19490976.2023.2249150, https://www.tandfonline.com/doi/abs/10.1080/19490976.2023.2249150.

Brehm, J. M., Schuemann, B., Fuhlbrigge, A. L., Hollis, B. W., Strunk, R. C., Zeiger, R. S., Weiss, S. T., & Litonjua, A. A. (2010). Serum vitamin D levels and severe asthma exacerbations in the Childhood Asthma Management Program study. *Journal of Allergy and Clinical Immunology, 126*(1), 52. https://doi.org/10.1016/J.JACI.2010.03.043.

Buondonno, I., Rovera, G., Sassi, F., Rigoni, M. M., Lomater, C., Parisi, S., Pellerito, R., Isaia, G. C., & D'Amelio, P. (2017). Vitamin D and immunomodulation in early rheumatoid arthritis: A randomized double-blind placebo-controlled study. *PLOS ONE, 12*(6), e0178463. https://doi.org/10.1371/JOURNAL.PONE.0178463, https://journals.plos.org/plosone/article?id=10.1371/journal.pone.0178463.

Carr, A. C., & Gombart, A. F. (2022). Multi-level immune support by vitamins C and D during the SARS-CoV-2 pandemic. *Nutrients, 14*(3), 689. https://doi.org/10.3390/NU14030689, https://www.mdpi.com/2072-6643/14/3/689/htm.

Carrelli, A., Bucovsky, M., Horst, R., Cremers, S., Zhang, C., Bessler, M., Schrope, B., Evanko, J., Blanco, J., Silverberg, S. J., & Stein, E. M. (2016). Vitamin D storage in adipose tissue of obese and normal weight women. *Journal of Bone and Mineral Research: The Official Journal of the American Society for Bone and Mineral Research, 32*(2), 237. https://doi.org/10.1002/JBMR.2979, https://pmc.ncbi.nlm.nih.gov/articles/PMC5577589/.

Cashman, K. D. (2018). Vitamin D requirements for the future—Lessons learned and charting a path forward. *Nutrients, 10*(5), 533. https://doi.org/10.3390/NU10050533, https://www.mdpi.com/2072-6643/10/5/533/htm.

Cassard, S. D., Fitzgerald, K. C., Qian, P., Emrich, S. A., Azevedo, C. J., Goodman, A. D., Sugar, E. A., Pelletier, D., Waubant, E., & Mowry, E. M. (2023). High-dose vitamin D3 supplementation in relapsing-remitting multiple sclerosis: A randomised clinical trial. *eClinicalMedicine, 59.* 101957. http://www.thelancet.com/article/S2589537023001347/fulltext https://doi.org/10.1016/j.eclinm.2023.101957.

Cervero, M., López-Wolf, D., Casado, G., Novella-Mena, M., Ryan-Murua, P., Taboada-Martínez, M. L., Rodríguez-Mora, S., Vigón, L., Coiras, M., & Torres, M. (2022). Beneficial effect of short-term supplementation of high dose of vitamin D3 in hospitalized patients with COVID-19: A multicenter, single-blinded, prospective randomized pilot clinical trial. *Frontiers in Pharmacology, 13.* https://doi.org/10.3389/FPHAR.2022.863587, https://pubmed.ncbi.nlm.nih.gov/35860019/.

Chang, J. H., Cha, H. R., Lee, D. S., Seo, K. Y., Mi, & Kweon, N. (2010). 1,25-Dihydroxyvitamin D3 inhibits the differentiation and migration of T(H)17 cells to protect against experimental autoimmune encephalomyelitis. *PloS One, 5*(9). https://doi.org/10.1371/JOURNAL.PONE.0012925, https://pubmed.ncbi.nlm.nih.gov/20886077/.

Chang, S. H., Chung, Y., & Dong, C. (2010). Vitamin D suppresses Th17 cytokine production by inducing C/EBP Homologous Protein (CHOP) expression. *Journal of Biological Chemistry, 285*(50), 38751–38755. https://doi.org/10.1074/jbc.C110.185777.

Chen, Y., Liu, W., Sun, T., Huang, Y., Wang, Y., Deb, D. K., Yoon, D., Kong, J., Thadhani, R., & Li, Y. C. (2013). 1,25-Dihydroxyvitamin D promotes negative feedback regulation of TLR signaling via targeting MicroRNA-155–SOCS1 in macrophages. *Journal of Immunology.* https://doi.org/10.4049/jimmunol.1203273.

Chen, J., Tang, Z., Slominski, A. T., Li, W., Zmijewski, M. A., Liu, Y., & Chen, J. (2020). Vitamin D and its analogs as anticancer and anti-inflammatory agents. *European Journal of Medicinal Chemistry, 207,* 112738. https://doi.org/10.1016/J.EJMECH.2020.112738.

Chen, J., Yun, C., He, Y., Piao, J., Yang, L., & Yang, X. (2017). Vitamin D status among the elderly Chinese population: A cross-sectional analysis of the 2010-2013 China national nutrition and health survey (CNNHS). *Nutrition Journal, 16*(1), 1–8. https://doi.org/10.1186/S12937-016-0224-3/TABLES/2, https://nutritionj.biomedcentral.com/articles/10.1186/s12937-016-0224-3.

Chun, R. F., Shieh, A., Gottlieb, C., Yacoubian, V., Wang, J., Hewison, M., & Adams, J. S. (2019). Vitamin D binding protein and the biological activity of vitamin D. *Frontiers in Endocrinology, 10,* 718. https://doi.org/10.3389/fendo.2019.00718, https://www.frontiersin.org/journals/endocrinology/articles/10.3389/fendo.2019.00718/full.

Clark, A., & Mach, N. (2016). Role of vitamin D in the hygiene hypothesis: The interplay between vitamin D, vitamin D receptors, gut microbiota, and immune response. *Frontiers in Immunology, 7*(DEC), 215942. https://doi.org/10.3389/FIMMU.2016.00627/BIBTEX, http://www.frontiersin.org.

Cooper, J. D., Smyth, D. J., Walker, N. M., Stevens, H., Burren, O. S., Wallace, C., Greissl, C., Ramos-Lopez, E., Hyppönen, E., Dunger, D. B., Spector, T. D., Ouwehand, W. H., Wang, T. J., Badenhoop, K., & Todd, J. A. (2011). Inherited variation in vitamin D genes is associated with predisposition to autoimmune disease type 1 diabetes. *Diabetes, 60*(5), 1624. https://doi.org/10.2337/DB10-1656, https://pmc.ncbi.nlm.nih.gov/articles/PMC3292339/.

Coussens, A., Timms, P. M., Boucher, B. J., Venton, T. R., Ashcroft, A. T., Skolimowska, K. H., Newton, S. M., Wilkinson, K. A., Davidson, R. N., Griffiths, C. J., Wilkinson, R. J., & Martineau, A. R. (2009). 1α,25-dihydroxyvitamin D3 inhibits matrix metalloproteinases induced by Mycobacterium tuberculosis infection. *Immunology, 127*(4), 539–548. https://doi.org/10.1111/J.1365-2567.2008.03024.X https://onlinelibrary.wiley.com/doi/full/10.1111/j.1365-2567.2008.03024.x.

Crowe, F. L., Steur, M., Allen, N. E., Appleby, P. N., Travis, R. C., & Key, T. J. (2011). Plasma concentrations of 25-hydroxyvitamin D in meat eaters, fish eaters, vegetarians and vegans: Results from the EPIC-Oxford study. *Public Health Nutrition, 14*(2), 340–346. https://doi.org/10.1017/S1368980010002454 https://pubmed.ncbi.nlm.nih.gov/20854716/.

Cusick, S. E., Opoka, R. O., Lund, T. C., John, C. C., & Polgreen, L. E. (2014). Vitamin D insufficiency is common in Ugandan children and is associated with severe malaria. *PLoS ONE, 9*(12), e113185. https://doi.org/10.1371/JOURNAL.PONE.0113185 https://pmc.ncbi.nlm.nih.gov/articles/PMC4254466/.

Cutolo, M., Otsa, K., Laas, K., Yprus, M., Lehtme, R., Secchi, M. E., Sulli, A., Paolino, S., & Seriolo, B. (2006). Circannual vitamin d serum levels and disease activity in rheumatoid arthritis: Northern versus Southern Europe. *Clinical and Experimental Rheumatology.*

Dankers, W., Colin, E. M., van Hamburg, J. P., & Lubberts, E. (2017). Vitamin D in autoimmunity: Molecular mechanisms and therapeutic potential.

Dehkordi, V. H., Dehkordi, E. H., Mohammad, S., Fatemi, R., & Zolfaghari, M. (2018). Effect of vitamin D supplement therapy on HbA1C and IGF-1 levels in children with type 1 diabetes mellitus and vitamin D deficiency. *Electronic Journal of General Medicine, 15*(4), 69. https://doi.org/10.29333/ejgm/93167, http://creativecommons.org/licenses/by/4.0/.

Deng, J., Yang, Y., He, J., Xie, Z., Luo, F., Xu, J., & Zhang, Z. (2021). Vitamin D receptor activated by vitamin D administration alleviates Mycobacterium tuberculosis-induced bone destruction by inhibiting NFκB-mediated aberrant osteoclastogenesis. *The FASEB Journal, 35*(6), e21543. https://doi.org/10.1096/FJ.202100135R, https://onlinelibrary.wiley.com/doi/full/10.1096/fj.202100135R.

Desai, N. S., Tukvadze, N., Frediani, J. K., Kipiani, M., Sanikidze, E., Nichols, M. M., Hebbar, G., Kempker, R. R., Mirtskhulava, V., Kalandadze, I., Seydafkan, S., Sutaria, N., Chen, T. C., Blumberg, H. M., Ziegler, T. R., & Tangpricha, V. (2012). Effects of sunlight and diet on vitamin D status of pulmonary tuberculosis patients in Tbilisi, Georgia. *Nutrition (Burbank, Los Angeles County, Calif.). 28*(4), 362. https://doi.org/10.1016/J.NUT.2011.08.012, https://pmc.ncbi.nlm.nih.gov/articles/PMC3303957/.

Deuster, E., Jeschke, U., Ye, Y., Mahner, S., & Czogalla, B. (2017). Vitamin D and VDR in gynecological cancers—A systematic review. *International Journal of Molecular Sciences, 18*(11), 2328. https://doi.org/10.3390/IJMS18112328, https://www.mdpi.com/1422-0067/18/11/2328/htm.

Dimitrov, V., Bouttier, M., Boukhaled, G., Salehi-Tabar, R., Avramescu, R. G., Memari, B., Hasaj, B., Lukacs, G. L., Krawczyk, C. M., & White, J. H. (2017). Hormonal vitamin D up-regulates tissue-specific PD-L1 and PD-L2 surface glycoprotein expression in humans but not mice. *The Journal of Biological Chemistry, 292*(50), 20657. https://doi.org/10.1074/JBC.M117.793885, https://pmc.ncbi.nlm.nih.gov/articles/PMC5733602/.

Dong, J. Y., Wei, Zhang, G., Chen, J. J., Zhang, Z. L., Han, S. F., & Qin, L. Q. (2013). Vitamin D intake and risk of type 1 diabetes: A meta-analysis of observational studies. *Nutrients, 5*(9), 3551. https://doi.org/10.3390/NU5093551, https://pmc.ncbi.nlm.nih.gov/articles/PMC3798920/.

Dragomir, R. E., Toader, D. O., Gheoca Mutu, D. E., Dogaru, I. A., Răducu, L., Tomescu, L.țiu C., Moleriu, L. C., Bordianu, A., Petre, I., & Stănculescu, R. (2024). Consequences of maternal vitamin D deficiency on newborn health. *Life, 14*(6), 714. https://doi.org/10.3390/LIFE14060714, https://www.mdpi.com/2075-1729/14/6/714/htm.

Driver, J. P., Foreman, O., Mathieu, C., Van Etten, E., & Serreze, D. V. (2007). Comparative therapeutic effects of orally administered 1,25-dihydroxyvitamin D3 and 1alpha-hydroxyvitamin D3 on type-1 diabetes in non-obese diabetic mice fed a normal-calcaemic diet. *Clinical and Experimental Immunology, 151*(1), 76–85. https://doi.org/10.1111/J.1365-2249.2007.03537.X, https://doi.org/10.1111/j.1365-2249.2007.03537.x.

Dwivedi, H., Singh, S. K., Singh Chauhan, B., Gunjan, S., & Tripathi, R. (2016). Potential cerebral malaria therapy: Intramuscular arteether and vitamin D co-administration. *Parasitology, 143*(12), 1557–1568. https://doi.org/10.1017/S0031182016001207 https://pubmed.ncbi.nlm.nih.gov/27440106/.

Earthman, C. P., Beckman, L. M., Masodkar, K., & Sibley, S. D. (2011). The link between obesity and low circulating 25-hydroxyvitamin D concentrations: Considerations and implications. *International Journal of Obesity, 36*(3), 387–396. https://doi.org/10.1038/ijo.2011.119, https://www.nature.com/articles/ijo2011119.

El-Sharkawy, A., & Malki, A. (2020). Vitamin D signaling in inflammation and cancer: Molecular mechanisms and therapeutic implications. *Molecules, 25*(14), 3219. https://doi.org/10.3390/MOLECULES25143219, https://pmc.ncbi.nlm.nih.gov/articles/PMC7397283/.

Engelsen, O. (2010). *The relationship between ultraviolet radiation exposure and vitamin D status.*

Fabri, M., Stenger, S., Shin, D. M., Yuk, J. M., Liu, P. T., Realegeno, S., Lee, H. M., Krutzik, S. R., Schenk, M., Sieling, P. A., Teles, R., Montoya, D., Iyer, S. S., Bruns, H., Lewinsohn, D. M., Hollis, B. W., Hewison, M., Adams, J. S., Steinmeyer, A., ... Modlin, R. L. (2011). Vitamin D is required for IFN-γ-mediated antimicrobial activity of human macrophages. *Science Translational Medicine, 3*(104). https://doi.org/10.1126/SCITRANSLMED.3003045/SUPPL_FILE/3-104RA102_SM.PDF, https://www.science.org/doi/10.1126/scitranslmed.3003045.

Feige, J., Moser, T., Bieler, L., Schwenker, K., Hauer, L., & Sellner, J. (2020). Vitamin D supplementation in multiple sclerosis: A critical analysis of potentials and threats. *Nutrients, 12*(3), 783. https://doi.org/10.3390/nu12030783, https://www.mdpi.com/2072-6643/12/3/783.

Ferrari, M., Schenk, K., Papadopoulou, C., Ferrari, P., Dalle Carbonare, L., & Bertoldo, F. (2011). Serum 25-hydroxy vitamin D and exercise capacity in COPD. *Thorax, 66*(6), 544–545. https://doi.org/10.1136/THX.2010.152785, https://thorax.bmj.com/content/66/6/544.2.

Forrest, K. Y. Z., & Stuhldreher, W. L. (2011). Prevalence and correlates of vitamin D deficiency in US adults. *Nutrition Research (New York, N.Y.). 31*(1), 48–54. https://doi.org/10.1016/J.NUTRES.2010.12.001, https://pubmed.ncbi.nlm.nih.gov/21310306/.

Gabbay, M. A. L., Sato, M. N., Finazzo, C., Duarte, A. J. S., & Dib, S. A. (2012). Effect of cholecalciferol as adjunctive therapy with insulin on protective immunologic profile and decline of residual β-cell function in new-onset type 1 diabetes mellitus. *Archives of Pediatrics & Adolescent Medicine, 166*(7), 601–607. https://doi.org/10.1001/ARCHPEDIATRICS.2012.164, https://pubmed.ncbi.nlm.nih.gov/22751874/.

Gallagher, J. C. (2013). Vitamin D and aging. *Endocrinology and Metabolism Clinics of North America, 42*(2), 319. https://doi.org/10.1016/J.ECL.2013.02.004, https://pmc.ncbi.nlm.nih.gov/articles/PMC3782116/.

Gasmi, A., Tippairote, T., Mujawdiya, P. K., Peana, M., Menzel, A., Dadar, M., Gasmi Benahmed, A., & Bjørklund, G. (2020). Micronutrients as immunomodulatory tools for COVID-19 management. *Clinical Immunology (Orlando, Fla.). 220*, 108545. https://doi.org/10.1016/J.CLIM.2020.108545, https://pmc.ncbi.nlm.nih.gov/articles/PMC7833875.

Ginde, A. A., Mansbach, J. M., & Camargo, C. A. (2009). Association between serum 25-hydroxyvitamin D level and upper respiratory tract infection in the third national health and nutrition examination survey. *Archives of Internal Medicine, 169*(4), 384–390. https://doi.org/10.1001/ARCHINTERNMED.2008.560, https://jamanetwork.com/journals/jamainternalmedicine/fullarticle/414815.

Gombart, A. F., Pierre, A., & Maggini, S. (2020). A review of micronutrients and the immune system–working in harmony to reduce the risk of infection. *Nutrients, 12*(1), 236. https://doi.org/10.3390/NU12010236, https://www.mdpi.com/2072-6643/12/1/236/htm.

Gregori, S., Giarratana, N., Smiroldo, S., Uskokovic, M., & Adorini, L. (2002). A 1alpha,25-dihydroxyvitamin D (3) analog enhances regulatory T-cells and arrests autoimmune diabetes in NOD mice. *Diabetes, 51*(5), 1367–1374. https://doi.org/10.2337/DIABETES.51.5.1367, https://pubmed.ncbi.nlm.nih.gov/11978632/.

Grimm, M., Cetindis, M., Biegner, T., Lehman, M., Munz, A., Teriete, P., & Reinert, S. (2015). Serum vitamin D levels of patients with oral squamous cell carcinoma (OSCC) and expression of vitamin D receptor in oral precancerous lesions and OSCC. *Medicina oral, patologia oral y cirugia bucal, 20*(2), e188. https://doi.org/10.4317/MEDORAL.20368, https://pubmed.ncbi.nlm.nih.gov/25662556/.

Haidari, F., Abiri, B., Iravani, M., Ahmadi-Angali, K., & Vafa, M. (2020). Effects of vitamin D and omega-3 fatty acids co-supplementation on inflammatory factors and tumor marker CEA in colorectal cancer patients undergoing chemotherapy: A randomized, double-blind, placebo-controlled clinical trial. *Nutrition and Cancer, 72*(6), 948–958. https://doi.org/10.1080/01635581.2019.1659380, https://pubmed.ncbi.nlm.nih.gov/32441198/.

Hansen, K. E., Bartels, C. M., Gangnon, R. E., Jones, A. N., & Gogineni, J. (2014). An evaluation of high-dose vitamin d for rheumatoid arthritis. *Journal of Clinical Rheumatology, 20*(2), 112–114. https://doi.org/10.1097/RHU.0000000000000072, https://journals.lww.com/jclinrheum/fulltext/2014/03000/an{_}evaluation{_}of{_}high{_}dose{_}vitamin{_}d{_}for.13.aspx.

Haque, U. J., & Bartlett, S. J. (2010). Relationships among vitamin D, disease activity, pain and disability in rheumatoid arthritis. *Clinical and Experimental Rheumatology*.

Harishankar, M., Anbalagan, S., & Selvaraj, P. (2016). Effect of vitamin D3 on chemokine levels and regulatory T-cells in pulmonary tuberculosis. *International Immunopharmacology, 34*, 86–91. https://doi.org/10.1016/J.INTIMP.2016.02.021.

Harrison, S. R., Li, D., Jeffery, L. E., Raza, K., & Hewison, M. (2019). Vitamin D, autoimmune disease and rheumatoid arthritis. *Calcified Tissue International, 106*(1), 58–75. https://doi.org/10.1007/S00223-019-00577-2, https://link.springer.com/article/10.1007/s00223-019-00577-2.

He, L., Chhantyal, K., Chen, Z., Zhu, R., & Zhang, L. (2024). The association of combined vitamin C and D deficiency with bone mineral density and vertebral fracture. *Journal of Orthopaedic Surgery and Research, 19*(1), 460. https://doi.org/10.1186/S13018-024-04953-Z, https://pmc.ncbi.nlm.nih.gov/articles/PMC11297575/.

Hedström, A. K., Olsson, T., Kockum, I., Hillert, J., & Alfredsson, L. (2019). Low sun exposure increases multiple sclerosis risk both directly and indirectly. *Journal of Neurology, 267*(4), 1045. https://doi.org/10.1007/S00415-019-09677-3, https://pmc.ncbi.nlm.nih.gov/articles/PMC7109160/.

Holick, M. F. (2005). Vitamin D for health and in chronic kidney disease. *Seminars in dialysis, 18*(4), 266–275. https://doi.org/10.1111/J.1525-139X.2005.18402.X, https://pubmed.ncbi.nlm.nih.gov/16076348/.

Holick, M. F. (2006). High prevalence of vitamin D inadequacy and implications for health.

Holick, M. F., & Chen, T. C. (2008). Vitamin D deficiency: A worldwide problem with health consequences. *The American Journal of Clinical Nutrition, 87*(4), 1080S. https://doi.org/10.1093/AJCN/87.4.1080S.

Holick, M. F. (2007). Vitamin D deficiency. *The New England journal of medicine, 357*(3), 266–281. https://doi.org/10.1056/NEJMRA070553, https://pubmed.ncbi.nlm.nih.gov/17634462/.

Hollis, B. W., & Wagner, C. L. (2004a). Assessment of dietary vitamin D requirements during pregnancy and lactation. *The American journal of clinical nutrition, 79*(5), 717–726. https://doi.org/10.1093/AJCN/79.5.717, https://pubmed.ncbi.nlm.nih.gov/15113709/.

Hollis, B. W., & Wagner, C. L. (2004b). Vitamin D requirements during lactation: High-dose maternal supplementation as therapy to prevent hypovitaminosis D for both the mother and the nursing infant. *The American journal of clinical nutrition, 80*(6 Suppl). https://doi.org/10.1093/AJCN/80.6.1752S https://pubmed.ncbi.nlm.nih.gov/15585800/.

Hu, J.-J., Lin, Y.-S., Zhang, J.-C., & Wang, Y.-H. (2024). Vitamin D improves Klebsiella-induced severe Pneumonia in rats by regulating intestinal microbiota. *Infection and Drug Resistance, Volume 17*, 475–484. https://doi.org/10.2147/IDR.S442330, https://www.dovepress.com/vitamin-d-improves-klebsiella-induced-severe-pneumonia-in-rats-by-regu-peer-reviewed-fulltext-article-IDR.

Huhtakangas, J. A., Veijola, J., Turunen, S., Karjalainen, A., Valkealahti, M., Nousiainen, T., Yli-Luukko, S., Vuolteenaho, O., & Lehenkari, P. (2017). 1,25(OH)2D3 and calcipotriol, its hypocalcemic analog, exert a long-lasting anti-inflammatory and anti-proliferative effect in synoviocytes cultured from patients with rheumatoid arthritis and osteoarthritis. *The Journal of Steroid Biochemistry and Molecular Biology, 173*, 13–22. https://doi.org/10.1016/J.JSBMB.2017.01.017, https://pubmed.ncbi.nlm.nih.gov/28167299/.

Hung, M., Almpani, K., Thao, B., Sudweeks, K., & Lipsky, M. S. (2023). Vitamin D in the prevention and treatment of oral cancer: A scoping review. *Nutrients, 15*(10), 2346. https://doi.org/10.3390/NU15102346, https://www.mdpi.com/2072-6643/15/10/2346/htm.

Infante, M., Ricordi, C., Sanchez, J., Clare-Salzler, M. J., Padilla, N., Fuenmayor, V., Chavez, C., Alvarez, A., Baidal, D., Alejandro, R., Caprio, M., & Fabbri, A. (2019). Influence of vitamin D on islet autoimmunity and beta-cell function in type 1 diabetes. *Nutrients, 11*(9), 2185. https://doi.org/10.3390/NU11092185, https://pubmed.ncbi.nlm.nih.gov/31514368/.

Ismiyati, A., Wiyasa, I. W. A., & Hidayati, D. Y. N. (2016). Protective effect of vitamins C and E on depot-medroxyprogesterone acetate-induced ovarian oxidative stress in vivo. *Journal of Toxicology, 2016*(1), 3134105. https://doi.org/10.1155/2016/3134105, https://onlinelibrary.wiley.com/doi/full/10.1155/2016/3134105.

Jacobo-Delgado, Y. M., Torres-Juarez, F., Rodríguez-Carlos, A., Santos-Mena, A., Enciso-Moreno, J. E., Rivas-Santiago, C., Diamond, G., & Rivas-Santiago, B. (2021). Retinoic acid induces antimicrobial peptides and cytokines leading to Mycobacterium tuberculosis elimination in airway epithelial cells. *Peptides, 142*, 170580. https://doi.org/10.1016/J.PEPTIDES.2021.170580.

Janssens, W., Bouillon, R., Claes, B., Carremans, C., Lehouck, A., Buysschaert, I., Coolen, J., Mathieu, C., Decramer, M., & Lambrechts, D. (2010). Vitamin D deficiency is highly prevalent in COPD and correlates with variants in the vitamin D-binding gene. *Thorax, 65*(3), 215–220. https://doi.org/10.1136/THX.2009.120659, https://thorax.bmj.com/content/65/3/215.

Janghorbani, M., Etemadifar, M., & Janghorbani, M. (2015). Efficacy of high-dose vitamin D3 supplementation in vitamin D deficient pregnant women with multiple sclerosis: Preliminary findings of a randomized-controlled trial. *Iranian Journal of Neurology, 14*(2), 67. https://pmc.ncbi.nlm.nih.gov/articles/PMC4449396/.

Janoušek, J., Pilařová, V., Macáková, K., Nomura, A., Veiga-Matos, J., da Silva, D. D., Remião, F., Saso, L., Malá-Ládová, K., Malý, J., Nováková, L., & Mladěnka, P. (2022). Vitamin D: Sources, physiological role, biokinetics, deficiency, therapeutic use, toxicity, and overview of analytical methods for detection of vitamin D and its metabolites. *Critical Reviews in Clinical Laboratory Sciences, 59*(8), 517–554. https://doi.org/10.1080/10408363.2022.2070595, https://www.tandfonline.com/doi/abs/10.1080/10408363.2022.2070595.

Jin, T., Guo, Y., Huang, Z., Zhang, Q., Huang, Z., Zhang, Y., & Huang, Z. (2020). Vitamin D inhibits the proliferation of oral squamous cell carcinoma by suppressing lncRNA LUCAT1 through the MAPK pathway. *Journal of Cancer, 11*(20), 5971–5981. https://doi.org/10.7150/JCA.45389, http://www.jcancer.org//creativecommons.org/licenses/by/4.0/.

Jolliffe, D. A., Camargo, C. A., Sluyter, J. D., Aglipay, M., Aloia, J. F., Ganmaa, D., Bergman, P., Bischoff-Ferrari, H. A., Borzutzky, A., Damsgaard, C. T., Dubnov-Raz, G., Esposito, S., Gilham, C., Ginde, A. A., Golan-Tripto, I., Goodall, E. C., Grant, C. C., Griffiths, C. J., Hibbs, A. M., ... Martineau, A. R. (2021). Vitamin D supplementation to prevent acute respiratory infections: a systematic review and meta-analysis of aggregate data from randomised controlled trials. *The Lancet Diabetes and Endocrinology, 9*(5), 276–292. https://doi.org/10.1016/S2213-8587(21)00051-6/ATTACHMENT/3D2D3E6A-7062-449B-BD43-D0755B586F3C/MMC1.PDF, http://www.thelancet.com/article/S2213858721000516/fulltext.

Jones, M. L., Martoni, C. J., & Prakash, S. (2013). Oral supplementation with probiotic L. reuteri NCIMB 30242 increases mean circulating 25-hydroxyvitamin D: A post hoc analysis of a randomized controlled trial. *The Journal of clinical endocrinology and metabolism, 98*(7), 2944–2951. https://doi.org/10.1210/JC.2012-4262, https://pubmed.ncbi.nlm.nih.gov/23609838/.

Joshi, L., Ponnana, M., Penmetsa, S. R., Nallari, P., Valluri, V., & Gaddam, S. (2014). Serum vitamin D levels and VDR polymorphisms (BsmI and FokI) in patients and their household contacts susceptible to tuberculosis. *Scandinavian Journal of Immunology, 79*(2), 113–119. https://doi.org/10.1111/SJI.12127, https://pubmed.ncbi.nlm.nih.gov/24219580/.

Kamen, D. L., & Tangpricha, V. (2010). Vitamin D and molecular actions on the immune system: Modulation of innate and autoimmunity. *Journal of Molecular Medicine, 88*(5), 441–450. https://doi.org/10.1007/S00109-010-0590-9/METRICS, https://link.springer.com/article/10.1007/s00109-010-0590-9.

Kassem, Z., Sitarik, A., Levin, A. M., Lynch, S. V., Havstad, S., Fujimura, K., Kozyrskyj, A., Ownby, D. R., Johnson, C. C., Yong, G. J. M., Wegienka, G., & Cassidy-Bushrow, A. E. (2020). Maternal and cord blood vitamin D level and the infant gut microbiota in a birth cohort study. *Maternal Health, Neonatology and*

Perinatology, 6(1), 1–10. https://doi.org/10.1186/S40748-020-00119-X, https://mhnpjournal.biomedcentral.com/articles/10.1186/s40748-020-00119-x.

Kerr, G. S., Sabahi, I., Richards, J. S., Caplan, L., Cannon, G. W., Reimold, A., Thiele, G. M., Johnson, D., & Mikuls, T. R. (2011). Prevalence of vitamin D insufficiency/deficiency in rheumatoid arthritis and associations with disease severity and activity. *The Journal of Rheumatology, 38*(1), 53–59. https://doi.org/10.3899/JRHEUM.100516, https://pubmed.ncbi.nlm.nih.gov/20952475/.

Kim, H., Baek, S., Hong, S. M., Lee, J., Jung, S. M., Lee, J., Cho, M. L., Kwok, S. K., & Park, S. H. (2020). 1,25-Dihydroxy vitamin D3 and interleukin-6 blockade synergistically regulate rheumatoid arthritis by suppressing interleukin-17 production and osteoclastogenesis. *Journal of Korean Medical Science, 35*(6), e40. https://doi.org/10.3346/JKMS.2020.35.E40, https://pmc.ncbi.nlm.nih.gov/articles/PMC7025907/.

Kim, Y., & Je, Y. (2014). Vitamin D intake, blood 25(OH)D levels, and breast cancer risk or mortality: A meta-analysis. *British Journal of Cancer, 110*(11), 2772–2784. https://doi.org/10.1038/bjc.2014.175, https://www.nature.com/articles/bjc2014175.

Klug-Micu, G. M., Stenger, S., Sommer, A., Liu, P. T., Krutzik, S. R., Modlin, R. L., & Fabri, M. (2013). CD40 ligand and interferon-γ induce an antimicrobial response against Mycobacterium tuberculosis in human monocytes. *Immunology.* https://doi.org/10.1111/imm.12062.

Kuznia, S., Zhu, A., Akutsu, T., Buring, J. E., Camargo, C. A., Cook, N. R., Chen, L. J., Cheng, T. Y. D., Hantunen, S., Lee, I. M., Manson, J. A. E., Neale, R. E., Scragg, R., Shadyab, A. H., Sha, S., Sluyter, J., Tuomainen, T. P., Urashima, M., Virtanen, J. K., ... Schöttker, B. (2023). Efficacy of vitamin D3 supplementation on cancer mortality: Systematic review and individual patient data meta-analysis of randomised controlled trials. *Ageing Research Reviews, 87*, 101923. https://doi.org/10.1016/J.ARR.2023.101923.

Kweder, H., & Eidi, H. (2018). Vitamin D deficiency in elderly: Risk factors and drugs impact on vitamin D status. *Avicenna Journal of Medicine, 8*(4), 139. https://doi.org/10.4103/AJM.AJM_20_18, https://pmc.ncbi.nlm.nih.gov/articles/PMC6178567/.

Lai, J. K. C., Lucas, R. M., Banks, E., Ponsonby, A.-l, Ausimmune Investigator Group, Correspondence, & Lai, K. J. C. (2012). Variability in vitamin D assays impairs clinical assessment of vitamin D status. *Internal Medicine Journal, 42*(1), 43–50. https://doi.org/10.1111/J.1445-5994.2011.02471.X, https://onlinelibrary.wiley.com/doi/full/10.1111/j.1445-5994.2011.02471.x.

Lai, X., Liu, X., Cai, X., & Zou, F. (2022). Vitamin D supplementation induces CatG-mediated CD4[+] T cell inactivation and restores pancreatic β-cell function in mice with type 1 diabetes. *American Journal of Physiology. Endocrinology and metabolism. 322*(1), E74. https://doi.org/10.1152/AJPENDO.00066.2021, https://pubmed.ncbi.nlm.nih.gov/34779254/.

Lappe, J., Watson, P., Travers-Gustafson, D., Recker, R., Garland, C., Gorham, E., Baggerly, K., & McDonnell, S. L. (2017). Effect of vitamin D and calcium supplementation on cancer incidence in older women: A randomized clinical trial. *JAMA, 317*(12), 1234–1243. https://doi.org/10.1001/JAMA.2017.2115, https://pubmed.ncbi.nlm.nih.gov/28350929/.

Larcombe, L., Orr, P., Turner-Brannen, E., Slivinski, C. R., Nickerson, P. W., & Mookherjee, N. (2012). Effect of vitamin D supplementation on Mycobacterium tuberculosis-induced innate immune responses in a Canadian Dené First Nations cohort. *PLoS ONE.* https://doi.org/10.1371/journal.pone.0040692.

Laursen, J. H., Søndergaard, H. B., Sørensen, P. S., Sellebjerg, F., & Oturai, A. B. (2016). Vitamin D supplementation reduces relapse rate in relapsing-remitting multiple sclerosis patients treated with natalizumab. *Multiple Sclerosis and Related Disorders, 10*, 169–173. https://doi.org/10.1016/J.MSARD.2016.10.005, https://pubmed.ncbi.nlm.nih.gov/27919484/.

Lemire, J. M., Ince, A., & Takashima, M. (1992). 1,25-dihydroxyvitamin d3 attenuates of expression of experimental murine lupus of MRL/1 mice. *Autoimmunity.* https://doi.org/10.3109/08916939209150321.

Lewis, E. D., Meydani, S. N., & Wu, D. (2018). Regulatory role of vitamin E in the immune system and inflammation. *IUBMB life, 71*(4), 487. https://doi.org/10.1002/IUB.1976, https://pmc.ncbi.nlm.nih.gov/articles/PMC7011499/.

Leyssens, C., Verlinden, L., & Verstuyf, A. (2014). The future of vitamin D analogs. *Frontiers in Physiology, 5*(APR), 85935. https://doi.org/10.3389/FPHYS.2014.00122/BIBTEX, http://www.frontiersin.org.

Li, P., Zhu, X., Cao, G., Wu, R., Li, K., Yuan, W., Chen, B., Sun, G., Xia, X., Zhang, H., Wang, X., Yin, Z., Lu, L., & Gao, Y. (2022). 1α,25(OH)2D3 reverses exhaustion and enhances antitumor immunity of human cytotoxic T cells. *Journal for ImmunoTherapy of Cancer, 10*(3), e003477. https://doi.org/10.1136/JITC-2021-003477, https://jitc.bmj.com/content/10/3/e003477.

Liggins, M. C., Li, F., Zhang, L.-juan, Dokoshi, T., & Gallo, R. L. (2019). Retinoids enhance the expression of cathelicidin antimicrobial peptide during reactive dermal adipogenesis. *The Journal of Immunology, 203*(6), 1589–1597. https://doi.org/10.4049/JIMMUNOL.1900520, https://doi.org/10.4049/jimmunol.1900520.

Lin, J., Liu, J., Davies, M. L., & Chen, W. (2016). Serum vitamin D level and rheumatoid arthritis disease activity: Review and meta-analysis. *PLOS ONE, 11*(1), e0146351. https://doi.org/10.1371/JOURNAL.PONE.0146351, https://journals.plos.org/plosone/article?id=10.1371/journal.pone.0146351.

Ling, S. F., Broad, E., Murphy, R., Pappachan, J. M., Pardesi-Newton, S., Kong, M. F., & Jude, E. B. (2020). High-dose cholecalciferol booster therapy is associated with a reduced risk of mortality in patients with COVID-19: A cross-sectional multi-centre observational study. *Nutrients, 12*(12), 1–16. https://doi.org/10.3390/NU12123799, https://pubmed.ncbi.nlm.nih.gov/33322317.

Lips, P. (2001). Vitamin D deficiency and secondary hyperparathyroidism in the elderly: Consequences for bone loss and fractures and therapeutic implications. *Endocrine Reviews, 22*(4), 477–501. https://doi.org/10.1210/EDRV.22.4.0437, https://pubmed.ncbi.nlm.nih.gov/11493580/.

Lira, F. S., Rosa, J. C., Cunha, C. A., Ribeiro, E. B., Oller Do Nascimento, C., Oyama, L. M., & Mota, J. F. (2011). Supplementing alpha-tocopherol (vitamin E) and vitamin D3 in high fat diet decrease IL-6 production in murine epididymal adipose tissue and 3T3-L1 adipocytes following LPS stimulation. *Lipids in Health and Disease, 10*, 37. https://doi.org/10.1186/1476-511X-10-37, https://pmc.ncbi.nlm.nih.gov/articles/PMC3050762.

Liu, D., Fang, Y. X., Wu, X., Tan, W., Zhou, W., Zhang, Y., Liu, Y. Q., & Li, G. Q. (2019). 1,25-(OH)2D3/Vitamin D receptor alleviates systemic lupus erythematosus by downregulating Skp2 and upregulating p27. *Cell Communication and Signaling.* https://doi.org/10.1186/s12964-019-0488-2.

Lo, C. W., Paris, P. W., & Clemens, T. L. (1985). Vitamin D absorption in healthy subjects and in patients with intestinal malabsorption syndromes. *The American Journal of Clinical Nutrition, 42*(4), 644–649. https://doi.org/10.1093/AJCN/42.4.644, https://pubmed.ncbi.nlm.nih.gov/4050723/.

Mahler, J. V., Solti, M., Apóstolos-Pereira, S. L., Adoni, T., Silva, G. D., & Callegaro, D. (2024). Vitamin D3 as an add-on treatment for multiple sclerosis: A systematic review and meta-analysis of randomized controlled trials. *Multiple Sclerosis and Related Disorders, 82*, 105433. https://doi.org/10.1016/j.msard.2024.105433, https://www.sciencedirect.com/science/article/pii/S2211034824000129.

Manson, J. A. E., Cook, N. R., Lee, I.-M., Christen, W., Bassuk, S. S., Mora, S., Gibson, H., Gordon, D., Copeland, T., D'Agostino, D., Friedenberg, G., Ridge, C., Bubes, V., Giovannucci, E. L., Willett, W. C., & Buring, J. E. (2019). Vitamin D supplements and prevention of cancer and cardiovascular disease. *New England Journal of Medicine, 380*(1), 33–44. https://doi.org/10.1056/NEJMOA1809944/SUPPL_FILE/NEJMOA1809944_DATA-SHARING.PDF, https://www.nejm.org/doi/full/10.1056/NEJMoa1809944.

Martineau, A. R., Jolliffe, D. A., Hooper, R. L., Greenberg, L., Aloia, J. F., Bergman, P., Dubnov-Raz, G., Esposito, S., Ganmaa, D., Ginde, A. A., Goodall, E. C., Grant, C. C., Griffiths, C. J., Janssens, W., Laaksi, I., Manaseki-Holland, S., Mauger, D., Murdoch, D. R., Neale, R., ... Camargo, C. A. (2017). Vitamin D supplementation to prevent acute respiratory tract infections: Systematic review and meta-analysis of individual participant data. *BMJ (Clinical research ed.). 356.* https://doi.org/10.1136/BMJ.I6583, https://pubmed.ncbi.nlm.nih.gov/28202713/.

Martineau, A. R., Wilkinson, R. J., Wilkinson, K. A., Newton, S. M., Kampmann, B., Hall, B. M., Packe, G. E., Davidson, R. N., Eldridge, S. M., Maunsell, Z. J., Rainbow, S. J., Berry, J. L., & Griffiths, C. J. (2012). A single dose of vitamin D enhances immunity to mycobacteria. https://doi.org/10.1164/rccm.200701-007OC. 176 (2) (2012), 208–213. https://doi.org/10.1164/RCCM.200701-007OC, http://www.deqas.

Martineau, A. R., Wilkinson, K. A., Newton, S. M., Floto, R. A., Norman, A. W., Skolimowska, K., Davidson, R. N., Sørensen, O. E., Kampmann, B., Griffiths, C. J., & Wilkinson, R. J. (2007). IFN-γ- and TNF-independent vitamin D-inducible human suppression of mycobacteria: The role of cathelicidin LL-37. *The Journal of Immunology.* https://doi.org/10.4049/jimmunol.178.11.7190.

Marusca, L. M., Reddy, G., Blaj, M., Prathipati, R., Rosca, O., Bratosin, F., Bogdan, I., Horhat, R. M., Tapos, G. F., Marti, D. T., Susan, M., Pingilati, R. A., Horhat, F. G., & Adelina, M. (2023). The effects of vitamin D supplementation on respiratory infections in children under 6 years old: A systematic review. *Diseases, 11*(3), 104. https://doi.org/10.3390/DISEASES11030104, https://www.mdpi.com/2079-9721/11/3/104/htm.

Mattner, F., Smiroldo, S., Galbiati, F., Muller, M., Di Lucia, P., Poliani, P. L., Martino, G., Panina-Bordignon, P., & Adorini, L. (2000). Inhibition of Th1 development and treatment of chronic-relapsing experimental allergic encephalomyelitis by a non-hypercalcemic analogue of 1,25-dihydroxyvitamin D3. *European Journal of Immunology.* https://doi.org/10.1002/1521-4141(200002)30:2<498::AID-IMMU498>3.0.CO;2-Q.

Mendes, M. M., Darling, A. L., Hart, K. H., Morse, S., Murphy, R. J., & Lanham-New, S. A. (2019). Impact of high latitude, urban living and ethnicity on 25-hydroxyvitamin D status: A need for multidisciplinary action? *The Journal of Steroid Biochemistry and Molecular Biology, 188*, 95–102. https://doi.org/10.1016/J.JSBMB.2018.12.012.

Mily, A., Rekha, R. S., Kamal, S. M. M., Arifuzzaman, A. S. M., Rahim, Z., Khan, L., Haq, M. A., Zaman, K., Bergman, P., Brighenti, S., Gudmundsson, G. H., Agerberth, B., & Raqib, R. (2015). Significant effects of oral phenylbutyrate and vitamin D3 adjunctive therapy in pulmonary tuberculosis: A randomized controlled trial. *PLOS ONE, 10*(9), e0138340. https://doi.org/10.1371/JOURNAL.PONE.0138340, https://journals.plos.org/plosone/article?id=10.1371/journal.pone.0138340.

Missailidis, C., Sørensen, N., Ashenafi, S., Amogne, W., Kassa, E., Bekele, A., Getachew, M., Gebreselassie, N., Aseffa, A., Aderaye, G., Andersson, J., Brighenti, S., & Bergman, P. (2019). Vitamin D and phenylbutyrate supplementation does not modulate gut derived immune activation in HIV-1. *Nutrients, 11*(7). https://doi.org/10.3390/NU11071675, https://pubmed.ncbi.nlm.nih.gov/31330899/.

Mohammadian, S., Fatahi, N., Zaeri, H., & Vakili, M. A. (2015). Effect of vitamin d3 supplement in glycemic control of pediatrics with type 1 diabetes mellitus and vitamin d deficiency. *Journal of Clinical and Diagnostic Research: JCDR, 9*(3), SC05. https://doi.org/10.7860/JCDR/2015/10053.5683, https://pubmed.ncbi.nlm.nih.gov/25954674/.

Mokry, L. E., Ross, S., Ahmad, O. S., Forgetta, V., Smith, G. D., Leong, A., Greenwood, C. M. T., Thanassoulis, G., & Richards, J. B. (2015). Vitamin D and risk of multiple sclerosis: A mendelian randomization study. *PLoS Medicine, 12*(8). https://doi.org/10.1371/JOURNAL.PMED.1001866, https://pubmed.ncbi.nlm.nih.gov/26305103/.

Mora, J. R., Iwata, M., & Von Andrian, U. H. (2008). Vitamin effects on the immune system: Vitamins A and D take centre stage. *Nature Reviews. Immunology, 8*(9), 685–698. https://doi.org/10.1038/NRI2378, https://pubmed.ncbi.nlm.nih.gov/19172691/.

Morcos, M. M., Gabr, A. A., Samuel, S., Kamel, M., Baz, M. E., Beshry, M. E., & Michail, R. R. (1998). Vitamin D administration to tuberculous children and its value. *Bollettino Chimico Farmaceutico, 137*(5), 157–164. https://europepmc.org/article/med/9689902.

Mori, H., Sawada, T., Nishiyama, S., Shimada, K., Tahara, K., Hayashi, H., Kato, E., Tago, M., Matsui, T., & Tohma, S. (2019). Influence of seasonal changes on disease activity and distribution of affected joints in rheumatoid arthritis. *BMC Musculoskeletal Disorders, 20*(1), 1–8. https://doi.org/10.1186/S12891-019-2418-2/FIGURES/2, https://bmcmusculoskeletdisord.biomedcentral.com/articles/10.1186/s12891-019-2418-2.

Mouchel, P. L., Bérard, E., Tavitian, S., Gadaud, N., Vergez, F., Rieu, J. B., Luquet, I., Sarry, A., Huguet, F., Largeaud, L., Delabesse, E., Huynh, A., Bertoli, S., & Récher, C. (2023). Vitamin C and D supplementation in acute myeloid leukemia. *Blood Advances, 7*(22), 6886–6897. https://doi.org/10.1182/BLOODADVANCES.2023010559, https://doi.org/10.1182/bloodadvances.2023010559.

Naderpoor, N., Mousa, A., Fernanda Gomez Arango, L., Barrett, H. L., Dekker Nitert, M., & de Courten, B. (2019). Effect of vitamin D supplementation on faecal microbiota: A randomised clinical trial. *Nutrients, 11*(12), 2888. https://doi.org/10.3390/NU11122888, https://www.mdpi.com/2072-6643/11/12/2888/htm.

Nesby-O'Dell, S., Scanlon, K. S., Cogswell, M. E., Gillespie, C., Hollis, B. W., Looker, A. C., Alien, C., Dougherty, C., Gunter, E. W., & Bowman, B. A. (2002). Hypovitaminosis D prevalence and determinants among African American and white women of reproductive age: Third National Health and Nutrition Examination Survey, 1988-1994. *The American Journal of Clinical Nutrition, 76*(1), 187–192. https://doi.org/10.1093/AJCN/76.1.187, https://pubmed.ncbi.nlm.nih.gov/12081833/.

Nessvi, S., Johansson, L., Jopson, J., Stewart, A., Reeder, A., McKenzie, R., & Scragg, R. K. (2011). Association of 25-hydroxyvitamin D3)levels in adult New Zealanders with ethnicity, skin color and self-reported skin sensitivity to sun exposure. *Photochemistry and Photobiology, 87*(5), 1173–1178. https://doi.org/10.1111/J.1751-1097.2011.00956.X, https://pubmed.ncbi.nlm.nih.gov/21679191/.

De Niet, S., Trémège, M., Coffiner, M., Rousseau, A. F., Calmes, D., Frix, A. N., Gester, F., Delvaux, M., Dive, A. F., Guglielmi, E., Henket, M., Staderoli, A., Maesen, D., Louis, R., Guiot, J., & Cavalier, E. (2022). Positive effects of vitamin D supplementation in patients hospitalized for COVID-19: A randomized, double-blind, placebo-controlled trial. *Nutrients, 14*(15). https://doi.org/10.3390/NU14153048, https://pubmed.ncbi.nlm.nih.gov/35893907/.

Ning, Z., Song, S., Miao, L., Zhang, P., Wang, X., Liu, J., Hu, Y., Xu, Y., Zhao, T., Liang, Y., Wang, Q., Liu, L., Zhang, J., Hu, L., Huo, M., & Zhou, Q. (2016). High prevalence of vitamin D deficiency in urban health checkup population. *Clinical Nutrition (Edinburgh, Scotland), 35*(4), 859–863. https://doi.org/10.1016/J.CLNU.2015.05.019, https://pubmed.ncbi.nlm.nih.gov/26093537/.

Nireeksha, Hegde, M. N., & Kumari N, S. (2024). Potential role of salivary vitamin D antimicrobial peptide LL-37 and interleukins in severity of dental caries: An exvivo study. *BMC Oral Health, 24*(1), 79. https://doi.org/10.1186/s12903-023-03749-7, https://bmcoralhealth.biomedcentral.com/articles/10.1186/s12903-023-03749-7.

Nnoaham, K. E., & Clarke, A. (2008). Low serum vitamin D levels and tuberculosis: a systematic review and meta-analysis. *International Journal of Epidemiology, 37*(1), 113–119. https://doi.org/10.1093/IJE/DYM247, https://doi.org/10.1093/ije/dym247.

Pham, H., Waterhouse, M., Rahman, S., Baxter, C., Duarte Romero, B., McLeod, D. S. A., Ebeling, P. R., English, D. R., Hartel, G., O'Connell, R. L., van der Pols, J. C., Venn, A. J., Webb, P. M., Whiteman, D. C., Huygens, F., & Neale, R. E. (2023). The effect of vitamin D supplementation on the gut microbiome in older Australians – Results from analyses of the D-Health Trial. *Gut Microbes, 15*(1), 2221429. https://doi.org/10.1080/19490976.2023.2221429, https://pmc.ncbi.nlm.nih.gov/articles/PMC10251798/.

Pieters, J. (2008). Mycobacterium tuberculosis and the macrophage: Maintaining a balance. *Cell Host & Microbe, 3*(6), 399–407. https://doi.org/10.1016/J.CHOM.2008.05.006.

Pilz, S., Trummer, C., Pandis, M., Schwetz, V., Aberer, F., Grübler, M., Verheyen, N., Tomaschitz, A., & März, W. (2018). Vitamin D: Current guidelines and future outlook. *Anticancer research, 38*(2), 1145–1151. https://doi.org/10.21873/ANTICANRES.12333, https://pubmed.ncbi.nlm.nih.gov/29374751/.

Powe, C. E., Evans, M. K., Wenger, J., Zonderman, A. B., Berg, A. H., Nalls, M., Tamez, H., Zhang, D., Bhan, I., Karumanchi, S. A., Powe, N. R., & Thadhani, R. (2013). Vitamin D-binding protein and vitamin D status of black Americans and white Americans. *The New England journal of medicine, 369*(21), 1991–2000. https://doi.org/10.1056/NEJMOA1306357, https://pubmed.ncbi.nlm.nih.gov/24256378/.

Qiu, F., Zhang, Z., Yang, L., Li, R., & Ma, Y. (2021). Combined effect of vitamin C and vitamin D3 on intestinal epithelial barrier by regulating Notch signaling pathway. *Nutrition & Metabolism, 18*(1). https://doi.org/10.1186/S12986-021-00576-X, https://pubmed.ncbi.nlm.nih.gov/33964955/.

Quesada-Gomez, J. M., Entrenas-Castillo, M., & Bouillon, R. (2020). Vitamin D receptor stimulation to reduce acute respiratory distress syndrome (ARDS) in patients with coronavirus SARS-CoV-2 infections: Revised Ms SBMB 2020_166. *The Journal of Steroid Biochemistry and Molecular Biology, 202*, 105719. https://doi.org/10.1016/J.JSBMB.2020.105719, https://pmc.ncbi.nlm.nih.gov/articles/PMC7289092/.

Raju, A., Luthra, G., Shahbaz, M., Almatooq, H., Foucambert, P., Esbrand, F. D., Zafar, S., Panthangi, V., Cyril Kurupp, A. R., & Khan, S. (2022). Role of vitamin D deficiency in increased susceptibility to respiratory infections among children: A systematic review. *Cureus, 14*(9), e29205. https://doi.org/10.7759/CUREUS.29205, https://pmc.ncbi.nlm.nih.gov/articles/PMC9573008/.

Reichrath, J. (2006). The challenge resulting from positive and negative effects of sunlight: How much solar UV exposure is appropriate to balance between risks of vitamin D deficiency and skin cancer? *Progress in Biophysics and Molecular Biology, 92*(1), 9–16. https://doi.org/10.1016/J.PBIOMOLBIO.2006.02.010.

Reider, C. A., Chung, R. Y., Devarshi, P. P., Grant, R. W., & Hazels Mitmesser, S. (2020). Inadequacy of immune health nutrients: Intakes in US Adults, the 2005–2016 NHANES. *Nutrients, 12*(6), 1735. https://doi.org/10.3390/NU12061735, https://www.mdpi.com/2072-6643/12/6/1735/htm.

Rhead, B., Bäärnhielm, M., Gianfrancesco, M., Mok, A., Shao, X., Quach, H., Shen, L., Schaefer, C., Link, J., Gyllenberg, A., Hedström, A. K., Olsson, T., Hillert, J., Kockum, I., Glymour, M. M., Alfredsson, L., & Barcellos, L. F. (2016). Mendelian randomization shows a causal effect of low vitamin D on multiple sclerosis risk. *Neurology. Genetics. 2*(5). https://doi.org/10.1212/NXG.0000000000000097, https://pubmed.ncbi.nlm.nih.gov/27652346/.

Rita, M., Young, I., & Xiong, Y. (2018). Influence of vitamin D on cancer risk and treatment: Why the variability? *Trends in Cancer Research, 13*, 43. https://pmc.ncbi.nlm.nih.gov/articles/PMC6201256/.

Robles-Vera, I., Callejo, M., Ramos, R., Duarte, J., & Perez-Vizcaino, F. (2019). Impact of vitamin D deficit on the rat gut microbiome. *Nutrients, 11*(11), 2564. https://doi.org/10.3390/NU11112564, https://www.mdpi.com/2072-6643/11/11/2564/htm.

Rockett, K. A., Brookes, R., Udalova, I., Vidal, V., Hill, A. V. S., & Kwiatkowski, D. (1998). 1,25-Dihydroxyvitamin D3 induces nitric oxide synthase and suppresses growth of Mycobacterium tuberculosis in a human macrophage-like cell line. *Infection and immunity, 66*(11), 5314–5321. https://doi.org/10.1128/IAI.66.11.5314-5321.1998, https://pubmed.ncbi.nlm.nih.gov/9784538/.

Rossini, M., Maddali Bongi, S., La Montagna, G., Minisola, G., Malavolta, N., Bernini, L., Cacace, E., Sinigaglia, L., Di Munno, O., & Adami, S. (2010). Vitamin D deficiency in rheumatoid arthritis: Prevalence, determinants and associations with disease activity and disability. *Arthritis Research & Therapy, 12*(6). https://doi.org/10.1186/AR3195, https://pubmed.ncbi.nlm.nih.gov/21114806/.

Salahuddin, N., Ali, F., Hasan, Z., Rao, N., Aqeel, M., & Mahmood, F. (2013). Vitamin D accelerates clinical recovery from tuberculosis: Results of the SUCCINCT Study [Supplementary Cholecalciferol in recovery from tuberculosis]. A randomized, placebo-controlled, clinical trial of vitamin D supplementation in patients with pulmonar. *BMC Infectious Diseases, 13*(1). https://doi.org/10.1186/1471-2334-13-22, https://pubmed.ncbi.nlm.nih.gov/23331510/.

Sanford, B. S., Aliano, J. L., Omary, C. S., McDonnell, S. L., Kimball, S. M., & Grant, W. B. (2023). Exposure to a vitamin D best practices toolkit, model, and E-tools increases knowledge, confidence, and the translation of research to public health and practice. *Nutrients, 15*(11), 2446. https://doi.org/10.3390/nu15112446, https://www.mdpi.com/2072-6643/15/11/2446.

Santana, K. Vd. Sd, Oliver, S. L., Mendes, M. M., Lanham-New, S., Charlton, K. E., & Ribeiro, H. (2022). Association between vitamin D status and lifestyle factors in Brazilian women: Implications of Sun Exposure Levels, Diet, and Health. *eClinicalMedicine, 47*. https://doi.org/10.1016/j.eclinm.2022.101400, https://www.thelancet.com/journals/eclinm/issue/current.

Sassi, F. (2018). Vitamin D: Nutrient, Hormone, and Immunomodulator. *Nutrients, 10*, 1656.

Schwalfenberg, G. (2008). Vitamin D and diabetes: Improvement of glycemic control with vitamin D3 repletion. *Canadian Family Physician.*

Scully, H., Laird, E., Healy, M., Crowley, V., Walsh, J. B., & McCarroll, K. (2022). Low socioeconomic status predicts vitamin D status in a cross-section of Irish children. *Journal of Nutritional Science, 11*, e61. https://doi.org/10.1017/JNS.2022.57, https://pmc.ncbi.nlm.nih.gov/articles/PMC9334117/.

Seura, T., & Fukuwatari, T. (2017). The relationship between habitual dietary intake and gut microbiota in young Japanese women. *Article in Journal of Nutritional Science and Vitaminology.* https://doi.org/10.3177/jnsv.63.396, https://www.researchgate.net/publication/322412094.

Siddiqee, M. H., Bhattacharjee, B., Siddiqi, U. R., & Rahman, M. M. (2021). High prevalence of vitamin D deficiency among the South Asian adults: A systematic review and meta-analysis. *BMC Public Health, 21*(1), 1–18. https://doi.org/10.1186/S12889-021-11888-1/FIGURES/5, https://bmcpublichealth.biomedcentral.com/articles/10.1186/s12889-021-11888-1.

Simpson, S., Taylor, B., Blizzard, L., Ponsonby, A. L., Pittas, F., Tremlett, H., Dwyer, T., Gies, P., & Van Der Mei, I. (2010). Higher 25-hydroxyvitamin D is associated with lower relapse risk in multiple sclerosis. *Annals of Neurology, 68*(2), 193–203. https://doi.org/10.1002/ANA.22043, https://onlinelibrary.wiley.com/doi/full/10.1002/ana.22043.

Singh, D. D., Digra, D. N., Verma, D. R., Shikha, D., Kaur, D. N., & Kaur Sarao, D. P. (2023). Assessment of disease activity score with respect to vitamin D in rheumatoid arthritis. *International Journal of Orthopaedics Sciences, 9*(2), 142–144. https://doi.org/10.22271/ORTHO.2023.V9.I2B.3363, https://www.orthopaper.com/archives/2023.v9.i2.3363/assessment-of-disease-activity-score-with-respect-to-vitamin-d-in-rheumatoid-arthritis.

Singh, P., Rawat, A., Alwakeel, M., Sharif, E., & Al Khodor, S. (2020). The potential role of vitamin D supplementation as a gut microbiota modifier in healthy individuals. *Scientific Reports, 10*(1), 1–14. https://doi.org/10.1038/s41598-020-77806-4, https://www.nature.com/articles/s41598-020-77806-4.

Sintzel, M. B., Rametta, M., & Reder, A. T. (2017). Vitamin D and multiple sclerosis: A comprehensive review. *Neurology and Therapy, 7*(1), 59. https://doi.org/10.1007/S40120-017-0086-4, https://pmc.ncbi.nlm.nih.gov/articles/PMC5990512/.

Staples, J. A., Ponsonby, A. L., Lim, L. L. Y., & McMichael, A. J. (2003). Ecologic analysis of some immune-related disorders, including type 1 diabetes, in Australia: Latitude, regional ultraviolet radiation, and disease prevalence. *Environmental Health Perspectives, 111*(4), 518–523. https://doi.org/10.1289/EHP.5941, https://pubmed.ncbi.nlm.nih.gov/12676609/.

Stevens, C. M., Bhusal, K., Levine, S. N., Dhawan, R., & Jain, S. K. (2023). The association of vitamin C and vitamin D status on bone mineral density and VCAM-1 levels in female diabetic subjects: Is combined supplementation with vitamin C and vitamin D potentially more successful in improving bone health than supplementation wit. *Human Nutrition & Metabolism, 34*, 200221. https://doi.org/10.1016/J.HNM.2023.200221.

Su, D., Nie, Y., Zhu, A., Chen, Z., Wu, P., Zhang, L., Luo, M., Sun, Q., Cai, L., Lai, Y., Xiao, Z., Duan, Z., Zheng, S., Wu, G., Hu, R., Tsukamoto, H., Lugea, A., Liu, Z., Pandol, S. J., & Han, Y. P. (2016). Vitamin D signaling through induction of paneth cell defensins maintains gut microbiota and improves metabolic disorders and hepatic steatosis in animal models. *Frontiers in Physiology, 7*(NOV), 226640. https://doi.org/10.3389/FPHYS.2016.00498/BIBTEX.

Suliman, H. A., Elkhawad, A. O., Babiker, O. O., Alhaj, Y. M., Eltom, K. H., & Elnour, A.A. (2024). Does vitamin D supplementation benefit patients with type 1 diabetes mellitus who are vitamin D deficient? A study was performed at the Sudan Childhood Diabetes Center from 2019 to 2022. **12**, https://doi.org/10.1177/20503121241242931, https://journals.sagepub.com/doi/10.1177/20503121241242931.

Svensson, D., Nebel, D., Voss, U., Ekblad, E., & Nilsson, B. O. (2016). Vitamin D-induced up-regulation of human keratinocyte cathelicidin anti-microbial peptide expression involves retinoid X receptor α. *Cell and Tissue Research*. https://doi.org/10.1007/s00441-016-2449-z.

Sommer, A., & Fabri, M. (2015). Vitamin D regulates cytokine patterns secreted by dendritic cells to promote differentiation of IL-22-Producing T cells. *PLoS One*. https://doi.org/10.1371/journal.pone.0130395.

Sørensen, I. M., Joner, G., Jenum, P. A., Eskild, A., Torjesen, P. A., & Stene, L. C. (2012). Maternal serum levels of 25-hydroxy-vitamin D during pregnancy and risk of type 1 diabetes in the offspring. *Diabetes, 61*(1), 175–178. https://doi.org/10.2337/DB11-0875, https://pubmed.ncbi.nlm.nih.gov/22124461/.

Talat, N., Perry, S., Parsonnet, J., Dawood, G., & Hussain, R. (2010). Vitamin D deficiency and tuberculosis progression. *Emerging Infectious Diseases, 16*(5), 853. https://doi.org/10.3201/EID1605.091693, https://pmc.ncbi.nlm.nih.gov/articles/PMC2954005/.

Taylor, P. N., & Davies, J. S. (2018). A review of the growing risk of vitamin D toxicity from inappropriate practice. *British Journal of Clinical Pharmacology, 84*(6), 1121. https://doi.org/10.1111/BCP.13573, https://pmc.ncbi.nlm.nih.gov/articles/PMC5980613/.

Thabet, R. H., Gomaa, A. A., Matalqah, L. M., & Shalaby, E. M. (2022). Vitamin D: An essential adjuvant therapeutic agent in breast cancer. *Journal of International Medical Research, 50*(7). https://doi.org/10.1177/

03000605221113800/ASSET/IMAGES/LARGE/10.1177_03000605221113800-FIG1.JPEG, https://journals.sagepub.com/doi/10.1177/03000605221113800.

Tiosano, D., Wildbaum, G., Gepstein, V., Verbitsky, O., Weisman, Y., Karin, N., & Eztioni, A. (2013). The role of vitamin D receptor in innate and adaptive immunity: A study in hereditary vitamin D–resistant rickets patients. *The Journal of Clinical Endocrinology & Metabolism, 98*(4), 1685–1693. https://doi.org/10.1210/JC.2012-3858, https://doi.org/10.1210/jc.2012-3858.

Tomei, S., Singh, P., Mathew, R., Mattei, V., Garand, M., Alwakeel, M., Sharif, E., & Al Khodor, S. (2020). The role of polymorphisms in vitamin D-related genes in response to vitamin D supplementation. *Nutrients, 12*(9), 2608. https://doi.org/10.3390/NU12092608, https://www.mdpi.com/2072-6643/12/9/2608/htm.

Torres-Juarez, F., Cardenas-Vargas, A., Montoya-Rosales, A., González-Curiel, I., Garcia-Hernandez, M. H., Enciso-Moreno, J. A., Hancock, R. E. W., & Rivas-Santiago, B. (2015). LL-37 immunomodulatory activity during Mycobacterium tuberculosis infection in macrophages. *Infection and Immunity, 83*(12), 4495–4503. https://doi.org/10.1128/IAI.00936-15, https://pubmed.ncbi.nlm.nih.gov/26351280/.

Treiber, G., Prietl, B., Fröhlich-Reiterer, E., Lechner, E., Ribitsch, A., Fritsch, M., Rami-Merhar, B., Steigleder-Schweiger, C., Graninger, W., Borkenstein, M., & Pieber, T. R. (2015). Cholecalciferol supplementation improves suppressive capacity of regulatory T-cells in young patients with new-onset type 1 diabetes mellitus - A randomized clinical trial. *Clinical Immunology (Orlando, Fla.). 161*(2), 217–224. https://doi.org/10.1016/J.CLIM.2015.08.002, https://pubmed.ncbi.nlm.nih.gov/26277548/.

Udeabor, S. E., Albejadi, A. M., Al-Shehri, W. A. K., Onwuka, C. I., Al-Fathani, S. Y., Al Nazeh, A. A., Aldhahri, S. F., & Alshahrani, F. A. (2020). Serum levels of 25-hydroxy-vitamin D in patients with oral squamous cell carcinoma: Making a case for chemoprevention. *Clinical and Experimental Dental Research, 6*(4), 428–432. https://doi.org/10.1002/CRE2.294, https://onlinelibrary.wiley.com/doi/full/10.1002/cre2.294.

Unal, A. D., Tarcin, O., Parildar, H., Cigerli, O., Eroglu, H., & Demirag, N. G. (2014). Vitamin D deficiency is related to thyroid antibodies in autoimmune thyroiditis. *Central European Journal of Immunology*. https://doi.org/10.5114/ceji.2014.47735.

Verway, M., Bouttier, M., Wang, T. T., Carrier, M., Calderon, M., An, B. S., Devemy, E., McIntosh, F., Divangahi, M., Behr, M. A., & White, J. H. (2013). Vitamin D induces interleukin-1β expression: Paracrine macrophage epithelial signaling controls *M. tuberculosis* infection. *PLoS Pathogens*. https://doi.org/10.1371/journal.ppat.1003407.

Vieira, V. M., Hart, J. E., Webster, T. F., Weinberg, J., Puett, R., Laden, F., Costenbader, K. H., & Karlson, E. W. (2010). Association between residences in U.S. northern latitudes and rheumatoid arthritis: A spatial analysis of the Nurses' Health Study. *Environmental Health Perspectives, 118*(7), 957–961. https://doi.org/10.1289/EHP.0901861, https://pubmed.ncbi.nlm.nih.gov/20338859/.

Waisberg, M., Vickers, B. K., Yager, S. B., Lin, C. K., & Pierce, S. K. (2012). Testing in mice the hypothesis that melanin is protective in malaria infections. *PLOS ONE, 7*(1), e29493. https://doi.org/10.1371/JOURNAL.PONE.0029493, https://journals.plos.org/plosone/article?id=10.1371/journal.pone.0029493.

Wallace, T. C., Reider, C., & Fulgoni, V. L. (2013). Calcium and vitamin D disparities are related to gender, age, race, household income level, and weight classification but not vegetarian status in the United States: Analysis of the NHANES 2001-2008 Data Set. *Journal of the American College of Nutrition, 32*(5), 321–330. https://doi.org/10.1080/07315724.2013.839905.

Wang, X., Li, X., & Dong, Y. (2020). Vitamin D decreases plasma trimethylamine-N-oxide level in mice by regulating gut microbiota. *BioMed Research International, 2020*(1), 9896743. https://doi.org/10.1155/2020/9896743, https://onlinelibrary.wiley.com/doi/full/10.1155/2020/9896743.

Wang, Y., Marling, S. J., Zhu, J. G., Severson, K. S., & DeLuca, H. F. (2012). Development of experimental autoimmune encephalomyelitis (EAE) in mice requires vitamin D and the vitamin D receptor. *Proceedings of the National Academy of Sciences of the United States of America, 109*(22), 8501–8504. https://doi.org/10.1073/PNAS.1206054109/ASSET/7423902B-3D17-41A3-AA53-06604801B9A9/ASSETS/GRAPHIC/PNAS.1206054109FIG04.JPEG, https://www.pnas.org/doi/abs/10.1073/pnas.1206054109.

Wayse, V., Yousafzai, A., Mogale, K., & Filteau, S. (2004). Association of subclinical vitamin D deficiency with severe acute lower respiratory infection in Indian children under 5 y. *European Journal of Clinical Nutrition, 58*(4), 563–567. https://doi.org/10.1038/sj.ejcn.1601845, https://www.nature.com/articles/1601845.

Wei, R., & Christakos, S. (2015). *Mechanisms underlying the regulation of innate and adaptive immunity by vitamin D.*

Welsh, P., Peters, M. J. L., McInnes, I. B., Lems, W. F., Lips, P. T., McKellar, G., Knox, S., Michael Wallace, A., Dijkmans, B. A. C., Nurmohamed, M. T., & Sattar, N. (2011). Vitamin D deficiency is common in patients with RA and linked to disease activity, but circulating levels are unaffected by TNFα blockade: results from a prospective cohort study. *Annals of the Rheumatic Diseases, 70*(6), 1165–1167. https://doi.org/10.1136/ARD.2010.137265, https://pubmed.ncbi.nlm.nih.gov/21047908/.

White, J. H. (2012). Macrophages vitamin D vitamin D receptor innate immunity adaptive immunity antimicrobial peptides pattern recognition receptors CYP27B1.

Wimalawansa, S. J. (2023). Infections and autoimmunity—The immune system and vitamin D: A systematic review. *Nutrients, 15*(17), 3842. https://doi.org/10.3390/nu15173842, https://www.mdpi.com/2072-6643/15/17/3842.

Wolden-Kirk, H., Overbergh, L., Christesen, H. T., Brusgaard, K., & Mathieu, C. (2011). Vitamin D and diabetes: Its importance for beta cell and immune function. *Molecular and Cellular Endocrinology, 347*(1-2), 106–120. https://doi.org/10.1016/J.MCE.2011.08.016.

Wortsman, J., Matsuoka, L. Y., Chen, T. C., Lu, Z., & Holick, M. F. (2000). Decreased bioavailability of vitamin D in obesity. *The American journal of clinical nutrition, 72*(3), 690–693. https://doi.org/10.1093/AJCN/72.3.690, https://pubmed.ncbi.nlm.nih.gov/10966885/.

Wu, S., & Sun, J. (2011). Vitamin D, Vitamin D receptor, and macroautophagy in inflammation and infection. *Discovery Medicine, 11*(59), 325. https://pmc.ncbi.nlm.nih.gov/articles/PMC3285235/.

Young, K., Beggs, M.R., Grimbly, C., & Alexander, R.T. (2022). Regulation of 1 and 24 hydroxylation of vitamin D metabolites in the proximal tubule..

Yuk, J. M., Shin, D. M., Lee, H. M., Yang, C. S., Jin, H. S., Kim, K. K., Lee, Z. W., Lee, S. H., Kim, J. M., & Jo, E. K. (2009). Vitamin D3 induces autophagy in human monocytes/macrophages via cathelicidin. *Cell Host and Microbe.* https://doi.org/10.1016/j.chom.2009.08.004.

Zelini, P., D'Angelo, P., Cereda, E., Klersy, C., Sabrina, P., Albertini, R., Grugnetti, G., Grugnetti, A. M., Marena, C., Cutti, S., Lilleri, D., Cassaniti, I., Fausto, B., & Caccialanza, R. (2022). Association between vitamin D serum levels and immune response to the BNT162b2 vaccine for SARS-CoV-2. *Biomedicines, 10*(8), 1993. https://doi.org/10.3390/BIOMEDICINES10081993, https://www.mdpi.com/2227-9059/10/8/1993/htm.

Zhen, D., Liu, L., Guan, C., Zhao, N., & Tang, X. (2015). High prevalence of vitamin D deficiency among middle-aged and elderly individuals in northwestern China: Its relationship to osteoporosis and lifestyle factors. *Bone, 71*, 1–6. https://doi.org/10.1016/J.BONE.2014.09.024, https://pubmed.ncbi.nlm.nih.gov/25284157/.

Zwerina, K., Baum, W., Axmann, R., Heiland, G. R., Distler, J. H., Smolen, J., Hayer, S., Zwerina, J., & Schett, G. (2011). Vitamin D receptor regulates TNF-mediated arthritis. *Annals of the Rheumatic Diseases, 70*(6), 1122–1129. https://doi.org/10.1136/ARD.2010.142331, https://ard.bmj.com/content/70/6/1122, https://ard.bmj.com/content/70/6/1122.abstract.

CHAPTER 7

The interplay of epigenetics and vitamin D: regulation, mechanisms, and implications for health and disease

Sofia Amjad[1,2], and Rehana Rehman[3]

[1]Department of Physiology, Faculty of Medical Sciences, Azra Naheed Medical College, The Superior University, Lahore, Pakistan [2]Department of Physiology, Ziaudin University, Karachi, Pakistan [3]Department of Biological & Biomedical Sciences, Aga Khan University, Karachi, Pakistan

7.1 Introduction

7.1.1 Epigenetics

Epigenetics is the study of heritable variations in gene expression that occur without changes in the DNA sequence (Forouhari et al., 2020). Epigenetics, which means "above genetics," was first introduced by Conrad Waddington to describe the mechanism of inheritance that goes beyond genetics (Waddington, 1942). He proposed the concept of epigenetics as the processes through which the genotype manifests the phenotype. Initially, epigenetics was thought to be a genetic process that involves development and cellular differentiation. However, it extends beyond cellular differentiation today and influences many physiological processes (Carlberg, 2017).

Epigenetics plays a crucial role in regulating DNA-related processes through chromatin-based events (Berger et al., 2009). Chromatin is a complex made up of DNA and histone proteins. The basic functional unit of chromatin is the "nucleosome, composed of 147 base pairs of DNA, wrapped around a histone octamer, comprising histones H2A, H2B, H3, and H4" (McGinty & Tan, 2015).

7.1.2 Role of vitamin D in epigenetics

The role of vitamin D (Vit. D) in epigenetics is an emerging research area. The Vit. D. controls many functions and explicitly regulates about 3% of the human genome (Snegarova & Naydenova, 2020). Epigenetics modulates both Vit. D metabolism and its functions. Thus, epigenetic mechanisms modulate the expression of target genes and genes involved in Vit. D synthesis and metabolism (Singla et al., 2023). Many diseases have shown disturbed

The Impact of Vitamin D on Health and Disease. DOI: https://doi.org/10.1016/B978-0-443-34037-6.00028-5

epigenetic regulatory systems of Vit. D. Thus, better knowledge of the role of Vit. D in epigenetics can aid in understanding its mechanistic role in disease and the development of therapeutic advances affecting the Vit. D signaling system (Khayami et al., 2022; Snegarova & Naydenova, 2020).

7.1.2.1   Genomic response of vitamin D

Vit. D induces both genomic and non-genomic responses (Szymczak-Pajor et al., 2022). In genomic response, Vit. D exerts its biological effects by binding to the "Vit. D receptor (VDR)," a member of the "steroid nuclear receptor superfamily" (Snegarova & Naydenova, 2020). VDR is a ligand-regulated transcription factor, activated by 1,25-dihydroxy vitamin D (1,25Vit. D) (Snegarova & Naydenova, 2020). VDR can bind their ligands at nanomolar concentrations within a conserved ligand-binding domain (LBD) (Saponaro et al., 2020). On activation, the VDR forms a complex with the "retinoid X receptor (RXR)" and binds to specific "Vitamin D response elements (VDREs)" in the promoter regions of target genes, influencing their expression. VDR primarily attaches to areas of open chromatin. This initiates the genomic action of Vit. D (Szymczak-Pajor et al., 2022). The VDR, when unliganded, can bind to genomic DNA and typically forms complexes with corepressor proteins that exhibit histone deacetylases (HDAC) activity. These corepressors disassociate upon binding of Vit. D with VDR and are substituted by coactivator complexes (Fetahu et al., 2014). Vit. D target genes are protein-coding genes transcribed by RNA polymerase II (Seuter et al., 2017).

7.1.2.2   Nongenomic response of vitamin D

The nongenomic effects are facilitated by a membrane receptor, that activates intracellular metabolic pathways (Szymczak-Pajor et al., 2022). These signals lead to the activation of transcription factors such as RXR and the binding of VDRE to the promoter region of genes. A crosstalk occurs between the genomic pathway, mediated directly by transcription factors, and the nongenomic pathway initiated by the second messenger. Studies on gene expression have shown that Vit. D signaling directly and indirectly controls over 1,000 genes in the human genome. Several enzymatic coregulatory complexes facilitate "histone epigenetic modification, chromatin remodeling, and the recruitment of local RNA polymerase II" (Szymczak-Pajor et al., 2022). The reversal of VDR epigenetic repression could increase cell sensitivity to the hormone's beneficial activity, which is potentially applicable in Vit. D-resistant diseases (Apprato et al., 2020). When it binds to VDREs, it controls the expression of target genes, which are involved in critical cellular processes such as immune response, inflammation, and cell differentiation.

7.1.2.3 Epigenetic modifications

Epigenetic modifications are "posttranslational heritable and reversible biochemical changes in chromatin structure" (He et al., 2023). These post-translational changes can occur in all nuclear proteins interacting with DNA and chromatin. In histone proteins, these are commonly known as "histone marks," which influence gene expression across generations (Carlberg, 2017). Vit. D can induce reversible epigenetic modifications, such as addition or removal of posttranslational DNA methylation or histone modification through chromatin-modifying and remodeling enzymes (Carlberg, 2019). These mechanisms can alter chromatin organization by regulating gene expression (Apprato et al., 2020). The first recognized epigenetic change was the methylation of cytosine in genomic DNA (Holliday & Pugh, 1975). Measuring such DNA methylation, particularly within "cytosine and guanine (CpG) islands, is the gold standard" to monitor the effects of epigenetics in clinical research, including oncology (Dawson & Kouzarides, 2012). Methylation of cytosine residues in CpG islands at the promoter region leads to gene silencing, while modifications to histone protein tails regulate chromatin accessibility to transcription factors (Forouhari et al., 2020). Epigenetic modifications influence both chromatin compaction and gene expression. Enzymes called "writers" add these modifications, which are recognized by proteins known as "readers." These modifications are reversible, removed by the enzymes called "erasers" (Dan & Chen, 2023). Vit. D deficiency can cause dysregulation of these epigenetic modifications, leading to abnormal DNA methylation patterns and changes in chromatin structure. Such alterations are commonly observed in cancerous cells (Fetahu et al., 2014).

7.1.3 Effect of vitamin D on epigenetic modifications

7.1.3.1 Vitamin D and DNA methylation

DNA methylation is a significant process in epigenetics, where "methyl groups from the methyl donor S-adenosylmethionine (SAM) are added to the 5′ carbon of the cytosine bases" (Moore et al., 2013). This transfer occurs at the "cytosine and guanine (CpG) dinucleotides by DNA methyltransferases (DNMTs) and ten-eleven translocation (TET) proteins" (Snegarova & Naydenova, 2020). CpG makes clusters called CpG islands, usually located within gene promoter regions. CpG islands in the promoter region are methylated, leading to gene repression and directly or indirectly influencing chromatin structure and condensation. Thus, DNA methylation is found in silenced genes' promoter regions, leading to transcriptional repression. The transcription initiation sites (CpG islands) are generally unmethylated in tissue-specific and "housekeeping" genes, which are expressed in all tissues (Fetahu et al., 2014).

It has been reported that a change in VDR signaling at the epigenetic level is a significant cause of the diminished responsiveness to Vit. D actions. These changes are primarily due to the DNA methylation of the Vit. D gene promoter region or the accumulation of VDR-associated corepressors, particularly at the promoters of genes that impede cell proliferation (Snegarova & Naydenova, 2020).

7.1.3.1.1 DNA methylation and cancer

Vit. D is crucial in safeguarding the body's normal physiological functions and defending against the onset and progression of neoplasms (Carlberg & Muñoz, 2022). Transforming a normal cell into a cancer cell involves epigenetic changes, resulting in more accessible chromatin regions (Klemm et al., 2019). The epigenome is dynamic and can be influenced by environmental signals, such as Vit. D. The epigenome undergoes significant changes in cancer, including loss of "global DNA methylation" and targeted methylation in specific gene promoters. This loss of Global methylation results in chromosomal instability, loss of imprinting, and activation of transposable elements, which disrupt the genome (Fetahu et al., 2014). Additionally, tumor suppressor gene promoter regions in cancer cells are hypermethylated, leading to the loss of expression of critical genes involved in the cell cycle, apoptosis, and DNA repair. Thus, hypermethylation at promoter regions leads to the suppression of tumor suppressor genes. Vit. D has been found to regulate DNA methylation in tumor suppressor genes, potentially inhibiting cancer progression by enhancing the expression of genes essential for cancer prevention and treatment (Snegarova & Naydenova, 2020). Vit. D deficiency is associated with an increased risk of causing certain types of cancers, such as colon, breast, prostate, and hematological cancers. Vit D's anticancer effects may be due to its role in regulating growth (Carlberg & Muñoz, 2022).

7.1.3.1.2 DNA methylation and metabolic diseases

Understanding the mechanism of epigenetic regulation in metabolic diseases is crucial for developing new strategies in clinical metabolic disease management (Wu et al., 2023). Vit. D significantly prevents hypermethylation of DNA and several gene inactivation, with other epigenetic alterations in pancreatic β cells and other insulin-sensitive peripheral tissues, the liver, adipose tissue, and muscle. Vit. D deficiency accelerates the process of insulin resistance and, consequently, the development of type 2 diabetes mellitus (Vondra & Hampl, 2021). The reversible and dynamically modulated effect of epigenetics makes Vit. D a potential target for novel therapeutic interventions in metabolic diseases.

7.1.3.1.3 DNA methylation and immunity

Vit. D affects the immune system, as immune cells express the VDR (Arora et al., 2022). Vit. D has significant epigenetic modulation of the immune system (Paubelle et al., 2020). Epigenetic modifications induced by Vit. D in immune cells have been linked to improved immune regulation and reduced inflammation by decreasing oxidative stress, normalizing the Ca^{2+} signaling, and reducing the expression of pro-inflammatory cytokines with a rise in anti-inflammatory cytokines (Ghaseminejad-Raeini et al., 2023). Upon binding to the VDR, Vit. D regulates the gene expression necessary for innate immune defense, including cytokines, chemokines, antimicrobial peptides, and pattern recognition receptors (Adams et al., 2014). Vit. D deficiency increases the risk of dental caries, inflammatory bowel diseases, and viral respiratory infections. The antiviral response of Vit. D is due to the expression of the antimicrobial peptide CAMP/LL37(Chow et al., 2018).

7.1.3.2 Vitamin D and histone modification

Vit. D also influences "covalent modifications of histones by methylation, acetylation, phosphorylation, or ubiquitination," which affects how tightly DNA is wound around histones and, consequently, gene expression is affected. Posttranslational histone modifications are crucial in chromatin remodeling (Snegarova & Naydenova, 2020). Histone modifications are associated with activation and repression of gene expression (Dawson & Kouzarides, 2012). By promoting or suppressing these histone modifications, Vit. D regulates chromatin accessibility to transcription factors and, hence, the transcription of target genes. The most widely recognized modifications involve "methylation and acetylation of lysine residues on histones H3 and H4, acetylation of histones H2A and H2B, and phosphorylation of serine and threonine residues" (Apprato et al., 2020). Histone acetyltransferases (HATs), histone deacetylases (HDACs), histone methyltransferases (HMTs), and histone demethylases (HDMs) mediate the process of histone acetylation and methylation (Apprato et al., 2020). Histone acetylases and deacetylases are involved in histone modifications of VDREs throughout the entire genome (Snegarova & Naydenova, 2020). Without Vit. D, the VDR/RXR complex binds corepressors, leading to gene repression by attracting HDACs. Upon binding with ligand, coactivators like HATs replace the corepressors. Histone acetylation relaxes chromatin and causes the transcription of the genes (Fetahu et al., 2014). Different histone modifications of VDR have various effects, such as histone H3 lysine 4 mono-methylation (H3K4me1) associated with transcriptional elongation, histone H3 lysine 4 tri-methylation (H3K4me3) with active transcription, histone H3 lysine 27 acetylation (H3K27ac) with active enhancers, and histone H3 lysine 27 tri-methylation (H3K27me3) with transcriptional inhibition when found in the VDR gene-body (Apprato et al., 2020).

7.1.3.2.1 Histone modification and disease

Research has demonstrated the impact of Vit. D on histone acetylation and methylation patterns in genes that regulate immune response and inflammation (Carlberg, 2017). Several histone modifications are seen in cancer. Vit. D increases H4 acetylation in VDR enhancers, indicating increased VDR expression. Treatment with the HDAC inhibitor trichostatin-A to resistant malignant melanoma cell lines has positively influenced VDR expression, suggesting a promising direction for future therapeutic strategies.

7.1.3.3 Vitamin D and noncoding RNAs

Noncoding RNAs (ncRNAs), including microRNAs (miRNAs), do not participate in protein translation. However, their participation in several physiological and pathological mechanisms by affecting different molecules has been reported. They are vital components in driving epigenetic modifications, effectively regulating gene expression, and facilitating crucial processes of cell growth and differentiation (He et al., 2023). Recently, miRNAs have emerged as essential mediators of Vit. D signaling. Vit. D transcriptionally regulates ncRNAs under the effect of RNA polymerase II. miRNAs regulate gene expression via Vit. D by regulating mRNA stability and translational levels (Kanemoto et al., 2022). Thus, they play critical roles in the post-transcriptional gene expression regulatory network. Vit. D controls miRNA systems during the processes of homeostasis and disease. These miRNAs are associated with cancer progression, immune response modulation, and metabolism regulation. Thus, miRNA-based transformative clinical applications provide a tool to develop new therapies for Vit D-associated disorders (Zhao et al., 2023). Long-coding RNAs (LncRNAs) can influence translation directly by interacting with mRNAs, leading to translational inhibition or activation through various mechanisms (Godet et al., 2024).

7.1.3.4 Vitamin D and chromatin remodeling

Chromatin remodeling complexes are crucial in altering chromatin structure by moving, sliding, disrupting, or reorganizing nucleosomes. These complexes have distinct functions and interactions with DNA and histones, contributing to the dynamic regulation of gene expression and other chromatin-related processes. Activation of the VDR with its ligand 1, 25Vit. D induces three dimensional (3D) chromatin changes, which are functionally important for regulating the primary and secondary vitamin D target genes. It has been reported that nuclear receptors with 3D chromatin structure lead to 3D epigenome remodeling. Thus, chromatin remodelers influence a number of physiological and pathological functions. Considering this, the regulatory chromatin domain for VDR fine-tunes the gene regulation by all nuclear receptor superfamily members. Thus, ligand-bound VDR affects chromatin remodelers and causes an increase in active histone marks and open chromatin (Warwick et al., 2022) (Fig. 7.1).

7.1.4 Effect of epigenetic modifications on vitamin D metabolism

Epigenetic mechanisms regulate the Vit. D metabolism. DNA methylation can silence Vit. D-regulated genes involved in its metabolism (Fetahu et al., 2014). Vit. D metabolism is influenced by epigenetic modifications of VDREs across the genome. These modifications are facilitated by both histone acetylases and histone deacetylases (Snegarova & Naydenova, 2020). The effect of epigenetic modifications on VDR–Vit. D can be mediated through complex processes involving Vit. D metabolizing enzymes, cytochrome P450 oxidase enzymes, CYP27A1, CYP27B1, and CYP24A1 (Saponaro et al., 2020). The resistance to Vit. D is crucial in various pathological conditions, impacting treatment and management (Apprato et al., 2020). This process also controls the expression of target genes, leading to the

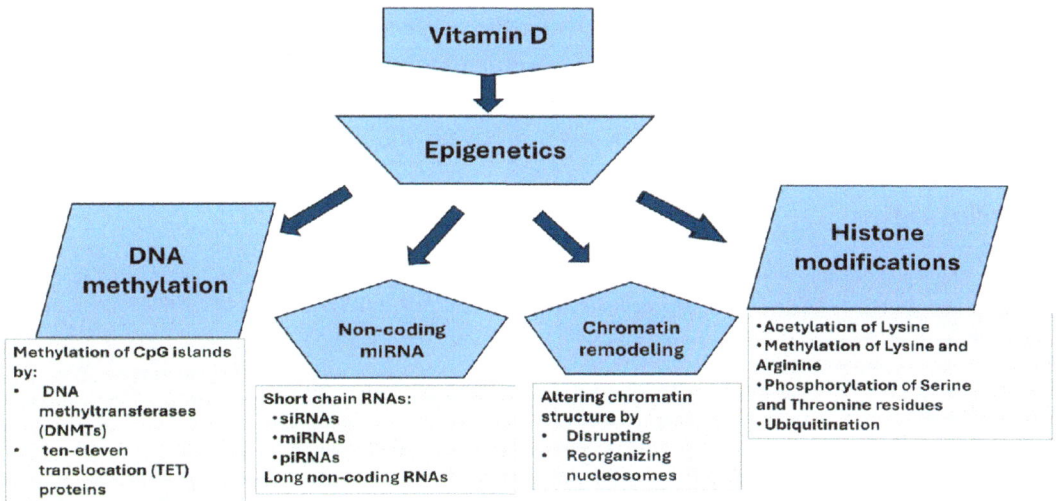

Figure 7.1
Role of vitamin D in epigenetic modification.

formation of enzymes that degrade and metabolize Vit. D. The CYP24A1 gene is significantly affected, encoding the enzyme 24-hydroxylase, which catabolizes Vit. D through a negative feedback loop (Ismailova & White, 2022). It has been demonstrated that pathologies showed an association of epigenetic effects with Vit. D metabolism, leading to epigenetic alterations of genes involved in Vit. D metabolism (Forouhari et al., 2020).

7.2 Clinical implication

Epigenetic regulation is reversible and dynamically modulated. The epigenetic repression of the VDR could be reversed, which causes an increased sensitivity of the cells to attain the beneficial effect of the hormone. Thus, Vit. D can be a potential target for novel therapeutic interventions in metabolic diseases, cancers, and immune disorders. Hence, epigenetics could be a cause of many Vit. D-resistant diseases (Apprato et al., 2020). miRNA-based effect of Vit. D and other epigenetic modifications can be used clinically to develop new therapeutic strategies for Vit. D-associated disorders.

7.3 Conclusion

Vit. D plays a critical role in gene regulation through epigenetic mechanisms, including DNA methylation, histone modification, the regulation of noncoding RNAs, and chromatin remodeling. Its potential to modulate gene expression in cancer-related pathways, immune function, and metabolic health opens new avenues for therapeutic interventions in chronic diseases. Further research will expand our understanding of the full extent of Vit. D's epigenetic impact on human health by knowing the epigenetic changes that can control the genes responsible for the pathogenesis of several cancers, immunological disorders, and metabolic diseases. This can help in assessing the body's response to therapeutic options and may benefit the condition with more effective management.

AI disclosure

During the preparation of this work the authors used an AI Chat Bot for grammar correction. After using this tool/service, the authors reviewed and edited the content as needed and took full responsibility for the content of the publication.

References

Adams, J. S., Rafison, B., Witzel, S., Reyes, R. E., Shieh, A., Chun, R., Zavala, K., Hewison, M., & Liu, P. T. (2014). Regulation of the extrarenal CYP27B1-hydroxylase. *Journal of Steroid Biochemistry and Molecular Biology, 144,* 22–27. https://doi.org/10.1016/j.jsbmb.2013.12.009, http://www.elsevier.com/locate/jsbmb.

Apprato, G., Fiz, C., Fusano, I., Bergandi, L., & Silvagno, F. (2020). Natural epigenetic modulators of vitamin D receptor. *Applied Sciences, 10*(12), 4096. https://doi.org/10.3390/app10124096.

Arora, J., Wang, J., Weaver, V., Zhang, Y., & Cantorna, M. T. (2022). Novel insight into the role of the vitamin D receptor in the development and function of the immune system. *The Journal of Steroid Biochemistry and Molecular Biology, 219,* 106084. https://doi.org/10.1016/j.jsbmb.2022.106084.

Berger, S. L., Kouzarides, T., Shiekhattar, R., & Shilatifard, A. (2009). An operational definition of epigenetics. *Genes and Development, 23*(7), 781–783. https://doi.org/10.1101/gad.1787609, http://genesdev.cshlp.org/content/23/7/781.full.pdf+html.

Carlberg, C. (2017). Molecular endocrinology of vitamin D on the epigenome level. *Molecular and Cellular Endocrinology, 453,* 14–21. https://doi.org/10.1016/j.mce.2017.03.016.

Carlberg, C., & Muñoz, A. (2022). An update on vitamin D signaling and cancer. *Seminars in Cancer Biology, 79,* 217–230. https://doi.org/10.1016/j.semcancer.2020.05.018.

Carlberg, C. (2019). Nutrigenomics of vitamin D. *Nutrients, 11*(3), 676. https://doi.org/10.3390/nu11030676.

Chow, K. T., Gale, M., & Loo, Y. M. (2018). RIG-I and other RNA sensors in antiviral immunity. *Annual Review of Immunology, 36,* 667–694. https://doi.org/10.1146/annurev-immunol-042617-053309 http://www.annualreviews.org/journal/immunol.

Dan, J., & Chen, T. (2023). Writers, erasers, and readers of DNA and histone methylation marks. In *Epigenetic cancer therapy, second edition.* China: Elsevier, 39–63. https://doi.org/10.1016/B978-0-323-91367-6.00012-X, https://www.sciencedirect.com/book/9780323913676.

Dawson, M. A., & Kouzarides, T. (2012). Cancer epigenetics: From mechanism to therapy. *Cell, 150*(1), 12–27. https://doi.org/10.1016/j.cell.2012.06.013, https://www.sciencedirect.com/journal/cell.

Fetahu, I. S., Höbaus, J., & Kállay, E. (2014). Vitamin D and the epigenome. *Frontiers in Physiology, 5.* https://doi.org/10.3389/fphys.2014.00164, http://journal.frontiersin.org/Journal/10.3389/fphys.2014.00164/full.

Forouhari, A., Heidari-Beni, M., Veisi, S., Poursafa, P., & Kelishadi, R. (2020). Effect of epigenetics on vitamin D levels: A systematic review until December. *Archives of Public Health, 81.*

Ghaseminejad-Raeini, A., Ghaderi, A., Sharafi, A., Nematollahi-Sani, B., Moossavi, M., Derakhshani, A., & Sarab, G. A. (2023). Immunomodulatory actions of vitamin D in various immune-related disorders: A comprehensive review. *Frontiers in Immunology, 14.* https://doi.org/10.3389/fimmu.2023.950465, https://www.frontiersin.org/journals/immunology#.

Godet, A. C., Roussel, E., Laugero, N., Morfoisse, F., Lacazette, E., Garmy-Susini, B., & Prats, A. C. (2024). Translational control by long non-coding RNAs. *Biochimie, 217,* 42–53. https://doi.org/10.1016/j.biochi.2023.08.015, https://www.sciencedirect.com/science/journal/03009084.

He, X., Cai, L., Tang, H., Chen, W., & Hu, W. (2023). Epigenetic modifications in radiation-induced non-targeted effects and their clinical significance. *Biochimica et Biophysica Acta (BBA) - General Subjects, 1867*(8), 130386. https://doi.org/10.1016/j.bbagen.2023.130386.

Holliday, R., & Pugh, J. E. (1975). DNA modification mechanisms and gene activity during development. *Science (New York, N.Y.), 187*(4173), 226–232. https://doi.org/10.1126/science.187.4173.226.

Ismailova, A., & White, J. H. (2022). Vitamin D, infections and immunity. *Reviews in Endocrine and Metabolic Disorders, 23*(2), 265–277. https://doi.org/10.1007/s11154-021-09679-5, https://www.springer.com/journal/11154.

Kanemoto, Y., Nishimura, K., Hayakawa, A., Sawada, T., Amano, R., Mori, J., Kurokawa, T., Murakami, Y., & Kato, S. (2022). A long non-coding RNA as a direct vitamin D target transcribed from the antisense strand of the human HSD17B2 locus. *Bioscience Reports, 42*(5). https://doi.org/10.1042/BSR20220321, https://portlandpress.com/bioscirep/article/42/5/BSR20220321/231267/A-long-non-coding-RNA-as-a-direct-vitamin-D-target.

Khayami, R., Goltzman, D., Rabbani, S. A., & Kerachian, M. A. (2022). Epigenomic effects of vitamin D in colorectal cancer. *Epigenomics, 14*(19), 1213–1228 https://doi.org/10.2217/epi-2022-0288, http://www.futuremedicine.com/loi/epi.

Klemm, S. L., Shipony, Z., & Greenleaf, W. J. (2019). Chromatin accessibility and the regulatory epigenome. *Nature Reviews. Genetics, 20*(4), 207–220. https://doi.org/10.1038/s41576-018-0089-8 http://www.nature.com/reviews/genetics.

McGinty, R. K., & Tan, S. (2015). Nucleosome structure and function. *Chemical Reviews, 115*(6), 2255–2273. https://doi.org/10.1021/cr500373h http://pubs.acs.org/journal/chreay.

Moore, L. D., Le, T., & Fan, G. (2013). DNA methylation and its basic function. *Neuropsychopharmacology: Official Publication of the American College of Neuropsychopharmacology, 38*(1), 23–38. https://doi.org/10.1038/npp.2012.112.

Paubelle, E., Zylbersztejn, F., Maciel, T. T., Carvalho, C., Mupo, A., Cheok, M., Lieben, L., Sujobert, P., Decroocq, J., Yokoyama, A., Asnafi, V., Macintyre, E., Tamburini, J., Bardet, V., Castaigne, S., Preudhomme, C., Dombret, H., Carmeliet, G., Bouscary, D., ... Moura, I. C. (2020). Vitamin D receptor controls cell stemness in acute myeloid leukemia and in normal bone marrow. *Cell Reports, 30*(3), 739. https://doi.org/10.1016/j.celrep.2019.12.055, http://www.sciencedirect.com/science/journal/22111247.

Saponaro, F., Saba, A., & Zucchi, R. (2020). An update on vitamin D metabolism. *International Journal of Molecular Sciences, 21*(18), 6573. https://doi.org/10.3390/ijms21186573.

Seuter, S., Neme, A., & Carlberg, C. (2017). Epigenomic PU.1-VDR crosstalk modulates vitamin D signaling. *Biochimica et Biophysica Acta (BBA) - Gene Regulatory Mechanisms, 1860*(4), 405–415. https://doi.org/10.1016/j.bbagrm.2017.02.005.

Singla, N., Thapa, R., Kulshrestha, R., Bhat, A. A., Gupta, S., Purohit, M., Singh, S. K., & Gupta, G. (2023). Introduction to epigenetics. In *Targeting Epigenetics in Inflammatory Lung Diseases*. India: Springer Nature, 17–42. https://doi.org/10.1007/978-981-99-4780-5_2 https://link.springer.com/book/10.1007/978-981-99-4780-5.

Snegarova, V., & Naydenova, D. (2020). Vitamin D: A review of its effects on epigenetics and gene regulation. *Folia Medica, 62*(4), 662–667. https://doi.org/10.3897/folmed.62.e50204.

Szymczak-Pajor, I., Miazek, K., Selmi, A., Balcerczyk, A., & Śliwińska, A. (2022). The action of vitamin D in adipose tissue: Is there the link between vitamin D deficiency and adipose tissue-related metabolic disorders? *International Journal of Molecular Sciences, 23*(2), 956. https://doi.org/10.3390/ijms23020956.

Vondra, K., & Hampl, R. (2021). Vitamin D and new insights into pathophysiology of type 2 diabetes. *Hormone Molecular Biology and Clinical Investigation, 42*(2), 203–208. https://doi.org/10.1515/hmbci-2020-0055.

Waddington, C. H. (1942). Canalization of development and the inheritance of acquired characters. *Nature, 150*(3811), 563–565. https://doi.org/10.1038/150563a0.

Warwick, T., Schulz, M. H., Gilsbach, R., Brandes, R. P., & Seuter, S. (2022). Nuclear receptor activation shapes spatial genome organization essential for gene expression control: lessons learned from the vitamin D receptor. *Nucleic Acids Research, 50*(7), 3745–3763. https://doi.org/10.1093/nar/gkac178 https://academic. oup.com/nar/issue.

Wu, Y. L., Lin, Z. J., Li, C. C., Lin, X., Shan, S. K., Guo, B., Zheng, M. H., Li, F., Yuan, L. Q., & Li, Z. H. (2023). Epigenetic regulation in metabolic diseases: Mechanisms and advances in clinical study. *Signal Transduction and Targeted Therapy, 8*(1). https://doi.org/10.1038/s41392-023-01333-7 https://www.nature.com/sigtrans.

Zhao, H., Forcellati, M., Buschittari, D., Heckel, J. E., Machado, C. J., Pullagura, S. R. N., & Lisse, T. S. (2023). Vitamin D and microRNAs. In *Feldman and Pike's vitamin D: Volume one: Biochemistry, physiology and diagnostics*. China: Elsevier, 261–290 https://doi.org/10.1016/B978-0-323-91386-7.00011-8, https://www. sciencedirect.com/book/9780323913867.

CHAPTER 8

Genetic variability in vitamin D metabolism: implications for health

Farzana Abubakar, and Khalid Ahmed

Department of Biological & Biomedical Sciences, Aga Khan University, Karachi, Pakistan

This chapter explores the multifactorial regulation of vitamin D metabolism and its association with the genetic variations in vitamin D-related genes that influence the serum 25(OH)D levels, which, in turn, predispose individuals to acquire various diseases and conditions, such as bone disorders, metabolic conditions, autoimmune diseases, cardiovascular diseases, and cancer. Vitamin D levels in the human body are affected by various factors, such as environmental factors (geographical latitude, sun exposure), genetic factors (skin pigmentation, vitamin D-related genes, e.g., *VDR, CYP27B1, GC*, and *CYP2R1*), dietary factors (vitamin D food intake, dietary supplements), physiological factors (age, body weight, obesity), and lifestyle and behavioral factors (outdoor activity, clothing, sunscreen cream, medication use) (Jiang et al., 2019; Krasniqi et al., 2021).

As per published literature, genetic factors have been shown to have a significant impact on human health and disease, which often involve the regulation of serum 25(OH)-D levels. It has been suggested that genetic components, for instance, vitamin D receptor gene allelic variations can account for up to 75% in terms of affecting bone density (Morrison et al., 1994). In studies on twins (either fraternal or identical), it has been revealed that hereditable genetic traits can account for up to 23%–80% for relationship between vitamin D status and common diseases (Dastani et al., 2013). Furthermore, a number of genetic mutations and polymorphisms affecting the genes that are related to the activation and production of vitamin D, as well as the proteins that are involved in the transport, for example, VDRs and the changes affecting proteins secondary to the regulation of vitamin D expression have been identified by genome-wide association studies as having veritable reproducible associations between vitamin D and various diseases such as diabetes, cancer, heart, and autoimmune diseases.

In this regard, several vitamin D-related genes are investigated, such as seven-dehydrocholesterol reductase (*DHCR7*), vitamin D-binding protein (*DBP/GC*), hydroxyvitamin D-1-α hydroxylase, cytochrome P450 family 27 subfamily B member 1 (*CYP27B1*), vitamin D 25-hydroxylase (*CYP2R1*), vitamin D receptor (*VDR*), retinoid X receptor (*RXR*), and vitamin D 24-hydroxylase

The Impact of Vitamin D on Health and Disease. **DOI:** https://doi.org/10.1016/B978-0-443-34037-6.00003-0

(*CYP24A1*). These genes are involved in various cellular and molecular pathways that are associated with vitamin D metabolism (Bahrami et al., 2018). Various regulatory pathways involving calcium (Ca^{2+}) levels are known to be affected by genetic polymorphisms of these genes, which involve either the upstream production of 25(OH)-D or the downstream activation of vitamin D to the active ligand 25(OH)-D, involving intermediate steps as such the binding of the carrier protein to the vitamin D and the active ligand 25(OH)-D, ligand-receptor interactions, such interaction either activate or inhibit various intermediary proteins (Ruiz-Ojeda et al., 2018).

8.1 Vitamin D receptor gene

The vitamin D receptor (*VDR*) gene has critical significance in mediating the effects of active vitamin D [1,25(OH)₂D] at the cellular level; therefore, the mutations or polymorphisms in this gene can affect influence calcium homeostasis, immune regulation, metabolic health, and the risk of several chronic diseases. The vitamin D receptor (VDR) is a nuclear receptor superfamily of transcriptional regulators (steroid receptor family). The VDR protein has two functional domains (the C-terminal ligand-binding activity domain and the N-terminal dual zinc finger DNA binding domain) and a connecting region that is crucial for the signaling of calcitriol or 1-α,25-dihidroxicolecalciferol (1α,25(OH)2D). After binding VDR, the 1α,25(OH)2D forms a heterodimer complex with the retinoid X receptor (RXR). To control the transcription of VDR-responsive genes, which carry out vitamin D effects such as calcium and phosphorous metabolism, the regulation of innate and adaptive immunity, and cell proliferation. VDR is extensively distributed throughout the body, as it is expressed in various places in the human body, including kidneys, bones, intestines, immunological cells, and other organs (Haroon & FitzGerald, 2012; Haussler et al., 2013; Karonova et al., 2018; Reschly & Krasowski, 2006).

The *VDR* gene, which has 11 exons and more than 900 allelic variations, has been documented on the long (q) arm of chromosome 12 (12q13.11). Taql (rs731236, exon 9, +65058 T > C), Apal (rs7975232, intron 8, +64978 C > A), BsmI (rs1544410, intron 8, +63980 G > A), and Fokl (rs10735810/ rs2228570, exon 2, +30920 C > T) are the most prevalent single nucleotide polymorphisms (SNPs) of the *VDR* gene. It has been demonstrated that the ApaI, TaqI, and BsmI are found in the 3′ untranslated region (UTR) of the *VDR* gene (silent genetic variations) and often affect the stability of the mRNA and the expression of the *VDR* gene. The *VDR* gene's 5' end contains the FokI, which is in linkage disequilibrium with other VDR variations, and the FokI SNP is found on exon 2 (close to the promoter region). The first translation initiation site (TIS) is eliminated as a result of the nucleotide substitution of T to C within the first codon of exon 2 (ATG to ACG, resulting in the allelic conversion of "f" to "F"). This produces a peptide that is shorter than the wild type of peptide (three amino acids absent), thereby generating a new form of VDR that is transcriptionally more active (Hoseinkhani et al., 2021; Sajjad et al., 2017). Chronic conditions like autoimmune diseases, cardiovascular disease, atherogenic lipid abnormalities, type 2 diabetes (T2DM), obesity, insulin resistance, rheumatic arthritis, cancer, metabolic syndrome, and metabolic bone diseases have all been reported to be linked with the VDR genetic variants (Karonova et al., 2018; Usategui-Martín et al., 2022).

8.2 Vitamin D-binding protein

Vitamin D-binding protein (DBP), which is encoded by the *GC* gene, is critical for transporting and regulating vitamin D bioavailability; therefore, the genetic variations in GC (*DBP* gene) are often linked to vitamin D insufficiency, immune function, and inflammatory responses. Hence, the mutations and the polymorphisms in the DBP gene can contribute to vitamin D deficiency and related disorders, including osteoporosis, autoimmune diseases, and inflammatory conditions.

Initially identified by Hirschfeld in 1959 as a group-specific component (Gc-globulin), DBP is a multifunctional serum glycoprotein of 51–58 kDa size that is synthesized in large quantities by hepatic parenchymal cells and is released into the bloodstream as a monomeric mature peptide of 458 residues. It was later identified in 1975 as the essential protein that transports vitamin D in the bloodstream and prevents its degradation. DBP is divided into structurally related domains, including two binding regions, for example, an actin-binding domain between residues 350 and 403 and a vitamin D/fatty acid-binding domain between residues 35 and 49. N-terminal and C-terminal domains (domains I and III) have recently been identified as the location of DBP cell surface binding sites, which may be required to mediate DBP cellular activities (Malik et al., 2013). In healthy people, 85% of the circulating vitamin D metabolites are DBP-bound, whereas 15% of those are albumin-bound. Glucocorticoids, inflammatory cytokines, and estrogen all influence DBP status, whereas the intestinal absorption of vitamin D depends on DBP levels. Pregnancy and the use of oral contraceptives boost the expression of DBP, which is overexpressed in the presence of estrogen hormone.

Although the precise mode of action of DBP is still unclear, however, DBP is not just a passive vitamin D carrier but DBP (also known as Gc protein) plays various physiological roles, including those associated with the scavenging extracellular G-actin and promoting macrophage activation, transporting and storing vitamin D, and enhancing neurotrophic chemotaxis via C5a during inflammation (Bikle & Schwartz, 2019; Nagasawa et al., 2005; Sorrenti et al., 2023). The single copy *GC* gene encodes for human DBP, which is 35 kb long with a single start site and is found on chromosome 4q12-q13 (as determined by in situ hybridization). With flanking untranslated areas at both ends and a critical enhancing motif (DNase hypersensitivity site IV) in intron 1, the gene is composed of 13 exons that encode 474 amino acids, including a 16-amino acid leader sequence that is cleaved before to release. The mature human DBP weighs about 58 kD, while the precise size varies depending on the allele's glycosylation of the protein. There have been reports linking vitamin D insufficiency to mutations in the *VDBP* gene.

DBP is divided into three structurally related domains. The binding location for the vitamin D metabolites is the first domain of DBP, which is located between amino acids 35 and 49. Only arachidonic acid competes with 25(OH)D for this binding site, while fatty acids, such as palmitic acid and arachidonic acid, bind with it using a single high-affinity site. A portion of the first domain is also implicated to be involved in this process, even though the actin binding site is situated at amino acid positions 373–403, which span portions of domains 2 and 3. The C5a/C5a des Arg-binding site is present at the amino acid positions 130–149, whereas membrane binding sites span the amino acids 150–172 and 379–402 (Bikle & Schwartz, 2019; Malik et al., 2013). A-albumin/afamin (*AFM*), a-fetoprotein (*AFP*), and albumin (*ALB*) are all members of the multigene family that includes the *DBP* gene. These genes are tandemly linked in the following order: centromere-*DBP-ALB-AFP-AFM*-telomere. *DBP* is subject to independent regulatory control, follows the opposite direction of gene transcription, and is distinguished from *albumin* by a 1.5 MB nontranscribed sequence (Malik et al., 2013). The most polymorphic gene is DBP, as based on its electrophoretic characteristics, over 120 gene variations have been identified, and the National Centre for Biotechnology Information (NCBI) database currently has 1,242 polymorphisms. The most prevalent polymorphisms of the *DBP* gene are Gc1f and Gc1s (located at rs7041) and Gc2 (located at rs4588). There are two polymorphisms in the Gc1f and Gc1s: one at position 432 (416 in the mature DBP) and another at position 436 (420 in the mature DBP). The amino acid sequence (432 and 436) is encoded as DATPT by the 1f allele (residues 432–436=Asp–Ala–Thr–Pro–Thr=-D–A–T–P–T), while EATPT is encoded by the 1s allele. During electrophoresis, the Gcf runs quicker than the Gcs due to this slight differential in charge. DATPK, which is encoded by the Gc2 allele, functions much more slowly. The Gc1 variations are further distinguished from the Gc2 variant by glycosylation. N-acetylgalactosamine is bound by the threonine (T) in Gc1, to which galactose and sialic acid bind simultaneously, whereas in Gc2, the lysine (K) in a similar location; however, it is not glycosylated. According to Bikle and Schwartz (2019), this has an impact on the conversion of DBP to DBP-MAF (macrophage activating factor), which entails a partial deglycosylation that eliminates the galactose and sialic acid by the successive activity of sialidase and b-galactosidase in T and B cells (Bikle & Schwartz, 2019).

8.3   25-Hydroxyvitamin D3 1-alpha-hydroxylase (cytochrome P450 family 27 subfamily B member 1(CYP27B1) gene

CYP27B1 gene, which encodes for 25-hydroxyvitamin D3 1α-hydroxylase is a critical enzyme that converts inactive vitamin D (25(OH)D3) into its biologically active form (1,25(OH)₂D3). 25-hydroxyvitamin D3 1α-hydroxylase is an enzyme that belongs to the cytochrome P450 superfamily that hydroxylates 25-hydroxyvitamin D3 at the 1alpha location is encoded by *CYP27B1* gene (1α-hydroxylase). The active form of vitamin D3 is produced by this reaction, 1alpha,25-dihydroxyvitamin D3, which binds to the vitamin D receptor and controls calcium metabolism by enhancing calcium absorption in the intestine and parathyroid glands, thereby preventing the transcription of the parathyroid hormone (*PTH*) gene, PTH secretion, and parathyroid cell growth, hence preserving homeostasis. Vitamin D-dependent rickets type I (VDDR I) is a rare autosomal recessive condition, or pseudo vitamin D deficiency rickets (PDDR), which can be caused by mutations in the *CYP27B1* gene (Demir et al., 2015; Lauter & Arnold, 2009). CYP27B1 has been found to be expressed in the proximal tubule of kidneys, parathyroid glands, pancreas, and colon. The chromosomal region 12q13.1–13.3 contains the *CYP27B1* gene. It is roughly 5 kb in size and has nine exons. 1-α-hydroxylase activity is reduced in pathogenic CYP27B1 variants, and it corresponds to low serum levels of 1,25(OH) 2D3 in affected individuals; however, 25(OH)D3 levels are either normal or high. The Human Gene Mutation Database (HGMD) currently has over 80 harmful variants that cover all *CYP27B1* exons, which have been shown to involve splice site alterations, insertions, deletions, duplications, and missense and nonsense mutations. In the French–Canadian population, two pathogenic variants have been identified, viz. c.1166 G > A (p. Arg389His) and c.1319_1325dup (p. Phe443Profs*24). Thus far, three pathogenic variants have been found in the Korean population: c.589+1 G > A, c.1319_1325dup, and c.983 G > A (p. Trp328*). Seven out of twelve Korean alleles exhibit the most prevalent pathogenic variation, c.589+1 G > A. The *CYP27B1* gene has six known splice site mutations, which are found in introns 1 and 7: c.195+2 T > G, c.386+1 G > A, c.589+1 G > A, c.1136+1 G > T, c.1215+1 G > A, and c.1215+2 T > A. Intron retention results from the mutations: c.195+2 T > G, c.386+1 G > A, and c.589+1 G > A. Splice site mutations disrupt normal mRNA processing and often lead to nonfunctional or dysfunctional CYP27B1 proteins. According to Demir et al. (2015), the effects of c.1136+1 G > T and c.1215+1 G > A have not yet been elucidated yet.

8.4   Vitamin D 24-hydroxylase (cytochrome P450 family 24 subfamily A member 1 (CYP24A1) gene

CYP24A1 plays a key role in vitamin D catabolism and calcium homeostasis, and its mutations can disrupt vitamin D metabolism. Vitamin D is catabolized in the kidneys. Through feedback regulation, the mitochondrial enzyme CYP24A1 can generate the inactive metabolite viz. 24,25-hydroxylated vitamin D (24,25(OH)D). The 24-hydroxylase enzyme is encoded by the *CYP24A1* gene, which is present on chromosome 20; it is principally in charge of breaking down calcitriol into the less active vitamin D metabolites, such as calcitroic acid and 1α,24,25-(OH)2D3. Additionally, 25-hydroxy vitamin D3 can be broken down by CYP24A1 to produce 24,25-dihydroxyvitamin D3, an inactive metabolite (Dauber et al., 2012). Infantile hypercalcemia 1 with loss of function mutations is associated with idiopathic infantile hypercalcemia and has been shown to be associated with more than 20 mutations in the *CYP24A1* gene. In adults, it not only causes severe hypercalciuric nephrolithiasis and nephrocalcinosis but also is associated with loss-of-function mutations of the *CYP24A1* gene, which results in chronic renal insufficiency (Dinour et al., 2013; Schlingmann et al., 2011). Recently, two pathogenic variants have been detected through genetic testing of the *CYP24A1* gene using Next Generation Sequencing Technology (NGS): c; 1186 C > T (p. Arg396Trp, rs114368325) and c; 428_430del (p. Glu143del, rs777676129); and as per the ClinVar NIH database (ClinVar archives, NIH), both variations as being shown to be linked to hypercalcemia (Leszczyńska et al., 2024).

8.5 Retinoid X receptor

The RXR binds with VDR in the nucleus, thereby regulates the expression of downstream vitamin D target genes, thereby acting as a ligand-dependent TF in the metabolism of vitamin D. There are three subtypes of *RXR* gene such as *RXRα*, *RXRβ*, and *RXRγ*, which are encoded by related genes (Germain et al., 2006). RXRα is expressed in the skin, kidney, intestine epithelium, and liver, while RXRβ has been found in all tissues. Whereas RXRγ is mostly found in the brain, skeletal muscle, and myocardium (Dollé et al., 1994). RXRs are involved in cell development, differentiation, cell growth, and apoptosis. When 1,25(OH)2D binds to the VDR, it results in allosteric conformational changes in RXR, thereby making it easier to recruit the coregulators. A significant association has been reported between RXR-A SNP rs3132299 and 1,25(OH)2D as well as rs877954 and 25(OH)D levels when studied in ursodeoxycholic acid (UDCA) population (Haussler et al., 2008; Wjst et al., 2006). In summary, genetic variations in *RXR* genes can disrupt vitamin D metabolism, leading to skeletal, immune, neurological, and metabolic diseases.

8.6 7-Dehydrocholesterol reductase (DHCR7) gene

DHCR7 is a key enzyme that is involved in the production of vitamin D precursor (7-DHC), and its mutations can affect vitamin D availability, leading to various vitamin D deficiencies associated with disorders. The 7-dehydrocholesterol reductase (*DHCR7*) gene is located on chromosome 11q12-q13 and is 14.02 kb in size. *DHCR7* encodes a reductase that converts 7-dehydrocholesterol into cholesterol in the epidermis. Nonetheless, because of its various gene mutations can result in the build-up of 7-dehydrocholesterol, which is associated with Smith–Lemli–Opitz syndrome, which is characterized by lower serum cholesterol levels and elevated serum 7-dehydrocholesterol levels and is phenotypically characterized by weak muscle tone, small head size, facial dysmorphism, cognitive impairment, syndactyly of second and third toes, and holoprosencephaly (Bahrami et al., 2018). In addition, *DHCR7* gene variants, that is, rs11234027, rs1790349, and rs12785878 are localized in the 5' edge region and have been shown to be associated with vitamin D insufficiency (Ahn et al., 2010), whereas the mutations such as rs1629220, rs11606033, rs7122671, rs1790329, rs2276360, rs2282618, and rs1790349, have been shown to protect against hypovitaminosis D (Zhang et al., 2013).

8.7 Vitamin D 25-hydroxylase (cytochrome P450 family 2 subfamily R member 1 CYP2R1) gene

To further understand the role of vitamin D metabolism and genetics, we focus on the *CYP2R1* gene, which is located on chromosome 11p15.2 and is 14.29 kb in size. *CYP2R1* encodes for a D-25 hydroxylase that converts cholecalciferol (vitamin D3) to 25(OH)D in the first step of the vitamin D activation pathway. However, genetic mutations of *CYP2R1* can impair this conversion; for instance, the SNP rs10741657 in the 50-edge region is found to be associated with lower levels of 25(OH)D. Additional gene mutations can affect vitamin D levels, such as rs12794714 (which causes a synonymous alteration in the *CYP2R1* exon and has an association with the altered levels of 25(OH)D), rs10766197 (5' flanking region SNP of the *CYP2R1* gene), rs1562902, rs7116978, rs2060793, rs1993116, rs11023332, and rs1007392. Vitamin D deficiency can be caused by a missense mutation in exon 2 of the *CYP2R1* gene. In addition, four SNPs, viz. rs10766197, rs10741657, rs7116978, and rs1562902 of *CYP2R1* were found to be significantly linked to alteration in the circulating 25(OH) levels in the Danish population (Bahrami et al., 2018). These findings explain how genetic abnormalities in CYP2R1 influence vitamin D levels, which, in turn, can lead to various disease conditions.

In conclusion, the regulation of vitamin D metabolism and serum 25(OH)D levels are deeply intertwined with genetic factors and have been shown to be associated with various kinds of diseases and conditions, as has been shown by the significant associations among the genetic variations in vitamin D-related genes, health and disease outcomes.

References

Ahn, J., Yu, K., Stolzenberg-Solomon, R., Simon, K. C., McCullough, M. L., Gallicchio, L., Jacobs, E. J., Ascherio, A., Helzlsouer, K., Jacobs, K. B., Li, Q., Weinstein, S. J., Purdue, M., Virtamo, J., Horst, R., Wheeler, W., Chanock, S., Hunter, D. J., Hayes, R. B., … Albanes, D. (2010). Genome-wide association study of circulating vitamin D levels. *Human Molecular Genetics, 19*(13), 2739–2745. https://doi.org/10.1093/hmg/ddq155.

Bahrami, A., Sadeghnia, H. R., Tabatabaeizadeh, S. A., Bahrami-Taghanaki, H., Behboodi, N., Esmaeili, H., Ferns, G. A., Mobarhan, M. G., & Avan, A. (2018). Genetic and epigenetic factors influencing vitamin D status. *Journal of Cellular Physiology, 233*(5), 4033–4043. https://doi.org/10.1002/jcp.26216, http://onlinelibrary.wiley.com/journal/10.1002/(ISSN)1097-4652.

Bikle, D. D., & Schwartz, J. (2019). Vitamin D binding protein, total and free Vitamin D levels in different physiological and pathophysiological conditions. *Frontiers in Endocrinology, 10*(MAY). https://doi.org/10.3389/fendo.2019.00317, https://www.frontiersin.org/journals/endocrinology#.

Dastani, Z., Li, R., & Richards, B. (2013). Genetic regulation of vitamin D levels. *Calcified Tissue International, 92*(2), 106–117. https://doi.org/10.1007/s00223-012-9660-z, https://www.link.springer.de/link/service/journals/00223/index.htm.

Dauber, A., Nguyen, T. T., Sochett, E., Cole, D. E. C., Horst, R., Abrams, S. A., Carpenter, T. O., & Hirschhorn, J. N. (2012). Genetic defect in CYP24A1, the vitamin D 24-hydroxylase gene, in a patient with severe infantile hypercalcemia. *Journal of Clinical Endocrinology and Metabolism, 97*(2), E268. https://doi.org/10.1210/jc.2011-1972, http://jcem.endojournals.org/content/97/2/E268.full.pdf+html.

Demir, K., Kattan, W. E., Zou, M., Durmaz, E., BinEssa, H., Nalbantoğlu, Ö., Al-Rijjal, R. A., Meyer, B., Özkan, B., Shi, Y., & Brusgaard, K. (2015). Novel CYP27B1 gene mutations in patients with vitamin D-dependent rickets type 1A. *PLoS One, 10*(7), e0131376. https://doi.org/10.1371/journal.pone.0131376.

Dinour, D., Beckerman, P., Ganon, L., Tordjman, K., Eisenstein, Z., & Holtzman, E. J. (2013). Loss-of-function mutations of CYP24A1, the vitamin D 24-hydroxylase gene, cause long-standing hypercalciuric nephrolithiasis and nephrocalcinosis. *Journal of Urology, 190*(2), 552–557. https://doi.org/10.1016/j.juro.2013.02.3188.

Dollé, P., Fraulob, V., Kastner, P., & Chambon, P. (1994). Developmental expression of murine retinoid X receptor (RXR) genes. *Mechanisms of Development, 45*(2), 91–104. https://doi.org/10.1016/0925-4773(94)90023-x.

Germain, P., Chambon, P., Eichele, G., Evans, R. M., Lazar, M. A., Leid, M., De Lera, A. R., Lotan, R., Mangelsdorf, D. J., & Gronemeyer, H. (2006). International union of pharmacology. LXIII. Retinoid X receptors. *Pharmacological Reviews, 58*(4), 760–772. https://doi.org/10.1124/pr.58.4.7France, http://pharmrev.aspetjournals.org/cgi/reprint/58/4/760.

Haroon, M., & FitzGerald, O. M. (2012). Vitamin D deficiency and its repletion: A review of current knowledge and consensus recommendations. *Journal of Arthritis, 1*, 1–11.

Haussler, M. R., Haussler, C. A., Bartik, L., Whitfield, G. K., Hsieh, J. C., Slater, S., & Jurutka, P. W. (2008). Vitamin D receptor: Molecular signaling and actions of nutritional ligands in disease prevention. *Nutrition Reviews, 66*(2), S98–S112S98. https://doi.org/10.1111/j.1753-4887.2008.00093.x.

Haussler, M. R., Whitfield, G. K., Kaneko, I., Haussler, C. A., Hsieh, D., Hsieh, J. C., & Jurutka, P. W. (2013). Molecular mechanisms of vitamin D action. *Calcified Tissue International, 92*(2), 77–98. https://doi.org/10.1007/s00223-012-9619-0, https://www.link.springer.de/link/service/journals/00223/index.htm.

Hoseinkhani, Z., Rastegari-Pouyani, M., Tajemiri, F., Yari, K., & Mansouri, K. (2021). Association of vitamin D receptor polymorphisms (Fok1 (rs2228570), ApaI (rs7975232), BsmI (rs1544410), and TaqI (rs731236)) with gastric cancer among Kurdish population from west of Iran. *Reports of Biochemistry and Molecular Biology, 9*(4), 435–441. https://doi.org/10.52547/rbmb.9.4.435.

Jiang, X., Dimou, N. L., Al-Dabhani, K., Lewis, S. J., Martin, R. M., Haycock, P. C., Gunter, M. J., Key, T. J., Eeles, R. A., Muir, K., Neal, D., Giles, G. G., Giovannucci, E. L., Stampfer, M., Pierce, B. L., Schildkraut, J. M., Andersen, S. W., Thompson, D., Zheng, W., ... Tsilidis, K. K. (2019). Circulating vitamin D concentrations and risk of breast and prostate cancer: A Mendelian randomization study. *International Journal of Epidemiology, 48*(5), 1416–1424. https://doi.org/10.1093/ije/dyy284, http://ije.oxfordjournals.org/.

Karonova, T., Grineva, E., Belyaeva, O., Bystrova, A., Jude, E. B., Andreeva, A., Kostareva, A., & Pludowski, P. (2018). Relationship between vitamin D status and vitamin D receptor gene polymorphisms with markers of metabolic syndrome among adults. *Federation Frontiers in Endocrinology, 9*. https://doi.org/10.3389/fendo.2018.00448, https://www.frontiersin.org/articles/10.3389/fendo.2018.00448/full.

Krasniqi, E., Boshnjaku, A., Wagner, K. H., & Wessner, B. (2021). Association between polymorphisms in vitamin d pathway-related genes, vitamin D status, muscle mass and function: A systematic review. *Nutrients, 13*(9). https://doi.org/10.3390/nu13093109, https://www.mdpi.com/2072-6643/13/9/3109/pdf.

Lauter, K., & Arnold, A. (2009). Analysis of CYP27B1, encoding 25-hydroxyvitamin D-1α-hydroxylase, as a candidate tumor suppressor gene in primary and severe secondary/tertiary hyperparathyroidism. *Journal of Bone and Mineral Research, 24*(1), 102–104. https://doi.org/10.1359/jbmr.080903.

Leszczyńska, D., Szatko, A., Latocha, J., Kochman, M., Duchnowska, M., Wójcicka, A., Misiorowski, W., Zgliczyński, W., & Glinicki, P. (2024). Persistent hypercalcaemia associated with two pathogenic variants in the CYP24A1 gene and a parathyroid adenoma—A case report and review. *Frontiers in Endocrinology, 15*. https://doi.org/10.3389/fendo.2024.1355916.

Malik, S., Fu, L., Juras, D. J., Karmali, M., Wong, B. Y. L., Gozdzik, A., & Cole, D. E. C. (2013). Common variants of the vitamin D binding protein gene and adverse health outcomes. *Critical Reviews in Clinical Laboratory Sciences, 50*(1), 1–22. https://doi.org/10.3109/10408363.2012.750262.

Morrison, N. A., Qi, J. C., Tokita, A., Kelly, P. J., Crofts, L., Nguyen, T. V., Sambrook, P. N., & Eisman, J. A. (1994). Prediction of bone density from vitamin D receptor alleles. *Nature, 367*(6460), 284–287. https://doi.org/10.1038/367284a0.

Nagasawa, H., Uto, Y., Sasaki, H., Okamura, N., Murakami, A., Kubo, S., Kirk, K. L., & Hori, H. (2005). Japan Gc protein (vitamin D-binding protein): Gc genotyping and GcMAF precursor activity. *Anticancer Research, 25*(6 A), 3689–3695.

Reschly, E. J., & Krasowski, M. D. (2006). Evolution and function of the NR1I nuclear hormone receptor subfamily (VDR, PXR, and CAR) with respect to metabolism of xenobiotics and endogenous compounds. *Current Drug Metabolism, 7*(4), 349–365. https://doi.org/10.2174/138920006776873526, http://www.ingentaconnect.com/content/ben/cdm/2006/00000007/00000004/art00002.

Ruiz-Ojeda, F. J., Anguita-Ruiz, A., Leis, R., & Aguilera, C. M. (2018). Genetic factors and molecular mechanisms of vitamin D and obesity relationship. *Annals of Nutrition and Metabolism, 73*(2), 89–99. https://doi.org/10.1159/000490669, https://www.karger.ch/journals/anm/anm_jh.htm.

Sajjad, S., Munir, S., Simeen-Ber-Rahman, N., Saba, S., & Rehman (2017). VDR polymorphisms ApaI (rs7975232), TaqI (rs731236) and FokI (rs2228570) in Pakistani vitiligo patients and controls. *Journal of Pakistan Association of Dermatologists, 27*(2), 102–109. http://jpad.com.pk/index.php/jpad/article/download/1074/968.

Schlingmann, K. P., Kaufmann, M., Weber, S., Irwin, A., Goos, C., John, U., Misselwitz, J., Klaus, G., Kuwertz-Bröking, E., Fehrenbach, H., Wingen, A. M., Güran, T., Hoenderop, J. G., Bindels, R. J., Prosser, D. E., Jones, G., & Konrad, M. (2011). Mutations in CYP24A1 and idiopathic infantile hypercalcemia. *New England Journal of Medicine, 365*(5), 410–421. https://doi.org/10.1056/NEJMoa1103864, http://www.nejm.org/doi/pdf/10.1056/NEJMoa1103864.

Sorrenti, V., Buriani, A., Davinelli, S., Scapagnini, G., & Fortinguerra, S. (2023). Vitamin D physiology, deficiency, genetic influence, and the effects of daily vs. bolus doses of vitamin D on overall health: A clinical approach. *Nutraceuticals, 3*(3), 403–420. https://doi.org/10.3390/nutraceuticals3030030.

Usategui-Martín, R., De Luis-Román, D. A., Fernández-Gómez, J. M., Ruiz-Mambrilla, M., & Pérez-Castrillón, J. L. (2022). Vitamin D receptor (VDR) gene polymorphisms modify the response to vitamin D supplementation: A systematic review and meta-analysis. *Nutrients, 14*(2). https://doi.org/10.3390/nu14020360, https://www.mdpi.com/2072-6643/14/2/360/pdf.

Wjst, M., Altmüller, J., Faus-Kessler, T., Braig, C., Bahnweg, M., & André, E. (2006). Asthma families show transmission disequilibrium of gene variants in the vitamin D metabolism and signalling pathway. *Respiratory Research, 7*(1). https://doi.org/10.1186/1465-9921-7-60.

Zhang, Z., He, J. W., Fu, W. Z., Zhang, C. Q., & Zhang, Z. L. (2013). An analysis of the association between the vitamin D pathway and serum 25-hydroxyvitamin D levels in a healthy Chinese population. *Journal of Bone and Mineral Research, 28*(8), 1784–1792. https://doi.org/10.1002/jbmr.1926, http://onlinelibrary.wiley.com/journal/10.1002/(ISSN)1523-4681.

CHAPTER 9

Vitamin D disorders: proteomic and metabolomic perspectives

Munazza Raza Mirza, Soma Vankwani, and Rabia Sultan

Dr. Panjwani Center for Molecular Medicine and Drug Research, International Center for Chemical and Biological Sciences, Karachi, Pakistan

9.1 Vitamin D and its essential roles in cellular function and metabolism

Vitamin D is a fat-soluble vitamin crucial for various biological processes, including immune system regulation, cellular function, and calcium and phosphorus homeostasis. The two main forms of vitamin D are D2 (ergocalciferol), and D3 (cholecalciferol), identified by their respective backbones: ergosterol and cholesterol. While animals primarily produce vitamin D3, both forms can be metabolized into their active forms.

9.1.1 Synthesis and activation

Vitamin D3 synthesis begins in the skin when UVB rays are absorbed by 7-dehydrocholesterol, a precursor in cholesterol metabolism. This precursor is photochemically converted to pre-vitamin D3, which is then isomerized to form cholecalciferol (D3) (Bikle, 2014). It is believed that 7-dehydrocholesterol, including whether it is synthesized de novo in the epidermis or produced via the action of 7-dehydrocholesterol reductase (DHCR7).

The metabolic activation of vitamin D involves two hydroxylation stages.

9.1.1.1 Liver hydroxylation

The main circulating form of vitamin D, 25-hydroxyvitamin D (25[OH]D), is produced when 25-hydroxylase (CYP2R1) breaks down vitamin D3.

9.1.2 Kidney hydroxylation

The kidney's 1α-hydroxylase (CYP27B1) further transforms 25(OH)D into the physiologically active form of vitamin D, 1,25-dihydroxyvitamin D (1,25[OH]$_2$D$_3$, calcitriol) (Jones et al., 2014).

The Impact of Vitamin D on Health and Disease. DOI: https://doi.org/10.1016/B978-0-443-34037-6.00020-0

These metabolites attach to vitamin D binding protein (GC) and are carried through the bloodstream (White & Cooke, 2000). A similar activation route occurs for vitamin D2, which is obtained through diet (Holick, 2017). The vitamin D receptor (VDR), found on various cell types, serves as the binding site for calcitriol. This receptor-ligand complex regulates the expression of genes involved in immunological regulation, cellular proliferation, and calcium absorption, underscoring the importance of these enzymes and receptors in vitamin D metabolism.

9.1.3   Regulation of vitamin D: proteins and pathways

Vitamin D exerts its effects through two primary pathways:

9.1.3.1   Pathway dependent on nuclear receptors

The retinoid X receptor (RXR) and vitamin D receptor (VDR) create a heterodimer when $1,25(OH)_2D_3$ binds to the VDR. This complex regulates genes mostly involved in calcium and phosphorus metabolism by interacting with vitamin D response elements (VDREs) in DNA. By regulating absorption in the kidneys, intestines, and bones, this mechanism preserves mineral homeostasis (Goltzman, 2018).

9.1.3.2   Pathway independent of nuclear receptors

The membrane-associated rapid response steroid-binding protein (PDIA3) mediates the quick actions of $1,25(OH)_2D_3$. This route impacts immune responses, cell proliferation, and survival (Hii & Ferrante, 2016).

9.2   Proteomic studies in vitamin D deficiency

Proteomic research on vitamin D deprivation has revealed significant protein changes associated with metabolism, inflammation, and cellular homeostasis. A variety of proteomic techniques, including 2D-PAGE, MALDI-TOF-MS, ESI-QTOF-MS, and various other mass spectrometric analyzers (e.g., ion trap, triple quadrupole, Orbitrap, etc.), have been used to identify key proteins affected by vitamin D deficiency. For example, MMP9, ICAM3, and PODXL play important roles in cell adhesion, inflammation, and tissue remodeling (Zhang et al., 2024). Disruptions in glycolysis are evident in the detection of metabolic enzymes such as 6-phosphofructokinase and pyruvate kinase, typically identified using 2D-PAGE (Keeney et al., 2013).

Additionally, iTRAQ-nanoLC-MS/MS has been employed to identify blood coagulation-related proteins, including fibrinogen gamma chain and vitamin K-dependent protein C, suggesting a connection between vitamin D and hemostasis (Al-Daghri et al., 2016). Proteins like FETUB and multimeric adiponectin have also been linked to regulating ectopic calcification and insulin sensitivity, further highlighting the broader metabolic effects of vitamin D deprivation (Walker et al., 2014). A list of proteins associated with vitamin D deficiency, along with the proteomic techniques used to identify these protein markers, are shown in Table 9.1.

9.2.1 Techniques employed in proteomics research of vitamin D research

Proteomics has provided valuable insights into the systemic effects of vitamin D. The development of proteomics platforms has highlighted their critical role in deciphering the intricate protein interactions influenced by vitamin D, leading to a better understanding of its physiological and pathological functions. By analyzing protein expression and modification patterns, researchers can elucidate pathways impacted by vitamin D and its deficiencies.

There are two main techniques widely used in this field: 2D gel electrophoresis (2DGE) and mass spectrometry (MS). Conventional techniques like 2DGE-MS and 2DGE provide expression profiles of biological samples (e.g., serum, tissue, and other samples), offering insights into the biological impact of vitamin D. However, these methods have become less common in modern proteomic research due to limitations in sensitivity and resolution. Despite this, they remain foundational for detecting differentially expressed proteins, particularly in vitamin D research.

Recent advancements in MS and nano-flow liquid chromatography have greatly enhanced the ability to explore previously uncharacterized protein networks regulated by vitamin D. Advanced protein analysis techniques such as MALDI-TOF, ESI, QTOF, and Orbitrap MS have significantly advanced the study of vitamin D's complex biological functions. MS is essential for identifying proteins in complex biological samples and understanding how vitamin D influences the proteomic landscape (Bromirski, 2018; Rochat, 2019).

The accurate quantification of designated proteins is made possible by triple quadrupole (QQQ) devices, which are particularly well-suited for targeted proteomics. However, compared to Orbitrap and TOF systems, QQQ devices have lower mass resolution and slower scan speeds, which makes them less appropriate for nontargeted proteomics (Rochat, 2019). Developments in MS and nano-flow liquid chromatography have expanded the depth of proteomic analysis, allowing the exploration of protein networks that were previously unknown to be regulated by vitamin D.

Among these, ESI Orbitrap is particularly notable due to its high mass resolution, sensitivity, and robustness, making it ideal for shotgun proteomics, a high-throughput approach for identifying large numbers of proteins in complex samples.

Table 9.1 Proteins identified in vitamin D deficiency and their detection techniques.

S.No	Proteins	ID	Technique	Functions	References
1	MMP9	H0XAI0	iTRAQ-coupled LC-MS/MS	Tissue remodeling, recruitment of proinflammatory agents	Zhang et al. (2024).
	ICAM3	H0XAH7		Cell adhesion, inflammation	
	PODXL(podocalyxin)	A0A5F9CFN3		Regulation and protection of podocytes against inflammation	
	ApoF (apolipoprotein F)	Q13790		Synthesis, secretion, metabolism of lipoproteins	
2	6-Phosphofructokinase	P17858	2D-PAGE	Glycolysis	Keeney et al. (2013)
	Triose phosphate isomerase	A0A6P5QYN2			
	Pyruvate kinase	A0A5F9CFN3			
	Peroxiredoxin-3	A0A5F9CFN3		Peroxidase activity, mitochondria	
	DJ-1/PARK7	A0A3Q7TWT6			
	Peptidyl–prolyl cis–trans isomerase A (cyclophilin A)	A0A5F9CFN3		Protein folding, regulation of protein kinases and phosphatases, immunoregulation, cell signaling, and redox status	
3	Vitamin K-dependent protein C	X5D5A9	iTRAQ-nano-LCMS/MS	Blood coagulation	Al-Daghri et al. (2016)
	Von Willebrand factor	X5D5A9			
	Fibrinogen gamma chain	A0A7L3L4Z6			
	Multimerin-1	H0XAI0			
4	Multimeric adiponectin	H0XAI0	2D-electrophoresis	Insulin-sensitizing effects, food intake, and body weight regulation, cardioprotective, antiinflammatory, antioxidant effect	Walker et al. (2014).
5	FETUB	A0A452RLE8	2D-Electrophoresis, LCMS/MS	Protein inhibitor of systemic ectopic calcification	Walker et al. (2018)

#	Protein	Method	UniProt ID	Function	Reference
6	Drebrin	2-DE, MALDI-TOF-MS	A0A3Q7TWT6	Dendritic spine formation	Almeras et al. (2007)
	Ox6a1		H0XAI0	Oxidative phosphorylation system	
	Pdx5		H0XAI0	Redox balance	
	Pdx6		H0XAI0		
	Vdac2		A0A6P5R0L9	Calcium homeostasis and ATP transport	
	Grp78		A0A3P8K320	Chaperone proteins, proteosomes	
	Hs7c, Hs70p5		A0A3P8K320		
	Uchl1		A0A6P5QYN2		
	Psa2, Psa5		A0A5F9CFN3		
	Tpm1		A0A8C7G4G5	Organelle transport	
	RhoA		A0A5F9CFN3		
7	ApoE	QBB using SOMAscan aptamer-based affinity proteomics platform	Q8TCZ8	Synthesis of apolipoproteins	(Mousa et al., 2024)
	LRP1B		H0XAH7	Tumor suppressor, regulation of blood-brain barrier integrity	
	PEBP1		H2L6B7	Inflammation	
	SOD1		P00441		
	ANXA2		P07355		
	CAMK2D		A0A3Q7THT9	Calcium and bone metabolism	
	IBSP		A0A852FHE6		
	TNFRSF17		A0A5F9CFN3	B-cell development and autoimmune response	
	LSAMP		H0XAI0	Tumor suppressor	
	GHRL		A0A7L3LSR2	Appetite regulation	

9.2.1.1   Examples of mass spectrometry-based studies

Vitamin D insufficiency is linked to a variety of systemic problems, including cardiovascular disease, cancer, and autoimmune issues. Proteomic studies have begun to reveal the complicated mechanisms that underpin these relationships. Proteomics is a great tool for correlating vitamin D status with disease pathophysiology because it identifies differentially expressed proteins and pathways.

9.2.1.1.1   Vitamin D associated with cardiovascular risk

Several studies explored the role of vitamin D in cardiovascular complications. The effects of vitamin D supplementation on cardiovascular risk proteins in overweight individuals, with a focus on sex-based differences, were observed in a study. Proteomic analyses revealed sex-specific changes in proteins related to coagulation, highlighting the need for tailored vitamin D interventions based on gender(Al-Daghri et al., 2016). Additionally, animal models of CVD and atherosclerosis (AS) showed significant alterations in protein expression related to oxidative stress, inflammation, and energy metabolism (Almofti et al., 2006; Wang et al., 2011). These findings suggest that vitamin D's role in cardiovascular health varies by sex and may be crucial in understanding CVD and AS progression, offering potential targets for diagnostics and treatments.

9.2.1.1.2   Vitamin D and calcium-binding proteins

Prenatal vitamin D deficiency was found to alter the expression of calcium-binding proteins in the brains of adult rats. These changes were associated with disruptions in pathways related to oxidative phosphorylation, calcium homeostasis, and synaptic plasticity. This dysfunction may contribute to neurodevelopmental disorders such as schizophrenia and multiple sclerosis. Vitamin D deficiency (DVD) induces long-term dysregulation of proteins essential for mitochondrial function, cytoskeleton maintenance, and neurotransmission. Proteomic analysis of the frontal cortex and hippocampus revealed significantly lower expression of 36 proteins, with 89% downregulated. As per mitochondrial dysfunction, three oxidative phosphorylation components and two redox balance regulators were downregulated, affecting ATP production and cellular homeostasis. While in cytoskeletal alterations, proteins linked to cytoskeletal stability and organelle transport, such as RhoA and Drebrin, were dysregulated. Four neurotransmission-related proteins and three synaptic plasticity regulators showed reduced expression in neurotransmission impairments. Similarly, pathological associations showed 15 dysregulated proteins, which were also downregulated in schizophrenia or multiple sclerosis, suggesting a potential link between DVD deficiency and neurological disorders (Almeras et al., 2007).

9.2.1.1.3 Proteomic study of maternal vitamin D deficiency

An important LCMS orbitrap-based proteomic study investigated the effect of prenatal vitamin D deprivation on mice lung development. This study analyzed fetal and postnatal lung tissues and discovered that proteome changes were more significant on postnatal day 7 than during fetal development. Key modulated proteins included those involved in lung maturation, demonstrating the significance of maternal vitamin D levels in postnatal organ development (Chen et al., 2016).

Although transcriptomics and proteomics provide useful information about the molecular mechanisms of 1,25(OH)$_2$D, more studies using different cell lines and experimental setups are required to fully understand the range of vitamin D's effects, particularly in cancer. More thorough research may be able to pinpoint a common molecular program that vitamin D modulates and its possible connection to carcinogenesis.

Many biological processes are significantly regulated by vitamin D, and the nuclear vitamin D receptor (VDR) is the primary mechanism via which it mediates its effects. A sequence of protein-protein interactions, such as the heterodimerization of VDR with retinoid X receptor (RXR), the recruitment of coactivators such as CBP/p300, SRC-16, and BAF57, and the activation of RNA polymerase II for transcription, change gene expression when 1,25-dihydroxyvitamin D (1,25(OH)$_2$D) binds to VDR. In addition to the traditional genomic pathway, 1,25(OH)$_2$D also triggers nongenomic signaling pathways, including MAP kinases JNK and ERK, protein kinase C (PKC), and phospholipase C (PLC). These quick effects of vitamin D have created new opportunities for proteomics research, especially in figuring out how vitamin D affects protein interactions and biological functions like apoptosis, and cell division.

9.2.2 *Broader implications of vitamin D research*

Vitamin D insufficiency is linked to various systemic disorders, including cardiovascular diseases, cancer, and autoimmune conditions. Proteomic studies have begun to uncover the complex molecular mechanisms that underlie these associations. Proteomics offers a powerful tool for correlating vitamin D status with disease pathophysiology by identifying differentially expressed proteins and signaling pathways. However, further research is needed to fully understand the range of vitamin D's effects on cellular functions, particularly in the context of cancer and other chronic diseases.

Proteomic techniques, including 2D gel electrophoresis and MS, are instrumental in advancing our understanding of how vitamin D influences protein interactions and biological functions. These studies provide insights into how vitamin D may modulate pathways related to apoptosis, cell division, and cellular signaling, offering potential therapeutic targets for various diseases (Zhang & Yao, 2000).

9.3 Metabolomics studies in vitamin D deficiency

Vitamin D metabolism is a complex process involving synthesis, conversion, and activation, resulting in several active and inactive forms, each with distinct physiological roles. Vitamin D is sourced through sunlight exposure, dietary intake, or supplements. When the skin is exposed to ultraviolet B (UVB) radiation, 7-dehydrocholesterol is converted into cholecalciferol (vitamin D_3). This precursor undergoes hydroxylation in the liver to form 25-hydroxyvitamin D (25(OH)D). In the kidneys, 25(OH)D is further hydroxylated to form 1,25-dihydroxyvitamin D (1,25(OH)$_2$D), the biologically active hormone with diverse physiological effects (Muscogiuri et al., 2014).

In addition to the primary metabolites 25(OH)D and 1,25(OH)$_2$D, other bioactive derivatives, such as 24,25-dihydroxy vitamin D and conjugated metabolites, contribute in maintaining balance within the vitamin D metabolic pathway. Vitamin D deficiency is associated with a wide range of health conditions, including primary diseases directly linked to vitamin D metabolism and secondary disorders indirectly related to cardiovascular diseases, cancers, autoimmune disorders, neuropsychiatric diseases, and endocrine dysfunctions. The below sections focus on metabolomics profiling of primary diseases related to vitamin D metabolism (Holick, 2017).

9.3.1 Techniques employed in metabolomics

Metabolomics is the study of metabolites—the small molecules involved in metabolic processes—in cells, tissues, and organisms. Unlike genomics, transcriptomics, and proteomics, which focus on DNA, RNA, and proteins, metabolomics emphasizes the end products of cellular processes (metabolites), providing a detailed insight into the biochemical state of an organism. Over the past two decades, advances in technology and data analysis have significantly expanded the field of metabolomics. Key techniques that have revolutionized this field include chromatography, MS, capillary electrophoresis, and nuclear magnetic resonance (NMR) spectroscopy.

Chromatographic techniques, including gas chromatography (GC) and liquid chromatography (LC), are commonly used to separate metabolites. LC is particularly suitable for polar metabolites (e.g., amino acids, organic acids), while GC is ideal for volatile compounds (e.g., fatty acids, alcohols). MS is a cornerstone of modern metabolomics due to its high sensitivity, specificity, and ability to measure a wide range of metabolites. When coupled with chromatographic techniques like LC–MS or GC–MS, MS enhances separation efficiency and detection sensitivity, making it critical for comprehensive metabolomics profiling. MS works by ionizing metabolites and measuring their mass-to-charge ratio (*m/z*). LC–MS is effective for polar and thermally labile compounds, while GC–MS is suitable for volatile or thermally stable metabolites.

Capillary electrophoresis (CE) is another advanced technique used in metabolomics, particularly for analyzing ionic and charged metabolites. CE offers high-resolution separation based on the size and charge of molecules, making it ideal for profiling amino acids, organic acids, and nucleotides. When integrated with MS (CE–MS), it enables precise identification and quantification of charged metabolites with minimal sample preparation. NMR spectroscopy, a nondestructive technique, provides structural information about metabolites based on their interaction with magnetic fields. Although NMR has lower sensitivity compared to MS, it is highly reproducible and can quantify metabolites without the need for complex sample preparation, making it ideal for profiling water-soluble metabolites such as amino acids, organic acids, and sugars.

Metabolomics generates vast amounts of data, requiring advanced bioinformatics tools for data processing, normalization, and analysis. Statistical techniques such as principal component analysis (PCA) and partial least squares discriminant analysis (PLS-DA) are used to identify patterns in metabolite profiles and correlate them with disease conditions. Machine learning algorithms are increasingly being used to predict metabolic trends, identify potential biomarkers, and interpret complex datasets, providing deeper insights into disease mechanisms and therapeutic interventions. The current chapter examines the connection between metabolomics and vitamin D metabolism, with a focus on studies linked to vitamin D and its associated metabolites using various metabolomics profiling techniques (Danzi et al., 2023; Meng et al., 2024).

9.3.2   *Metabolomics profiling of primary diseases of vitamin D metabolism*

Metabolomics profiling provides valuable insights into how vitamin D impacts broader metabolic pathways, helping to identify potential biomarkers for early diagnosis and targeted therapies. Primary diseases related to vitamin D metabolism arise from abnormalities in synthesis, activation, or physiological functions of vitamin D, leading to imbalances in calcium and phosphate homeostasis—critical for bone health and overall metabolic stability. These diseases can be broadly categorized into those caused by vitamin D deficiency (hypovitaminosis) and those resulting from vitamin D excess (hypervitaminosis).

Vitamin D deficiency diseases, such as rickets and osteomalacia, are classic examples of conditions associated with vitamin D deficiency, affecting children and adults, respectively. These conditions arise from impaired calcium and phosphate absorption, leading to defective bone mineralization. Metabolomics studies have revealed key biomarkers for rickets, including metabolites involved in energy metabolism, amino acid metabolism, and the tricarboxylic acid (TCA) cycle, which could potentially enable non-invasive diagnostic approaches. In animal models, such as calcium-deficient rats, metabolomics analyses using UPLC/Q-TOF MS/MS have identified disruptions in amino acid metabolism, lipid metabolism, and the TCA cycle, providing deeper insight into the systemic impact of calcium deficiency (Meng et al., 2020).

In a study of Hong Kong, Chinese individuals, serum metabolomics profiling with LC-MS identified 102 metabolites significantly correlating with serum 25-hydroxyvitamin D (25(OH)

D) levels, with 27 metabolites validated during follow-up. A meta-analysis confirmed 13 metabolites, primarily lipids, that strongly correlated with vitamin D levels, with docosahex-aenoylcarnitine and eicosapentaenoylcholine showing the most significant association. These findings highlight the link between vitamin D status and lipid metabolism, suggesting lipid-related metabolites as valuable markers for assessing vitamin D's role in health.

Osteoporosis, a chronic manifestation of vitamin D deficiency, shows a metabolomic signature marked by reduced bone turnover markers and lower vitamin D metabolites, suggesting a need for targeted interventions. A study in Shanghai involving 320 participants (males and postmenopausal females) used serum metabolomic profiling and bone turnover markers (BTMs) to examine their association with bone mineral density (BMD) and osteoporosis. Key metabolites identified included valerylcarnitine, lysophosphatidylcholine (16:0), lysophosphatidylcholine (18:1), and glycine in males, and phosphatidylcholine (36:4), lysophosphatidylcholine (18:2), sphingomyelin (34:1), and serine in postmenopausal females. These metabolites improved the sensitivity of osteoporosis detection models, with random forest-based feature selection revealing their diagnostic potential.

Research on vitamin D supplementation has revealed its complex, dose-dependent effects on metabolic and musculoskeletal health. One study highlighted significant variability in genomic and metabolomic responses to different doses of vitamin D3, suggesting that higher doses of vitamin D significantly alter serum 25(OH)D levels, parathyroid hormone (PTH) levels, and gene expression (Shirvani et al., 2020). Another study on postmenopausal women with vitamin D insufficiency showed that a daily dose of 70 μg of vitamin D3 raised serum levels of 25(OH)D and 1,25(OH)2D, while also increasing metabolites such as carnitine, choline, urea, and creatinine. However, these metabolites showed a negative correlation with muscle strength and physical performance, indicating that despite improved vitamin D status, supplementation may adversely affect skeletal muscle health (Bislev et al., 2020).

9.3.3 Metabolomics-based biomarkers in vitamin D diseases

Accurately assessing vitamin D status is crucial for diagnosing and monitoring its levels, which can be categorized as deficiency, sufficiency, or excess. Traditionally, the total serum concentration of 25-hydroxyvitamin D [25(OH)D] has been the gold standard for evaluating vitamin D status due to its ability to reflect both dietary intake and sunlight-derived vitamin D. 25(OH)D is a reliable marker because it has a relatively long half-life of 15–20 days and is independent of the body's calcium and phosphate homeostasis mechanisms. As a result, it provides a stable and consistent measure of vitamin D exposure over time, making it invaluable in clinical practice for assessing deficiency, sufficiency, or intoxication (Seamans & Cashman, 2009).

However, the relationship between 25(OH)D levels and health outcomes is complex, influenced by factors like the time of day, seasonal changes, and individual metabolic variability. Additionally, 25(OH)D offers a limited view of the broader metabolic activity of vitamin D, prompting interest in identifying complementary biomarkers for a more comprehensive understanding of vitamin D's role in health.

One promising candidate is the vitamin D metabolite ratio (VMR), the ratio of 24,25-dihydroxyvitamin D to 25(OH)D. The VMR has shown a stronger correlation with parathyroid hormone (PTH) levels than 25(OH)D alone, making it a sensitive biomarker for vitamin D deficiency. Studies have also found that a low VMR ($< 4\%$) is associated with higher all-cause mortality, further emphasizing its clinical relevance (Ladang et al., 2024).

References

Al-Daghri, N. M., Alokail, M. S., Manousopoulou, A., Heinson, A., Al-Attas, O., Al-Saleh, Y., Sabico, S., Yakout, S., Woelk, C. H., Chrousos, G. P., & Garbis, S. D. (2016). Sex-specific vitamin D effects on blood coagulation among overweight adults. *European Journal of Clinical Investigation, 46*(12), 1031–1040. https://doi.org/10.1111/eci.12688, http://www3.interscience.wiley.com/journal/118482631/home.

Almeras, L., Eyles, D., Benech, P., Laffite, D., Villard, C., Patatian, A., Boucraut, J., Mackay-Sim, A., McGrath, J., & Féron, F. (2007). Developmental vitamin D deficiency alters brain protein expression in the adult rat: Implications for neuropsychiatric disorders. *Proteomics, 7*(5), 769–780. https://doi.org/10.1002/pmic.200600392.

Almofti, M. R., Huang, Z., Yang, P., Rui, Y., & Yang, P. (2006). Proteomic analysis of rat aorta during atherosclerosis induced by high cholesterol diet and injection of vitamin D3. *Clinical and Experimental Pharmacology and Physiology, 33*(4), 305–309. https://doi.org/10.1111/j.1440-1681.2006.04366.x.

Bikle, D. D. (2014). Vitamin D metabolism, mechanism of action, and clinical applications. *Chemistry & Biology, 21*(3), 319–329. https://doi.org/10.1016/j.chembiol.2013.12.016.

Bislev, L. S., Sundekilde, U. K., Kilic, E., Dalsgaard, T. K., Rejnmark, L., & Bertram, H. C. (2020). Circulating levels of muscle-related metabolites increase in response to a daily moderately high dose of a vitamin d3 supplement in women with vitamin d insufficiency—secondary analysis of a randomized placebo-controlled trial. *Nutrients, 12*(5). https://doi.org/10.3390/nu12051310, https://www.mdpi.com/2072-6643/12/5/1310/pdf.

Bromirski, M. (2018). First choice in high resolution mass spectrometry with Orbitrap mass analyzer technology for screening, confirmative and quantitative analyses. Thermo Scientific. White Paper, Thermo Scientific. White Paper.

Chen, L., Wilson, R., Bennett, E., & Zosky, G. R. (2016). Identification of vitamin D sensitive pathways during lung development. *Respiratory Research, 17*(1). https://doi.org/10.1186/s12931-016-0362-3, http://respiratory-research.com/home/.

Danzi, F., Pacchiana, R., Mafficini, A., Scupoli, M. T., Scarpa, A., Donadelli, M., & Fiore, A. (2023). To metabolomics and beyond: A technological portfolio to investigate cancer metabolism. *Signal Transduction and Targeted Therapy, 8*(1). https://doi.org/10.1038/s41392-023-01380-0, https://www.nature.com/sigtrans.

Goltzman, D. (2018). Functions of vitamin D in bone. *Histochemistry and Cell Biology, 149*(4), 305–312. https://doi.org/10.1007/s00418-018-1648-y.

Hii, C. S., & Ferrante, A. (2016). The non-genomic actions of vitamin D. *Nutrients, 8*(3). https://doi.org/10.3390/nu8030135, http://www.mdpi.com/2072-6643/8/3/135/pdf.

Holick, M. F. (2017). The vitamin D deficiency pandemic: Approaches for diagnosis, treatment and prevention. *Reviews in Endocrine and Metabolic Disorders, 18*(2), 153–165. https://doi.org/10.1007/s11154-017-9424-1.

Jones, G., Prosser, D. E., & Kaufmann, M. (2014). Cytochrome P450-mediated metabolism of vitamin D. *Journal of Lipid Research, 55*(1), 13–31. https://doi.org/10.1194/jlr.R031534, http://www.jlr.org/content/55/1/13.full.pdf+html.

Keeney, J. T. R., Förster, S., Sultana, R., Brewer, L. D., Latimer, C. S., Cai, J., Klein, J. B., Porter, N. M., & Butterfield, D. A. (2013). Dietary vitamin D deficiency in rats from middle to old age leads to elevated tyrosine nitration and proteomics changes in levels of key proteins in brain: Implications for low vitamin D-dependent age-related cognitive decline. *Free Radical Biology and Medicine, 65*, 324–334. https://doi.org/10.1016/j.freeradbiomed.2013.07.019.

Ladang, A., Gendebien, A. S., Kovacs, S., Demonceau, C., Beaudart, C., Peeters, S., Alokail, M. S., Al-Daghri, N. M., Le Goff, C., Reginster, J. Y., Bruyere, O., & Cavalier, E. (2024). Investigation of the vitamin D metabolite ratio (VMR) as a marker of functional vitamin D deficiency: Findings from the SarcoPhAge cohort. *Nutrients, 16*(19). https://doi.org/10.3390/nu16193224, http://www.mdpi.com/journal/nutrients/.

Meng, F., Fan, L., Sun, L., Yu, Q., Wang, M., & Sun, C. (2020). Serum biomarkers of the calcium-deficient rats identified by metabolomics based on UPLC/Q-TOF MS/MS. *Nutrition & Metabolism, 17*(1). https://doi.org/10.1186/s12986-020-00507-2.

Meng, X., Liu, Y., Xu, S., Yang, L., & Yin, R. (2024). Review on analytical technologies and applications in metabolomics. *Biocell, 48*(1), 65–78. https://doi.org/10.32604/biocell.2023.045986.

Mousa, H., Al saei, A., Razali, R. M., & Zughaier, S. M. (2024). Vitamin D status affects proteomic profile of HDL-associated proteins and inflammatory mediators in dyslipidemia. *Journal of Nutritional Biochemistry, 123*. https://doi.org/10.1016/j.jnutbio.2023.109472, www.elsevier.com/locate/jnutbio.

Muscogiuri, G., Mitri, J., Mathieu, C., Badenhoop, K., Tamer, G., Orio, F., Mezza, T., Vieth, R., Colao, A., & Pittas, A. (2014). Mechanisms in endocrinology: Vitamin D as a potential contributor in endocrine health and disease. *European Journal of Endocrinology, 171*(3), R101. https://doi.org/10.1530/eje-14-0158.

Rochat, B. (2019). *Quantitative and qualitative LC-high-resolution MS: The technological and biological reasons for a shift of paradigm.* IntechOpen. https://doi.org/10.5772/intechopen.81285.

Seamans, K. M., & Cashman, K. D. (2009). Existing and potentially novel functional markers of vitamin D status: A systematic review. *The American Journal of Clinical Nutrition, 89*(6), 1997S. https://doi.org/10.3945/ajcn.2009.27230d.

Shirvani, A., Kalajian, T. A., Song, A., Allen, R., Charoenngam, N., Lewanczuk, R., & Holick, M. F. (2020). Variable genomic and metabolomic responses to varying doses of vitamin D supplementation. *Anticancer Research, 40*(1), 535–543. https://doi.org/10.21873/anticanres.13982, http://ar.iiarjournals.org/content/40/1/535.full.pdf.

Walker, G. E., Follenzi, A., Bruscaggin, V., Manfredi, M., Bellone, S., Marengo, E., Maiuri, L., Prodam, F., & Bona, G. (2018). Fetuin B links vitamin D deficiency and pediatric obesity: Direct negative regulation by vitamin D. *Journal of Steroid Biochemistry and Molecular Biology, 182*, 37–49. https://doi.org/10.1016/j.jsbmb.2018.04.009, www.elsevier.com/locate/jsbmb.

Walker, G. E., Ricotti, R., Roccio, M., Moia, S., Bellone, S., Prodam, F., Bona, G., & Palau, F. (2014). Pediatric obesity and vitamin D deficiency: A proteomic approach identifies multimeric adiponectin as a key link between these conditions. *PLoS ONE, 9*(1), e83685. https://doi.org/10.1371/journal.pone.0083685.

Wang, Q. Q., Zhao, X., & Pu, X. P. (2011). Proteome analysis of the left ventricle in the vitamin D 3 and nicotine-induced rat vascular calcification model. *Journal of proteomics, 74*(4), 480–489. https://doi.org/10.1016/j.jprot.2010.12.010.

White, P., & Cooke, N. (2000). The multifunctional properties and characteristics of vitamin D-binding protein. *Trends in Endocrinology & Metabolism, 11*(8), 320–327. https://doi.org/10.1016/s1043-2760(00)00317-9.

Zhang, J., & Yao, Z. (2000). Effect of 1,25(OH)2D3 on the growth and apoptosis of breast cancer cell line MCF-7. *Chinese Medical Journal, 113*(2), 124–128.

Zhang, L., Wang, Z., Wang, X., Wei, L., Zhang, B., & Yang, L. (2024). Comparative proteomic exploration of plasma proteins in different levels of vitamin D with type 2 diabetes mellitus using iTRAQ-coupled LC-MS/MS. *Journal of Diabetes & Metabolic Disorders, 23*(2), 2001–2010. https://doi.org/10.1007/s40200-024-01456-w.

CHAPTER 10

Global perspectives on vitamin D

Tarek Arabi[1], Belal Nedal Sabbah[1], and Dileep Kumar Rohra[2]
[1]*College of Medicine, Alfaisal University, Riyadh, Saudi Arabia* [2]*Department of Pharmacology, College of Medicine, Alfaisal University, Riyadh, Saudi Arabia*

10.1 Introduction

Vitamin D, frequently called the sunshine vitamin, is essential for human well-being, well beyond its most commonly recognized role in bone strength. Recently, public health experts worldwide have recognized that vitamin D deficiency is widespread and may significantly impact overall health (Palacios & Gonzalez, 2014). Here, we take a global look at vitamin D—exploring how common deficiency is in different regions and what is being done about it, with attention to regional differences in vitamin D status, assessment, and treatment.

We now know vitamin D's importance cannot be overstated. While its role in bone health is well known, research has linked vitamin D to many other processes—from supporting the immune system to influencing heart and mental health (Hossein-Nezhad & Holick, 2013). A key discovery was finding vitamin D receptors in many different tissues (Bikle, 2016). This means vitamin D is not just a calcium regulator, but acts like a hormone with effects throughout the body. Studies suggest it helps control cell growth, keeps muscles and nerves working properly, supports immunity, and reduces inflammation (Aranow, 2011). Furthermore, there are data that support the role of vitamin D in preventing chronic diseases, including certain cancers, autoimmune conditions, and heart disease (Wang et al., 2017).

Despite vitamin D's importance, deficiency remains a persistent global issue. Many factors determine a person's vitamin D level: where they live, their lifestyle, and what they eat. The main source of vitamin D is sunlight—our skin makes vitamin D when exposed to UVB rays. But modern life often means less time in the sun. In many places, sunlight alone is not enough to maintain healthy vitamin D levels year-round (Srivastava, 2021). People may spend most of their day indoors or live in northern regions where the winter sun is too weak, which contributes to widespread vitamin D insufficiency.

The worldwide prevalence of vitamin D deficiency is striking. One review called vitamin D deficiency a global pandemic, affecting people of all ages and regions (Hilger et al., 2014). Surprisingly, even some very sunny places have high deficiency rates due to factors like

The Impact of Vitamin D on Health and Disease. DOI: https://doi.org/10.1016/B978-0-443-34037-6.00026-1

cultural dress (covering most of the skin), darker skin pigmentation, and indoor lifestyles (Hilger et al., 2014).

In this overview, we examine the complex mix of factors influencing vitamin D status around the world. We will see how deficiency rates vary across regions, how latitude, cultural habits, and diet contribute to those differences, and why it is challenging to set one global "normal" range for vitamin D. We will also discuss the ongoing debate about what optimal vitamin D levels should be since different organizations recommend different cutoffs. Finally, we will explore public health efforts to combat vitamin D deficiency, from fortifying foods and supplement programs to education campaigns, and consider their successes and challenges.

Conclusively, one thing becomes clear: addressing vitamin D deficiency is not a one-size-fits-all task. The interplay between physiology, environment, and culture means we need nuanced, culturally sensitive approaches to combat vitamin D deficiency worldwide. By understanding these global perspectives, we can better inform future research, policies, and health strategies.

10.2   Varied prevalence of vitamin D deficiency worldwide

10.2.1   The vitamin D paradox: unexpected deficiencies

It might seem intuitive that vitamin D deficiency occurs mostly in places with little sun. In reality, even some of the sunniest regions have surprisingly high rates of vitamin D deficiency (Szalay et al., 2011). This counterintuitive trend shows that sunlight alone is not the whole story.

A prime example comes from the Middle East and North Africa. Despite abundant year-round sunshine, these regions report some of the highest vitamin D deficiency rates in the world. A systematic review found that in this region, between 12% and 96% of children and adolescents and 44%–96% of adults had vitamin D levels below 20 ng/mL—a common threshold for deficiency (Chakhtoura et al., 2018). These extreme ranges indicate that factors other than sunlight (such as clothing that limits sun exposure, spending time indoors, or diet) heavily influence vitamin D status.

Likewise, India enjoys plenty of sunlight but still has widespread vitamin D deficiency. In India, about 80%–90% of people were found to be vitamin D deficient (Aparna et al., 2018), likely due to a combination of indoor lifestyles, air pollution, and skin pigmentation factors. Even Australia—known for its sunshine and outdoor lifestyle—faces this issue. A national study found that 31% of Australian adults over 25 had vitamin D levels below 50 nmol/L, indicating deficiency (Daly et al., 2012). Conclusively, no population is deemed safe from vitamin D deficiency, even if its environment receives frequent, ample sunshine.

10.2.2   Factors influencing vitamin D levels

Why do so many people lack vitamin D, even in sunny places? Several factors are at play:

* Geography (latitude and season): Location matters. Above roughly 33° latitude (north or south), the winter sun's UVB rays are too weak to trigger vitamin D production in the skin, creating a "vitamin D winter" (Holick et al., 2011; O'Neill et al., 2016).
* Urban living: City dwellers often have lower vitamin D levels than rural residents. For example, a study in Belgium found urban residents had lower vitamin D than those in the countryside at the same latitude, likely because air pollution in cities (like ozone) blocks some UVB sunlight (Manicourt & Devogelaer, 2008).
* Skin pigmentation: Melanin, which makes skin darker, reduces the skin's ability to produce vitamin D from sunlight. Thus, individuals with darker skin generally need more sun exposure to make adequate vitamin D compared to those with lighter skin (Raymond-Lezman & Riskin, 2023). This can put darker-skinned populations at higher risk of deficiency, especially in low-sunlight environments.
* Modern lifestyles: Many people spend much of their time indoors (at work, school, etc.), which dramatically cuts down sun exposure. A systematic review found vitamin D deficiency in roughly 80% of shift workers and 78% of indoor workers, compared to about 48% of outdoor workers (Sowah et al., 2017). This shows how our work and lifestyle habits contribute to the vitamin D gap.

10.2.3   The elusive "normal" range

Defining a "normal" or sufficient vitamin D level in the blood is surprisingly complicated. Different health organizations have set different benchmarks, leading to some confusion.

In the United States, the Institute of Medicine (IOM) considers a blood 25(OH)D level below 20 ng/mL (50 nmol/L) as vitamin D deficient (Ross et al., 2011). Meanwhile, the Endocrine Society's recent guidelines avoid strict cutoffs altogether, suggesting that context matters and no single number fits all (Demay et al., 2024).

Emerging research also indicates that vitamin D needs may vary between groups of people. For example, a study found Black Americans tend to have lower measured 25(OH)D levels and lower vitamin D–binding protein levels than White Americans, yet the Black participants had higher bone density and calcium levels. This implies that a "low" vitamin D level on a lab test may have different health implications in different ethnic groups (Powe et al., 2013). In other words, the clinical significance of a given vitamin D level can depend on genetic and ethnic background.

Regional differences highlight the same issue. One national study found that people living in certain northern parts of a country had a higher risk of vitamin D deficiency than those in the south (Hu et al., 2022). And broadly, the Middle East has a higher prevalence of deficiency compared to many other parts of the world (Cui et al., 2023). All of this suggests that a one-size-fits-all standard for "normal" vitamin D may not be appropriate worldwide.

10.2.4   Toward a consensus: challenges and opportunities

Experts are exploring ways to develop more tailored vitamin D guidelines to account for these differences. A few ideas have been proposed:

• Population-specific recommendations: Some countries set their own vitamin D intake guidelines based on local needs. For instance, the United Kingdom recommends 400 IU per day for most adults up to age 65, while France recommends 200 IU/day for nonpregnant adults (Battault et al., 2013). These differences reflect attempts to tailor advice to local diet, sun exposure, and lifestyle factors.

• Genetic insights: Research has identified genetic variations that affect vitamin D status. Certain gene variants influence how vitamin D is synthesized and transported in the body, and these variants are more common in some ethnic groups (Wang et al., 2010). Such findings show that genetics can influence vitamin D levels and may need to be considered in the future.

• Functional measures: Instead of relying only on vitamin D blood levels, some scientists look at functional indicators of health. One study examined how much vitamin D was needed to suppress parathyroid hormone (PTH), which rises when vitamin D is low. It turned out about 20 ng/mL of 25(OH)D was enough for African-American women, whereas about 30 ng/mL was needed for Caucasian women to achieve the same effect (Wright et al., 2012). This suggests that optimal vitamin D levels might differ among groups when judged by physiological outcomes.

10.3   Public health initiatives

Recognizing the scope of vitamin D deficiency, many countries have launched public health initiatives to improve vitamin D status. These efforts vary but generally include food fortification, supplementation programs, education campaigns, and international collaborations. Here are some key strategies and how they're working:

10.3.1   Food fortification

Fortifying foods with vitamin D has been a cornerstone strategy in several countries. In the United States, adding vitamin D to milk (a practice since the 1930s) significantly reduced the incidence of rickets, a bone disease caused by severe deficiency (Itkonen et al., 2018). Today, many staple foods like milk, orange juice, cereals, and bread are fortified with vitamin D in the United States.

Fortification policies differ across the globe. In Europe, for example, some countries aggressively fortify foods while others do very little. Finland has a comprehensive program that adding vitamin D to various foods, whereas other European nations have more limited fortification (Spiro & Buttriss, 2014). These differences lead to varying dietary vitamin D intakes between countries.

The effectiveness of fortification depends on doing it wisely. It matters which foods are fortified and how much vitamin D is added. A UK modeling study suggested that adding vitamin D to everyday staples like milk and bread could significantly boost vitamin D levels in the population, though the benefits might vary among age and ethnic groups (Allen et al., 2015). In short, fortification can help, but it should be tailored—ensuring the fortified foods reach those who need them most.

10.3.2 Supplementation programs

Vitamin D supplementation programs target groups who are most at risk of deficiency. Infants, pregnant women, and the elderly are often the focus since they have higher vitamin D needs or risk of bone problems.

In the United Kingdom, for example, the Healthy Start program provides free vitamin D supplements to low-income pregnant women and young children (Moonan et al., 2022). However, making supplements available is only half the battle; they have to be taken. An evaluation found that many eligible families were not actually using the free vitamins consistently due to factors like low awareness or difficulty accessing them (Jessiman et al., 2013). This shows that even when supplements are provided, public health officials need to promote and facilitate their use.

In countries with long, dark winters (such as the Nordic nations), health authorities often recommend everyone take vitamin D during those sunless months. Finland provides a success story: after issuing new national guidelines for wintertime vitamin D supplements, vitamin D levels in the Finnish population improved significantly (Jääskeläinen et al., 2017). This indicates that clear guidance, combined with making supplements accessible, can raise a population's vitamin D status.

10.3.3 Education and awareness campaigns

Public health campaigns spread information on why vitamin D matters and how to get it—for example, promoting safe sun exposure, vitamin D-rich foods, or taking supplements during low-sunlight periods. Such campaigns have had mixed results. They can increase awareness (in the United Kingdom, public awareness of vitamin D's importance rose after national campaigns); however, knowledge does not always turn into action, as many people still do not change their habits or start supplements.

To bridge this gap, a comprehensive approach is needed. Combining broad awareness with targeted outreach tends to be most effective. For instance, educating healthcare providers can amplify the message: in Australia, improving general practitioners' knowledge about vitamin D led to better management of vitamin D deficiency in patients (Bonevski et al., 2012). The most successful campaigns pair general public messaging with specific interventions for high-risk groups and ensure that healthcare professionals are also engaged in promoting vitamin D.

10.3.4   International and collaborative efforts

International organizations contribute by setting broad agendas and supporting countries in their vitamin D initiatives. WHO provides broad guidelines on vitamin D (often emphasizing pregnant women, infants, and the elderly), but implementing these recommendations locally can be challenging due to differences in resources, culture, and priorities.

UNICEF includes vitamin D in its maternal and child nutrition programs, often combining it with other micronutrient interventions to tackle multiple deficiencies at once. This integrated approach can be efficient, but it requires careful coordination so that vitamin D supplementation does not get overlooked among other health priorities.

10.3.5   Evaluating impact and addressing challenges

Monitoring and evaluating these public health efforts is crucial. Some countries have improved vitamin D status significantly, while others still see high deficiency rates despite programs. This highlights the need for ongoing research and flexible strategies (Pilz et al., 2018).

One challenge in evaluation is the lack of standardization in vitamin D measurements. Different studies or laboratories might measure vitamin D levels in slightly different ways or at different times of year, making comparisons difficult. International efforts to standardize vitamin D testing techniques are underway and could greatly improve our ability to assess and compare the effectiveness of interventions (Sempos et al., 2012).

Economics play a role too. Vitamin D programs—fortifying foods and providing supplements—cost money, but they can also save money by preventing illnesses associated with deficiency. For example, an analysis in Germany suggested that adding vitamin D (and calcium) to foods could result in substantial healthcare savings by reducing fractures and other health issues in the population (Sandmann et al., 2017). Such cost–benefit insights are important for governments deciding whether to implement large-scale vitamin D interventions.

10.3.6 Emerging and tailored approaches

Looking ahead, more nuanced and innovative approaches are being explored to fight vitamin D deficiency:

- Culturally tailored strategies: There is a growing awareness that strategies must fit local cultures and lifestyles. If a community has traditional clothing that limits sun exposure or diets low in vitamin D, interventions might focus more on supplements or fortified foods. Tailoring programs to local practices helps improve acceptance and effectiveness.
- Biofortification: This is a cutting-edge idea of increasing the vitamin D content of foods through agricultural methods. For instance, scientists have found that exposing certain foods like mushrooms to UV light can dramatically boost their vitamin D levels. Research has shown the feasibility of producing vitamin D–enriched mushrooms as a potential source of the vitamin (Malik et al., 2022). Such biofortified foods could benefit people who have limited access to supplements or who prefer dietary solutions.
- Technology and personalization: Mobile apps and wearable devices are emerging tools for nutrition. Apps can estimate how much vitamin D you might be getting based on your location (sun exposure potential), skin type, and habits, then give personalized advice (like suggesting a supplement or a bit of sun exposure on a given day). While these tech solutions are promising and can engage people in managing their health, we need more evidence on how much they improve actual vitamin D levels (Lee et al., 2014). Still, they represent an innovative way to raise awareness and encourage individuals to take charge of their vitamin D intake.

10.4 Conclusion

Even sunshine-rich regions can face high vitamin D deficiency rates due to cultural, environmental, or lifestyle factors. Public health efforts have made progress, from fortifying foods to educating communities, yet challenges persist.

One clear lesson is that there is no single fix for vitamin D deficiency globally. Effective strategies must combine broad measures with targeted ones. Food fortification and supplementation guidelines provide a safety net for populations while tailored outreach and education address specific local needs. Keeping up with the science is also vital: as we learn more about how vitamin D works and what different populations need, guidelines and programs should adapt accordingly.

By staying flexible and evidence-based in our approach, we can continue to improve vitamin D status around the world. Ensuring people get enough of this "sunshine vitamin" will pay dividends in better health outcomes.

AI disclosure

During the preparation of this work the authors used Claude in order to improve writing. After using this tool/service, the authors reviewed and edited the content as needed and took full responsibility for the content of the publication.

References

Allen, R. E., Dangour, A. D., Tedstone, A. E., & Chalabi, Z. (2015). Does fortification of staple foods improve vitamin D intakes and status of groups at risk of deficiency? A United Kingdom modeling study. *American Journal of Clinical Nutrition, 102*(2), 338–344. https://doi.org/10.3945/ajcn.115.107409, http://ajcn.nutrition.org/content/102/2/338.full.pdf+html.

Aparna, P., Muthathal, S., Nongkynrih, B., & Gupta, S. K. (2018). Vitamin D deficiency in India. *Journal of Family Medicine and Primary Care, 7*(2), 324. https://doi.org/10.4103/jfmpc.jfmpc_78_18.

Aranow, C. (2011). Vitamin D and the immune system. *Journal of Investigative Medicine, 59*(6), 881–886. https://doi.org/10.2310/jim.0b013e31821b8755.

Battault, S., Whiting, S. J., Peltier, S. L., Sadrin, S., Gerber, G., & Maixent, J. M. (2013). Vitamin D metabolism, functions and needs: From science to health claims. *European Journal of Nutrition, 52*(2), 429–441. https://doi.org/10.1007/s00394-012-0430-5.

Bikle, D. D. (2016). Extraskeletal actions of vitamin D. *Annals of the New York Academy of Sciences, 1376*(1), 29–52. https://doi.org/10.1111/nyas.13219, http://www.blackwellpublishing.com/0077-8923.

Bonevski, B., Girgis, A., Magin, P., Horton, G., Brozek, I., & Armstrong, B. (2012). Prescribing sunshine: A cross-sectional survey of 500 Australian general practitioners' practices and attitudes about vitamin D. *International Journal of Cancer, 130*(9), 2138–2145. https://doi.org/10.1002/ijc.26225.

Chakhtoura, M., Rahme, M., Chamoun, N., & El-Hajj Fuleihan, G. (2018). Vitamin D in the Middle East and North Africa. *Bone Reports, 8*, 135–146. https://doi.org/10.1016/j.bonr.2018.03.004.

Cui, A., Zhang, T., Xiao, P., Fan, Z., Wang, H., & Zhuang, Y. (2023). Global and regional prevalence of vitamin D deficiency in population-based studies from 2000 to 2022: A pooled analysis of 7.9 million participants. *Frontiers in Nutrition, 10*. https://doi.org/10.3389/fnut.2023.1070808.

Daly, R. M., Gagnon, C., Lu, Z. X., Magliano, D. J., Dunstan, D. W., Sikaris, K. A., Zimmet, P. Z., Ebeling, P. R., & Shaw, J. E. (2012). Prevalence of vitamin D deficiency and its determinants in Australian adults aged 25 years and older: A national, population-based study. *Clinical Endocrinology, 77*(1), 26–35. https://doi.org/10.1111/j.1365-2265.2011.04320.x.

Demay, M. B., Pittas, A. G., Bikle, D. D., Diab, D. L., Kiely, M. E., Lazaretti-Castro, M., Lips, P., Mitchell, D. M., Murad, M. H., Powers, S., Rao, S. D., Scragg, R., Tayek, J. A., Valent, A. M., Walsh, J. M. E., & McCartney, C. R. (2024). Vitamin D for the prevention of disease: An endocrine society clinical practice guideline. *Journal of Clinical Endocrinology and Metabolism, 109*(8), 1907–1947. https://doi.org/10.1210/clinem/dgae290, https://academic.oup.com/jcem.

Hilger, J., Friedel, A., Herr, R., Rausch, T., Roos, F., Wahl, D. A., Pierroz, D. D., Weber, P., & Hoffmann, K. (2014). A systematic review of vitamin D status in populations worldwide. *British Journal of Nutrition, 111*(1), 23–45. https://doi.org/10.1017/S0007114513001840.

Holick, M. F., Binkley, N. C., Bischoff-Ferrari, H. A., Gordon, C. M., Hanley, D. A., Heaney, R. P., Murad, M. H., & Weaver, C. M. (2011). Evaluation, treatment, and prevention of vitamin D deficiency: An endocrine society clinical practice guideline. *Journal of Clinical Endocrinology and Metabolism, 96*(7), 1911–1930. https://doi.org/10.1210/jc.2011-0385, http://jcem.endojournals.org/content/96/7/1911.full.pdf+html.

Hossein-Nezhad, A., & Holick, M. F. (2013). Vitamin D for health: A global perspective. *Mayo Clinic Proceedings, 88*(7), 720–755. https://doi.org/10.1016/j.mayocp.2013.05.011, http://www.journals.elsevier.com/mayo-clinic-proceedings.

Hu, Y., Jiang, S., Lu, J., Yang, Z., Yang, X., & Yang, L. (2022). Vitamin D status for Chinese children and adolescents in CNNHS 2016–2017. *Nutrients, 14*(22), 4928. https://doi.org/10.3390/nu14224928.

Itkonen, S. T., Erkkola, M., & Lamberg-Allardt, C. J. E. (2018). Vitamin D fortification of fluid milk products and their contribution to vitamin D intake and vitamin D status in observational studies—A review. *Nutrients, 10*(8). https://doi.org/10.3390/nu10081054, http://www.mdpi.com/2072-6643/10/8/1054/pdf.

Jessiman, T., Cameron, A., Wiggins, M., & Lucas, P. J. (2013). A qualitative study of uptake of free vitamins in England. *Archives of Disease in Childhood, 98*(8), 587–591. https://doi.org/10.1136/archdischild-2013-303838.

Jääskeläinen, T., Itkonen, S. T., Lundqvist, A., Erkkola, M., Koskela, T., Lakkala, K., Dowling, K. G., Hull, G. L. J., Kröger, H., Karppinen, J., Kyllönen, E., Härkänen, T., Cashman, K. D., Männistö, S., & Lamberg-Allardt, C. (2017). The positive impact of general Vitamin D food fortification policy on Vitamin D status in a representative adult Finnish population: Evidence from an 11-y follow-up based on standardized 25-hydroxyVitamin D data. *American Journal of Clinical Nutrition, 105*(6), 1512–1520. https://doi.org/10.3945/ajcn.116.151415, http://ajcn.nutrition.org/content/105/6/1512.full.pdf+html.

Lee, S., Oncescu, V., Mancuso, M., Mehta, S., & Erickson, D. (2014). A smartphone platform for the quantification of vitamin D levels. *Lab on a Chip, 14*(8), 1437–1442. https://doi.org/10.1039/c3lc51375k.

Malik, M. A., Jan, Y., Al-Keridis, L. A., Haq, A., Ahmad, J., Adnan, M., Alshammari, N., Ashraf, S. A., & Panda, B. P. (2022). Effect of vitamin-D-enriched edible mushrooms on vitamin D status, bone health and expression of CYP2R1, CYP27B1 and VDR gene in Wistar Rats. *Journal of Fungi, 8*(8). https://doi.org/10.3390/jof8080864, http://www.mdpi.com/journal/jof.

Manicourt, D. H., & Devogelaer, J. P. (2008). Urban tropospheric ozone increases the prevalence of vitamin d deficiency among belgian postmenopausal women with outdoor activities during summer. *Journal of Clinical Endocrinology and Metabolism, 93*(10), 3893–3899. https://doi.org/10.1210/jc.2007-2663, http://jcem.endojournals.org/cgi/reprint/93/10/3893.

Moonan, M., Maudsley, G., Hanratty, B., & Whitehead, M. (2022). An exploration of the statutory Healthy Start vitamin supplementation scheme in North West England. *BMC Public Health, 22*(1). https://doi.org/10.1186/s12889-022-12704-0.

O'Neill, C. M., Kazantzidis, A., Ryan, M. J., Barber, N., Sempos, C. T., Durazo-Arvizu, R. A., Jorde, R., Grimnes, G., Eiriksdottir, G., Gudnason, V., Cotch, M. F., Kiely, M., Webb, A. R., & Cashman, K. D. (2016). Seasonal changes in vitamin D-effective UVB availability in Europe and associations with population serum 25-hydroxyvitamin D. *Nutrients, 8*(9). https://doi.org/10.3390/nu8090533, http://www.mdpi.com/2072-6643/8/9/533/pdf.

Palacios, C., & Gonzalez, L. (2014). Is vitamin D deficiency a major global public health problem? *The Journal of Steroid Biochemistry and Molecular Biology, 144*, 138–145. https://doi.org/10.1016/j.jsbmb.2013.11.003.

Pilz, S., März, W., Cashman, K. D., Kiely, M. E., Whiting, S. J., Holick, M. F., Grant, W. B., Pludowski, P., Hiligsmann, M., Trummer, C., Schwetz, V., Lerchbaum, E., Pandis, M., Tomaschitz, A., Grübler, M. R., Gaksch, M., Verheyen, N., Hollis, B. W., Rejnmark, L., ... Zittermann, A. (2018). Rationale and plan for vitamin D food fortification: A review and guidance paper. *Frontiers in Endocrinology, 9*(JUL). https://doi.org/10.3389/fendo.2018.00373.

Powe, C. E., Evans, M. K., Wenger, J., Zonderman, A. B., Berg, A. H., Nalls, M., Tamez, H., Zhang, D., Bhan, I., Karumanchi, S. A., Powe, N. R., & Thadhani, R. (2013). Vitamin D-binding protein and vitamin D status of black Americans and white Americans. *New England Journal of Medicine, 369*(21), 1991–2000. https://doi.org/10.1056/NEJMoa1306357, http://www.nejm.org/doi/pdf/10.1056/NEJMoa1306357.

Raymond-Lezman, J. R., & Riskin, S. I. (2023). Benefits and risks of sun exposure to maintain adequate vitamin D levels. *Cureus, 15*(5). https://doi.org/10.7759/cureus.38578.

Ross, A. C., Manson, J. A. E., Abrams, S. A., Aloia, J. F., Brannon, P. M., Clinton, S. K., Durazo-Arvizu, R. A., Gallagher, J. C., Gallo, R. L., Jones, G., Kovacs, C. S., Mayne, S. T., Rosen, C. J., & Shapses, S. A. (2011). The 2011 report on dietary reference intakes for calcium and vitamin D from the Institute of Medicine: What clinicians need to know. *Journal of Clinical Endocrinology and Metabolism, 96*(1), 53–58. https://doi.org/10.1210/jc.2010-2704, http://jcem.endojournals.org/cgi/reprint/96/1/53.

Sandmann, A., Amling, M., Barvencik, F., König, H. H., & Bleibler, F. (2017). Economic evaluation of vitamin D and calcium food fortification for fracture prevention in Germany. *Public Health Nutrition, 20*(10), 1874–1883. https://doi.org/10.1017/S1368980015003171, http://journals.cambridge.org/PHN.

Sempos, C. T., Vesper, H. W., Phinney, K. W., Thienpont, L. M., & Coates, P. M. (2012). Vitamin D status as an international issue: National surveys and the problem of standardization. *Scandinavian Journal of Clinical and Laboratory Investigation, 72*(SUPPL. 243), 32–40. https://doi.org/10.3109/00365513.2012.681935.

Sowah, D., Fan, X., Dennett, L., Hagtvedt, R., & Straube, S. (2017). Vitamin D levels and deficiency with different occupations: A systematic review. *BMC Public Health, 17*(1). https://doi.org/10.1186/s12889-017-4436-z.

Spiro, A., & Buttriss, J. L. (2014). Vitamin D: An overview of vitamin D status and intake in E urope. *Nutrition Bulletin, 39*(4), 322–350. https://doi.org/10.1111/nbu.12108.

Srivastava, S. B. (2021). Vitamin D: Do we need more than sunshine? *American Journal of Lifestyle Medicine, 15*(4), 397–401. https://doi.org/10.1177/15598276211005689, http://www.sagepub.com/journalsProdDesc.nav?prodId=Journal201781.

Szalay, E. A., Tryon, E. B., Pleacher, M. D., & Whisler, S. L. (2011). Pediatric vitamin D deficiency in a southwestern luminous climate. *Journal of Pediatric Orthopaedics, 31*(4), 469–473. https://doi.org/10.1097/BPO.0b013e31821e10c5.

Wang, H., Chen, W., Li, D., Yin, X., Zhang, X., Olsen, N., & Zheng, S. G. (2017). Vitamin D and chronic diseases. *Aging and Disease, 8*(3), 346–353. https://doi.org/10.14336/AD.2016.1021, http://www.aginganddisease.org/EN/article/downloadArticleFile.do?attachType=PDF&id=147579.

Wang, T. J., Zhang, F., Richards, J. B., Kestenbaum, B., Van Meurs, J. B., Berry, D., Kiel, D. P., Streeten, E. A., Ohlsson, C., Koller, D. L., Peltonen, L., Cooper, J. D., O'Reilly, P. F., Houston, D. K., Glazer, N. L., Vandenput, L., Peacock, M., Shi, J., Rivadeneira, F., ... Spector, T. D. (2010). Common genetic determinants of vitamin D insufficiency: A genome-wide association study. *The Lancet, 376*(9736), 180–188. https://doi.org/10.1016/S0140-6736(10)60588-0, http://www.journals.elsevier.com/the-lancet/.

Wright, N. C., Chen, L., Niu, J., Neogi, T., Javaid, K., Nevitt, M. A., Lewis, C. E., & Curtis, J. R. (2012). Defining physiologically "normal" vitamin D in African Americans. *Osteoporosis International, 23*(9), 2283–2291. https://doi.org/10.1007/s00198-011-1877-6.

CHAPTER 11

Vitamin D deficiency

Faiza Alam[1], Samar Zaki[2], and Maah Amir[3]

[1]Pengiran-Anak-Puteri-Rashidah-Sa'adatul-Bolkiah Institute of Health Sciences, Universiti Brunei Darussalam, Bandar Seri Begawan, Brunei Darussalam [2]Department of Family Medicine, Aga Khan University Hospital, Karachi, Sindh, Pakistan [3]Medical College, Aga Khan University, Karachi, Pakistan

11.1 Introduction

Vitamin D is a fat-soluble vitamin, which plays an important role in maintaining calcium homeostasis and bone metabolism. It can be obtained from food and dietary supplements and is produced in the skin when exposed to sunlight. It was discovered in the early 20th century, and it is commonly recognized as a prohormone (Mavar et al., 2024). In addition to supporting bone health, it helps to reduce inflammation and regulates various processes in the body, such as the growth of cells, neuromuscular function, immune modulation, and metabolism of glucose. It also affects genes that control cell multiplication, growth, differentiation, and programmed death. Many tissues have vitamin D receptors (VDRs), and some can convert 25(OH) D into its active form, 1, 25(OH) 2 D.

Diagnosis of vitamin D deficiency (VDD) is made by determining the concentration of the 25-hydroxycholecalciferol in the serum, which is the most reliable indicator of vitamin D stores in the body. Several leading organizations, including the Endocrine Society and the National and International Osteoporosis Foundation, define VDD as serum vitamin D levels < 30 ng/mL. An optimal range of 40–60 ng/mL is suggested by the Endocrine Society (Grygorieva et al., 2024). To reduce the risk of falls and fractures in the geriatric population, the International Osteoporosis Foundation recommends minimum serum levels of 25-hydroxycholecalciferol of 30 ng/mL (Chang & Lee, 2019).

The classification of VDD is as follows:
Vitamin D insufficiency: 25-hydroxycholecalciferol of 20–29 ng/mL=50–75nmol/L.
Vitamin D deficiency: 25-hydroxycholecalciferol of less than 20 ng/mL ≤ 50 nmol/L.
Vitamin D severe deficiency: 25-hydroxycholecalciferol < 12 ng/mL ≤30 nmol/L (Amrein et al., 2020).

There is a lack of consensus about the maximum safe upper level of serum vitamin D; however, the risk of toxicity is increased at high levels > 100 ng/mL as a result of secondary hypercalcemia (Chang & Lee, 2019).

The Impact of Vitamin D on Health and Disease. DOI: https://doi.org/10.1016/B978-0-443-34037-6.00016-9

VDD has become a global public health issue, and this situation is referred to by some authors as an epidemic or pandemic. According to one estimate, about one billion of the world's population has VDD, while vitamin D insufficiency is present in 50% of the population. The prevalence is highest in elderly, hospitalized patients, nursing home residents, and obese patients. VDD in the United States is prevalent in African-American (47%) and Caucasian infants (56%), while over 90% of infants in Iran, Turkey, and India suffer from VDD. In the adult population, 35% of the American population and more than 80% of the adult population of Pakistan, India, and Bangladesh are suffering from VDD. In the elderly group, 61% in the United States while 90% in Turkey, 96% in India, 72% in Pakistan, and 67% in Iran are vitamin D deficient (Chang & Lee, 2019). VDD has a significant impact on health, affecting physical as well as mental well-being. The deficiency has been linked to various health-related issues, including cardiovascular and autoimmune diseases, cancer, and depression. Research has also shown an association of VDD with increased susceptibility to infectious diseases, including respiratory tract infections like COVID-19. Vitamin D is also involved in controlling inflammation during sepsis, potentially lessening organ damage and improving survival rates (Chang & Lee, 2019).

11.2   Causes of vitamin D deficiency (discussed in more detail in Chapter 2)

VDD can result from several causes. Some of the important factors are as follows:

1. Geographic and seasonal factors

Literature shows that geographic location plays a significant role in VDD. In regions such as Latin America and Australia, vitamin D levels are generally sufficient, while areas in the Middle East and parts of Asia have lower levels. Research on populations at different latitudes shows that those living away from the equator are more likely to get VDD due to less exposure to sunlight. In the Arctic, where sunlight is weak in winter as well as summer, VDD is prevalent because the skin receives less ultraviolet B (UVB) radiation, which is required for vitamin D production. In tropical regions where sunlight is strong, individuals with darker skin, which blocks UVB rays, may have difficulty synthesizing vitamin D. This is true for populations inhabiting sub-Saharan Africa and southern India. Studies also highlight that people in Eastern Mediterranean regions and lower-middle-income countries are at a greater chance for VDD. Seasonal changes in sunlight exposure have a major effect on vitamin D levels. Deficiency rates are generally higher during the winter and spring months compared to summer and autumn (Lips et al., 2021). The reason could be because the amount of exposure to sunlight varies significantly through the seasons (Herdea et al., 2024).

2. Cultural and lifestyle factors

Cultural and lifestyle factors have also been found to contribute to VDD. These include cultural practices such as wearing veils or long-sleeved clothing, which limit sun exposure, as well as lifestyle factors such as dietary habits, failure to consume vitamin supplements or fortified foods, prolonged indoor activity, reduced physical activity, and frequent use of sunscreens (Lips et al., 2021; Frost, 2022).

3. Decreased dietary intake and/or absorption

Lower intake of vitamin D-rich diets is an important cause of VDD, especially in the elderly population. Certain gastrointestinal diseases causing malabsorption can also lead to VDD (Matsui, 2020).

4. Decreased sun exposure

The body meets part of its vitamin D needs through sunlight exposure. The skin synthesizes vitamin D3 when it is exposed to a certain type of ultraviolet light (UVB, with wavelength between 290 and 320 nanometers). This light converts 7-dehydrocholesterol in the skin into previtamin D3, which then changes into vitamin D3. Vitamin D production is influenced by several factors, including season, time of day, daylight hours, cloud cover, air pollution, and skin pigmentation. The ability to synthesize vitamin D from sunlight is diminished in older adults and individuals with darker skin tones. Maintaining adequate vitamin D levels often involves exposing at least 40% of the skin to sunlight for a minimum of 20 minutes each day. Individuals who are hospitalized or living in long-term care facilities frequently experience VDD due to restricted sun exposure. The regular application of sunscreen may interfere with the cutaneous synthesis of vitamin D due to reduced UV radiation exposure (Chang & Lee, 2019).

5. Decreased endogenous synthesis

In chronic liver failure, such as patients with cirrhosis, active vitamin D is deficient because of defective 25-hydroxylation. Defect in 1-alpha hydroxylation occurs in diseases like hyperparathyroidism, renal failure, and 1-alpha hydroxylase deficiency (Chang & Lee, 2019).

6. Medications causing increased hepatic catabolism

Certain medicines like phenobarbital, carbamazepine, dexamethasone, nifedipine, spironolactone, clotrimazole, and rifampin can stimulate the hepatic 450 enzymes, which activate the degradation of vitamin D, thereby leading to VDD (Matsui, 2020).

11.3 Pathophysiology

VDD poses a substantial threat to global well-being, impacting bone health and a variety of other bodily functions. Vitamin D performs a very critical role in calcium homeostasis involving bone health. It can be obtained from sunlight, food, or supplements, but it must be activated in the body through two steps. First, the liver converts vitamin D into calcidiol. Second, the kidneys convert it into calcitriol. Calcitriol, the active form of vitamin D, regulates calcium absorption and bone metabolism. It promotes intestinal calcium uptake and maintains calcium and phosphate levels which are vital for bone health, including growth and remodeling of bones. VDD impairs calcium and phosphorus absorption in small intestines. This results in reduced levels of ionized calcium levels and produces secondary hyperparathyroidism as a compensatory response. Parathyroid hormone (PTH) is fundamental for maintaining serum calcium levels. It increases calcium reabsorption in the kidneys and triggers bone resorption to release calcium into the bloodstream. PTH also reduces phosphate reabsorption, which can lead to phosphate depletion and, consequently, osteomalacia and osteoporosis in adults, and rickets in children. Rickets disrupts bone mineralization in children whose skeletons are still developing. Osteomalacia, on the other hand, affects adults and is characterized by impaired bone mineralization after the growth plates (epiphyses) have closed. Despite some controversy surrounding the connection between vitamin D and osteoporosis, there is broad agreement that vitamin D contributes to bone density. Insufficient vitamin D can impair calcium absorption, resulting in lower bone mineral density and an increased risk of fractures (Charoenngam et al., 2019).

Vitamin D preserves endothelial function, and its deficiency can lead to endothelial dysfunction, a key precursor to atherosclerosis and other cardiovascular pathologies. Insufficient vitamin D levels are also linked to elevated vascular inflammation and the development of atherosclerotic plaques, which facilitate the progression of coronary artery disease. Furthermore, VDD may activate the renin–angiotensin–aldosterone system, contributing to the development of hypertension and other cardiovascular complications. Additionally, VDD has been associated with left ventricular hypertrophy, which impairs cardiac function. Vitamin D insufficiency promotes the proliferation of vascular smooth muscle cells, causing increased vascular stiffness and eventually elevated blood pressure (Haider et al., 2023).

Vitamin D influences both the innate and adaptive immune systems. It is crucial for the innate immune response, which serves as the first line of defense against pathogens. Vitamin D promotes the synthesis of antimicrobial peptides and enhances the activity of immune cells such as macrophages and dendritic cells. The VDR is expressed in various immune cells, hence modulating their function. This includes promoting the maturation of dendritic cells and activation of T cells, a process essential for an effective immune response. Vitamin D also regulates T-cell differentiation and supports the development of regulatory T cells (Tregs), which are essential for maintaining immune tolerance and preventing autoimmunity. This modulation shifts the immune response by promoting a transition from pro-inflammatory T helper cell profiles (Th1/Th17) to antiinflammatory Th2 profiles, thereby reducing inflammation (Athanassiou et al., 2022).

11.3.1   Clinical manifestations of vitamin D deficiency

Recent research has underscored the clinical characteristics of VDD in various age groups, uncovering notable trends and health implications. Many individuals with VDD may not exhibit clear symptoms or may experience vague, nonspecific ones. Recent studies have highlighted several key symptoms and conditions linked to insufficient vitamin D levels.

11.3.1.1   Rickets and osteomalacia

VDD in children can lead to rickets, which typically manifests before 18 months of age. Rickets affects areas of rapid bone growth, including the costochondral junctions and epiphyses of long bones. The deficiency disrupts normal cartilage cell maturation, causing these cells to enlarge and the growth plates to widen. This leads to characteristic signs like rachitic rosary (beading of the ribs), a protruding sternum, and rib cage deformities. In severe cases, rickets can cause pelvic flattening, skull deformities (like craniotabes), and a prominent forehead (frontal bossing). Affected infants may also experience bone pain, irritability, and excessive sweating. If the condition progresses, low calcium levels can trigger muscle spasms, seizures, heart problems, and even death. Developmental delays, such as in sitting and crawling, are also common. In adolescents, VDD increases the risk of delayed growth, tooth decay, and fractures.

In adults, VDD can cause osteomalacia, which manifests as the characteristic throbbing, aching bone pain. Tenderness when pressing on the sternum can aid in diagnosis. Individuals often experience muscle weakness, particularly in the proximal muscles, making it hard to rise from a sitting position. In severe cases, shoulder muscle weakness can even prevent them from lifting their head. Generalized fatigue is another common symptom, which can sometimes lead to misdiagnosis as fibromyalgia, chronic fatigue syndrome, or polymyalgia rheumatica. A waddling gait, often due to weakness in the thighs and hip pain, may also occur.[9] Patients with rickets or osteomalacia typically have 25(OH)D levels below 15 ng/mL, elevated serum alkaline phosphatase, normal serum calcium, and low-normal to low serum phosphate (Charoenngam et al., 2019).

11.3.2 Complications

VDD can lead to several complications, particularly affecting bone strength and stability. A major concern is the increased risk of fractures since vitamin D is crucial for absorbing calcium, which is essential in maintaining bone strength. Without enough vitamin D, bones can weaken and break more easily. VDD is also linked to a greater risk of falls, particularly in older adults because it can cause muscle weakness and poor coordination (Charoenngam et al., 2019).

Vitamin D is also fundamentally involved in dental health. During childhood growth as well as in adulthood, VDD is related to a variety of dental health issues, with impaired vitamin D synthesis potentially accelerating some of these forms. Severe deficiency can lead to improper tooth mineralization, causing dentin and enamel defects. As a result, these defects may elevate the risk of developing and advancing dental caries. Additionally, VDD has been linked to the predominance of periodontitis and gingival inflammation (Botelho et al., 2020).

11.3.3 Associated conditions

11.3.3.1 Cardiovascular diseases

Sufficient vitamin D levels are crucial for the health of the cardiovascular system, as low levels have been linked to several negative cardiovascular outcomes. VDD is increasingly recognized as a significant risk factor for heart diseases, including increased susceptibility to heart attacks, strokes, and heart failure. The deficiency also interacts with other known risk factors like hypertension, diabetes, and abnormalities in lipid metabolism, making heart disease even more likely (Haider et al., 2023).

11.3.3.2   *Cognitive decline and depression*

VDD has been associated with declining cognitive function and an increased risk of dementia and Alzheimer's disease. Low vitamin D levels are also linked to depression, suggesting it may play a role in mood regulation. This connection to mood disorders is thought to be related to VDR and the VDR gene. A mutation in this gene can interfere with vitamin D's ability to bind to its receptor and be converted into its active form (calcitriol), which is needed for producing neurotrophic factors—essential substances for brain health. Without these factors, brain function can be impaired, potentially contributing to mood disorder symptoms. Furthermore, VDD is linked to several mental health issues, including major depression, seasonal affective disorder, suicidal thoughts, postpartum depression, premenstrual syndrome, ADHD, schizophrenia, and depressive symptoms in older adults (Shah & Gurbani, 2020).

11.3.3.3   *Immune disorders and chronic diseases*

Vitamin D plays a crucial role in preventing chronic diseases linked to immune dysfunction. A growing body of research suggests that VDD may play a significant role in increasing the risk as well as exacerbating the symptoms of autoimmune disorders like lupus, rheumatoid arthritis, and multiple sclerosis (Álvarez-Mercado et al., 2023).

VDD is strongly linked to the development and progression of various chronic diseases. The deficiency is frequently seen in people with obesity and metabolic syndrome, contributing to these conditions. Research also suggests a connection between low vitamin D and several types of cancer, raising the possibility that sufficient vitamin D may play a role in cancer prevention. Vitamin D may help lower cancer risk through several mechanisms, including promoting normal cell development, slowing tumor growth, triggering cancer cell death, and reducing the formation of new blood vessels that feed tumors. Numerous studies suggest that vitamin D can help control the growth of breast, colon, and prostate cancer cells (Nasri, 2017; Álvarez-Mercado et al., 2023).

11.3.4   *Diagnosis*

11.3.4.1   *Screening guidelines and laboratory tests*

Vitamin D deficiency is a growing global health concern, leading to a significant rise in Vitamin D testing worldwide. Recent consensus guidelines identify measuring total serum 25-hydroxyvitamin D [25(OH)D] levels as the most reliable method for assessing an individual's vitamin D status (Pludowski et al., 2022). Targeted screening plays a crucial role in the early detection and prevention of vitamin D deficiency, particularly in high-risk groups. These individuals at high risk include those with osteoporosis or osteomalacia, as well as individuals with chronic kidney disease or malabsorption conditions like Crohn's disease and celiac disease. Autoimmune disorders such as multiple sclerosis and rheumatoid arthritis also increase susceptibility. Additional high-risk groups include pregnant women, the elderly, and people with limited sun exposure. Patients taking medications that impact vitamin D metabolism, such as corticosteroids and anticonvulsants, may also need careful monitoring. For further details, refer to Chapter 29.

Moreover, vitamin D supplementation has been shown to enhance muscle strength and decrease fall frequency by nearly 50%. Therefore, individuals with low bone mineral density, a history of low-impact (fragility) fractures, or a high risk of falls should be assessed for VDD to minimize the risk of various skeletal fractures (Kennel et al., 2010). Additionally, periodic testing is also recommended in certain cases to monitor the efficacy of vitamin D supplementation and treatment (Grygorieva et al., 2024).

11.3.4.2 Definition and interpretation of vitamin D levels

The definition of vitamin D deficiency varies across medical organizations, leading to differences in screening and treatment recommendations. The various threshold values are outlined in the Table 11.1 below:

Table 11.1 Vitamin D deficiency cut-offs across various medical organizations.

Organization	Deficiency (ng/mL)	Insufficiency (ng/mL)	Optimal Range (ng/mL)	References
Endocrine Society	≤ 20	21–29	≥ 30	Pludowski et al. (2022)
Institute of Medicine (National Academies of Sciences, Engineering, and Medicine)	< 12	12–20	≥ 20	Pludowski et al. (2022)
Mayo Clinic	Severe: < 10 mild–moderate: 10–24	Not specified	25–80	Han et al. (2023)
American Association of Clinical Endocrinologists	< 30	Not specified	30–50	Grygorieva et al. (2024)
Polish Guidelines (2023)	< 20	20–30	30–50	Płudowski et al. (2023)
Ukrainian Guidelines (2024)	< 30	30–50	75–125 (30–50)	Grygorieva et al. (2024)

These variations highlight the ongoing debate in the medical community regarding the ideal vitamin D levels necessary for overall health and disease prevention. While there is no universal standard, most guidelines agree on the need for targeted screening rather than widespread population testing, ensuring that high-risk and pregnant individuals receive appropriate diagnosis and intervention.

11.3.4.3   Laboratory testing for vitamin D deficiency

The measurement of serum 25-hydroxyvitamin D [25(OH)D] is widely recognized as the gold standard for evaluating vitamin D status. It is the most accurate indicator of vitamin D levels as it reflects both dietary intake and endogenous production from sun exposure. Advanced methods such as liquid chromatography–mass spectrometry (LC–MS) are considered the most precise for measuring 25(OH)D in serum samples (Yin et al., 2020).

11.3.4.4   Potential limitations of vitamin D testing

Despite being the preferred diagnostic method, serum 25(OH)D testing has some limitations, including:

- **Assay variability**: Different laboratories use different testing methods (e.g., immunoassays, LC–MS), which can lead to variations in results (Anusha et al., 2022).
- **Seasonal fluctuations**: Vitamin D levels naturally fluctuate throughout the year, often peaking in late summer and dropping in winter due to changes in sun exposure (Cao et al., 2021).
- **Geographic and lifestyle factors**: People living at higher latitudes or with limited sun exposure due to indoor lifestyles, clothing choices, or sunscreen use may have persistently lower levels, influencing interpretation and treatment decisions (Krist et al., 2021).

11.3.4.5   Differential diagnosis—distinguishing from other causes of bone pain and muscle weakness

While VDD commonly presents with diffuse musculoskeletal pain and proximal muscle weakness (Charoenngam et al., 2019). A similar clinical presentation may also result from various metabolic, inflammatory, and neurological conditions. Therefore, differential diagnoses should encompass disorders such as fibromyalgia, inflammatory myopathies, chronic kidney disease, and endocrine abnormalities, including primary hyperparathyroidism and hypothyroidism (D'Amuri et al., 2024). Thus, careful evaluation of clinical features, laboratory findings, and imaging studies is required to reach an accurate diagnosis in patients presenting with similar symptoms.

Patients with low serum levels of vitamin D may present with a spectrum of clinical manifestations ranging from asymptomatic states to severe skeletal complications, such as frequent or pathological fractures. The severity and extent of symptoms typically correlate with the degree of vitamin D deficiency. To investigate the underlying cause and confirm the diagnosis, a comprehensive assessment is essential.

Key laboratory investigations include measuring serum 25-hydroxyvitamin D [25(OH)D], which is the most reliable indicator of vitamin D status. Additionally, serum parathyroid hormone (PTH) levels are often elevated in response to hypocalcemia induced by vitamin D deficiency. Evaluation of serum calcium and phosphorus levels provides insight into mineral metabolism, while elevated alkaline phosphatase (ALP) levels may indicate increased bone turnover secondary to osteomalacia or rickets (Holick, 2006).

Imaging studies play a critical role in the diagnostic process. Dual-energy X-ray absorptiometry (DEXA) scans are utilized to assess bone mineral density (BMD) and evaluate for osteoporosis, a common complication of prolonged vitamin D deficiency. Radiographic imaging, including X-rays, may reveal characteristic findings such as Looser's zones (pseudofractures) in cases of osteomalacia (Sangondimath et al., 2023; Zimmerman, Anastasopoulou and McKeon, 2024).

In clinical practice, a thorough evaluation combining biochemical markers and imaging studies is fundamental for diagnosing VDD and differentiating it from other metabolic bone disorders. Early identification and appropriate management are essential to mitigate complications and restore skeletal health.

11.3.5 Management and treatment of vitamin D deficiency

VDD is predominantly managed through supplementation, with cholecalciferol (vitamin D3) rather than ergocalciferol (vitamin D2) as it is more efficient in elevating serum 25-hydroxyvitamin D [25(OH)D] concentrations. Standard treatment for adults involves high-dose supplementation, typically 6,000 IU daily or 50,000 IU weekly for eight weeks, followed by a maintenance regimen of 1,000–2,000 IU daily once serum 25(OH)D exceeds 30 ng/mL. Higher initial doses, such as 10,000 IU daily, may be necessary for individuals with obesity, malabsorption disorders, or increased skin pigmentation, with maintenance doses ranging from 3,000 to 6,000 IU daily. In pediatric patients, deficiency is commonly addressed with 2,000 IU daily or 50,000 IU weekly for six weeks, transitioning to a maintenance dose of 1,000 IU daily. For breastfed infants and children with insufficient intake of vitamin D-fortified milk (< 1 L/day), the American Academy of Pediatrics recommends prophylactic supplementation of 400 IU daily.

In cases where conventional supplementation fails to achieve target serum levels, calcitriol (active vitamin D) may be indicated, necessitating close monitoring of serum calcium due to the risk of hypercalcemia. Additionally, calcidiol (25-hydroxyvitamin D) serves as an alternative for individuals with fat malabsorption syndromes or severe hepatic dysfunction.

11.3.6 Prevention of vitamin D deficiency

Preventative strategies emphasize adequate daily intake, adjusted for age and risk factors. Adults younger than 65 years require 600–800 IU daily, whereas those aged 65 years and older should consume 800–1000 IU daily to mitigate the risk of fractures and falls. Maintaining serum 25(OH)D levels ≥30 ng/mL is essential for musculoskeletal health, as evidence suggests an association between optimal vitamin D status and improved muscle function, reduced fall incidence, and enhanced bone mineral density. Epidemiological analyses, including data from NHANES III, demonstrate a dose-dependent relationship between vitamin D intake and skeletal outcomes. A 2009 meta-analysis of randomized controlled trials (RCTs) found that daily doses below 400 IU were ineffective, whereas supplementation in the range of 482–770 IU significantly reduced the risk of non-vertebral fractures by 20% and hip fractures by 18%. Long-term supplementation is particularly beneficial for older adults, contributing to sustained skeletal health and fall prevention (Bischoff-Ferrari, 2009).

Optimizing vitamin D levels through lifestyle modifications, including sun exposure and dietary intake, is also an effective strategy for preventing deficiency. Sunlight remains the primary natural source, as ultraviolet B (UVB) radiation stimulates vitamin D synthesis in the skin. Literature suggests that individuals with regular sun exposure tend to have higher serum vitamin D levels than those who rely solely on dietary sources. Additionally, eating vitamin D-rich foods helps to maintain adequate levels, particularly in regions or seasons with limited sunshine (McAdler, 2013; Sahota & Shaw, 2014). Combining moderate sun exposure with a well-balanced diet offers a practical and sustainable approach to preventing vitamin D deficiency.

11.3.7   Monitoring and follow-up

Effective management of VDD requires continuous monitoring beyond the initial correction phase. Physicians should establish structured follow-up protocols to facilitate patients' transition from corrective therapy to a long-term maintenance regimen. Regular evaluation of serum 25-hydroxyvitamin D [25(OH)D] levels is particularly important for individuals at increased risk of recurrent deficiency, including elders, those with limited sun exposure, and individuals with chronic conditions that impair vitamin D metabolism. Maintaining serum 25(OH)D concentrations above 30 ng/mL is recommended, as this threshold has been linked to enhanced calcium absorption, suppression of parathyroid hormone (PTH) levels, and a reduced risk of secondary hyperparathyroidism and bone mineral loss. Patients with conditions affecting vitamin D absorption, such as renal disease or gastrointestinal disorders, may require tailored monitoring and dosage adjustments to maintain adequate levels.

Consideration of vitamin D supplements must also weigh the potential risk of toxicity, although this remains rare. Prolonged intake exceeding 10,000 IU/day can lead to hypervitaminosis D, but standard high-dose regimens, such as 1600 IU daily or 50,000 IU monthly, have not been consistently associated with toxicity. Effective monitoring should go beyond serum 25(OH)D levels to include markers like serum calcium and PTH to detect early signs of hypercalcemia indicative of excessive vitamin D activity. For patients with severe malabsorption disorders, UVB phototherapy may offer an alternative means of stimulating endogenous vitamin D synthesis. Additionally, patients on enteral nutrition should avoid vitamin D2 in oil-based formulations due to the risk of tube occlusion, favoring vitamin D3 in powder or tablet form. An individualized and comprehensive approach to monitoring and supplementation is essential for optimizing outcomes and ensuring the safe management of VDD in diverse patient populations (Kennel et al., 2010).

References

Álvarez-Mercado, A. I., Mesa, M. D., & Gil, Á. (2023). Vitamin D: Role in chronic and acute diseases. *Encyclopedia of Human Nutrition: Volume 1-4, Fourth Edition, 1-4*, 535–544. https://doi.org/10.1016/B978-0-12-821848-8.00101-3, https://www.sciencedirect.com/book/9780323908160.

Amrein, K., Scherkl, M., Hoffmann, M., Neuwersch-Sommeregger, S., Köstenberger, M., Tmava Berisha, A., Martucci, G., Pilz, S., & Malle, O. (2020). Vitamin D deficiency 2.0: an update on the current status worldwide. *European Journal of Clinical Nutrition, 74*(11), 1498–1513. https://doi.org/10.1038/s41430-020-0558-y.

Anusha, T., Bhavani, K. S., Shanmukha Kumar, J. V., Brahman, P. K., & Hassan, R. Y. A. (2022). Fabrication of electrochemical immunosensor based on GCN-β-CD/Au nanocomposite for the monitoring of vitamin D deficiency. *Bioelectrochemistry (Amsterdam, Netherlands), 143*. https://doi.org/10.1016/j.bioelechem.2021.107935, www.elsevier.com/locate/bioelechem.

Athanassiou, L., Mavragani, C. P., & Koutsilieris, M. (2022). The immunomodulatory properties of vitamin D. *Mediterranean Journal of Rheumatology, 33*(1), 7–13. https://doi.org/10.31138/MJR.33.1.7, http://www.mjrheum.org/.

Bischoff-Ferrari, H. (2009). Vitamin D: What is an adequate vitamin D level and how much supplementation is necessary? *Best Practice & Research. Clinical Rheumatology, 23*(6), 789–795. https://doi.org/10.1016/j.berh.2009.09.005.

Botelho, J., Machado, V., Proença, L., Delgado, A. S., & Mendes, J. J. (2020). Vitamin D Deficiency and Oral Health: A Comprehensive Review. *Nutrients, 12*(5), 1471. https://doi.org/10.3390/nu12051471.

Cao, X., Ying, Z., Li, X., Zhang, J., Hoogendijk, E. O., & Liu, Z. (2021). Serum 25-hydroxyvitamin D in relation to disability in activities of daily living, mobility, and objective physical functioning among Chinese older adults. *Experimental Gerontology, 148*. https://doi.org/10.1016/j.exger.2021.111290, www.elsevier.com/locate/expgero.

Chang, S.-W., & Lee, H.-C. (2019). Vitamin D and health - The missing vitamin in humans. *Pediatrics & Neonatology, 60*(3), 237–244. https://doi.org/10.1016/j.pedneo.2019.04.007.

Charoenngam, N., Shirvani, A., & Holick, M. F. (2019). Vitamin D for skeletal and non-skeletal health: What we should know. *Journal of Clinical Orthopaedics and Trauma, 10*(6), 1082–1093. https://doi.org/10.1016/j.jcot.2019.07.004, http://www.elsevier.com/wps/find/journaldescription.cws_home/724754/description#description.

D'Amuri, A., Greco, S., Pagani, M., Presciuttini, B., Ciaffi, J., & Ursini, F. (2024). Common non-rheumatic medical conditions mimicking fibromyalgia: A simple framework for differential diagnosis. *Diagnostics, 14*(16), 1758. https://doi.org/10.3390/diagnostics14161758.

Frost, P. (2022). The problem of vitamin D scarcity: Cultural and genetic solutions by indigenous arctic and tropical peoples. *Nutrients, 14*(19), 4071. https://doi.org/10.3390/nu14194071.

Grygorieva, N., Tronko, M., Kovalenko, V., Komisarenko, S., Tatarchuk, T., Dedukh, N., Veliky, M., Strafun, S., Komisarenko, Y., Kalashnikov, A., Orlenko, V., Pankiv, V., Shvets, O., Gogunska, I., & Regeda, S. (2024). Ukrainian consensus on diagnosis and management of vitamin D deficiency in adults. *Nutrients, 16*(2), 270. https://doi.org/10.3390/nu16020270.

Haider, F., Ghafoor, H., Hassan, O. F., Farooqui, K., Bel Khair, A. O. M., & Shoaib, F. (2023). Vitamin D and cardiovascular diseases: An update. *Cureus, 15*(11). https://doi.org/10.7759/cureus.49734.

Han, F., Wang, Y., Li, J., Li, Z., Mu, D., He, L., & Zhang, J. (2023). [Determination of 25-hydroxyvitamin D in serum by pre-column derivatization-stable isotope labeling-ultra performance liquid chromatography-quadrupole electrostatic field orbitrap high-resolution mass spectrometry]. Wei Sheng Yan Jiu =. *Journal of Hygiene Research, 52*(1), 129–135. https://doi.org/10.19813/J.CNKI.WEISHENGYANJIU.2023.01.022.

Herdea, A., Marie, H., Ionescu, A., Sandu, D.-M., Pribeagu, S.-T., & Ulici, A. (2024). Vitamin D Deficiency-A Public Health Issue in Children. *Children (Basel, Switzerland), 11*(9), 1061. https://doi.org/10.3390/CHILDREN11091061.

Holick, M. F. (2006). Resurrection of vitamin D deficiency and rickets. *Journal of Clinical Investigation, 116*(8), 2062–2072. https://doi.org/10.1172/JCI29449.

Kennel, K. A., Drake, M. T., & Hurley, D. L. (2010). Vitamin D deficiency in adults: When to test and how to treat. *Mayo Clinic Proceedings, 85*(8), 752–758. https://doi.org/10.4065/mcp.2010.0138, http://www.mayoclinicproceedings.com/content/85/8/752.full.pdf+html.

Krist, A. H., Davidson, K. W., Mangione, C. M., Cabana, M., Caughey, A. B., Davis, E. M., Donahue, K. E., Doubeni, C. A., Epling, J. W., Kubik, M., Li, L., Ogedegbe, G., Owens, D. K., Pbert, L., Silverstein, M., Stevermer, J., Tseng, C. W., & Wong, J. B. (2021). Screening for vitamin D deficiency in adults: US preventive services task force recommendation statement. *JAMA - Journal of the American Medical Association, 325*(14), 1436–1442. https://doi.org/10.1001/jama.2021.3069, http://jama.jamanetwork.com/journal.aspx.

Lips, P., de Jongh, R. T., & van Schoor, N. M. (2021). Trends in vitamin D status around the world. *JBMR Plus, 5*, 12. https://doi.org/10.1002/jbm4.10585, https://asbmr.onlinelibrary.wiley.com/journal/24734039.

Matsui, M. S. (2020). Vitamin D update. *Current Dermatology Reports, 9*(4), 323–330. https://doi.org/10.1007/s13671-020-00315-0, http://www.springer.com/medicine/dermatology/journal/13671.

McAdler, M. M. (2013). The Relationship Between Vitamin D Status of Adult Women and Diet, Sun Exposure, Skin Reflectance, Body Composition, and Insulin Sensitivity. Master's Theses. https://doi.org/10.15368/theses.2013.31.

Mavar, M., Sorić, T., Bagarić, E., Sarić, A., & Matek Sarić, M. (2024). The Power of Vitamin D: Is the Future in Precision Nutrition through Personalized Supplementation Plans? *Nutrients, 16*(8). https://doi.org/10.3390/NU16081176.

Nasri, H. (2017). The adverse effects of vitamin D deficiency on health. *Journal of Renal Endocrinology, 3*(1).

Płudowski, P., Kos-Kudła, B., Walczak, M., Fal, A., Zozulińska-Ziółkiewicz, D., Sieroszewski, P., Peregud-Pogorzelski, J., Lauterbach, R., Targowski, T., Lewiński, A., Spaczyński, R., Wielgoś, M., Pinkas, J., Jackowska, T., Helwich, E., Mazur, A., Ruchała, M., Zygmunt, A., Szalecki, M., ... Misiorowski, W. (2023). Guidelines for Preventing and Treating Vitamin D Deficiency: A 2023 Update in Poland. *Nutrients, 15*(3), 695. https://doi.org/10.3390/NU15030695.

Pludowski, P., Takacs, I., Boyanov, M., Belaya, Z., Diaconu, C. C., Mokhort, T., Zherdova, N., Rasa, I., Payer, J., & Pilz, S. (2022). Clinical practice in the prevention, diagnosis and treatment of vitamin D deficiency: A Central and Eastern European Expert Consensus Statement. *Nutrients, 14*(7). https://doi.org/10.3390/nu14071483, https://www.mdpi.com/2072-6643/14/7/1483/pdf.

Sahota, J. K., & Shaw, N. (2014). Preventing vitamin D deficiency in children in the UK. *Nurse Prescribing, 12*(12), 596–602. https://doi.org/10.12968/npre.2014.12.12.596.

Sangondimath, G., Sen, R. K., & F.R., T. (2023). DEXA and imaging in osteoporosis. *Indian Journal of Orthopaedics, 57*, 82–93. https://doi.org/10.1007/s43465-023-01059-2, https://www.springer.com/journal/43465.

Shah, J., & Gurbani, S. (2020). *Association of vitamin D deficiency and mood disorders: A systematic review.* IntechOpen. https://doi.org/10.5772/intechopen.90617.

Yin, D., Hu, J., Zhao, J., Qiao, H., & Zhao, Y. (2020). Simultaneous determination of 25-hydroxyvitamin D and vitamin K_1 in serum by ultra-performance liquid chromatography-tandem mass spectrometry. *Wei Sheng Yan Jiu=Journal of Hygiene Research.* https://doi.org/10.19813/J.CNKI.WEISHENGYANJIU.2020.04.013.

Zimmerman, L., Anastasopoulou, C., & McKeon, B. (2024). *Osteomalacia. In StatPearls [Internet].* StatPearls Publishing.

The health matrix: vitamin D and the many systems it touches

CHAPTER 12

Vitamin D and chronic respiratory diseases: a complex relationship

Muhammad Irfan[1], Midrar Ullah[1], Amna Ansari[2], and Nousheen Iqbal[1,3]

[1]*Department of Medicine, Aga Khan University, Karachi, Pakistan* [2]*Medical College, Aga Khan University, Karachi, Pakistan* [3]*Department of Medicine, Jinnah Medical and Dental College, Karachi, Pakistan*

12.1 Introduction

Vitamin D is one of the fat-soluble vitamins important for calcium and phosphate absorption and has emerged as a crucial player in various biological processes beyond bone health. In recent years, interest has been growing in the potential role of vitamin D regarding the pathogenesis and management of chronic respiratory diseases (CRDs), such as asthma, chronic obstructive pulmonary disease (COPD), pulmonary fibrosis, and chronic pulmonary infections.

This chapter will look at the evidence supporting an association of vitamin D deficiency with CRDs, discussing the basic mechanisms and its therapeutic implications.

12.2 Vitamin D implications in chronic pulmonary infections

12.2.1 Tuberculosis

From an infectious disease point of view, tuberculosis (TB) remains the major cause of death worldwide, and TB has resulted in significant mortality and morbidity despite the available chemotherapy for more than 50 years. Globally, TB has resulted in the death of 1.6 million people in 2021 (Who, 2022). Furthermore, mycobacterium TB latently infects 25% of the world's population, placing them at a 5%–10% lifetime chance of acquiring active illness (Houben et al., 2016; Who, 2022).

In 1834 the British physician C.J.B. Williams described the role of cod liver oil in patients with phthisis, a progressive wasting and consumptive condition mainly from TB. He reported that among 234 patients who had TB, 206 had significant improvement, ranging in severity from a brief delay in the illness's progression to a reduction in uncomfortable symptoms (Williams, 1849). Niels Finsen received the Nobel Prize in 1903 in Medicine for his research demonstrating the potential therapeutic benefits of ultraviolet (UV) radiation for those

The Impact of Vitamin D on Health and Disease. DOI: https://doi.org/10.1016/B978-0-443-34037-6.00011-X

suffering from lupus vulgaris, TB of the skin. Hermann Brehmer founded the first sanatorium dedicated to treating TB in the late 1800s (Liu et al., 2007). These sanitariums offered healthy food and lots of fresh air, even at high altitudes. There have been suggestions that the benefits that TB patients in these sanatoriums enjoyed might have resulted from their exposure to UV light, which may have increased the skin's generation of vitamin D precursors.

12.2.1.1 Pathophysiology

Vitamin D modulates various functions of the body, cellular and regulatory processes, which include host defense against various infections, inflammation, and plays a role in innate immunity by modulating monocyte and macrophage activity.

The process of conversion of inactive pro-vitamin 25-hydroxyvitamin D3 into the active form 1,25-dihydroxy-vitamin D3 is accomplished by 1,alpha-hydroxylase (CYP27B1) mainly presents in the kidney. But various studies concluded that the CYP27B1 is not only present in the kidney but also synthesized in pulmonary macrophages and monocytes as well resulting in local activation of vitamin D3 (Pike & Christakos, 2017). The monocytes and macrophages play an important role in innate immunity, which provides a rapid response against microbial pathogens. Toll-like receptors on monocytes and macrophages mainly recognize and attach to the ligand derived from the pathogens, including lipopeptides. The stimulation of TLRs on monocytes and macrophages activates an antimicrobial response by stimulating downstream signaling pathways in the cells (Fig. 12.1). Activation of TLRs in monocytes and macrophages results in increased expression of mRNA for vitamin D receptors and CYP27b1, an enzyme capable of catalyzing the conversion of inactive pro-vitamin D3 (25-hydroxyl-vitamin D3) into the active form 1, 25-dihydroxy-vitamin D3. Expression of vitamin D receptors and vitamin D-hydroxylase gene results in the induction of antimicrobial peptides, including cathelicidin, resulting in killing of intracellular mycobacterium (Holick, 2007; Liu et al., 2006; Ralph et al., 2008) (Fig. 12.1).

In the meanwhile, Vit-D has an immune-modulatory function in treating TB by inducing the formation of molecules which has antimicrobial activity including methyl glycol and β-Fenin 2, which bring neutrophils, monocytes, and T cells to the area of infection (Rivas-Santiago et al., 2009).

12.2.1.2 Correlation of vitamin D with pulmonary tuberculosis

The mycobacterium is involved in phagocytic activity, and this activity of phagocytosis is correlated with those patients who are suffering from rickets (Ströder & Kasal, 1970). Research has shown a correlation between the vitamin D level and the susceptibility of hosts to mycobacterium TB. Three observations were listed by researchers as potential examples of its association: First, the cold winter months when sun exposure reduces the formation of vitamin D in the body are correlated with

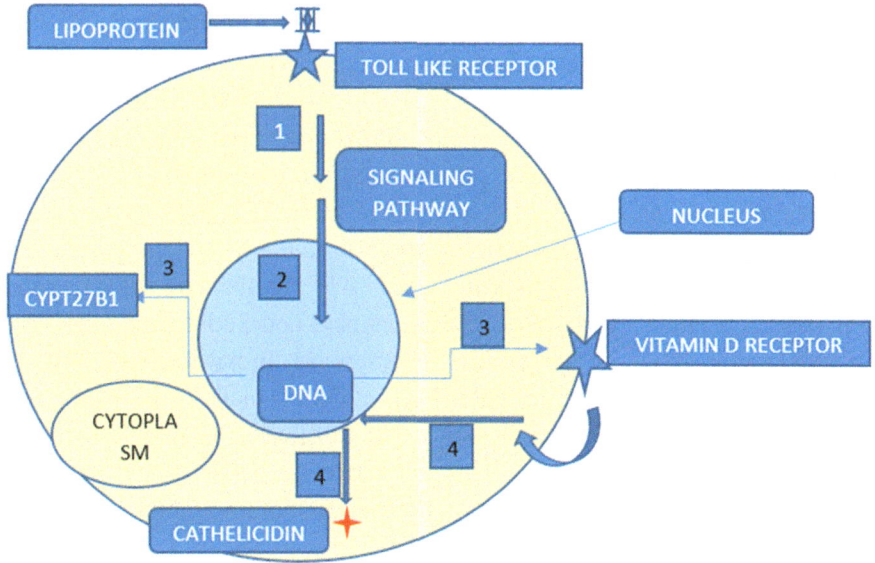

Figure 12.1
Vitamin D and the induction of cathelicidin.
Lipoprotein attached to the toll-like receptor on the cell membrane activates a signaling pathway, resulting in increased expression of vitamin D receptors and CYP7B1. CYP7B1 and the vitamin D receptor cause increased expression of cathelicidin. Cathelicidin then kills intracellular organisms.

higher incidence of TB; second, certain demographic groups (for instance, children, uremic patients, the elders, and Asian immigrants in the United Kingdom) are more likely to have lower serum vit-D levels and higher incidence of TB (Cai et al., 2022; Chan, 2000).

According to Hewison, innate and adaptive immunity are strongly correlated with vitamin D level, making such individuals more vulnerable to TB (Hewison, 2012).

The metaanalysis which included seven case–control studies from different ethnic populations concluded that decreased serum vitamin D levels are linked with increased risk of active TB compared to healthy individuals matched for factors like age, gender, race, nutrition, and geographical place (Nnoaham & Clarke, 2008).

Due to higher melanin content in the skin of African Americans, they have a reduced ability to produce vitamin D through exposure to ultraviolet light. As a result, they often have lower levels of 25-hydroxyvitamin D3 (25-OH vitamin D3), which increases their susceptibility to infections caused by mycobacterium even resulting in a rapid worsening of the disease. Research indicates that in the African American, the expression of cathelicidin mRNA, an antimicrobial peptide, is significantly lower compared to Caucasians. However, when African American serum is supplemented with 25-OH vitamin D to reach physiological levels, the response was an increase in the Toll-like receptor (TLR) mediated induction of cathelicidin mRNA.

12.2.1.3 Role of vitamin D in time-to-sputum smear and culture conversion

A significant inverse connection exists between serum 25 (OH) D levels and the time to acquire consecutive negative sputum smears or cultures, which signifies that decreased vitamin D levels could be associated with poor treatment outcome in addition to raising the risk of getting active TB. Consequently, patients with active pulmonary TB, insufficient vitamin D levels may be indicative of a prolonged clinical course (Sato et al., 2012). Similarly, a systematic review focused on case–control research to find out the possibilities of vitamin D. The study concluded that giving vitamin D supplements to TB patients can enhance their clinical results (Sutaria et al., 2014). Jahnavi and Sudha separated 100 patients receiving antitubercular drugs at Anganwadi Centers in India into two groups for a case–control study. The control group did not receive dietary plans or supplements, and the experimental group was given food supplements that fulfilled daily targets for vitamin and mineral intake. Compared to the control group, the experimental group showed greater rates of sputum conversion and treatment completion after three months (Jahnavi & Sudha, 2010).

One of the randomized control studies showed that the intramuscular vitamin D supplementation to TB medication significantly increased sputum smear conversion rates in pulmonary TB patients, albeit with certain drawbacks. However, it was not double-blinded, and the randomized group for anti-TB therapy alone did not receive a placebo. These factors may have contributed to the risk of a "false positive," and the noted differences between the groups may be due to the psychological impact of the intramuscular vitamin D injection in the intervention group (Afzal et al., 2018).

In a metaanalysis of 1850 participants across eight studies, the factors influencing the outcomes were analyzed. The researchers focused on randomized controlled trials (RCTs) on vitamin D supplementation among individuals receiving antimicrobial treatment for pulmonary TB. The primary as well as secondary outcomes of interest were the time-to-sputum culture and time-to-sputum smear conversion. The findings revealed that, overall, supplementation with vitamin D did not show an evident impact on the time it took for sputum cultures to convert (indicating the clearance of TB bacteria from the sputum). However, among patients who had multidrug-resistant pulmonary TB, vitamin D had accelerated the time-to-sputum culture conversion. The study also showed that supplementation with vitamin D accelerated the time-to-sputum smear conversion across the entire patient group, suggesting a faster clearance of bacteria from the sputum when examined under a microscope (Jolliffe et al., 2019).

12.2.1.4 Role of vitamin D in treatment outcome

A randomized double-blinded, multicenter, placebo-controlled clinical trial from Pakistan showed rapid improvement in clinical and radiographic parameters in all TB patients and enhanced host immunity predicted by an increase in the interferon gamma secretion among patients who have decrease baseline deficient vitamin D levels when administered with 600,000 IU of vitamin D3. The clinical improvement results in significant weight gain in patients receiving higher supplementation of vitamin D, and radiological response was greater than 50% or more decrease in the TB cavity size and resulting in lesser residual disease and zones involvements. These may suggest a potential role of vitamin D for the treatment of TB (Salahuddin et al., 2013).

However, recent studies on vitamin D supplementation did not demonstrate any advantage (Martineau et al., 2011; Wejse et al., 2009).

Furthermore, a two-by-two factorial study carried out in Tanzania showed that giving vitamin and mineral supplements to sputum-positive TB patients who were also coinfected with HIV greatly increased their survival rates. These results may highlight the potential advantages of nutritional supplementation in improving treatment outcomes for individuals with TB, especially those who also have coinfections (Range et al., 2006).

12.2.1.5 Role of vitamin D in latent tuberculosis

In regard to latent TB infection (LTBI), metaanalysis found a substantial correlation between the deficiency of vitamin D and increased risk of having LTBI or active TB development among people with LTBI or those who interact closely with TB patients. Moreover, vitamin D deficiency was linked to a higher chance of having TB infection conversion (TBIC) or converting a tuberculin skin test (TST). Interestingly, although there was a tendency for active TB patients to have lower vitamin D levels than LTBI participants or active TB patients' household contacts, the difference did not reach statistical significance. This concludes that vitamin D deficiency (VDD) may not simply be a consequence of malnutrition, often seen in active TB patients. If VDD were purely a result of malnutrition associated with TB, a more noticeable difference in vitamin D levels would be expected between the groups. Overall, the study suggests that VDD is more likely a risk factor for the development of TB instead of a consequence of the disease. The lack of a noticeable difference in vitamin D levels between the patients who have active TB and those with LTBI or household contacts implies that VDD likely contributes to the risk of developing TB rather than being a result of the disease itself. This distinction is crucial for understanding the vitamin D role in TB pathogenesis and may have implications for preventive strategies in at-risk populations (Nnoaham & Clarke, 2008).

This was also supported by the study that showed the effects of vitamin D administration on the conversion rate of tuberculin skin test (TST), which is an indicator of TB infection in a group of Mongolian schoolchildren. The children received either 800 IU of vitamin D per day or a placebo for six months. The results showed that there was a 59% greater reduction in the TST conversion rate among those who received vitamin D as compared to the placebo group (Ganmaa et al., 2012).

In another randomized controlled trial (RCT), it was shown that the innate immunity among the vitamin D group against mycobacterium was much better that of placebo group but there was no improvement in the acquired immunity (Martineau et al., 2007). The antimicrobial immunity of TB contacts was markedly improved in vitro by administering a single dose of vitamin D (Martineau et al., 2007).

12.2.2 Role of vitamin D in COVID-19 and acute respiratory distress syndrome

Acute respiratory distress syndrome (ARDS) is the severe form of acute lung injury resulting in respiratory failure, characterized by the development of hypoxemia, noncardiac pulmonary edema, and the need for ventilator support. Around 10% of patients in intensive care units worldwide are diagnosed with to have ARDS. In most studies, mortality stays high at 30–40% despite some improvements (Matthay et al., 2018). The deficiency of vitamin D is associated with worse outcomes for individuals suffering from ARDS. According to research, patients with ARDS frequently have vitamin D insufficiency (Dancer et al., 2015). In vitro, insufficient vitamin D caused inflammation in the alveoli, hypoxia, and harm to lung epithelial cells. These results are supported by clinical evidence that individuals with vitamin D deficiency who took supplements prior to esophagectomy had reduced alveolar capillary damage (Parekh et al., 2018). Evidence suggests that vitamin D increases the proliferation of alveolar epithelial type II (AT-II) cells by PI3K/Akt signaling pathway. This pathway is necessary for regulating cell growth and survival. Thus vitamin D stimulates the replication and growth of AT-II cells, maintaining healthy lung tissue and repairing damage. Vitamin D has been found to reduce epithelial-mesenchymal transition (EMT) by TGF-β (Transforming Growth Factor Beta) molecular signaling pathway. Epithelial cells go through a transformation process called EMT, which may exacerbate lung injury and fibrosis. Vitamin D aids in preventing this shift by blocking the TGF-β pathway, which lessens fibrosis and preserves improved lung function (Zheng et al., 2020).

These insights have prompted researchers to investigate the effect of vitamin D in COVID-19, which has led to a global pandemic. ARDS is well-known complication of COVID-19 and has resulted in significant mortality and morbidity. SARS-CoV-2 attaches to the angiotensin-converting enzyme 2 (ACE2) on the membrane of respiratory epithelial cells. Increased activation of the dual rennin-angiotensin system (RAS) has been related to vitamin D deficiency, and ACE2 is an important regulator of this process (Getachew & Tizabi, 2021). Additionally, it is suggested that vitamin D aids in the suppression of the ACE/Angiotensin II/AT1 receptor (AT1R) signaling pathway in the RAS. Acute Respiratory Distress Syndrome (ARDS) and other disorders may benefit from this inhibition's ability to balance the body and lessen inflammation and damage caused by overactivation of the RAS (Getachew & Tizabi, 2021; Xiao et al., 2021).

The effect of vitamin D levels on COVID-19 outcomes is still a subject of debate. A number of observational and experimental studies have found a negative correlation between the supplementation of vitamin D and the severity or mortality of COVID-19, implying a possible benefit (Abdulateef et al., 2021; Alcala-diaz et al., 2021; Annweiler et al., 2020; Entrenas

Castillo et al., 2020; Ling et al., 2020). Other studies have reported no significant outcome, indicating that the effects of vitamin D on COVID-19 are inconclusive (Cereda et al., 2021; Murai et al., 2021; Oristrell et al., 2021).

Vitamin D insufficiency was linked to increased illness severity and mortality in a 2021 systematic review and metaanalysis, which included 27 observational data, but no notable correlation was observed with the probability of contracting COVID-19 infection. Nevertheless, in this metaanalysis, 74% of the contributing studies were categorized as having a high risk of bias (Pereira et al., 2022).

The most extensive metaanalysis covering 13 intervention studies has reported decrease in the ICU admissions and death rates when supplemented with vitamin D (Pal et al., 2022).

In another metaanalysis, vitamin D supplementation when given to hospitalized COVID-19 patients was linked to a decrease in ICU admission, the need for invasive ventilation, and a reduction in death rate. However, this metaanalysis did not show convincing evidence for preventing COVID-19 as primary prevention (Hosseini et al., 2022).

Vitamin D upregulates the production of cathelicidin. Cathelicidin is then broken down to generate LL37, which is an innate antimicrobial and demonstrates effectiveness against a diverse array of microbes, including enveloped viruses, including coronavirus family. The link of vitamin D deficiency with weak immune response may be due to decreased activity of LL37 (Crane-Godreau et al., 2020).

12.2.3   Vitamin D and fungal infections

Vitamin D shapes the immune system and regulates the transcription of cathelicidin. The influence of vitamin D on fungal infection is not well studied, and more research is required to draw a conclusion. In an in vitro study on mice with invasive aspergillosis, statistical significance between groups treated with Amphotericin only and those who were treated with Amphotericin and vitamin D was not observed. Vitamin D on its own demonstrated neither positive nor negative effects on the life expectancy of mice with aspergillosis (Sirivoranankul et al., 2014).

In another study done on the mice nurtured on a deficient vitamin D or a sufficient diet were infected with *Aspergillus fumigatus*, intratracheally, and were observed. Mice with Vitamin D deficiency experienced increased mortality, increased fungal burden, and greater weight reduction compared to vitamin D-sufficient mice. The deficiency led to more severe and prolonged inflammation of lung, along with elevated broncho-alveolar-lavage cell counts, mainly neutrophils, following infection. Vitamin D-deficient mice exhibited higher resting levels of proinflammatory cytokines in their lungs with alveolar macrophages (Li et al., 2014).

A study showed from single-center, high occurrence of vitamin D insufficiency in patient with chronic pulmonary aspergillosis. However, no difference was observed in mortality and morbidity in subjects with vitamin D or without deficiency (Sehgal et al., 2020).

12.2.3.1 Vitamin D and pneumocystis

Interestingly, the importance of vitamin D in regard to the treatment of Pneumocystis murinum (major form of Pneumocystis in rats) in an in vitro study showed a promising result. In a study in which immunodeficient mice were inoculated with Pneumocystis murinum were followed and treated with for 3 weeks with Vit-D3 alone, Primaquine alone, a combination of Primaquine and Vit-D3, or a combination of trimethoprim and sulfamethoxazole. In this study, vitamin D had a synergistic effect with primaquine. This property is similar to Al trans retinoic acid, which is used in combination with primaquine for Pneumocystis. The combination also resulted in the reduction of inflammatory cells in the lung (Lei et al., 2016).

12.2.4 Vitamin D supplementation to reduce pulmonary infections

The Endocrine Society of Clinical Practice Guidelines creates clinical practice guidelines for using the active form of vitamin D to reduce the disease risk in individuals who do not have specific indications for 25-(OH)D testing or vitamin D treatment. And they suggest empirical vitamin D supplementation from aged 1–18 years to decrease the incidence of nutritional rickets and to potentially decrease the risk of respiratory infections. Empirical vitamin D may involve the daily consumption of fortified (supplemented) foods, vitamin preparations containing vitamin D, and daily use of vitamin D. In the clinical trials incorporated in the systematic review, vitamin D doses regarding respiratory infections varied from 300 to 2000 IU daily equivalent. The guidelines were based on 12 RCTs. The relative risk (RR) of acquiring TB (from 2 trials with 10,533 participants) was 0.67 (95% CI, 0.14–3.11) in individual who received vitamin D (10 000 and 14 000 IU weekly) with an absolute effect size of 1 fewer case per 1000 (ranging from 2 fewer to 6 more). This data suggests a potential mitigation of the risk of developing TB with vitamin D supplementation, but the evidence is not strong enough to be conclusive due to the wide confidence interval (Ganmaa et al., 2020; Middelkoop et al., 2023). The actual impact could vary widely, and more research may be needed to clarify the effect. The combined data from three trials show that vitamin D supplementation significantly reduces the rate of respiratory infections. This finding is further supported by another trial where the incidence of multiple respiratory infections (three or more) was considerably lower in the vitamin D group compared to the control group (Camargo et al., 2012; Di Mauro et al., 2018; Marusca et al., 2023; Singh et al., 2019). This suggests that vitamin D may be effective in reducing both the incidence and severity of respiratory infections.

Vitamin D is affordable, easily accessible, and has a low risk of side effects, even at higher doses. However, additional research is needed to know the effectiveness in vivo, to diminish confounding variables, and to establish the doses, duration, and the method of administration for preventing and treating various diseases related to pulmonary infections.

12.3 Vitamin D implications in obstructive airway diseases a chronic

12.3.1 Obstructive pulmonary disease

COPD is a chronic inflammatory disease linked with increased morbidity and mortality (GBD, 2015). Vitamin D deficiency, popularly recognized in the context of bone diseases, is being associated increasingly with other chronic conditions, and it is also being studied in the context of a possible factor that may influence the course of disease in COPD (Brøndum-Jacobsen et al., 2012; Forouhi et al., 2012; Gandini et al., 2011; Ginde et al., 2009).

12.3.1.1 Vitamin D and lung functions

Results from numerous cross-sectional studies indicate that patients with a higher level of vitamin D have concomitantly better lung functions based on their FEV1 (Afzal et al., 2014; Choi et al., 2013; Kunisaki et al., 2011; Wannamethee et al., 2021). Wannamethee et al. investigated the relationship between vitamin D deficiency and its negative impact on restrictive and obstructive lung function in older men aged 60–75 in the United Kingdom. They also studied the long-term mortality associated with vitamin D deficiency-induced impaired lung function. They report that elevated lung function parameters (both FEV1 and FVC) were observed in those with higher 25(OH)D levels. COPD was more prevalent in men with Vitamin D deficiency. Moreover, the odds of having vitamin D deficiency were increased in men with moderate or severe COPD versus men with normal lung function, postadjustment for confounders, including age, season, smoking, physical activity, social class, heavy drinking, BMI, diabetes, and preexisting CVD. There was an additional increased risk of respiratory mortality (Wannamethee et al., 2021).

Data analysis from three National Health and Nutrition Examination Surveys (2007–12) discovered a positive correlation between serum 25-hydroxyvitamin D [25(OH)D] concentrations and lung function markers, namely, FVC and FEV1, in US adults. Individuals with higher vitamin D levels had markedly improved FVC and FEV1. This association persisted even after stratification by gender and smoking status. However, no association was observed between vitamin D and the prevalence of asthma, chronic bronchitis, or emphysema (Ganji et al., 2020).

Afzal et al. carried out a cross-sectional study on the association of decreased vitamin D levels with diminished lung function, increased rate of lung function decline, and higher risk of COPD. They analyzed data from 10 116 white participants from the Copenhagen City Heart Study, tracked for up to 20 years, and 8391 white participants from the Copenhagen General

Population Study. Lower plasma vitamin D levels were linked with decreased FEV1 and FVC, as well as an increased risk of COPD diagnosed with spirometry (Afzal et al., 2014).

A South Korean investigated the relationship between Vitamin D levels and lung function in adult Koreans using data from the KNHANES survey (2008–2010). Increased vitamin D levels were linked to improved lung function (FEV1 and FVC), independent of age, sex, height, and season. The results maintained significance even after stratifying against BMI, lifestyle, socioeconomic factors, and respiratory illness. However, the association between vitamin D and lung function was particularly strong in subjects with a history of pulmonary TB (Choi et al., 2013).

12.3.1.2 Vitamin D and chronic obstructive pulmonary disease

Prospective studies exploring the relationship between baseline vitamin D levels and lung function decline, along with the onset of COPD, have produced mixed results. Smokers with vitamin D deficiency have been linked with decreased lung function and rapid decline in lung function with the hypothesis that sufficient vitamin D levels might play a protective role in combating the adverse effects of smoking on the lung parenchyma (Lange et al., 2012). The prospective component of the study based on the Danish population corroborated these results by reporting that greater decline in lung function (FEV1 and FVC) and increased risk of COPD diagnosed on spirometric information was found in those with a lower level of vitamin D. This finding was consistent irrespective of the smoking status of the patient, however, compared to the two groups there was a stronger association with smokers (Afzal et al., 2014). Similarly, higher mortality was linked with lower vitamin D levels in COPD (Færk et al., 2018). Other prospective studies, however, report no significant association between vitamin D levels and decline in lung function or incidence of COPD (Kunisaki et al., 2011; Skaaby et al., 2014).

A study, conducted between January 2014 and September 2015, on the Turkish population investigated the association of vitamin D deficiency (VDD) with lung function in COPD patients. The study included 216 participants with measured vitamin D levels, excluding those with certain comorbidities or a history of smoking fewer than 10 pack-years. Significantly more annual exacerbations and hospitalizations along with lower FEV1 and FVC were found in patients with vitamin D deficiency. Additionally, significantly lower mMRC dyspnea scores were seen with decreased vitamin D levels. The study concluded that vitamin D deficiency led to worse lung function in COPD patients, and the deficiency increased with the increasing severity of COPD.

12.3.1.2.1 Pathogenesis

Proposed possible pathways by which vitamin D could influence the development and prognosis of COPD heavily focus on the vitamin D receptor (VDR). Expression of over 900 genes related to immune functions is controlled by the VDR by its function as nuclear transcription factor. Research has demonstrated that a stronger innate immune response against airway infections is linked to vitamin D. It promotes the production of antimicrobial peptides (AMPs) and enhances the phagocytic and chemotactic activity of macrophages. Additionally, vitamin D has been related to enhanced lung development and tissue repair. It is reported that vitamin D, in its forms 25(OH)D and 1,25(OH)2D, can lower the levels of PGE2—a substance involved in inflammation—in lung cells. This happens because vitamin D reduces the activity of a protein that makes PGE2 and boosts the activity of another protein that breaks it down. It uses the VDR for this purpose in both fetal and adult lung cells. VDR carries the vitamin D signal into the cell nucleus and affects how genes are turned on or off (Baeke et al., 2010; Kongsbak et al., 2013; Li et al., 2014). Conversely, vitamin D may reduce inflammation by decreasing T-cell reactivity and the proinflammatory response. This is also due to its effect on VDR, which is present in various inflammatory and structural cells. When vitamin D is deficient, it is unable to regulate the maturation of dendritic cells and macrophages by controlling major histocompatibility complex class II molecules. This deficiency also reduces the generation of proinflammatory cytokines and chemokines, promotes the recruitment of monocytes and neutrophils via the NFκB-mediated pathway, and shifts Th1 T cells towards Th2 and regulatory T cells. This disrupted immune-inflammatory reaction may result in prolonged inflammation and damage to lung structure, ultimately contributing to the development and progression of COPD. However, it is also theorized that vitamin D might not be directly implicated in the progression of COPD but since it prevents respiratory infections, it may prevent COPD deaths through prevention of pulmonary infections. Since morbidity and mortality in COPD are highly linked to respiratory infections, reduced risk due to supplementing vitamin D could lead to a better prognosis in COPD (Barragan et al., 2015; Cantorna et al., 2008; Trujillo et al., 2013; Wei & Christakos, 2015; Zhang et al., 2012).

12.3.1.2.2 Effect of vitamin D supplementation on chronic obstructive pulmonary disease

Despite several associations of COPD and vitamin D deficiency, supplementation has not led to a conclusive result. A randomized, double-blind, placebo-controlled trial investigated the impact of vitamin D3 supplementation on COPD exacerbations and upper respiratory infections in 240 participants. The study found that supplementing vitamin D did not significantly reduce the time to initial moderate or severe exacerbation or first upper respiratory infection overall. A predefined subgroup analysis, however, showed that vitamin D supplementation reduced the risk of moderate or severe exacerbations in patients with baseline serum 25-hydroxyvitamin D levels below 50 nmol/L, but had no effect in those with levels of 50 nmol/L or higher. The intervention did not affect the risk of upper respiratory tract infection regardless of baseline vitamin D status. These results suggested that supplementing vitamin D in patients with COPD may reduce the risk of moderate or severe exacerbations (Martineau et al., 2015).

Another randomized, single-center, placebo-controlled, double-blind trial investigated the role of supplementing standard COPD treatment with vitamin D and its effect on C-reactive protein and pulmonary function tests in 135 patients with moderate-to-severe COPD exacerbations. The primary outcomes were FEV1, FVC, and MMRC scale. The study found no significant difference in FEV1 or FEV1/FVC ratio in the treatment groups and placebo. However, patients who received calcitriol showed significant clinical improvement. No side effects were reported. The study concluded that a short course of calcitriol or 25(OH)2 vitamin D did not change FEV1 or FVC in vitamin D-sufficient patients with COPD exacerbation but may provide clinical benefits (Sanjari et al., 2015).

Another recent double-blind, randomized, multicenter trial assessed the impact of vitamin D supplementation on exacerbation rates in COPD patients with vitamin D deficiency. The study included 155 participants with a known history of exacerbations and vitamin D levels between 15 and 50 nmol/L. They were assigned randomly to receive either 16,800 IU of vitamin D3 or placebo weekly for one year. The primary outcome was the exacerbation rate. Despite significantly improving vitamin D levels in the treatment cohort, supplementation did not reduce exacerbation rates. Additionally, no significant differences were observed in secondary outcomes, including time to exacerbations, hospitalizations, antibiotic use, pulmonary function, physical performance, and quality of life. It was concluded that vitamin D supplementation had no role in reducing the rate of exacerbation in COPD patients with vitamin D deficiency (Rafiq et al., 2022).

In contrast, an earlier placebo-controlled, double-blind, randomized clinical trial assessed the impact of vitamin D supplementation on COPD exacerbations and FEV1 in patients with severe and very severe COPD. A total of 88 patients were allocated randomly to receive a 6-month regimen of either routine treatment plus 100,000 IU of oral vitamin D monthly for 6 months or routine treatment plus placebo. The study found significant improvements in FEV1 with a decrease in the number of exacerbations in the vitamin D group versus the placebo group. The authors concluded that in the severe and very severe COPD cohorts, vitamin D supplementation led to reduced COPD exacerbations and improved FEV1 (Zendedel et al., 2015).

A metaanalysis using individual participant data from randomized controlled trials examined the effect of vitamin D supplementation on COPD exacerbations. Four eligible RCTs with 560 patients were located, and information from 469 participants in three RCTs was analyzed. Overall, vitamin D supplementation had no significant effect on the rate of moderate/severe COPD exacerbations. However, in the subgroup analysis, it was revealed that vitamin D supplementation reduced exacerbations in participants with baseline vitamin D levels <25 nmol/L but not in those with levels ≥25 nmol/L. There was no increase in the serious adverse events with vitamin D supplementation. It was concluded that vitamin D supplementation safely and significantly reduced COPD exacerbations in patients with baseline vitamin D deficiency but not in those with higher levels (Jolliffe et al., 2019).

12.3.1.3   Vitamin D and asthma

Multiple studies have associated vitamin D deficiency with a higher risk of developing asthma and experiencing its symptoms.

A cross-sectional study of 5011 Caucasian adults between ages of 45–69 years examined the association between vitamin D levels and respiratory diseases. Low vitamin D levels (<50 nmol/L) were significantly associated with a higher prevalence of asthma, bronchitis, wheezing, and chest tightness even after adjusting for confounders. Conversely, better lung function, as measured by forced vital capacity (FVC), was seen in patients with vitamin D levels >100 nmol/L than those with levels between 50–100 nmol/L. The study concluded that decreased vitamin D levels were independently related to asthma, while higher levels were linked to improved lung function (Mulrennan et al., 2018).

Another study looked at the association between serum vitamin D levels and asthma in adults, hypothesizing a stronger link in nonatopic individuals. Using data from the 1958 birth cohort, Cherrie et al. designed a measure of atopic status based on total and specific IgE values and history of eczema and allergic rhinitis. A nested case–control analysis was conducted, stratified by atopic status, to examine the relationship between vitamin D levels at age 46 and the prevalence of asthma and wheezy bronchitis at age 50, excluding those with a history of these conditions before age 42. Fully adjusted models revealed that an increase in serum vitamin D by 10 nmol/L was significantly associated with a decreased prevalence of asthma. Depending on the atopic status, the association between vitamin D levels and asthma varied. Initially, lower atopy scores were associated with stronger links to asthma. However, these associations were no longer statistically significant after adjusting for adiposity (Cherrie et al., 2018).

Another study using data from the National Health and Nutrition Examination Survey (2001–2010) examined the association between vitamin D insufficiency (serum 25-hydroxyvitamin D <30 ng/mL) and asthma or wheeze in 10,860 children (6–17 years) and 24,115 adults (18–79 years), as well as lung function in a subset of participants. Vitamin D insufficiency was associated with current asthma and wheeze in children, and with current wheeze in adults, particularly in non-Hispanic whites. Additionally, lower lung function (FEV1 and FVC) in both children and adults was linked to vitamin D insufficiency. The prevalence of vitamin D insufficiency decreased from 2007 to 2010, paralleling a decrease in asthma prevalence during the same period. The study concluded that there are associations between vitamin D insufficiency and asthma or wheeze specific to certain racial/ethnic groups and noted the concurrent decreases in vitamin D insufficiency and asthma prevalence (Han et al., 2017).

Similarly, a cross-sectional study, including 3937 participants aged 13–69 years enrolled in the Canadian Health Measures Survey—Cycle 1, analyzed the association between vitamin D levels and asthma prevalence and lung function. Participants were categorized into low (≤49 nmol/L), moderate (50–74 nmol/L), and high (≥75 nmol/L) vitamin D levels. The study found that lower vitamin D levels were associated with a higher prevalence of current and ever asthma. The study concluded that vitamin D levels <50 nmol/L were associated with a higher risk of current and ever asthma, warranting additional exploration of this association for optimal asthma management (Niruban et al., 2015).

A metaanalysis was conducted to investigate the association between serum vitamin D levels and lung function in asthma patients. The study reported that asthma patients with low vitamin D levels had lower FEV1 and FEV1% versus those with optimum vitamin D levels. Additionally, there was a positive correlation of vitamin D levels and various lung function measures, including FEV1, FEV1%, FVC, FEV1/FVC, and the asthma control test (ACT). These associations remained significant for both children and adults. The metaanalysis suggests that better lung function in asthma patients might be associated with higher serum vitamin D levels. Additional research is required to validate these findings and explore the underlying mechanisms (Liu et al., 2019).

12.3.1.3.1 Effect of vitamin D supplementation on asthma

The therapeutic effects of vitamin D have been a subject of considerable interest, particularly in the context of chronic conditions such as asthma. Vitamin D supplementation exhibits antiinflammatory effects in the lungs by inhibiting the activity of nuclear factor-κB and mitogen-activated protein kinase, leading to reduced release of inflammatory cytokines and chemokines like IL-1β, IL-6, and IL-8, and causing decreased infiltration of inflammatory cells into the interstitial space. Additionally, vitamin D diminishes oxidative stress since it inhibits antiprotease activity and activates nuclear factor erythroid-related factor 2, a regulator of antioxidant genes. It enhances immune function by promoting monocyte-to-macrophage proliferation and upregulating cathelicidin in airway epithelial cells. Furthermore, in airway smooth muscle cells and alveolar macrophages, vitamin D inhibits metalloproteinases, affecting the airway remodeling and extracellular matrix deposition (Amrein et al., 2020; Leclair et al., 2019).

In allergic asthma, vitamin D reduces inflammation, increases IL-10 levels, decreases mast cell activation, eosinophil count, and lung tissue infiltration, and inhibits B cell proliferation and differentiation. It also decreases phospholipase A2 production, which contributes to asthma pathogenesis. In nonallergic asthma, vitamin D reduces oxidative stress and IL-6 response in bronchial epithelial cells, decreasing proliferation, proinflammatory cytokines, and matrix metalloproteinase in airway smooth muscle cells. Moreover, vitamin D may benefit severe asthmatics with steroid-resistant asthma linked to IL-17 by shifting Th17 effector cells towards a Treg phenotype, causing decreased IL-17 production and increased IL-10 levels. It also inhibits neutrophilic inflammation by reducing the production of proinflammatory cytokines and enhancing antibacterial activity in neutrophils. These findings highlight the prospects of vitamin D as a therapeutic option in asthma management (Gaudet et al., 2022).

An updated metaanalysis, published in 2023, evaluated the effectiveness and safety of vitamin D supplementation in causing less exacerbations and controlling symptoms. The review included 20 studies with 1155 children and 1070 adults. The incidence of severe asthma exacerbations requiring systemic corticosteroids was the primary outcome. The analysis found no significant effect of vitamin D supplementation on decreasing or increasing the rate of exacerbations, or the time to first exacerbation. Subgroup analyses showed no effect modification based on baseline vitamin D status, dosage, dosing regimen, or age. The authors concluded that, contrary to previous findings, this updated review does not provide evidence that vitamin D supplementation helps reduce asthma exacerbations or improve asthma control (Williamson et al., 2023).

Older studies, however, contradict this finding. Individual participant data from randomized controlled trials were used in a systematic review and metaanalysis to investigate the role of vitamin D supplementation in reducing asthma exacerbations requiring systemic corticosteroids, and whether this effect is influenced by baseline vitamin D status. The analysis included 955 participants from seven eligible trials. Vitamin D supplementation reduced the rate of asthma exacerbations overall. Subgroup analyses revealed that this protective effect was significant in patients with baseline vitamin D levels <25 nmol/L. No significant differences were found in other subgroup analyses. The study concluded that there was a reduction in the number of asthma exacerbations with vitamin D supplementation, with some evidence suggesting a greater benefit for those with lower baseline vitamin D levels (Jolliffe et al., 2017).

A randomized, double-blind, placebo-controlled trial assessed the impact of high-dose vitamin D3 supplementation (400,000 IU) on airway inflammation in 44 patients with nonatopic asthma characterized by neutrophilic and/or eosinophilic inflammation. After 9 weeks, vitamin D supplementation significantly reduced sputum eosinophils in patients with high baseline eosinophil levels but not in the total group or those with predominantly neutrophilic inflammation. Additionally, a small improvement in Asthma Control Questionnaire scores was seen. The study concluded that vitamin D supplementation may be beneficial as an add-on treatment for patients with nonatopic asthma and severe eosinophilic airway inflammation (De Groot et al., 2015).

12.3.1.4 Cystic fibrosis

Cystic fibrosis (CF) is an autosomal-recessive disorder and is usually caused by CF transmembrane conductance regulator (CFTR) gene polymorphism. It commonly affects the pancreas and lungs. Vitamin D deficiency is common in CF patients because of pancreatic insufficiency and fat malabsorption. Vitamin D levels in 40–90% of CF patients are below 30 ng/mL (Mangas-Sánchez et al., 2021). Recent guidelines recommend increased doses of vitamin D supplementation in patients with CF (Gaudet et al., 2022).

Pulmonary infections like *nontuberculous mycobacteria* (NTM) and *Pseudomonas aeruginosa* are also more common in these patients (Richter et al., 2021; Wood et al., 2021). *In one of a randomized trials, researchers showed an* antiinflammatory effect of vitamin D by reducing the level of IL-17A and IL-23 in the airway of these patients with chronic *P. aeruginosa* infection (Olszowiec-Chlebna et al., 2019). So, vitamin D deficiency causes recurrent exacerbations and progressive lung function decline due to respiratory infections in CF patients. Owing to its immune-modulation effects of vitamin D, its supplementation during exacerbation can result in improvement in lung functions and reduction in exacerbation rate (Abu-Fraiha et al., 2019). DiFranco et al. (2017) showed that topical administration can be converted to the active form in the airway by increasing CFTR levels in these patients. That can be used as adjunctive therapy in CF patients, and the result of this study can help in the development of future therapies.

There should be an aim to keep serum 25-hydroxyvitamin D levels above the normal level in these patients. Cholecalciferol is preferred over ergocalciferol. Daily or once weekly dosing regimens can be chosen according to patient preference and compliance (Wood et al., 2021).

12.4 Vitamin D implications in restrictive lung diseases

12.4.1 Idiopathic pulmonary fibrosis

Idiopathic pulmonary fibrosis (IPF) is caused by excessive accumulation of extracellular matrix (ECM) proteins triggered by lung fibroblasts and myofibroblasts, a pro-fibrotic state improvised by different elements like genetic susceptibility, oxidative stress, impaired regenerative responses, chronic injury, and aging (Chanda et al., 2019). Like other CRDs, vitamin D has an impact on IPF but data are limited (Gaudet et al., 2022). A study showed that vitamin D dosing inhibited bleomycin-induced lung fibrosis, by declining hydroxyproline concentration. Lack of vitamin D is also found to be linked with enhanced disease severity in addition to a higher mortality rate in IPF (Tzilas et al., 2019). Chang J, et al. found in the mouse model of IPF that therapy with paricalcitol (a compound similar to vitamin D) prohibited mouse body weight loss and improved lung fibrosis, by impending the stimulation of the lung renin–angiotensin system (RAS) (Chang et al., 2021). Another study findings suggested that during pulmonary fibrosis, fibroblast vitamin D receptors (VDR) upregulation limits fibroblast production and stimulation by suppressing the JAK1/STAT3/ER stress pathway (J. Wei et al., 2023). VDRs are abundant in lung and have antiinflammatory effect in lung tissues (Kong et al., 2013).

In Contrast, a study from UK population discovered no relationship between vitamin D deficiency and prevalence of restrictive lung impairment. However, vitamin D deficiency was related to increased all-cause mortality in normal as well as in restrictive lung disorder or patients with mild/moderate COPD (Wannamethee et al., 2021). Further studies are mandatory to assess vitamin D's role in IPF.

12.4.2 Sarcoidosis

Compared to Caucasians in the United States, Afro-Americans are likely to suffer from sarcoidosis and severe vitamin D deficiency (Gallagher & Sai, 2010; Judson et al., 2012).

Prior research has demonstrated a negative association between serum vitamin D 25-(OH)D levels and the degree of sarcoidosis activity. Lower serum vitamin D levels are linked with more severe sarcoidosis symptoms (Burke et al., 2010; Kamphuis et al., 2014).

The perception of excess vitamin D has been negatived mostly due to concern of hypercalcemia. But 1,25-(OH)2D overproduction in sarcoidosis might be an adaptive immune response to reduce granulomatous inflammation by encouraging elimination triggering antigen to preserve overall tissue health. There is also a concern over complications from vitamin D supplementation as doses that are typically too low can cause changes in calcium levels both in the blood and urine of healthy people. This concern has slowed down research interested in the effects of vitamin D supplementation in sarcoidosis, as the condition already involves calcium imbalances, and researchers are cautious about possible adverse effects (Baughman et al., 2013; Saidenberg-Kermanac'h et al., 2014; Sodhi & Aldrich, 2016). Nonetheless, there is a broad variation in the prevalence of hypercalcemia in sarcoidosis among various groups. According to recent studies, among sarcoidosis patients receiving vitamin D therapy, the incidence of hypercalcemia ranged from 5.2% to 7.7% (Bolland et al., 2013; Capolongo et al., 2016; Kamphuis et al., 2014).

Vitamin D therapy did not modify the mean serum calcium or urine calcium in a randomized, placebo-controlled trial conducted in New Zealand on 27 normocalcemic patients with sarcoidosis and vitamin D insufficiency. In this study, 7.7% experienced significant hypercalcemia at an accumulative dose of 250,000 IU of cholecalciferol over a 6-week period. The other patients received 50,000 IU weekly cholecalciferol or a placebo for 11 months (Bolland et al., 2013).

A significant negative relationship was detected between serum 25-(OH)D levels and disease activity. This was determined by somatostatin receptor scintigraphy in a retrospective study involving 301 patients with sarcoidosis over a period of 23 years. Five out of 104 (4.8%) patients experienced hypercalcemia as a result of calcium and vitamin D supplementation (500 mg and 400 IU, respectively) (Kamphuis et al., 2014).

In another study, there was no change in the incidence of vitamin D insufficiency between the patients and the correspondingly matched general population 12. When 16 African American patients with sarcoidosis and low vitamin D were given oral ergocalciferol (50,000 IU) once a week for 12 weeks, the mean serum calcium level did not change; however, one patient experienced hypercalcemia (6.25%) (Capolongo et al., 2016). This study also showed that the 1,25-(OH)2D decreased after vitamin D replacement. The reasons behind the decrease are yet unknown, but it is possible that extra-renal 1,25-(OH)2D synthesis by immune cells in sarcoidosis is heightened in the context of vitamin D deficiency as an adaptive reaction to lessen antigen-stimulated granuloma development. A study on rodents has shown that the locally produced 1,25-(OH)2D increases 24-hydroxylase, which in turn promotes the inactive 1,24,25(OH)D from 25-(OH)D and/or 1,25-(OH)2D (Hewison, 2010).

As steroids are the first-line treatment of sarcoidosis, these patients are at risk of steroid-induced osteoporosis. The calcium and vitamin D dosage should be cautiously amended to avoid hypercalcemia. If serum calcium or urinary calcium rises to a maximum, the dose of the calcium supplements should be adjusted. Various studies have shown reversal of hypercalcemia after withdrawal of supplements (Capolongo et al., 2016; Crouser et al., 2020; Kamphuis et al., 2014). If hypercalcemia persists, then the dose of vitamin D should be amended.

Vitamin D and calcium imbalances perform a key position in sarcoidosis, but the management of vitamin D supplementation remains controversial due to concerns over worsening calcium metabolism. This caution has limited research into vitamin D in sarcoidosis, though a recent study in two ethnic groups suggests that restoring vitamin D levels may reduce disease activity by lowering markers like ACE and γ-globulin (Capolongo et al., 2016). While promising, these small studies emphasize the requirement for larger trials to fully evaluate the risks and benefits of vitamin D supplementation in sarcoidosis patients.

References

Abdulateef, D. S., Rahman, H. S., Salih, J. M., Osman, S. M., Mahmood, T. A., Omer, S. H. S., & Ahmed, R. A. (2021). COVID-19 severity in relation to sociodemographics and vitamin D use. *Open Medicine (Poland), 16*(1), 591–609. https://doi.org/10.1515/med-2021-0273, https://www.degruyter.com/view/j/med.

Abu-Fraiha, Y., Elyashar-Earon, H., Shoseyov, D., Cohen-Cymberknoh, M., Armoni, S., Kerem, E., & Wilschanski, M. (2019). Increasing vitamin D serum levels is associated with reduced pulmonary exacerbations in patients with cystic fibrosis. *Journal of Pediatric Gastroenterology and Nutrition, 68*(1), 110–115. https://doi.org/10.1097/mpg.0000000000002126.

Afzal, A., Rathore, R., Butt, N. F., & Randhawa, F. A. (2018). Efficacy of vitamin D supplementation in achieving an early sputum conversion in smear positive pulmonary tuberculosis. *Pakistan Journal of Medical Sciences, 34*(4), 849–854. https://doi.org/10.12669/pjms.344.14397, http://www.pjms.com.pk/index.php/pjms/article/viewFile/14397/6195.

Afzal, S., Lange, P., Bojesen, S. E., Freiberg, J. J., & Nordestgaard, B. G. (2014). Plasma 25-hydroxyvitamin D, lung function and risk of chronic obstructive pulmonary disease. *Thorax, 69*(1), 24–31. https://doi.org/10.1136/thoraxjnl-2013-203682, http://thorax.bmj.com/content/69/1/24.full.pdf.

Alcala-diaz, J. F., Limia-perez, L., Gomez-huelgas, R., Martin-escalante, M. D., Cortes-rodriguez, B., Zambrana-garcia, J. L., Entrenas-castillo, M., Perez-caballero, A. I., López-carmona, M. D., Garcia-alegria, J., Rodríguez-mancheño, A. L., Arenas-De Larriva, M. D. S., Pérez-belmonte, L. M., Jungreis, I., Bouillon, R., Quesada-gomez, J. M., & Lopez-miranda, J. (2021). Calcifediol treatment and hospital mortality due to covid-19: A cohort study. *Nutrients, 13*(6). https://doi.org/10.3390/nu13061760, https://www.mdpi.com/2072-6643/13/6/1760/pdf.

Amrein, K., Scherkl, M., Hoffmann, M., Neuwersch-Sommeregger, S., Köstenberger, M., Tmava Berisha, A., Martucci, G., Pilz, S., & Malle, O. (2020). Vitamin D deficiency 2.0: an update on the current status worldwide. *European Journal of Clinical Nutrition, 74*(11), 1498–1513. https://doi.org/10.1038/s41430-020-0558-y.

Annweiler, C., Hanotte, B., Grandin de l'Eprevier, C., Sabatier, J.-M., Lafaie, L., & Célarier, T. (2020). Vitamin D and survival in COVID-19 patients: A quasi-experimental study. *The Journal of Steroid Biochemistry and Molecular Biology, 204*, 105771. https://doi.org/10.1016/j.jsbmb.2020.105771.

Baeke, F., Takiishi, T., Korf, H., Gysemans, C., & Mathieu, C. (2010). Vitamin D: modulator of the immune system. *Current Opinion in Pharmacology, 10*(4), 482–496. https://doi.org/10.1016/j.coph.2010.04.001.

Barragan, M., Good, M., & Kolls, J. K. (2015). Regulation of dendritic cell function by vitamin D. *Nutrients, 7*(9), 8127–8151. https://doi.org/10.3390/nu7095383, http://www.mdpi.com/2072-6643/7/9/5383/pdf.

Baughman, R. P., Janovcik, J., Ray, M., Sweiss, N., & Lower, E. E. (2013). Calcium and vitamin D metabolism in sarcoidosis. *Sarcoidosis, Vasculitis, and Diffuse Lung Diseases, 30*(2), 113–120.

Bolland, M. J., Wilsher, M. L., Grey, A., Horne, A. M., Fenwick, S., Gamble, G. D., & Reid, I. R. (2013). Randomised controlled trial of vitamin D supplementation in sarcoidosis. *BMJ Open, 3*(10). https://doi.org/10.1136/bmjopen-2013-003562NewZealand, http://bmjopen.bmj.com/content/3/10/e003562.full.pdf+html.

Brøndum-Jacobsen, P., Benn, M., Jensen, G. B., & Nordestgaard, B. G. (2012). 25-hydroxyvitamin D levels and risk of ischemic heart disease, myocardial infarction, and early death: Population-based study and meta-analyses of 18 and 17 studies. *Arteriosclerosis, Thrombosis, and Vascular Biology, 32*(11), 2794–2802. https://doi.org/10.1161/ATVBAHA.112.248039.

Burke, R. R., Rybicki, B. A., & Rao, D. S. (2010). Calcium and vitamin D in sarcoidosis: How to assess and manage. *Seminars in respiratory and critical care medicine, 31*(4), 474–484. https://doi.org/10.1055/s-0030-1262215, http://www.thieme-connect.com/ejournals/toc/srccm.

Cai, L., Wang, G., Zhang, P., Hu, X., Zhang, H., Wang, F., & Tong, Y. (2022). The progress of the prevention and treatment of vitamin D to tuberculosis. *Frontiers in Nutrition, 9*. https://doi.org/10.3389/fnut.2022.873890.

Camargo, C. A., Ganmaa, D., Frazier, A. L., Kirchberg, F. F., Stuart, J. J., Kleinman, K., Sumberzul, N., & Rich-Edwards, J. W. (2012). Randomized trial of vitamin D supplementation and risk of acute respiratory infection in Mongolia. *Pediatrics, 130*(3), e561. https://doi.org/10.1542/peds.2011-3029, http://pediatrics.aappublications.org/content/130/3/e561.full.pdf+html.

Cantorna, M. T., Yu, S., & Bruce, D. (2008). The paradoxical effects of vitamin D on type 1 mediated immunity. *Molecular Aspects of Medicine, 29*(6), 369–375. https://doi.org/10.1016/j.mam.2008.04.004.

Capolongo, G., Xu, L. H. R., Accardo, M., Sanduzzi, A., Stanziola, A. A., Colao, A., Agostini, C., Zacchia, M., Capasso, G., Adams-Huet, B., Moe, O. W., Maalouf, N. M., Sakhaee, K., & Hsia, C. C. W. (2016). Vitamin-D status and mineral metabolism in two ethnic populations with sarcoidosis. *Journal of Investigative Medicine, 64*(5), 1025–1034. https://doi.org/10.1136/jim-2016-000101, http://jim.bmj.com/content/about-us.

Cereda, E., Bogliolo, L., Lobascio, F., Barichella, M., Zecchinelli, A. L., Pezzoli, G., & Caccialanza, R. (2021). Vitamin D supplementation and outcomes in coronavirus disease 2019 (COVID-19) patients from the outbreak area of Lombardy, Italy. *Nutrition, 82*, 111055. https://doi.org/10.1016/j.nut.2020.111055.

Chan, T. Y. K. (2000). Vitamin D deficiency and susceptibility to tuberculosis. *Calcified Tissue International, 66*(6), 476–478. https://doi.org/10.1007/s002230010095.

Chanda, D., Otoupalova, E., Smith, S. R., Volckaert, T., De Langhe, S. P., & Thannickal, V. J. (2019). Developmental pathways in the pathogenesis of lung fibrosis. *Molecular Aspects of Medicine, 65*, 56–69. https://doi.org/10.1016/j.mam.2018.08.004, http://www.elsevier.com/locate/mam.

Chang, J., Nie, H., Ge, X., Du, J., Liu, W., Li, X., Sun, Y., Wei, X., Xun, Z., & Li, Y. C. (2021). Vitamin D suppresses bleomycin-induced pulmonary fibrosis by targeting the local renin–angiotensin system in the lung. *Scientific Reports, 11*(1). https://doi.org/10.1038/s41598-021-96152-7, http://www.nature.com/srep/index.html.

Cherrie, M. P. C., Sarran, C., & Osborne, N. J. (2018). Association between serum 25-hydroxy vitamin D levels and the prevalence of adult-onset asthma. *International journal of environmental research and public health, 15*(6). https://doi.org/10.3390/ijerph15061103, http://www.mdpi.com/1660-4601/15/6/1103/pdf.

Choi, C. J., Seo, M., Choi, W. S., Kim, K. S., Youn, S. A., Lindsey, T., Choi, Y. J., & Kim, C. M. (2013). Relationship between serum 25-hydroxyvitamin D and lung function among Korean adults in Korea National Health and Nutrition Examination Survey (KNHANES), 2008-2010. *Journal of Clinical Endocrinology and Metabolism, 98*(4), 1703–1710. https://doi.org/10.1210/jc.2012-3901SouthKorea, http://jcem.endojournals.org/content/98/4/1703.full.pdf+html.

Crane-Godreau, M. A., Clem, K. J., Payne, P., & Fiering, S. (2020). Vitamin D deficiency and air pollution exacerbate COVID-19 through suppression of antiviral peptide LL37. *Frontiers in Public Health, 8.* https://doi.org/10.3389/fpubh.2020.00232, http://journal.frontiersin.org/journal/public-health/section/public-health-education-and-promotion#archive.

Crouser, E. D., Maier, L. A., Wilson, K. C., Bonham, C. A., Morgenthau, A. S., Patterson, K. C., Abston, E., Bernstein, R. C., Blankstein, R., Chen, E. S., Culver, D. A., Drake, W., Drent, M., Gerke, A. K., Ghobrial, M., Govender, P., Hamzeh, N., James, W. E., Judson, M. A., ... Baughman, R. P. (2020). Diagnosis and detection of sarcoidosis. An official american thoracic society clinical practice guideline. *American Journal of Respiratory and Critical Care Medicine, 201*(8), e26. https://doi.org/10.1164/rccm.202002-0251st.

Dancer, R. C. A., Parekh, D., Lax, S., D'Souza, V., Zheng, S., Bassford, C. R., Park, D., Bartis, D. G., Mahida, R., Turner, A. M., Sapey, E., Wei, W., Naidu, B., Stewart, P. M., Fraser, W. D., Christopher, K. B., Cooper, M. S., Gao, F., Sansom, D. M., ... Thickett, D. R. (2015). Vitamin D deficiency contributes directly to the acute respiratory distress syndrome (ARDS). *Thorax, 70*(7), 617–624. https://doi.org/10.1136/thoraxjnl-2014-206680.

De Groot, J. C., Van Roon, E. N. H., Storm, H., Veeger, N. J. G. M., Zwinderman, A. H., Hiemstra, P. S., Bel, E. H. D., & Ten Brinke, A. (2015). Vitamin D reduces eosinophilic airway inflammation in nonatopic asthma. *Journal of Allergy and Clinical Immunology, 135*(3), 670. https://doi.org/10.1016/j.jaci.2014.11.033, http://www.elsevier.com/inca/publications/store/6/2/3/3/6/8/index.htt.

Di Mauro, A., Baldassarre, M. E., Capozza, M., Nicolardi, A., Tafuri, S., Di Mauro, F., Ferorelli, D., Laforgia, N., & Grosso, R. (2018). The impact of vitamin D supplementation in paediatric primary care on recurrent respiratory infections: A randomized controlled trial. *EuroMediterranean Biomedical Journal, 13*(44), 194–199. https://doi.org/10.3269/1970-5492.2018.13.44, http://www.embj.org/2018/.

DiFranco, K. M., Mulligan, J. K., Sumal, A. S., & Diamond, G. (2017). Induction of CFTR gene expression by 1,25(OH)2 vitamin D3, 25OH vitamin D3, and vitamin D3 in cultured human airway epithelial cells and in mouse airways. *Journal of Steroid Biochemistry and Molecular Biology, 173*, 323–332. https://doi.org/10.1016/j.jsbmb.2017.01.013, http://www.elsevier.com/locate/jsbmb.

Entrenas Castillo, M., Entrenas Costa, L. M., Vaquero Barrios, J. M., Alcalá Díaz, J. F., López Miranda, J., Bouillon, R., & Quesada Gomez, J. M. (2020). Effect of calcifediol treatment and best available therapy versus best available therapy on intensive care unit admission and mortality among patients hospitalized for COVID-19: A pilot randomized clinical study. *Journal of Steroid Biochemistry and Molecular Biology, 203.* https://doi.org/10.1016/j.jsbmb.2020.105751, http://www.elsevier.com/locate/jsbmb.

Færk, G., Çolak, Y., Afzal, S., & Nordestgaard, B. G. (2018). Low concentrations of 25-hydroxyvitamin d and long-term prognosis of copd: A prospective cohort study. *European Journal of Epidemiology, 33*(6), 567–577. https://doi.org/10.1007/s10654-018-0393-9, http://www.wkap.nl/journalhome.htm/0393-2990.

Forouhi, N. G., Ye, Z., Rickard, A. P., Khaw, K. T., Luben, R., Langenberg, C., & Wareham, N. J. (2012). Circulating 25-hydroxyvitamin D concentration and the risk of type 2 diabetes: Results from the European Prospective Investigation into Cancer (EPIC)-Norfolk cohort and updated meta-analysis of prospective studies. *Diabetologia, 55*(8), 2173–2182. https://doi.org/10.1007/s00125-012-2544-y.

Gallagher, J. C., & Sai, A. J. (2010). Vitamin D insufficiency, deficiency, and bone health. *Journal of Clinical Endocrinology and Metabolism, 95*(6), 2630–2633. https://doi.org/10.1210/jc.2010-0918, http://jcem.endojournals.org/cgi/reprint/95/6/2630.

Gandini, S., Boniol, M., Haukka, J., Byrnes, G., Cox, B., Sneyd, M. J., Mullie, P., & Autier, P. (2011). Meta-analysis of observational studies of serum 25-hydroxyvitamin D levels and colorectal, breast and prostate cancer and colorectal adenoma. *International Journal of Cancer, 128*(6), 1414–1424. https://doi.org/10.1002/ijc.25439.

Ganji, V., Al-Obahi, A., Yusuf, S., Dookhy, Z., & Shi, Z. (2020). Serum vitamin D is associated with improved lung function markers but not with prevalence of asthma, emphysema, and chronic bronchitis. *Scientific Reports, 10*(1). https://doi.org/10.1038/s41598-020-67967-7.

Ganmaa, D., Giovannucci, E., Bloom, B. R., Fawzi, W., Burr, W., Batbaatar, D., Sumberzul, N., Holick, M. F., & Willett, W. C. (2012). Vitamin D, tuberculinskin test conversion, and latent tuberculosis in Mongolian school-age children: A randomized, double-blind, placebo-controlled feasibility trial. *American Journal of Clinical*

Nutrition, 96(2), 391–396. https://doi.org/10.3945/ajcn.112.034967, http://www.ajcn.org/content/96/2/391. full.pdf+html.

Ganmaa, D., Uyanga, B., Zhou, X., Gantsetseg, G., Delgerekh, B., Enkhmaa, D., Khulan, D., Ariunzaya, S., Sumiya, E., Bolortuya, B., Yanjmaa, J., Enkhtsetseg, T., Munkhzaya, A., Tunsag, M., Khudyakov, P., Seddon, J. A., Marais, B. J., Batbayar, O., Erdenetuya, G., ... Martineau, A. R. (2020). Vitamin D supplements for prevention of tuberculosis infection and disease. *New England Journal of Medicine, 383*(4), 359–368. https://doi.org/10.1056/NEJMoa1915176, http://www.nejm.org/medical-index.

Gaudet, M., Plesa, M., Mogas, A., Jalaleddine, N., Hamid, Q., & Al Heialy, S. (2022). Recent advances in vitamin D implications in chronic respiratory diseases. *Respiratory Research, 23*(1). https://doi.org/10.1186/s12931-022-02147-x.

GBD. (2015). Global, regional, and national deaths, prevalence, disability-adjusted life years, and years lived with disability for chronic obstructive pulmonary disease and asthma, 1990-2015: A systematic analysis for the Global Burden of Disease Study. *Lancet Respir Med, 5*(9). https://doi.org/10.1016/s2213-2600.

Getachew, B., & Tizabi, Y. (2021). Vitamin D and COVID-19: Role of ACE2, age, gender, and ethnicity. *Journal of Medical Virology, 93*(9), 5285–5294. https://doi.org/10.1002/jmv.27075.

Ginde, A. A., Mansbach, J. M., & Camargo, C. A. (2009). Association between Serum 25-hydroxyvitamin D level and upper respiratory tract infection in the Third National Health and Nutrition Examination Survey. *Archives of Internal Medicine, 169*(4), 384–390. https://doi.org/10.1001/archinternmed.2008.560, http://archinte.ama-assn.org/cgi/reprint/169/4/384.

Han, Y. Y., Forno, E., & Celedón, J. C. (2017). Vitamin D Insufficiency and Asthma in a US Nationwide Study. *Journal of Allergy and Clinical Immunology: In Practice, 5*(3), 790. https://doi.org/10.1016/j.jaip.2016.10.013, http://www.elsevier.com/journals/the-journal-of-allergy-and-clinical-immunology-in-practice/2213-2198.

Hewison, M. (2010). Vitamin D and the intracrinology of innate immunity. *Molecular and Cellular Endocrinology, 321*(2), 103–111. https://doi.org/10.1016/j.mce.2010.02.013.

Hewison, M. (2012). Vitamin D and immune function: An overview. *Proceedings of the Nutrition Society, 71*(1), 50–61. https://doi.org/10.1017/s0029665111001650.

Holick, M. F. (2007). Vitamin D Deficiency. *New England Journal of Medicine, 357*(3), 266–281. https://doi.org/10.1056/nejmra070553.

Hosseini, B., El Abd, A., & Ducharme, F. M. (2022). Effects of Vitamin D Supplementation on COVID-19 related outcomes: A systematic review and meta-analysis. *MDPI, Canada Nutrients, 14*(10). https://doi.org/10.3390/nu14102134, https://www.mdpi.com/2072-6643/14/10/2134/pdf?version=1653033949.

Houben, R. M. G. J., Dodd, P. J., & Metcalfe, J. Z. (2016). The global burden of latent tuberculosis infection: A re-estimation using mathematical modelling. *PLoS medicine, 13*(10), e1002152. https://doi.org/10.1371/journal.pmed.1002152.

Jahnavi, G., & Sudha, C. H. (2010). Randomised controlled trial of food supplements in patients with newly diagnosed tuberculosis and wasting. *Singapore Medical Journal, 51*(12), 957–962. http://smj.sma.org.sg/5112/5112a8.pdf.

Jolliffe, D. A., Greenberg, L., Hooper, R. L., Griffiths, C. J., Camargo, C. A., Kerley, C. P., Jensen, M. E., Mauger, D., Stelmach, I., Urashima, M., & Martineau, A. R. (2017). Vitamin D supplementation to prevent asthma exacerbations: A systematic review and meta-analysis of individual participant data. *The Lancet Respiratory Medicine, 5*(11), 881–890. https://doi.org/10.1016/S2213-2600(17)30306-5, http://www.elsevier.com/journals/the-lancet-respiratory-medicine/2213-2600.

Jolliffe, D. A., Ganmaa, D., Wejse, C., Raqib, R., Haq, M. A., Salahuddin, N., Daley, P. K., Ralph, A. P., Ziegler, T. R., & Martineau, A. R. (2019). Adjunctive vitamin D in tuberculosis treatment: Meta-analysis of individual participant data. *European Respiratory Journal, 53*(3). https://doi.org/10.1183/13993003.02003-2018, https://erj.ersjournals.com/content/53/3/1802003.

Judson, M. A., Boan, A. D., & Lackland, D. T. (2012). The clinical course of sarcoidosis: Presentation, diagnosis, and treatment in a large white and black cohort in the United States. *Sarcoidosis, Vasculitis, and Diffuse Lung Diseases, 29*(2), 119–127.

Kamphuis, L. S., Bonte-Mineur, F., Van Laar, J. A., Van Hagen, P. M., & Van Daele, P. L. (2014). Calcium and vitamin D in sarcoidosis: Is supplementation safe? *Journal of Bone and Mineral Research, 29*(11), 2498–2503. https://doi.org/10.1002/jbmr.2262, http://onlinelibrary.wiley.com/journal/10.1002/(ISSN)1523-4681.

Kong, J., Zhu, X., Shi, Y., Liu, T., Chen, Y., Bhan, I., Zhao, Q., Thadhani, R., & Li, Y. C. (2013). VDR attenuates acute lung injury by blocking Ang-2-Tie-2 pathway and renin-angiotensin system. *Molecular Endocrinology, 27*(12), 2116–2125. https://doi.org/10.1210/me.2013-1146.

Kongsbak, M., Levring, T. B., Geisler, C., & von Essen, M. R. (2013). The vitamin D receptor and T cell function. *Frontiers in immunology, 4.* https://doi.org/10.3389/fimmu.2013.00148, http://www.frontiersin.org/Journal/FullText.aspx?ART_DOI=10.3389/fimmu.2013.00148&name=T_Cell_Biology&x=y.

Kunisaki, K. M., Niewoehner, D. E., Singh, R. J., & Connett, J. E. (2011). Vitamin D status and longitudinal lung function decline in the Lung Health Study. *European Respiratory Journal, 37*(2), 238–243. https://doi.org/10.1183/09031936.00146509.

Lange, N. E., Sparrow, D., Vokonas, P., & Litonjua, A. A. (2012). Vitamin D deficiency, smoking, and lung function in the normative aging study. *American Journal of Respiratory and Critical Care Medicine, 186*(7), 616–621. https://doi.org/10.1164/rccm.201110-1868OC, http://ajrccm.atsjournals.org/content/186/7/616.full.pdf+html.

Leclair, T. R., Zakai, N., Bunn, J. Y., Gianni, M., Heyland, D. K., Ardren, S. S., & Stapleton, R. D. (2019). Vitamin D supplementation in mechanically ventilated patients in the medical intensive care unit. *Journal of Parenteral and Enteral Nutrition, 43*(8), 1037–1043. https://doi.org/10.1002/jpen.1520, http://onlinelibrary.wiley.com/journal/10.1002/(ISSN)1941-2444.

Lei, G.-S., Zhang, C., Zimmerman, M. K., & Lee, C.-H. (2016). Vitamin D as supplemental therapy for pneumocystis pneumonia. *Antimicrobial Agents and Chemotherapy, 60*(3), 1289–1297. https://doi.org/10.1128/aac.02607-15.

Li, P., Xu, X., Cao, E., Yu, B., Li, W., Fan, M., Huang, M., Shi, L., Zeng, R., Su, X., Shi, Y., & Sturtevan, J. (2014). Vitamin D deficiency causes defective resistance to *Aspergillus fumigatus* in mice via aggravated and sustained inflammation. *PLoS ONE, 9*(6), e99805. https://doi.org/10.1371/journal.pone.0099805.

Ling, S. F., Broad, E., Murphy, R., Pappachan, J. M., Pardesi-Newton, S., Kong, M. F., & Jude, E. B. (2020). High-dose cholecalciferol booster therapy is associated with a reduced risk of mortality in patients with covid-19: A cross-sectional multi-centre observational study. *Nutrients, 12*(12), 1–16. https://doi.org/10.3390/nu12123799, https://www.mdpi.com/2072-6643/12/12/3799.

Liu, J., Dong, Y. Q., Yin, J., Yao, J., Shen, J., Sheng, G. J., Li, K., Lv, H. F., Fang, X., & Wu, W. F. (2019). Meta-analysis of vitamin D and lung function in patients with asthma. *Respiratory Research, 20*(1). https://doi.org/10.1186/s12931-019-1072-4, http://respiratory-research.com/home/.

Liu, P. T., Stenger, S., Li, H., Wenzel, L., Tan, B. H., Krutzik, S. R., Ochoa, M. T., Schauber, J., Wu, K., Meinken, C., Kamen, D. L., Wagner, M., Bals, R., Steinmeyer, A., Zügel, U., Gallo, R. L., Eisanberg, D., Hewison, M., Hollis, B. W., ... Modlin, R. L. (2006). Toll-like receptor triggering of a vitamin D-mediated human antimicrobial response. *Science, 311*(5768), 1770–1773. https://doi.org/10.1126/science.1123933.

Liu, P. T., Krutzik, S. R., & Modlin, R. L. (2007). Therapeutic implications of the TLR and VDR partnership. *Trends in Molecular Medicine, 13*(3), 117–124. https://doi.org/10.1016/j.molmed.2007.01.006.

Mangas-Sánchez, C., Garriga-García, M., Serrano-Nieto, M. J., García-Romero, R., Álvarez-Beltrán, M., Crehuá-Gaudiza, E., Muñoz-Codoceo, R., Suárez-Cortina, L., Vicente-Santamaría, S., Martínez-Costa, C., Díaz-Martin, J. J., Bousoño-García, C., & González-Jiménez, D. (2021). Vitamin d status in pediatric and young adult cystic fibrosis patients. Are the new recommendations effective? *Nutrients, 13*(12). https://doi.org/10.3390/nu13124413, https://www.mdpi.com/2072-6643/13/12/4413/pdf.

Martineau, A. R., Wilkinson, R. J., Wilkinson, K. A., Newton, S. M., Kampmann, B., Hall, B. M., Packe, G. E., Davidson, R. N., Eldridge, S. M., Maunsell, Z. J., Rainbow, S. J., Berry, J. L., & Griffiths, C. J. (2007). A single dose of vitamin D enhances immunity to mycobacteria. *American Journal of Respiratory and Critical Care Medicine, 176*(2), 208–213. https://doi.org/10.1164/rccm.200701-007OC, http://ajrccm.atsjournals.org/cgi/reprint/176/2/208.pdf.

Martineau, A. R., Timms, P. M., Bothamley, G. H., Hanifa, Y., Islam, K., Claxton, A. P., & Griffiths, C. J. (2011). High-dose vitamin D(3) during intensive-phase antimicrobial treatment of pulmonary tuberculosis: a double-blind randomised controlled trial. *Lancet, 377*(9761). https://doi.org/10.1016/s0140-6736 61889–2.

Martineau, A. R., James, W. Y., Hooper, R. L., Barnes, N. C., Jolliffe, D. A., Greiller, C. L., Islam, K., McLaughlin, D., Bhowmik, A., Timms, P. M., Rajakulasingam, R. K., Rowe, M., Venton, T. R., Choudhury, A. B., Simcock, D. E., Wilks, M., Degun, A., Sadique, Z., Monteiro, W. R., ... Griffiths, C. J. (2015). Vitamin D3 supplementation in patients with chronic obstructive pulmonary disease (ViDiCO): A multicentre, double-blind, randomised controlled trial. Lancet Publishing Group, United Kingdom. *The Lancet Respiratory Medicine, 3*(2), 120–130. https://doi.org/10.1016/S2213-2600(14)70255-3, http://www.elsevier.com/journals/the-lancet-respiratory-medicine/2213-2600.

Marusca, L. M., Reddy, G., Blaj, M., Prathipati, R., Rosca, O., Bratosin, F., Bogdan, I., Horhat, R. M., Tapos, G. F., Marti, D. T., Susan, M., Pingilati, R. A., Horhat, F. G., & Adelina, M. (2023). The effects of vitamin D supplementation on respiratory infections in children under 6 years old: A systematic review. *Diseases, 11*(3). https://doi.org/10.3390/diseases11030104, http://www.mdpi.com/journal/diseases.

Matthay, M. A., Zemans, R. L., Zimmerman, G. A., Arabi, Y. M., Beitler, J. R., Mercat, A., Herridge, M., Randolph, A. G., & Calfee, C. S. (2018). Acute respiratory distress syndrome. *Nature Reviews Disease Primers, 5*(1). https://doi.org/10.1038/s41572-019-0069-0, http://www.nature.com/nrdp/.

Middelkoop, K., Stewart, J., Walker, N., Delport, C., Jolliffe, D. A., Coussens, A. K., Nuttall, J., Tang, J. C. Y., Fraser, W. D., Griffiths, C. J., Kumar, G. T., Filteau, S., Hooper, R. L., Wilkinson, R. J., Bekker, L. G., & Martineau, A. R. (2023). Vitamin D supplementation to prevent tuberculosis infection in South African schoolchildren: multicenter phase 3 double-blind randomized placebo-controlled trial (ViDiKids). *International Journal of Infectious Diseases, 134*, 63–70. https://doi.org/10.1016/j.ijid.2023.05.010, https://www.journals.elsevier.com/international-journal-of-infectious-diseases.

Mulrennan, S., Knuiman, M., Walsh, J. P., Hui, J., Hunter, M., Divitini, M., Zhu, K., Cooke, B. R., Musk, A. W. B., & James, A. (2018). Vitamin D and respiratory health in the Busselton Healthy Ageing Study. *Respirology, 23*(6), 576–582. https://doi.org/10.1111/resp.13239, http://onlinelibrary.wiley.com/journal/10.1111/(ISSN)1440-1843.

Murai, I. H., Fernandes, A. L., Sales, L. P., Pinto, A. J., Goessler, K. F., Duran, C. S. C., Silva, C. B. R., Franco, A. S., MacEdo, M. B., Dalmolin, H. H. H., Baggio, J., Balbi, G. G. M., Reis, B. Z., Antonangelo, L., Caparbo, V. F., Gualano, B., & Pereira, R. M. R. (2021). Effect of a single high dose of vitamin D3 on hospital length of stay in patients with moderate to severe COVID-19: A randomized clinical trial. *JAMA - Journal of the American Medical Association, 325*(11), 1053–1060. https://doi.org/10.1001/jama.2020.26848, http://jama.jamanetwork.com/journal.aspx.

Niruban, S. J., Alagiakrishnan, K., Beach, J., & Senthilselvan, A. (2015). Association between vitamin D and respiratory outcomes in *Canadian adolescents* and adults. *Journal of Asthma, 52*(7), 653–661. https://doi.org/10.3109/02770903.2015.1004339.

Nnoaham, K. E., & Clarke, A. (2008). Low serum vitamin D levels and tuberculosis: a systematic review and meta-analysis. *International Journal of Epidemiology, 37*(1), 113–119. https://doi.org/10.1093/ije/dym247.

Olszowiec-Chlebna, M., Koniarek-Maniecka, A., Brzozowska, A., Błauż, A., Rychlik, B., & Stelmach, I. (2019). Vitamin D inhibits pro-inflammatory cytokines in the airways of cystic fibrosis patients infected by Pseudomonas aeruginosa- pilot study. *Italian Journal of Pediatrics, 45*(1). https://doi.org/10.1186/s13052-019-0634-x.

Oristrell, J., Oliva, J. C., Subirana, I., Casado, E., Domínguez, D., Toloba, A., Aguilera, P., Esplugues, J., Fafián, P., & Grau, M. (2021). Association of calcitriol supplementation with reduced covid-19 mortality in patients with chronic kidney disease: A population-based study. *Biomedicines, 9*(5). https://doi.org/10.3390/biomedicines9050509, https://www.mdpi.com/2227-9059/9/5/509/pdf.

Pal, R., Banerjee, M., Bhadada, S. K., Shetty, A. J., Singh, B., & Vyas, A. (2022). Vitamin D supplementation and clinical outcomes in COVID-19: A systematic review and meta-analysis. *Journal of Endocrinological Investigation, 45*(1), 53–68. https://doi.org/10.1007/s40618-021-01614-4.

Parekh, D., Dancer, R. C. A., Scott, A., D'Souza, V. K., Howells, P. A., Mahida, R. Y., Tang, J. C. Y., Cooper, M. S., Fraser, W. D., Tan, L. C., Gao, F., Martineau, A. R., Tucker, O., Perkins, G. D., & Thickett, D. R. (2018). Vitamin D to prevent lung injury following esophagectomy—A randomized, placebo-controlled trial. *Critical Care Medicine, 46*(12), E1128. https://doi.org/10.1097/CCM.0000000000003405, http://journals.lww.com/ccmjournal/pages/default.aspx.

Pereira, M., Dantas Damascena, A., Galvão Azevedo, L. M., de Almeida Oliveira, T., & da Mota Santana, J. (2022). Vitamin D deficiency aggravates COVID-19: Systematic review and meta-analysis. *Critical Reviews in Food Science and Nutrition, 62*(5), 1308–1316. https://doi.org/10.1080/10408398.2020.1841090, https://www.tandfonline.com/loi/bfsn20.

Pike, J. W., & Christakos, S. (2017). Biology and mechanisms of action of the vitamin D hormone. *Endocrinology and Metabolism Clinics of North America, 46*(4), 815–843. https://doi.org/10.1016/j.ecl.2017.07.001, http://www.endo.theclinics.com/.

Rafiq, R., Aleva, F. E., Schrumpf, J. A., Daniels, J. M., Bet, P. M., Boersma, W. G., Bresser, P., Spanbroek, M., Lips, P., van den Broek, T. J., Keijser, B. J. F., van der Ven, A. J. A. M., Hiemstra, P. S., den Heijer, M., de Jongh, R. T., den Heijer, M., de Jongh, R. T., Lips, P., Rafiq, R., ... Braunstahl, G. J. (2022). Vitamin D supplementation in chronic obstructive pulmonary disease patients with low serum vitamin D: a randomized controlled trial. *American Journal of Clinical Nutrition, 116*(2), 491–499. https://doi.org/10.1093/ajcn/nqac083, http://www.ajcn.org/contents-by-date.2005.shtml.

Ralph, A. P., Kelly, P. M., & Anstey, N. M. (2008). L-arginine and vitamin D: novel adjunctive immunotherapies in tuberculosis. *Trends in Microbiology, 16*(7), 336–344. https://doi.org/10.1016/j.tim.2008.04.003.

Range, N., Changalucha, J., Krarup, H., Magnussen, P., Andersen, A. B., & Friis, H. (2006). The effect of multivitamin/mineral supplementation on mortality during treatment of pulmonary tuberculosis: A randomised two-by-two factorial trial in Mwanza, Tanzania. *British Journal of Nutrition, 95*(4), 762–770. https://doi.org/10.1079/BJN20051684.

Richter, W. J., Sun, Y., Psoter, K. J., Santos, M. N., Nguyen, J. A., Sidhaye, A., Lechtzin, N., Jennings, M. T., & Cohen, K. A. (2021). Vitamin D deficiency is associated with increased nontuberculous mycobacteria risk in cystic fibrosis. *Annals of the American Thoracic Society, 18*(5), 913–916. https://doi.org/10.1513/AnnalsATS.202003-216RL, https://www.atsjournals.org/doi/pdf/10.1513/AnnalsATS.202003-216RL.

Rivas-Santiago, B., Serrano, C. J., & Enciso-Moreno, J. A. (2009). Susceptibility to infectious diseases based on antimicrobial peptide production. *Infection and Immunity, 77*(11), 4690–4695. https://doi.org/10.1128/IAI.01515-08, http://iai.asm.org/cgi/reprint/77/11/4690.

Saidenberg-Kermanac'h, N., Semerano, L., Nunes, H., Sadoun, D., Guillot, X., Boubaya, M., Naggara, N., Valeyre, D., & Boissier, M. C. (2014). Bone fragility in sarcoidosis and relationships with calcium metabolism disorders: A cross sectional study on 142 patients. *Arthritis Research and Therapy, 16*(2). https://doi.org/10.1186/ar4519, http://arthritis-research.com/content/16/2/R78.

Salahuddin, N., Ali, F., Hasan, Z., Rao, N., Aqeel, M., & Mahmood, F. (2013). Vitamin D accelerates clinical recovery from tuberculosis: results of the SUCCINCT Study [Supplementary Cholecalciferol in recovery from tuberculosis]. A randomized, placebo-controlled, clinical trial of vitamin D supplementation in patients with pulmonary tuberculosis. *BMC infectious diseases, 13*(1). https://doi.org/10.1186/1471-2334-13-22.

Sanjari, M., Soltani, A., Habibi Khorasani, A., & Zareinejad, M. (2015). The effect of vitamin D on COPD exacerbation: A double blind randomized placebo-controlled parallel clinical trial. *Journal of Diabetes & Metabolic Disorders, 15*(1). https://doi.org/10.1186/s40200-016-0257-3.

Sato, S., Tanino, Y., Saito, J., Nikaido, T., Inokoshi, Y., Fukuhara, A., Fukuhara, N., Wang, X., Ishida, T., & Munakata, M. (2012). The relationship between 25-hydroxyvitamin D levels and treatment course of pulmonary tuberculosis. *Respiratory Investigation, 50*(2), 40–45. https://doi.org/10.1016/j.resinv.2012.05.002.

Sehgal, I. S., Dhooria, S., Prasad, K. T., Muthu, V., Sachdeva, N., Bhadada, S. K., Aggarwal, A. N., Garg, M., Chakrabarti, A., & Agarwal, R. (2020). Prevalence of vitamin d deficiency in treatment-naïve subjects with chronic pulmonary aspergillosis. *Journal of Fungi, 6*(4), 1–8. https://doi.org/10.3390/jof6040202, https://www.mdpi.com/2309-608X/6/4/202/pdf.

Singh, N., Kamble, D., & Mahantshetti, N. S. (2019). Effect of vitamin D supplementation in the prevention of recurrent pneumonia in under-five children. *Indian Journal of Pediatrics, 86*(12), 1105–1111. https://doi.org/10.1007/s12098-019-03025-z. http://www.springerlink.com/content/0019-5456.

Sirivoranankul, C., Martinez, M., Chen, V., Clemons, K. V., & Stevens, D. A. (2014). Vitamin D and experimental invasive aspergillosis. *Medical Mycology, 52*(8), 847–852. https://doi.org/10.1093/mmy/myu048, https://mmy.oxfordjournals.org/.

Skaaby, T., Husemoen, L. L. N., Thuesen, B. H., Pisinger, C., Jørgensen, T., Fenger, R. V., & Linneberg, A. (2014). Vitamin D status and chronic obstructive pulmonary disease: A prospective general population study. *PLoS ONE, 9*(3). https://doi.org/10.1371/journal.pone.0090654, http://www.plosone.org/article/fetchObject.action?uri=info%3Adoi%2F10.1371%2Fjournal.pone.0090654&representation=PDF.

Sodhi, A., & Aldrich, T. (2016). Vitamin D supplementation: Not so simple in sarcoidosis. *The American Journal of the Medical Sciences, 352*(3), 252–257. https://doi.org/10.1016/j.amjms.2016.05.027.

Ströder, J., & Kasal, P. (1970). Evaluation of phagocytosis in rickets. *Acta Paediatrica, 59*(3), 288–292. https://doi.org/10.1111/j.1651-2227.1970.tb09005.x.

Sutaria, N., Liu, C. T., & Chen, T. C. (2014). Vitamin D status, receptor gene polymorphisms, and supplementation on tuberculosis: A systematic review of case-control studies and randomized controlled trials. *Journal of Clinical and Translational Endocrinology, 1*(4), 151–160. https://doi.org/10.1016/j.jcte.2014.08.001, http://www.journals.elsevier.com/journal-of-clinical-and-translational-endocrinology/.

Trujillo, G., Habiel, D. M., Ge, L., Ramadass, M., Cooke, N. E., & Kew, R. R. (2013). Neutrophil recruitment to the lung in both C5a- and CXCL1-induced alveolitis is impaired in vitamin D-binding protein-deficient mice. *Journal of Immunology, 191*(2), 848–856. https://doi.org/10.4049/jimmunol.1202941, http://www.jimmunol.org/content/191/2/848.full.pdf+html.

Tzilas, V., Bouros, E., Barbayianni, I., Karampitsakos, T., Kourtidou, S., Ntassiou, M., Ninou, I., Aidinis, V., Bouros, D., & Tzouvelekis, A. (2019). Vitamin D prevents experimental lung fibrosis and predicts survival in patients with idiopathic pulmonary fibrosis. *Pulmonary Pharmacology & Therapeutics, 55*, 17–24. https://doi.org/10.1016/j.pupt.2019.01.003.

Wannamethee, S. G., Welsh, P., Papacosta, O., Lennon, L., & Whincup, P. (2021). Vitamin D deficiency, impaired lung function and total and respiratory mortality in a cohort of older men: cross-sectional and prospective findings from The British Regional Heart Study. *BMJ Open, 11*(12), e051560. https://doi.org/10.1136/bmjopen-2021-051560.

Wei, J., Zhan, J., Ji, H., Xu, Y., Xu, Q., Zhu, X., & Liu, Y. (2023). Fibroblast upregulation of vitamin D receptor represents a self-protective response to limit fibroblast proliferation and activation during pulmonary fibrosis. *Antioxidants, 12*(8), 1634. https://doi.org/10.3390/antiox12081634.

Wei, R., & Christakos, S. (2015). Mechanisms underlying the regulation of innate and adaptive immunity by vitamin D. *Nutrients, 7*(10), 8251–8260. https://doi.org/10.3390/nu7105392.

Wejse, C., Gomes, V. F., Rabna, P., Gustafson, P., Aaby, P., Lisse, I. M., Andersen, P. L., Glerup, H., & Sodemann, M. (2009). Vitamin D as supplementary treatment for tuberculosis: A double-blind, randomized, placebo-controlled trial. *American Journal of Respiratory and Critical Care Medicine, 179*(9), 843–850. https://doi.org/10.1164/rccm.200804-567OC, http://ajrccm.atsjournals.org/cgi/reprint/179/9/843.

Who, Global Tuberculosis Report 2022. (2022).

Williams, C. J. B. (1849). Cod-liver oil in phthisis. *British Medical Journal, s2-1*(1), 1–18. https://doi.org/10.1136/bmj.s2-1.1.1.

Williamson, A., Martineau, A. R., Sheikh, A., Jolliffe, D., & Griffiths, C. J. (2023). Vitamin D for the management of asthma. *Cochrane Database of Systematic Reviews, 2023*(2). https://doi.org/10.1002/14651858.CD011511.pub3, https://www.cochranelibrary.com/cdsr/table-of-contents.

Wood, C., Hasan, S., Darukhanavala, A., & Tangpricha, V. (2021). A Clinician's guide to vitamin D supplementation for patients with cystic fibrosis. *Journal of Clinical & Translational Endocrinology, 26*, 100273. https://doi.org/10.1016/j.jcte.2021.100273.

Xiao, D., Li, X., Su, X., Mu, D., & Qu, Y. (2021). Could SARS-CoV-2-induced lung injury be attenuated by vitamin D? *International Journal of Infectious Diseases, 102*, 196–202. https://doi.org/10.1016/j.ijid.2020.10.059.

Zendedel, A., Gholami, M., Anbari, K., Ghanadi, K., Bachari, E. Ce, & Azargon, A. (2015). Effects of vitamin D intake on FEV1 and COPD exacerbation: A randomized clinical trial study. *Global Journal of Health Science, 7*(4), 243–248. https://doi.org/10.5539/gjhs.v7n4p243.

Zhang, Y., Leung, D. Y. M., Richers, B. N., Liu, Y., Remigio, L. K., Riches, D. W., & Goleva, E. (2012). Vitamin D inhibits monocyte/macrophage proinflammatory cytokine production by targeting MAPK phosphatase-1. *Journal of Immunology, 188*(5), 2127–2135. https://doi.org/10.4049/jimmunol.1102412, http://www.jimmunol.org/content/188/5/2127.full.pdf+html.

Zheng, S. X., Yang, J. X., Hu, X., Li, M., Wang, Q., Dancer, R. C. A., Parekh, D., Gao-Smith, F., Thickett, D. R., & Jin, S. W. (2020). Vitamin D attenuates lung injury via stimulating epithelial repair, reducing epithelial cell apoptosis and inhibits TGF-β induced epithelial to mesenchymal transition. *Biochemical Pharmacology, 177*. https://doi.org/10.1016/j.bcp.2020.113955, http://www.elsevier.com/locate/biochempharm.

CHAPTER 13

Vitamin D and cardiovascular health: a vital connection

Rabiya Ali[1], Nazra Remtulla[2], and Faiza Alam[3]

[1]Karachi Institute of Medical Sciences, National University of Medical Sciences, Islamabad, Punjab, Pakistan [2]Department of Biology, Western University, London, ON, Canada [3]Pengiran-Anak-Puteri-Rashidah-Sa'adatul-Bolkiah Institute of Health Sciences, Universiti Brunei Darussalam, Bandar Seri Begawan, Brunei Darussalam

13.1 Background

Though vitamin D's positive effects on cardiovascular health were first confirmed by epidemiological data, recent well-conducted longitudinal observational trials have failed to clearly connect serum vitamin D levels to cardiovascular mortality (Van Der Schueren et al., 2012). The results proved that a vitamin D deficiency raises the mortality rate from cardiovascular diseases (CVDs). Further investigation is recommended to independently analyze the impact of vitamin D level on CVD in men and women due to the paucity research on patients of both genders (Gholami et al., 2019). True vitamin D inadequacy is still prevalent and connected to negative health effects despite these inconsistent findings.

13.2 Association between vitamin D and cardiovascular disease

Approximately 30%–50% of people worldwide suffer from "Vitamin D" deficiency. Concurrently, according to the World Health Organization (WHO), CVDs appear to represent the main cause of fatalities and morbidity, accounting for 17.9 million global deaths annually (Ghodeshwar et al., 2023). These overlapping global health crises have prompted extensive research into whether inadequate levels of "vitamin D" are linked to CVD.

Numerous observational studies have established a negative correlation between serum concentration of vitamin D and risk of developing CVDs (Zhang et al., 2017). The Framingham Offspring study demonstrated that people with serum vitamin D under 15 ng/mL at a 60% greater probability of CVDs, compared to those with sufficient levels (Manson & Bassuk, 2017). The "National Health and Nutrition Examination Survey" revealed, individuals with vitamin D deficit (≤20 ng/mL) had a strong prevalence of "hypertension," "coronary artery disease," and "heart failure" in contrast to those with adequate levels in blood (Dwyer et al., 2015; Mozos & Marginean, 2015).

The Impact of Vitamin D on Health and Disease. DOI: https://doi.org/10.1016/B978-0-443-34037-6.00004-2

"Randomized Controlled Trials" (RCTs) examining how vitamin D administration affects CVDs, these outcomes produced mixed findings. Some experiments suggest modest benefits, while others report no significant effect (Chin et al., 2017). A vitamin D and omega-3 large supplementation trial with a large sample size in the general population had observed no significant improvement in major cardiovascular events (Manson et al., 2012). However, subgroup analyses suggested potential benefits for individuals with severe deficiency at baseline (Bouillon et al., 2022). When the study was focused solely on older adults, there was no significant impact of vitamin D supplementation on blood pressure or cardiovascular events (Giustina et al., 2023). This highlighted the complexity of the relationship between vitamin D and CVDs. The discrepancies between observational studies and RCTs may arise from differences in the research framework, demographic details of participants, initial vitamin D levels, and the administered supplementation dosage.

Elderly populations are particularly susceptible to hypovitaminosis D, which coincides with "CVDs" (Pirrotta et al., 2023).

Vitamin D contributes to blood pressure regulation by influencing the renin–angiotensin–aldosterone system (RAAS). Reduced levels have been linked to elevated "systolic" and "diastolic" "blood pressure" (McMullan et al., 2017). Studies have not demonstrated a decrease in blood pressure with vitamin D supplementation thus far (Beveridge et al., 2015). Large-scale "metaanalyses" have highlighted the relationship among "vitamin D" deficiency and hypertension (Qi et al., 2017).

"Vitamin D" deficiency is associated with active calcification of "coronary arteries," a key marker of atherosclerosis (Young et al., 2011). People with vitamin D deficiency are more likely to have "coronary artery disease" (CAD) and greater plaque burden. In patients with existing CAD, "vitamin D" insufficiency is associated with worse clinical outcomes, involving higher rates of recurrent myocardial infarction (Milazzo et al., 2017). Moreover, prospective cohort studies suggest that vitamin D reduced levels may speed up the development of atherosclerosis, highlighting its role as a potentially modifiable risk factor for CAD (Khanolkar et al., 2023). "Vitamin D" effects in cardiac muscle function have been studied extensively. Epidemiological research, such as the Rotterdam Study, has demonstrated that "vitamin D" shortage is an independent predictor of heart failure (HF). These findings emphasize the need for targeted interventions in high-risk groups (Ikram et al., 2017).

Recent investigation indicates a possible association between "vitamin D" deficiency and arrhythmias, particularly atrial fibrillation (AF) (Bie, 2019). "Vitamin D" function in "calcium homeostasis" may influence electrical activity in the heart (Barsan et al., 2022).

"Antiinflammatory" and vascular-protective properties of "vitamin D" are implicated in PAD. In both general and high-risk populations, a higher prevalence of PAD is linked to low "vitamin D" levels (Melamed et al., 2008). Longitudinal research studies mentioned that "vitamin D" reduced levels may exacerbate progression PAD, underscoring the importance of early detection and intervention (Mascitelli et al., 2010).

"Vitamin D" deficiency has been involved in the pathogenesis of stroke. Individuals with low "vitamin D" insufficiency are more prone to develop both "ischemic" and "hemorrhagic stroke." Deficient patients tend to have worse recovery trajectories and higher rates of poststroke complications (Cui et al., 2024).

13.3 Pathophysiological mechanisms linking vitamin D deficiency to cardiovascular disease

"Vitamin D" deficiency has been involved in the pathophysiology of CVDs, with evidence pointing to specific pathophysiological mechanisms. This subchapter explores the critical roles of endothelial dysfunction, inflammation, atherosclerosis, oxidative stress, dysregulation of the RAAS, cardiac remodeling fibrosis, and failure in mediating these effects.

13.4 Vitamin D and endothelial dysfunction

An essential function of endothelial cells is to preserve vascular homeostasis by regulating vasodilation, inflammation, and thrombosis. Deficiency of "vitamin D" is a potential contributor to endothelial dysfunction, a hallmark of atherosclerosis and CVD. Vitamin D, acting through its receptor "VDR" in vascular cells, stimulates "endothelial nitric oxide synthase" (eNOS) influences production of "nitric oxide" (NO), a key molecule that relaxes blood vessels (Legarth et al., 2018), facilitating the synthesis and release of NO, a critical biomarker for vasodilation and vascular health. Deficiency in vitamin D reduces NO bioavailability, leading to impaired vasodilation and increased vascular resistance. Studies demonstrate that people with low vitamin D levels have less endothelial function and stiffer arteries (Al Mheid et al., 2011; Kerr et al., 2011). Vitamin D exerts antiinflammatory effects by inhibiting the action of "pro-inflammatory" cytokines like tumor necrosis factor-alpha (TNF-α) and interleukin-6 (IL-6). Deficiency in vitamin D fosters a pro-inflammatory state, exacerbating "endothelial damage" and promoting atherosclerotic plaques formation (Khanolkar et al., 2023). Vitamin D also reduces endothelial apoptosis by modulating oxidative stress and inflammation. Experimental models indicate that vitamin D supplementation restores endothelial integrity and improves vascular function in deficiency states (Kim et al., 2020).

There is an associated link between low levels of vitamin D and higher oxidative stress, or a reduced antioxidant capacity, according to observational research (Victor et al., 2009). A negative association among circulating levels of "vitamin D" and arterial caliber was identified in cases of "chronic kidney disease" acquiring conservative therapies. This study discovered a correlation between artery dilatation, which was assessed by a measurement of brachial artery flow, and serum "vitamin D" levels. Furthermore, this study revealed that patients with hypovitaminosis D have greater plasma levels of pro-atherosclerosis cytokines.

Particularly, compared to participants with normal serum "vitamin D," cases with "vitamin D" deficiency had greater concentration of "soluble vascular cell adhesion molecule-I" (sVCAM-I) and "soluble E-selectin" (Napoli et al., 2006; Zhang et al., 2015). Further mechanisms involve the endothelial 1-α-hydroxylase (Napoli et al., 2006) and the activated version of "vitamin D" that can control the proliferation of both kinds of cells (Cardús et al., 2006; Zehnder et al., 2002). The activation of "vitamin D" maintains several functional alterations, including gene programs that are vasodilatory and antithrombotic. When coronary vascular smooth muscle cells are exposed to "vitamin D," they express more "fibrinolytic" and "vasodilatory genes" and fewer "thrombogenic genes" (Wu-Wong et al., 2006).

13.5   Vitamin D and hypercoagulability

There is evidently a correlation between hypercoagulability and genetic models of VDR-/- mice. ADP-induced aggregation of platelets was shown to be enhanced in VDR-deficient animals and in mice with normal calcium plasma levels. Several chemicals involved in hemostasis were changed in this model. Specifically, the pro-thrombotic tissue factor's gene expression was elevated, whereas antithrombin and thrombomodulin's gene expression was downregulated. The same study examined the differences between VDR null animals and wild-type mice under both low and normal calcium concentration in plasma using a "pro-thrombotic" stimulus. "Exogenous lipopolysaccharide" was the pro-thrombotic agent that, independent of plasma calcium levels, increased tissue factor levels and decreased antithrombin and thrombomodulin levels, exacerbating multiorgan thrombosis. This evidence supports the hypothesis that vitamin D, acting directly on endothelial cells through its receptor, affects the endothelial system by modifying the production of pro- and antithrombotic substances (Aihara et al., 2004; Condoleo et al., 2021).

13.6   Vitamin D, inflammation, and atherosclerosis

Oxidative stress and chronic inflammation play a key role in the pathophysiology of CVD. Both processes are dynamically modulated by vitamin D. Vitamin D inhibits the synthesis of inflammatory cytokines and stimulates the expression of antiinflammatory mediators by acting on the "vitamin D receptor" (VDR) present in immune cells (Ao et al., 2021). For instance, it inhibits "nuclear factor-kappa B" (NF-κB), a "transcription factor" that drives inflammation (Liu et al., 2017). The "c-reactive protein" (CRP) along with different indicators of systemic inflammation are correlated with low "vitamin D" levels. An imbalance between the generation of "reactive oxygen species" (ROS) and "antioxidant defenses" leads to oxidative stress. By upregulating "antioxidant enzymes" like "glutathione peroxidase" and "superoxide dismutase (SOD)," vitamin D lowers oxidative stress. Excess "ROS" in "vitamin D" deficiency can harm proteins, lipids, and DNA, contributing to vascular dysfunction and atherosclerosis (Batty et al., 2022).

Vitamin D, through its receptor (VDR), exhibits several antiatherosclerotic effects independent of systemic calcium and parathyroid hormone levels. It reduces macrophage scavenger receptor expression, limiting foam cell formation and preventing the "LDL cholesterol" from building up in the foam cells and avoiding vascular atherosclerosis. VDR activation also curbs inflammation and thrombosis by modulating NF-κB signaling, decreasing pro-inflammatory cytokines (like IL-6), and increasing protective factors (like thrombomodulin and IL-10). These local effects may explain why vitamin D supplementation trials have yielded inconsistent cardiovascular benefits, despite observed associations between the in vivo plaque load and "VDR" expression (Condoleo et al., 2021).

Studies in rats showed the overexpression of "24-hydroxylase," an enzyme that inhibits the active "vitamin D," facilitating the pathogenesis of atherosclerosis. Human plaque analysis revealed a correlation between intraplaque VDR levels and M1 macrophage expression. Critically, low intraplaque VDR, not serum vitamin D, predicts major adverse cardiovascular events (MACE) in carotid stenosis patients. Furthermore, vitamin D's influence on fat deposition may perform a role in cardiometabolic dysfunction. In fact, findings from certain clinical trials indicate that combined supplementation of vitamin D and calcium may help lower fat accumulation and reduce the risk of cardiovascular and metabolic disorders (Condoleo et al., 2021; Neeland et al., 2018).

13.7   Vitamin D, renin–angiotensin–aldosterone system dysregulation, and hypertension

The RAAS, a critical mechanism of "blood pressure" monitoring and fluid balance, and its dysregulation is a key factor connecting "vitamin D" deficiency to "hypertension" and other CVDs. Vitamin D inhibits renin gene expression directly, thereby inhibiting the RAAS (Ajabshir et al., 2014). Deficiency in vitamin D results in unchecked renin activity, resulting in a rise in "angiotensin II" in blood. "Angiotensin II" facilitates vasoconstriction, sodium retention, and vascular remodeling, contributing to hypertension and end-organ damage. Elevated angiotensin II levels in vitamin D deficiency stimulate vascular smooth muscle proliferation and fibrosis, exacerbating arterial stiffness and increasing afterload on the heart (McMullan et al., 2017). These changes are associated with left ventricular hypertrophy and impaired cardiac function.

13.8   Vitamin D, cardiac remodeling, and ventricular dilatation

"Vitamin D" deficiency is associated with adverse structural and functional changes in heart, collectively termed cardiac remodeling. Vitamin D influences the expression of 'matrix metalloproteinases' (MMPs) and their suppressors, which regulate extracellular matrix turnover. Deficiency in vitamin D increases MMP activity, leading to extracellular matrix degradation, ventricular dilation, and pathological remodeling. Clinical research studies have documented that "vitamin D" deficient individuals exhibit greater left ventricular mass and reduced ejection fraction (Hassanzadeh-Makoui et al., 2020). Vitamin D modulates fibroblast activity, preventing excessive collagen deposition in the myocardium. In states of deficiency, fibroblast activation leads to myocardial fibrosis, reduced compliance, and diastolic dysfunction (Humeres & Frangogiannis, 2019). Animal studies demonstrated that "vitamin D" dosage reduces the cardiac fibrosis and improves myocardial function in models of deficiency (Tappia et al., 2023).

13.9   Vitamin D and heart failure

Studies have demonstrated that "vitamin D" plays a key role in regulating hypertension and CVDs, including HF. HF remains the primary cause of death globally. Low "vitamin D" levels have been associated with worse outcomes in HF patients, according to recognized clinical variables and biomarkers analysis. These patients are also more likely to develop "atherosclerosis," "diabetes," "hypertension," and other HF-related conditions. Recent experiments indicate that "vitamin D" may have cardio-protective benefits. Although its efficacy is still unknown, vitamin D supplementation might improve ventricular remodeling in HF patients; however, its mechanism is still unknown (Hazique et al., 2022). Furthermore, less serum "vitamin D" and high parathormone concentrations are linked with more advanced stages of chronic HF (Belen et al., 2017).

Ventricular cardiomyocytes express both "VDR" and the "hydroxylases" required to produce the active form of "vitamin D." "Vitamin D" deficiency alters the structural, functional, molecular, and genetic areas of myocardium leading to cardiac hypertrophy and dysfunction that result in HF with preserved ejection fraction (HF-PEF). The active form of "vitamin D" may either prevent or lessen the remodeling of cardiomyocytes and the extracellular matrix that is caused by the interruption in vitamin D signal transmission, according to current in vivo evidence. Increased filling pressure, cardiac hypertrophy, and diastolic dysfunction are the hallmarks of HF-PEF, but the ejection fraction remains normal. More evidence suggests activation of the vitamin D pathway improves diastolic function, boosts calcium absorption, and increases contractility in wild-type mice but not in VDR mutant/knockout animals. VDR knockout mice show hypertrophy and cardiomegaly in the cardiomyocytes (Condoleo et al., 2021).

Recent randomized intervention trials and Mendelian randomization studies, however, refute the idea that vitamin D supplements cause CVDs. This disparity has been attributed to observational studies' inability to control for confounding factors or reverse causation, genetic studies' nonlinear connections, and the improper recruitment of vitamin D-replete people for vitamin D supplementation trials (Afzal & Nordestgaard, 2017) (Fig. 13.1).

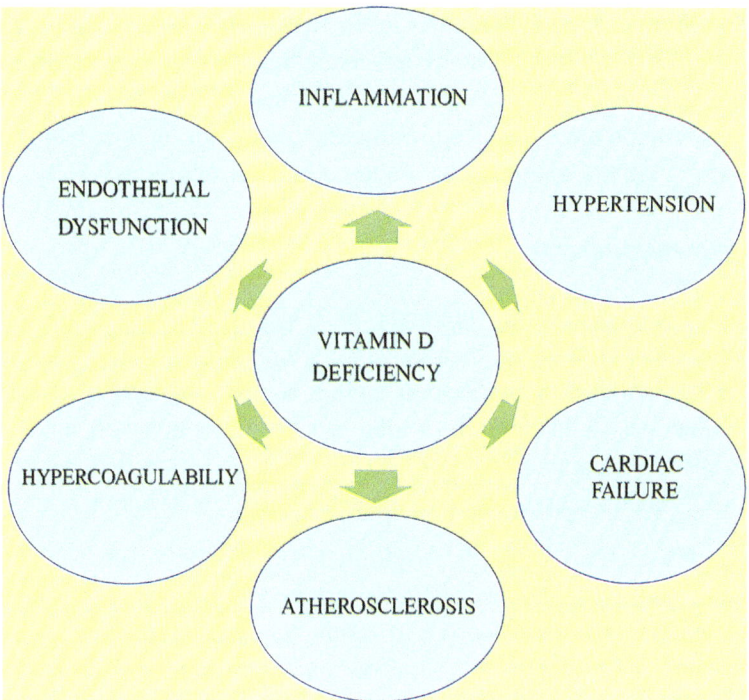

Figure 13.1
Mechanisms linking vitamin D deficiency to cardiovascular disease.

13.10 Calcium, phosphates, and cardiovascular diseases

"Vitamin D" has a central role in calcium and phosphate homeostasis, and it is reasonable to develop a link between these mineral levels and cardiovascular risk. Numerous experimental and clinical trials demonstrated a role for "calcium," "phosphate," and "vitamin D" in CVDs pathogenesis. These three elements form an interconnected biological axis, requiring consideration of all elements and their interactions. However, their interconnected roles in CVDs pathophysiology and progression remain unclear. Despite this complexity, appropriately designed clinical trials have yet to definitively establish the impact of deficiencies or supplementation within this axis on overall cardiovascular risk (Condoleo et al., 2021).

13.11 Conclusions

"Vitamin D" is essential for the metabolism of "calcium" and "phosphate" and needs to be consumed in sufficient amounts and exposed to sunlight. Hypovitaminosis D is linked to CVDs. "Vitamin D" deficiency in animal models worsens "endothelial dysfunction," which in turn promotes atherosclerosis. Through the dysregulation of RAAS, which is reversible with "vitamin D" replacement, this deficit also leads to hypertension. Moreover, hypertrophic cardiac remodeling that resembles HF with preserved "ejection fraction" (HFpEF) is linked to "vitamin D" deficiency. Human trials and metaanalyses on the cardiovascular benefits of vitamin D supplementation have produced conflicting results for major adverse cardiovascular events, despite strong animal and patients' data, calling for additional study.

13.12 Future perspective

"Vitamin D" deficiency is a strong predictor of CVDs through multiple epidemiological pathways and correlations with specific cardiovascular conditions. While observational studies frequently highlighted a negative association among serum "vitamin D" concentrations and CVDs risk, interventional studies present a more nuanced picture, with mixed outcomes for "vitamin D" dosage administration. Complexity of this association underscores the need for further research to establish causal relationships and optimal intervention strategies.

Given the strong associations between "vitamin D" deficiency and CVDs, public health initiatives aimed at improving "vitamin D" status may yield significant benefits. Necessary fortification of food has proven effective in reducing deficiency rates. High-risk groups, including the elderly, individuals with limited sun exposure, and dark skin, should be prioritized for supplementation. Public education on the significance of "vitamin D" for cardiovascular health can drive behavioral changes, such as increased outdoor activity and dietary adjustments.

References

Afzal, S., & Nordestgaard, B. G. (2017). Vitamin D and risk of cardiovascular disease. *Arteriosclerosis, Thrombosis, and Vascular Biology, 37*(11), 1981–1982. https://doi.org/10.1161/ATVBAHA.117.310204, http://atvb.ahajournals.org/.

Aihara, K. I., Azuma, H., Akaike, M., Ikeda, Y., Yamashita, M., Sudo, T., Hayashi, H., Yamada, Y., Endoh, F., Fujimura, M., Yoshida, T., Yamaguchi, H., Hashizume, S., Kato, M., Yoshimura, K., Yamamoto, Y., Kato, S., & Matsumoto, T. (2004). Disruption of nuclear vitamin D receptor gene causes enhanced thrombogenicity in mice. *Journal of Biological Chemistry, 279*(34), 35798–35802. https://doi.org/10.1074/jbc.M404865200.

Ajabshir, S., Asif, A., & Nayer, A. (2014). The effects of vitamin D on the renin-angiotensin system. *Journal of Nephropathology, 3*(2), 41–43. https://doi.org/10.12860/jnp.2014.09, http://nephropathol.com/PDF/jnp-3-41.pdf.

Al Mheid, I., Patel, R., Murrow, J., Morris, A., Rahman, A., Fike, L., Kavtaradze, N., Uphoff, I., Hooper, C., Tangpricha, V., Alexander, R. W., Brigham, K., & Quyyumi, A. A. (2011). Vitamin D status is associated with arterial stiffness and vascular dysfunction in healthy humans. *Journal of the American College of Cardiology, 58*(2), 186–192. https://doi.org/10.1016/j.jacc.2011.02.051.

Ao, T., Kikuta, J., & Ishii, M. (2021). The effects of vitamin D on immune system and inflammatory diseases. *Biomolecules, 11*(11), 1624. https://doi.org/10.3390/biom11111624.

Barsan, M., Brata, A. M., Ismaiel, A., Dumitrascu, D. I., Badulescu, A. V., Duse, T. A., Dascalescu, S., Popa, S. L., Grad, S., Muresan, L., Maerescu, C. M., Cismaru, G., & Brata, V. D. (2022). The pathogenesis of cardiac arrhythmias in vitamin D deficiency. *Biomedicines, 10*(6). https://doi.org/10.3390/biomedicines10061239, https://www.mdpi.com/2227-9059/10/6/1239/pdf?version=1653554269.

Batty, M., Bennett, M. R., & Yu, E. (2022). The role of oxidative stress in atherosclerosis. *Cells, 11*(23). https://doi.org/10.3390/cells11233843, https://www.mdpi.com/journal/cells.

Belen, E., Tıpı, F. F., Aykan, A.Ç., Findikçioğlu, U., Karakuş, G., Yeşil, A., Helvaci, A., Kalaycioğlu, E., & Çetın, M. (2017). Clinical staging in chronic heart failure associated with low vitamin D and elevated parathormone levels. *Acta Cardiologica, 69*(6), 665–671. https://doi.org/10.1080/AC.69.6.1000009.

Beveridge, L. A., Struthers, A. D., Khan, F., Jorde, R., Scragg, R., Macdonald, H. M., Alvarez, J. A., Boxer, R. S., Dalbeni, A., Gepner, A. D., Isbel, N. M., Larsen, T., Nagpal, J., Petchey, W. G., Stricker, H., Strobel, F., Tangpricha, V., Toxqui, L., Vaquero, M. P., ... Witham, M. D. (2015). Effect of vitamin D supplementation on blood pressure a systematic review and meta-analysis incorporating individual patient data. *JAMA Internal Medicine, 175*(5), 745–754. https://doi.org/10.1001/jamainternmed.2015.0237, http://archinte.jamanetwork.com/article.aspx?articleid=2195120.

Bie, L. (2019). The status and research progress on vitamin d deficiency and atrial fibrillation. *Brazilian Journal of Cardiovascular Surgery, 34*(5), 605–609. https://doi.org/10.21470/1678-9741-2018-0322, http://www.bjcvs.org/pdf/3242/v34n5a16.pdf.

Bouillon, R., Manousaki, D., Rosen, C., Trajanoska, K., Rivadeneira, F., & Richards, J. B. (2022). The health effects of vitamin D supplementation: Evidence from human studies. *Nature Reviews Endocrinology, 18*(2), 96–110. https://doi.org/10.1038/s41574-021-00593-z, http://www.nature.com/nrendo/index.html.

Cardús, A., Parisi, E., Gallego, C., Aldea, M., Fernández, E., & Valdivielso, J. M. (2006). 1,25-Dihydroxyvitamin D3 stimulates vascular smooth muscle cell proliferation through a VEGF-mediated pathway. *Kidney International, 69*(8), 1377–1384. https://doi.org/10.1038/sj.ki.5000304.

Chin, K., Appel, L. J., & Michos, E. D. (2017). Vitamin D, calcium, and cardiovascular disease: A"D"vantageous or "D"etrimental? An era of uncertainty. *Current Atherosclerosis Reports, 19*(1). https://doi.org/10.1007/s11883-017-0637-2, https://www.springer.com.

Condoleo, V., Pelaia, C., Armentaro, G., Severini, G., Clausi, E., Cassano, V., Miceli, S., Fiorentino, T. V., Succurro, E., Arturi, F., Andreozzi, F., Sesti, G., & Sciacqua, A. (2021). Role of vitamin D in cardiovascular diseases. *Endocrines, 2*(4), 417–426. https://doi.org/10.3390/endocrines2040037.

Cui, P., Hou, H., Song, B., Xia, Z., & Xu, Y. (2024). Vitamin D and ischemic stroke - Association, mechanisms, and therapeutics. *Ageing Research Reviews, 96*, 102244. https://doi.org/10.1016/j.arr.2024.102244.

Dwyer, J. T., Wiemer, K. L., Dary, O., Keen, C. L., King, J. C., Miller, K. B., Philbert, M. A., Tarasuk, V., Taylor, C. L., Gaine, P. C., Jarvis, A. B., & Bailey, R. L. (2015). Fortification and health: Challenges and opportunities. *Advances in Nutrition, 6*(1), 124–131. https://doi.org/10.3945/an.114.007443, http://advances.nutrition.org/content/6/1/124.full.pdf.

Ghodeshwar, G. K., Dube, A., & Khobragade, D. (2023). Impact of lifestyle modifications on cardiovascular health: A narrative review. *Cureus, 15*(7). https://doi.org/10.7759/cureus.42616.

Gholami, F., Moradi, G., Zareei, B., Rasouli, M. A., Nikhoo, B., Roshani, D., & Ghaderi, E. (2019). The association between circulating 25-hydroxyvitamin D and cardiovascular diseases: A meta-analysis of prospective cohort studies. *BMC Cardiovascular Disorders, 19*(1). https://doi.org/10.1186/s12872-019-1236-7, http://www.biomedcentral.com/bmccardiovascdisord/.

Giustina, A., Bouillon, R., Dawson-Hughes, B., Ebeling, P. R., Lazaretti-Castro, M., Lips, P., Marcocci, C., & Bilezikian, J. P. (2023). Vitamin D in the older population: A consensus statement. *Endocrine, 79*(1), 31–44. https://doi.org/10.1007/s12020-022-03208-3, https://www.springer.com/journal/12020.

Hassanzadeh-Makoui, R., Jamei, M., Hassanzadeh-Makoui, M., & K004erlou, H. (2020). Effects of vitamin D on left ventricular ejection fraction in patients with systolic heart failure: A double-blind randomized clinical trial. *International Journal of Endocrinology and Metabolism, 18*(3). https://doi.org/10.5812/ijem.103528.

Hazique, M., Khan, K. I., Ramesh, P., Kanagalingam, S., Zargham Ul Haq, F. N. U., Victory Srinivasan, N., Khan, A. I., Mashat, G. D., & Khan, S. (2022). A study of vitamin D and its correlation with severity and complication of congestive heart failure: A systematic review. *Cureus, 14*(9). https://doi.org/10.7759/cureus.28873.

Humeres, C., & Frangogiannis, N. G. (2019). Fibroblasts in the infarcted, remodeling, and failing heart. *JACC: Basic to Translational Science, 4*(3), 449–467. https://doi.org/10.1016/j.jacbts.2019.02.006, http://www.journals.elsevier.com/jacc-basic-to-translational-science.

Ikram, M. A., Brusselle, G. G. O., Murad, S. D., van Duijn, C. M., Franco, O. H., Goedegebure, A., Klaver, C. C. W., Nijsten, T. E. C., Peeters, R. P., Stricker, B. H., Tiemeier, H., Uitterlinden, A. G., Vernooij, M. W., & Hofman, A. (2017). The Rotterdam study: 2018 update on objectives, design and main results. *European Journal of Epidemiology, 32*(9), 807–850. https://doi.org/10.1007/s10654-017-0321-4, https://www.wkap.nl/journalhome.htm/0393-2990.

Kerr, P., Tam, R., & Plane, F. (2011). Endothelium. Mechanisms of vascular disease: A reference book for vascular specialists.

Khanolkar, S., Hirani, S., Mishra, A., Vardhan, S., Hirani, S., Prasad, R., & Wanjari, M. (2023). Exploring the role of vitamin D in atherosclerosis and its impact on cardiovascular events: A comprehensive review. *Cureus, 15*(7). https://doi.org/10.7759/cureus.42470.

Kim, D. H., Meza, C. A., Clarke, H., Kim, J. S., & Hickner, R. C. (2020). Vitamin D and endothelial function. *Nutrients, 12*(2). https://doi.org/10.3390/nu12020575, https://www.mdpi.com/2072-6643/12/2/575/pdf.

Legarth, C., Grimm, D., Wehland, M., Bauer, J., & Krüger, M. (2018). The impact of vitamin D in the treatment of essential hypertension. *International Journal of Molecular Sciences, 19*(2), 455. https://doi.org/10.3390/ijms19020455.

Liu, H., Zhang, Y., Li, L., & Zou, H. C. (2017). The application of sonication in diagnosis of periprosthetic joint infection. *European Journal of Clinical Microbiology & Infectious Diseases, 36*(1), 1–9. https://doi.org/10.1007/s10096-016-2778-6.

Manson, J. A. E., Bassuk, S. S., Lee, I. M., Cook, N. R., Albert, M. A., Gordon, D., Zaharris, E., MacFadyen, J. G., Danielson, E., Lin, J., Zhang, S. M., & Buring, J. E. (2012). The VITamin D and OmegA-3 TriaL (VITAL): Rationale and design of a large randomized controlled trial of vitamin D and marine omega-3 fatty acid supplements for the primary prevention of cancer and cardiovascular disease. *Contemporary Clinical Trials, 33*(1), 159–171. https://doi.org/10.1016/j.cct.2011.09.009.

Manson, J. E., & Bassuk, S. S. (2017). Invited commentary: The framingham offspring study-A pioneering investigation into familial aggregation of cardiovascular risk. *American Journal of Epidemiology, 185*(11), 1103–1108. https://doi.org/10.1093/aje/kwx068, http://aje.oxfordjournals.org/.

Mascitelli, L., Goldstein, M. R., & Grant, W. B. (2010). Does vitamin D have a role in reducing the risk of peripheral artery disease. *Mayo Clinic Proceedings, 85*(11), 1058–1059. https://doi.org/10.4065/mcp.2010.0508, http://www.mayoclinicproceedings.com/content/85/11/1058.full.pdf+html.

McMullan, C. J., Borgi, L., Curhan, G. C., Fisher, N., & Forman, J. P. (2017). The effect of vitamin D on renin–angiotensin system activation and blood pressure. *Journal of Hypertension, 35*(4), 822–829. https://doi.org/10.1097/hjh.0000000000001220.

Melamed, M. L., Muntner, P., Michos, E. D., Uribarri, J., Weber, C., Sharma, J., & Raggi, P. (2008). Serum 25-hydroxyvitamin D levels and the prevalence of peripheral arterial disease results from NHANES 2001 to 2004. *Arteriosclerosis, Thrombosis, and Vascular Biology, 28*(6), 1179–1185. https://doi.org/10.1161/ATVBAHA.108.165886.

Milazzo, V., De Metrio, M., Cosentino, N., Marenzi, G., & Tremoli, E. (2017). Vitamin D and acute myocardial infarction. *World Journal of Cardiology, 9*(1), 14. https://doi.org/10.4330/wjc.v9.i1.14.

Mozos, I., & Marginean, O. (2015). Links between vitamin D deficiency and cardiovascular diseases. *BioMed Research International, 2015*, 1–12. https://doi.org/10.1155/2015/109275.

Napoli, C., de Nigris, F., Williams-Ignarro, S., Pignalosa, O., Sica, V., & Ignarro, L. J. (2006). Nitric oxide and atherosclerosis: An update. *Nitric Oxide: Biology and Chemistry / Official Journal of the Nitric Oxide Society, 15*(4), 265–279. https://doi.org/10.1016/j.niox.2006.03.011.

Neeland, I. J., Poirier, P., & Després, J. P. (2018). Cardiovascular and metabolic heterogeneity of obesity: Clinical challenges and implications for management. *Circulation, 137*(13), 1391–1406. https://doi.org/10.1161/CIRCULATIONAHA.117.029617, http://circ.ahajournals.org.

Pirrotta, F., Cavati, G., Mingiano, C., Merlotti, D., Nuti, R., Gennari, L., & Palazzuoli, A. (2023). Vitamin D deficiency and cardiovascular mortality: Retrospective analysis "Siena Osteoporosis" cohort. *Nutrients, 15*(15), 3303. https://doi.org/10.3390/nu15153303.

Qi, D., Nie, X.-l, Wu, S., Cai, J., & Slominski, A. T. (2017). Vitamin D and hypertension: Prospective study and meta-analysis. *PLoS One, 12*(3), e0174298. https://doi.org/10.1371/journal.pone.0174298.

Tappia, P. S., Lopez, R., Fitzpatrick-Wong, S., & Ramjiawan, B. (2023). Understanding the role of vitamin D in heart failure. *Reviews in Cardiovascular Medicine, 24*(4). https://doi.org/10.31083/j.rcm2404111, https://www.imrpress.com/journal/RCM/24/4/10.31083/j.rcm2404111.

Van Der Schueren, B. J., Verstuyf, A., & Mathieu, C. (2012). Straight from D-Heart: Vitamin D status and cardiovascular disease. *Current Opinion in Lipidology, 23*(1), 17–23. https://doi.org/10.1097/MOL.0b013e32834d7357.

Victor, V., Rocha, M., Sola, E., Banuls, C., Garcia-Malpartida, K., & Hernandez-Mijares, A. (2009). Oxidative stress, endothelial dysfunction and atherosclerosis. *Current Pharmaceutical Design, 15*(26), 2988–3002. https://doi.org/10.2174/138161209789058093.

Wu-Wong, J. R., Nakane, M., Ma, J., Ruan, X., & Kroeger, P. E. (2006). Effects of Vitamin D analogs on gene expression profiling in human coronary artery smooth muscle cells. *Atherosclerosis, 186*(1), 20–28. https://doi.org/10.1016/j.atherosclerosis.2005.06.046.

Young, K. A., Snell-Bergeon, J. K., Naik, R. G., Hokanson, J. E., Tarullo, D., Gottlieb, P. A., Garg, S. K., & Rewers, M. (2011). Vitamin D deficiency and coronary artery calcification in subjects with type 1 diabetes. *Diabetes Care, 34*(2), 454–458. https://doi.org/10.2337/dc10-0757, http://care.diabetesjournals.org/content/34/2/454.full.pdf+html.

Zehnder, D., Bland, R., Chana, R. S., Wheeler, D. C., Howie, A. J., Williams, M. C., Stewart, P. M., & Hewison, M. (2002). Synthesis of 1,25-dihydroxyvitamin D3 by human endothelial cells is regulated by inflammatory cytokines: A novel autocrine determinant of vascular cell adhesion. *Journal of the American Society of Nephrology, 13*(3), 621–629. https://journals.lww.com/jasn/pages/default.aspx.

Zhang, Qy, Jiang, Cm, Sun, C., Tang, Tf, Jin, B., Cao, Dw, He, Js, & Zhang, M. (2015). Hypovitaminosis D is associated with endothelial dysfunction in patients with non-dialysis chronic kidney disease. *Journal of Nephrology, 28*(4), 471–476. https://doi.org/10.1007/s40620-014-0167-8, http://www.springer.com/medicine/nephrology/journal/40620.

Zhang, R., Li, B., Gao, X., Tian, R., Pan, Y., Jiang, Y., Gu, H., Wang, Y., Wang, Y., & Liu, G. (2017). Serum 25-hydroxyvitamin D and the risk of cardiovascular disease: dose-response meta-analysis of prospective studies. *The American Journal of Clinical Nutrition, 105*(4), 810–819. https://doi.org/10.3945/ajcn.116.140392.

CHAPTER 14

Vitamin D: illuminating the shadows of pancreatic dysfunction

Faiza Alam[1], Fasiha Fatima[2], and Ihsan Nazurah Zulkipli[1]

[1]*Pengiran-Anak-Puteri-Rashidah-Sa'adatul-Bolkiah Institute of Health Sciences, Universiti Brunei Darussalam, Bandar Seri Begawan, Brunei Darussalam* [2]*Karachi Institute of Medical Sciences, National University of Medical Sciences, Punjab, Pakistan*

14.1 Vitamin D and pancreatitis

Vitamin D is a steroid hormone found in trace amounts in food and is mostly produced internally by the skin in response to the sun's ultraviolet (UV) radiation. Maintaining a healthy mineralized skeleton and regulating calcium homeostasis are the primary roles of vitamin D. Vitamin D's many important roles include its ability to regulate the immune system, inhibit tumor growth, maintain metabolic balance, and reduce inflammation (Cai et al., 2022).

Recent research suggests a correlation between vitamin D and pancreatitis (Huh et al., 2019). Most individuals who develop pancreatitis have alterations in their dietary patterns before disease onset, typically resulting from excessive alcohol intake or fat intolerance. Due to maldigestion and malabsorption, compounded by additional variables such as a low dietary vitamin uptake, low exposure to sunshine, and exocrine dysfunction, nutritional deficiencies, especially in fat-soluble vitamins (vitamins A, D, E, and K), have been demonstrated in patients with AP and CP (Cai et al., 2022).

14.2 Vitamin D receptors and pancreatic cells

A relationship between vitamin D status and β-cell function has been established. Where vitamin D deficiency is related to impaired insulin secretion and increased risk of type 2 diabetes, adequate vitamin D levels are linked to improved β-cell function and insulin sensitivity (Zhao et al., 2021). Vitamin D receptors (VDRs) are nuclear receptors expressed in pancreatic cells along with other tissues and have a fundamental role in modulating insulin secretion and maintaining glucose homeostasis. Activation of VDR by its ligand, 1,25-dihydroxyvitamin D3, enhances insulin secretion, suggesting a direct influence on β-cell function (Lee et al., 1994). Thus, VDR activation in pancreatic β-cells is essential for optimal insulin secretion and β-cell function. Maintaining sufficient vitamin D levels may support β-cell health and contribute to the prevention and management of diabetes.

In pancreatic cancer cells, VDR stimulation has been involved in stromal reprograming. Usage of VDR ligand reduces inflammatory markers and fibrosis in pancreatitis and human tumor stroma, proposing VDR to be capable of transcriptionally regulating the pancreatic stellate cells, fostering an inactive state and potentially enhancing the effectiveness of chemotherapeutic agents (Sherman et al., 2014). Moreover, VDR activation prompts the transcription of peptide YY (PYY) in the pancreas, a hormone involved in regulating digestive processes, indicating VDR's influence on pancreatic endocrine functions beyond insulin secretion (Choi et al., 2012). These findings highlight the multifaceted role of VDR in pancreatic physiology and pathology, influencing both endocrine and exocrine functions, as well as tumor microenvironment dynamics.

14.3 Vitamin D receptor activation and pancreatic gene expression

Vitamin D, through its active form 1,25-dihydroxyvitamin D3 (calcitriol), modulates gene expression in pancreatic cells by activating the VDR. Upon activation, VDR binds to specific DNA sequences known as vitamin D response elements (VDREs), influencing the transcription of various genes involved in pancreatic function.

14.3.1 Influence on pancreatic stellate cells

In pancreatic stellate cells, which play a crucial role in the pancreatic tumor microenvironment, VDR activation has been shown to suppress stromal activation. Treatment with VDR ligands leads to the inhibition of genes associated with PSC activation, thereby modulating the tumor stroma and potentially enhancing the efficacy of pancreatic cancer therapies (Sherman et al., 2014).

Research indicates that VDR activation induces the transcription of the peptide YY (PYY) gene in the pancreas. PYY is a hormone involved in digestive processes, and its expression in pancreatic islets suggests a role in the regulation of insulin secretion and glucose homeostasis (Choi et al., 2012).

14.3.2 Interaction with FOXM1 pathway

In pancreatic ductal adenocarcinoma (PDAC), inactivation of vitamin D/VDR signaling has been linked to elevated expression and function of Forkhead Box M1 (FOXM1), a transcription factor associated with cancer progression. Restoring VDR activity can down-regulate FOXM1 expression, thereby inhibiting PDAC cell stemness, invasion, and metastasis (Li et al., 2015).

In summary, VDR activation in pancreatic cells influences gene expression by modulating pathways involved in cellular differentiation, hormone secretion, and tumor progression. These regulatory effects underscore the potential therapeutic applications of vitamin D analogs in pancreatic disorders.

14.4 Antiinflammatory effects of vitamin D in pancreatic tissue

Vitamin D, particularly in its active form 1,25-dihydroxyvitamin D3 (calcitriol), exhibits notable antiinflammatory effects within pancreatic tissue. These effects are primarily mediated through the activation of the VDR, which modulates various cellular pathways to mitigate inflammation.

14.4.1 Modulation of pancreatic stellate cells

In the context of pancreatic inflammation and cancer, PSCs play a pivotal role in the development of fibrosis and the tumor microenvironment. Activation of VDR in PSCs by calcitriol or its analogs, such as calcipotriol, has been shown to suppress their activation. This suppression leads to a reduction in the fibrotic and inflammatory responses within the pancreatic tissue, thereby exerting antiinflammatory and anticancer effects (Zheng & Gao, 2022).

14.4.2 Regulation of cytokine production

Vitamin D influences the production of various cytokines involved in inflammatory processes. By binding to VDRs in pancreatic cells, calcitriol can modulate the expression of genes responsible for cytokine production, leading to a decrease in proinflammatory cytokines and an increase in antiinflammatory cytokines. This shift helps in reducing inflammation within the pancreatic tissue (Krajewska et al., 2022).

14.5 Cellular pathways influenced by vitamin D

Vitamin D, through its active form, exerts significant influence on various cellular pathways within pancreatic cells, particularly affecting β-cell function and insulin secretion.

14.5.1 AMPK pathway activation

Calcitriol enhances the activity of AMP-activated protein kinase (AMPK) in pancreatic β-cells. Activation of AMPK leads to the suppression of the NLRP3 inflammasome, a component implicated in inflammatory responses and β-cell dysfunction. This mechanism helps protect β-cells from high-glucose-induced damage, thereby preserving their function and viability.

14.5.2   mTOR pathway inhibition

VDR signaling has been shown to inhibit the mammalian target of the rapamycin (mTOR) pathway in β-cells. The mTOR pathway is involved in cell growth and proliferation, and its overactivation can lead to β-cell apoptosis. By inhibiting this pathway, calcitriol helps prevent β-cell death, contributing to the maintenance of adequate insulin secretion (Ozcan et al., 2023).

14.5.3   Modulation of apoptosis and proliferation

Vitamin D influences apoptosis signaling pathways in pancreatic cells. In pancreatic cancer cells, activation of VDR signaling has been observed to modulate pathways involved in cell proliferation and apoptosis, suggesting a role in tumor suppression (Moz et al., 2020).

14.5.4   Interaction with transforming growth factor-beta pathway

VDR activation affects the transforming growth factor-beta (TGF-β) pathway in pancreatic cells. This interaction can influence processes such as epithelial-mesenchymal transition (EMT), which is relevant in the context of pancreatic cancer progression (Li et al., 2015).

In summary, vitamin D, through VDR-mediated mechanisms, regulates key signaling pathways in pancreatic cells, including AMPK and mTOR, thereby influencing β-cell survival, insulin secretion and potentially modulating pancreatic cancer cell behavior.

14.5.5   Potential therapeutic implications

The antiinflammatory properties of vitamin D in pancreatic tissue suggest its potential as a therapeutic agent in conditions characterized by pancreatic inflammation, such as chronic pancreatitis and pancreatic cancer. Vitamin D supplementation or the use of VDR agonists could serve as adjunctive treatments aimed at modulating inflammatory responses and improving clinical outcomes in these disorders (Cai et al., 2022).

14.6   Populations at risk and the implications for pancreatic function

Vitamin D deficiency is a global health concern, affecting diverse populations due to factors such as limited sun exposure, dietary insufficiency, genetic predisposition, and chronic illnesses. High-risk groups include individuals with darker skin, the elderly, obese individuals, those with malabsorption disorders (e.g., celiac disease and Crohn's disease), and people living in regions with minimal sunlight exposure.

The implications of vitamin D deficiency extend beyond bone health, significantly impacting pancreatic function. Vitamin D plays a vital role in insulin synthesis and secretion, influencing glucose metabolism and pancreatic β-cell function. Deficiency has been associated with an increased risk of insulin resistance, type 2 diabetes, and pancreatic inflammation. Besides, VD's immunomodulatory properties may add to the deterrence of pancreatic autoimmunity, emphasizing its possible role in conditions such as type 1 diabetes.

Given the crucial role of vitamin D in maintaining pancreatic health, addressing deficiencies through dietary supplementation, increased sun exposure, and lifestyle interventions is essential. Public health strategies should focus on high-risk populations to prevent the metabolic and inflammatory complications associated with pancreatic dysfunction.

Recent studies have highlighted the significant role of vitamin D in pancreatic health. A narrative review published in 2022 emphasized that vitamin D deficiency is prevalent among patients with both acute and chronic pancreatitis. The review discussed the molecular mechanisms of vitamin D and its receptor signaling in pancreatic cells, suggesting that vitamin D assessment and supplementation could be beneficial strategies in managing pancreatitis (Cai et al., 2022).

Additionally, a 2021 study explored the relationship between vitamin D status and islet function in individuals with prediabetes. The findings indicated that vitamin D plays a role in regulating calcium flux in pancreatic cells, which is crucial for insulin secretion and overall pancreatic function (Pittas et al., 2007).

Addressing vitamin D deficiency through supplementation, dietary modifications, and lifestyle interventions is crucial for reducing the risk of metabolic disorders and preserving pancreatic health. Understanding the populations at risk and the physiological impact of vitamin D can aid in the development of targeted public health strategies to mitigate associated complications.

14.7   Role of vitamin D in pancreatitis

The classical, hormonally active dihydroxy form of VD3, 1,25(OH)2D3, regulates target genes through the VDR pathway, fulfilling various functions. VDR is a member of the nuclear receptor superfamily and is an endocrine receptor. The VDR is present not just in the skeletal system but is also extensively dispersed in many tissues, including the small intestine, kidneys, heart, lungs, pancreas, liver, immune cells, and other cell types (Zheng & Gao, 2022). Recent research indicates that vitamin D signaling may have a role in maintaining pancreatic homeostasis through its antiinflammatory and antifibrotic effects. The influence of vitamin D may be corroborated by the expression of VDR and signaling in pancreatic cells.

14.8   Vitamin D and pancreatic diseases beyond diabetes

14.8.1   Vitamin D's potential role in pancreatitis: acute and chronic

Pancreatitis is a progressive, intricate, deleterious inflammatory illness of the pancreas, associated with a significant risk of morbidity and mortality. Various aetiologies may lead to an unexpected progression that can encompass acute (AP), recurrent acute (RAP), and chronic (CP) pancreatitis. This series generally commences with a sentinel AP event (Pérez et al., 2024). Approximately 20% of patients experiencing their initial attack of acute pancreatitis (AP) will have recurrent episodes. Furthermore, 35% of individuals with recurrent acute pancreatitis (RAP) progress to end-stage chronic pancreatitis (CP). There is significant variability in the progression rate and disease severity, potentially influenced by underlying etiology, environmental exposures, and genetic factors (Spagnolo et al., 2022).

14.9   Etiology of pancreatitis

14.9.1   Acute pancreatitis

Acute pancreatitis is a common inflammatory disease of the exocrine pancreas that causes severe abdominal pain and multiple organ dysfunction that may lead to pancreatic necrosis and persistent organ failure, with a mortality of 1%–5% (Petrov & Yadav, 2019).

- Cholelithiasis.
- Ethanol.
- Hypertriglyceridemia.
- Drugs (antiretroviral, chemotherapeutics, antiepileptics, steroids, antihypertensives, and thiopurines).
- Endoscopic retrograde cholangiopancreatography (ERCP).
- Others [trauma, hypercalcemia, viral infections (e.g., mumps, cytomegalovirus, coxsackie B virus, severe acute respiratory syndrome coronavirus 2 (SARS-CoV-2))], tumors, anatomical variants (pancreas divisum, pancreaticobiliary ductal malunion), cardiac bypass surgery, scorpion bites (notably from Tityus trinitatis), and organophosphate poisoning (Szatmary et al., 2022).

It has been suggested that dysregulation of vitamin D (VD) is linked to the generation of acute pancreatitis. The imbalance in active vitamin D levels is a primary cause of hypercalcemia, a risk factor for acute pancreatitis. Polymorphisms in the VDR gene can significantly disrupt the balance of circulating vitamin D levels and its physiological function in the body. Furthermore, the level of serum 25-hydroxyvitamin D3 (25-(OH) D3) exhibited an inverse correlation with the severity of acute pancreatitis and inflammatory markers, including C-reactive protein. VD also influences both innate and adaptive immune responses and diminishes oxidative stress, potentially triggering AP (Li et al., 2021). The severity of AP and inflammatory indicators, such as C-reactive protein, were inversely associated with serum 25-(OH) D3 levels. Apart from the usual suspects, a lower serum 25-(OH) D3 level is associated with an increased risk of severe acute pancreatitis and intensive care unit admission (Huh et al., 2019). It is uncertain whether vitamin D deficiency is a causative factor or a result of severe disease; nonetheless, evidence indicates that the extent of vitamin D deficiency may correlate with disease prognosis.

14.9.2   Chronic pancreatitis

Chronic pancreatitis is the progressive and irreversible destruction of the pancreas as characterized by permanent loss of endocrine and exocrine function (Muniraj et al., 2014).

• Alcohol.
• Autoimmune diseases.
• Smoking.
• Idiopathic.
• Genetic mutation (Munnelly et al., 2024).

Chronic pancreatitis is defined as a progressive malabsorptive disorder that impairs the body's digestive and absorptive functions, leading to malnutrition over time. The primary mechanisms contributing to vitamin D insufficiency are likely associated with steatorrhea and the malabsorption of vitamin D resulting from chronic pancreatitis. Additional risk factors for vitamin D deficiency encompass African-American race, diminished dietary status, and diabetes mellitus, among others (Cai et al., 2022). Impaired exocrine pancreatic function disrupts vitamin D metabolism. In chronic pancreatitis, structural atrophy and ductal-related characteristics were correlated with vitamin D insufficiency (Frøkjær et al., 2013). These not only influence vitamin D synthesis and absorption but also disrupt bone metabolism, potentially leading to reduced bone mass density and consequent conditions such as osteopenia and osteoporosis, resulting in heightened bone fragility and increased vulnerability to fractures (Vujasinovic et al., 2021). The onset of diabetes mellitus in chronic pancreatitis primarily results from the destruction of islet cells due to pancreatic inflammation. The loss of pancreatic islet cells transpires later in the disease progression, as endocrine cells are diffusely located within the pancreatic parenchyma. Patients may develop type 3c (pancreatogenic) diabetes mellitus (T3cDM), which is further complicated by concurrent diminished glucagon secretion (Mohapatra et al., 2020).

14.9.3   Pathophysiology of pancreatitis

Ischemia/reperfusion damage is widely acknowledged as a prevalent and significant mechanism in the pathophysiology of acute pancreatitis, particularly in the transition from moderate edematous to severe necrotizing forms. Elevated intracellular calcium levels also contribute to acinar cell injury. Oxygen-derived free radicals and other cytokines (e.g., interleukin [IL]-1, IL-6, IL-8, tumor necrosis factor-α, platelet-activating factor) are regarded as key mediators in the progression of acute pancreatitis from a localized inflammatory response to systemic multiorgan disease (Sakorafas & Tsiotou, 2000). Chronic pancreatitis is considered to be a consequence of recurring acute pancreatitis episodes (Klöppel & Maillet, 1992). An imbalance in pancreatic juice, excessive protein secretion, diminished fluid or bicarbonate secretion, and altered lithostatine levels can result in protein plugs within ducts and ductuli, culminating in calcium carbonate precipitates and intraductal stones. Lithostatine, synthesized in acinar cells, impedes the formation of calcium carbonate precipitation. Protein plugs are present in the majority of chronic pancreatitis cases, but ductal stones are mostly associated with alcohol-induced chronic pancreatitis (Strate et al., 2002).

14.9.4   Diagnosis of pancreatitis

For an AP diagnosis, two out of three of the following must be satisfied:
• Abnormally high levels of serum lipase activity (three times the upper limit of normal).
• Classic abdominal pain (immediate onset of chronic upper abdomen discomfort, frequently spreading to the back).
• Imaging results demonstrating distinctive morphology (high agreement).

It is advised to measure serum lipase solely because serum amylase has a lower specificity (Beyer et al., 2022).

14.10   Linking vitamin deficiency to pancreatic dysfunction

14.10.1   Effects of vitamin D deficiency on beta-cell function

The control of blood glucose levels requires the proper functioning of pancreatic beta-cells, which, in turn, requires sufficient amounts of vitamin D. This section will explore the mechanisms through which vitamin D contributes to the secretion of insulin, homeostasis of blood glucose levels, and overall metabolic health.

Indeed, the main function of pancreatic beta-cells is to secrete insulin in response to increased blood glucose levels—after a meal, for example. Insulin causes cells, particularly skeletal muscle cells, to take glucose in and reduce blood glucose levels to a healthy range.

Vitamin D is intricately linked with the efficacy of beta-cell function. Beta-cells express VDRs, which bind to 1,25-dihydroxyvitamin D (1,25(OH)D), the active metabolite of vitamin D (Morró et al., 2020). VDRs are crucial in the function of beta-cells as they regulate calcium signaling, which will be discussed in the next section. Ultimately, vitamin D deficiency will compromise beta-cell function and indirectly impact glucose metabolism (Fleet, 2004).

14.10.2   The connection between vitamin D and insulin secretion

Pancreatic beta-cells need calcium to carry out their function of insulin secretion (Idevall-Hagren & Tengholm, 2020; Klec et al., 2019; Trexler & Taraska, 2017). Their membranes contain voltage-gated calcium channels that control the entry of calcium into the beta-cell. When these channels open, the increase of intracellular calcium ions triggers the release of insulin from the beta-cells by exocytosis. This implies that the amount of calcium ions in the beta-cell cytosol will directly influence the amount of insulin that can be secreted. To ensure that beta-cells can respond effectively to the body's metabolic demands, these voltage-gated calcium channels are regulated in multiple ways. First, a rise in blood glucose levels, for example, after a meal, causes glucose to enter the beta-cells via GLUT transporters in the membrane. The glucose molecules will be metabolized, leading to an increase in ATP production. The rise in ATP levels will inhibit ATP-sensitive potassium channels, subsequently leading to the depolarization of the beta-cell membrane. This will open the voltage-gated calcium channels, allowing an influx of calcium into the beta-cell and causing the release of insulin by exocytosis. Second, vitamin D in the form of 1,25(OH)D will modulate the activity of the calcium channels by binding to VDRs on the beta-cell membrane. This will also increase the extent of membrane depolarization, further promoting calcium influx. As the amount of intracellular calcium present in the beta-cell cytosol will dictate the amount of insulin released, this will cause even more insulin to be released (Bourlon et al., 1999).

Vitamin D further enhances this process by upregulating the expression of genes associated with calcium homeostasis and insulin granule movement, mediated through the activation of VDRs on beta-cells. For example, 1,25(OH)D regulates the transcription of transient potential vanilloid type 6 (TRPV6), an epithelial calcium channel found in the intestines (Christakos et al., 2016; Khammissa et al., 2018; Meyer et al., 2006). Additionally, vitamin D influences the expression of calbindin, a calcium-binding protein that helps maintain stable intracellular calcium levels (Acharya et al., 2024; Doroudi et al., 2015; Ellison et al., 2005). Indeed, it appears that the primary function of vitamin D in calcium homeostasis is to increase calcium absorption.

In vitamin D-deficiency, the expression of VDRs on the beta-cell surface is reduced (Morró et al., 2020). This will diminish insulin secretion, which is a hallmark of diabetes mellitus. Chiu et al. (2004) showed a positive correlation between 1,25(OH)D concentration (as an indicator of vitamin D status) and the insulin sensitivity index, suggesting that individuals with lower vitamin D levels tend to experience reduced insulin sensitivity and highlighting the impact of vitamin D deficiency on beta-cell function. Vitamin D deficiency will also dysregulate calcium homeostasis and impair calcium absorption in the intestines (Chiu et al., 2004).

Both animal and human studies demonstrate that restoring vitamin D levels improves glucose metabolism. For instance, overexpression of VDRs in a mouse model rescued the diabetic phenotype (Morró et al., 2020). In rodent models of diabetes, vitamin D supplementation protects against beta-cell dysfunction (Wu et al., 2022). Human studies corroborate these findings; for example, a human study found that vitamin D supplementation improved fasting blood glucose, insulin, and insulin resistance in individuals with T2DM (Talaei et al., 2013). Additionally, Zhang et al. (2020) highlighted that vitamin D supplementation reduced markers of T2DM in their meta-analysis of randomized controlled trials for vitamin D supplementation in patients with prediabetes or new-onset diabetes (Zheng & Gao, 2022). Another meta-analysis also showed the beneficial effects of vitamin D supplementation in poorly controlled diabetes (Krul-Poel et al., 2017).

Furthermore, vitamin D modulates inflammatory pathways, reducing beta-cell stress and apoptosis, which indirectly supports insulin secretion, which we will discuss in the subsequent sections (Hashim et al., 2022). This evidence underscores the critical role of vitamin D in maintaining beta-cell function and highlights its therapeutic potential for managing diabetes.

14.10.3   Influence on insulin sensitivity and glucose metabolism

Vitamin D deficiency contributes to insulin resistance by reducing the responsiveness of various tissues to insulin, which is critical for lowering blood glucose levels. Vitamin D modulates skeletal muscle metabolism, composition, and insulin sensitivity (Ryan et al., 2016). In the liver, vitamin D deficiency will enhance gluconeogenesis, contributing to glycemia (Leung, 2016). Low vitamin D levels in adipose tissue will impair lipid metabolism and promote proinflammatory cytokine release(Abbas, 2017; Luo et al., 2020; Park & Han, 2021). All these disruptions will exacerbate insulin resistance.

Reduced vitamin D levels will also trigger secondary hormonal responses, particularly through parathyroid hormone (PTH) elevation, which, in turn, will also increase the risk of insulin resistance. Studies suggest that PTH might decrease the number of glucose transporters (GLUT1 and GLUT4) available on cell membranes, hindering glucose uptake and promoting insulin resistance (Sung et al., 2012). PTH may also suppress insulin secretion, further reducing glucose uptake by cells and aggravating the insulin-resistant state (Chang et al., 2009; Thomas et al., 1995).

One of the primary drivers of insulin resistance is chronic inflammation and oxidative stress, both of which will decrease cellular integrity and induce beta-cell apoptosis, ultimately resulting in decreased beta-cell function. A deficiency in vitamin D will result in an increase in proinflammatory cytokines such as TNF-α and IL-6, which interfere with insulin signaling pathways in peripheral tissues (Chagas et al., 2012; Fenercioglu, 2024; Wang et al., 2019). Therefore, the use of vitamin D supplementation to alleviate vitamin D deficiencies can reduce various markers of oxidative stress and inflammation due to its antiinflammatory properties as well as its role in boosting the production of antiinflammatory cytokines (Cojic et al., 2020; Hernandez et al., 2021; Wu et al., 2022; Zbaar, 2023). This multifaceted role of vitamin D in modulating inflammation results in improved insulin sensitivity due to improved beta cell function and emphasizes its therapeutic potential in diabetes management.

Epidemiological and cohort studies have provided additional strong evidence linking vitamin D deficiency to impaired glucose tolerance, insulin resistance, and eventual diabetes. Musazadeh et al. (2023) demonstrated a significant inverse relationship between serum vitamin D levels and insulin resistance markers such as HOMA-IR and fasting glucose levels in their recent meta-analysis. A Nigerian cohort study also illustrated that T2DM patients with higher serum vitamin D levels tend to have better insulin sensitivity and glycaemic control compared to individuals with lower levels (Adeleye et al., 2023). Indeed, prospective studies consistently show that individuals with vitamin D deficiency are at higher risk for developing T2DM. All these lines of evidence reinforce the importance of maintaining adequate vitamin D status, particularly in those at higher risk of T2DM.

14.11   Mechanistic insights and research gaps

Vitamin D has been shown to be linked to glucose metabolism and insulin sensitivity by modulating processes such as immune function, systemic inflammation, and intracellular calcium balance. The relationship between vitamin D and the immune response has been discussed in detail in Chapter 7. However, as mentioned in the previous section, vitamin D promotes a less inflammatory response by boosting antiinflammatory cytokines as well as suppressing proinflammatory cytokines. VDRs also have a multifaceted role with the pancreatic beta-cells. Activation of the VDRs not only regulates the entry of calcium ions in the beta-cells but also facilitates the transcription of genes involved in insulin production, calcium homeostasis, and inflammatory control, as detailed in the previous section. This gives vitamin D a comprehensive role in metabolic health (Argano et al., 2023).

Despite these extensive insights on the link between vitamin D and glucose metabolism, some inconsistencies are still seen in the effects of vitamin D supplementation between studies, particularly in dose-response relationships between vitamin D and alleviation of T2DM markers. Although some studies show significant improvements in insulin sensitivity and glycaemic control, other studies report minimal or no effect after vitamin D supplementation. While factors such as age, ethnicity, and baseline vitamin D status may cause inconsistent results, standardization of intervention protocols between studies is also required while also taking into account these population differences. For instance, populations with darker skin pigmentation or lower sun exposure may require different strategies to achieve optimal vitamin D levels after supplementation. Variables such as age-related differences in vitamin D metabolism and other comorbidities may also complicate the interpretation of any results obtained. This will be further examined in the next section of this chapter.

The long-term effects of vitamin D on glucose metabolism and diabetes prevention also have not been fully studied. It is unclear whether sustained supplementation with vitamin D can halt the progression from prediabetes to diabetes, especially in populations that tend to have lower vitamin D levels. The link between vitamin D and other metabolic pathologies, such as obesity and lipid dysregulation, if any, also needs to be investigated further. By addressing these research gaps, we may eventually be able to develop targeted and effective vitamin D-based interventions for metabolic disorders.

14.12 Vitamin D and diabetes mellitus

14.12.1 Role of vitamin D in type 1 diabetes: immune modulation and beta-cell protection

Type 1 diabetes mellitus (T1DM) is characterized by an autoimmune reaction that causes the immune-mediated destruction of pancreatic beta cells, leading to insulin deficiency. As detailed in Chapter 7, vitamin D can modulate immune responses, from the proinflammatory Th1 response to a more regulatory state, by increasing the activity of regulatory T cells (Tregs). The suppression of the autoimmune response will then reduce the destruction of beta-cells. The presence of 1,25(OH)D has been shown to enhance the production of antiinflammatory cytokines and inhibit the production of proinflammatory cytokines, which provides a protective effect against beta-cell damage (Cojic et al., 2020; Hernandez et al., 2021; Wu et al., 2022; Zbaar, 2023).

In a genetically predisposed population, adequate vitamin D levels may reduce the risk of T1DM. Miettinen et al. (2020) investigated the association between serum 1,25(OH)D concentrations and the development of islet autoimmunity (IA) and T1DM in children with increased genetic risk (Miettinen et al., 2020). The study found that children who developed IA had lower mean serum 1,25(OH)D levels 18 months prior to seroconversion compared to control children, suggesting that higher vitamin D levels may confer protection against the development of T1D.

In contrast, the Diabetes Autoimmunity Study in the Young (DAISY) found no significant association between vitamin D intake or 1,25(OH)D levels and the risk of IA or progression to T1DM (Barker et al., 2004). These differing outcomes highlight the complexity of vitamin D's role in T1DM development and underscore the need for further research to clarify these associations.

Preclinical studies in nonobese diabetic (NOD) mice have shown that vitamin D supplementation promotes Treg activity, which may decrease autoimmune triggers. Although it did not lower gut permeability, diabetes onset was still reduced. Furthermore, dietary vitamin D supplementation significantly lowered T1DM incidence and improved immune tolerance in these animal models (Martens et al., 2022).

Preclinical research also highlights vitamin D's direct protective effects on beta-cells. For instance, vitamin D supplementation reduced cathepsin G (CatG)-mediated CD4+ T-cell activation, which drives autoimmune beta-cell destruction. This effect was associated with restored beta-cell function and improved glycemic control in T1DM mice. In addition, Lai et al. (2022) show that vitamin D stabilizes the islet microenvironment, reduces oxidative stress, and preserves beta-cell viability (Lai et al., 2022). Despite these findings, gaps remain in understanding optimal dosing and the long-term impact of supplementation on disease progression, especially in diverse genetic and environmental contexts.

14.12.2 Type 2 diabetes: vitamin D's impact on insulin resistance

Vitamin D influences T2DM by enhancing insulin receptor sensitivity and modulating skeletal muscle and adipocyte function, as discussed in the previous section. It facilitates the activation of insulin receptors by regulating calcium-dependent signaling pathways critical for glucose uptake and metabolism. Vitamin D also improves adipocyte function by reducing inflammation and lipid accumulation, which are key contributors to insulin resistance. It modulates the expression of genes involved in adipogenesis, thereby improving the metabolic profile of adipose tissue. This dual action on muscle and adipose tissue enhances systemic insulin sensitivity (Argano et al., 2023).

Large cohort studies have consistently shown that individuals with vitamin D deficiency are at a higher risk of developing T2DM, suggesting a significant inverse correlation between vitamin D levels and T2DM risk (Pittas et al., 2019; Tobias et al., 2024). Indeed, a meta-analysis of observational studies suggests that each 10 ng/mL increase in serum vitamin D levels was associated with a 10%–15% reduced risk of T2DM onset (Lei et al., 2023). Furthermore, the study authors concluded that studies conducted in diverse populations indicate that vitamin D deficiency is prevalent among T2DM patients and strongly correlates with higher levels of insulin resistance markers, such as HOMA-IR, and worse glycemic control (Lei et al., 2023).

Interventional studies provide additional evidence of vitamin D's role in improving glycemic parameters, which we will discuss in the next section. In short, trials have shown that vitamin D supplementation reduces insulin resistance, fasting glucose, and HbA1c levels in patients with T2D or prediabetes.

14.12.3 Vitamin D supplementation in diabetes management

Clinical trials assessing vitamin D supplementation for diabetes management show varying efficacy in improving glycemic control across both T1DM and T2DM populations. In T2DM, meta-analyses demonstrate that vitamin D supplementation reduces fasting blood glucose (FBG), HbA1c, and insulin resistance (HOMA-IR), particularly in patients with baseline vitamin D deficiency. For instance, a randomized controlled trial demonstrated that daily vitamin D supplementation significantly lowered HbA1c and fasting blood glucose levels over 6 months compared to a placebo group (Alvina et al., 2023). However, the magnitude of these benefits varies across studies, likely due to differences in baseline vitamin D status, dosage, and patient demographics. While some studies show modest improvements, others report no significant effects, underscoring the need for personalized approaches in supplementation. Systematic reviews of randomized controlled trials found substantial improvements in HbA1c (−0.30%) and FBG (−0.49 mmol/L) with high-dose vitamin D supplementation, particularly in short-term interventions targeting overweight patients with poor glycemic control (Hu et al., 2019; Lei et al., 2023; Musazadeh et al., 2023). However, the results are less consistent for T1DM, where vitamin D is often explored as an immunomodulatory therapy to preserve beta-cell function rather than directly lowering glucose levels (He et al., 2022).

Optimal dosing and duration of supplementation remain areas of active investigation. Higher doses of vitamin D (≥2000 IU/day) have shown greater efficacy in reducing HbA1c and improving insulin sensitivity, especially in patients with severe deficiency. Yet, some trials report minimal effects in patients with normal or mildly deficient vitamin D levels, suggesting a threshold effect. Genetic factors such as polymorphisms in VDR genes and metabolic conditions like obesity may also influence patient response to vitamin D supplementation. A meta-analysis carried out by Zheng et al. (2022) indicated that in patients with prediabetes, nonobese patients showed a more pronounced reduction in diabetes risk compared to obese patients when supplemented with vitamin D (Zheng & Gao, 2022).

Vitamin D supplementation may also act synergistically with other diabetes therapies. For example, combining vitamin D with metformin may enhance insulin sensitivity and glycemic outcomes by addressing different mechanisms. Dietary interventions rich in calcium and vitamin D amplify these effects, which may further improve glycemic control and metabolic health. Emerging evidence suggests that personalized supplementation strategies based on baseline vitamin D status, genetic predisposition, and metabolic conditions could optimize outcomes for patients with T1D and T2D.

14.13 Pancreatic cancer: insights into vitamin D as a therapeutic agent

Pancreatic cancer can be recognized as a life-threatening condition and one of the most aggressive and lethal (Luo et al., 2020). At the time of diagnosis, pancreatic cancer frequently manifests at an advanced stage and has typically metastasized to other regions of the body. Pancreatic cancer clinically refers to malignant tumors originating in the epithelial cells of glandular structures within the pancreatic ductal cells, specifically termed adenocarcinoma, with pancreatic ductal adenocarcinoma (PDAC) constituting over 90% of pancreatic cancer cases (Aier et al., 2019). Despite being the tenth most prevalent cancer, PDAC ranks as the seventh greatest cause of cancer-related mortality worldwide due to its dismal survival rates. Other rarer exocrine pancreatic malignancies comprise adenosquamous carcinoma, squamous cell carcinoma, giant cell carcinoma, acinar cell carcinoma, and small cell carcinoma. Currently, pancreatic cancer persists as a catastrophic illness, with its prognosis virtually unchanged over the past twenty years (Siegel et al., 2019) (Table 14.1).

Table 14.1 Risk factors for pancreatic cancer.

Modifiable	Nonmodifiable
Age (over 55 years)	Human microflora
Sex (more in males)	Smoking
Area (more in African-Americans)	Alcohol
Blood group (A, AB, or B)	Chronic pancreatitis
Genetic factors	Obesity
Diabetes mellitus	

14.14 Vitamin D and pancreatic cancer

14.14.1 Anticancer properties

Vitamin D, upon activation to its active form calcitriol, regulates cancer growth via many routes. It restrains cell proliferation, encourages apoptosis, induces differentiation, curtails food supply and growth, and inhibits metastasis by diminishing the expression of matrix metalloproteinases, enzymes that facilitate cancer cell invasion and metastasis (El-Sharkawy & Malki, 2020).

14.14.2 Immune modulation

The immune system, which vitamin D aids in regulating, is a crucial component of the pancreatic cancer tumor microenvironment. Vitamin D enhances the efficacy of cytotoxic T lymphocytes and stimulates a reduction in regulatory T-cells and myeloid-derived suppressor cells, which inhibit the immune system. Decreases the production of cytokines that facilitate inflammation, such as IL-6 and TNF-α, which are linked to tumor progression (Moz et al., 2020).

14.14.3 Remodeling of tumor microenvironment

The tumor microenvironment in pancreatic cancer is dense and fibrotic (desmoplastic), impeding medication delivery. Vitamin D remodels stroma by activating VDR in pancreatic stellate cells, hence decreasing fibrosis and facilitating a more conducive environment for therapeutic drugs to access the tumor. Preclinical studies indicate that vitamin D analogs may augment the effectiveness of chemotherapy by facilitating medication infiltration into the tumor (Sherman et al., 2014).

14.15 Role of vitamin D treatment in pancreatic cancer

Vitamin D decreases cancer risk via its biologically active metabolite, $1\alpha,25(OH)2D3$, which governs cellular proliferation and differentiation, inhibits angiogenesis, and promotes apoptosis. The antiproliferative effects of $1\alpha,25(OH)2D3$ primarily result from modifications in numerous critical cell cycle regulators, leading to the dephosphorylation of retinoblastoma protein and the arrest of cells in the G0/G1 phase.

In adenocarcinoma, diminished vitamin D levels at diagnosis correlated with increased inflammatory biomarkers (IL-6, chitinase-3-like protein 1, CHI3L1, and CRP) across all disease stages; patients exhibiting adequate vitamin D levels in the initial stages of cancer demonstrated prolonged survival compared to those with insufficient vitamin D levels (Azzini et al., 2024). Another study indicates that pancreatic human primary cancer-associated fibroblasts (CAFs) respond to the vitamin D3 analog, calcipotriol, facilitating differentiation toward a less tumor-promoting CAF phenotype. Calcipotriol exerts an immunosuppressive effect on T cells, which is amplified in the presence of CAFs. While VDR activation may positively influence the phenotype of pancreatic CAFs, it may concurrently suppress a T cell-mediated response against tumor cells due to vitamin D3 (Gorchs et al., 2020).

14.16 Emerging research on vitamin D and exocrine pancreatic function

Vitamin D is becoming acknowledged for its functions beyond skeletal health, especially in regulating immunological response, inflammation, and cellular integrity. Recent studies indicate that it may also affect exocrine pancreatic function, which entails the release of digestive enzymes essential for nutrient absorption. Exocrine pancreatic insufficiency (EPI) is a disorder characterized by diminished or inadequate secretion or function of pancreatic juice and its digesting enzymes, particularly pancreatic lipase. EPI may lead to clinical manifestations, including steatorrhea, weight loss, and metabolic changes associated with the malabsorption and maldigestion of lipids and liposoluble micronutrients. Chronic pancreatitis, cystic fibrosis, genetic disorders, diabetes mellitus, acute severe pancreatitis, infections, and medication contribute to the development of exocrine pancreatic insufficiency (Capurso et al., 2019). Impaired exocrine pancreatic function disrupts vitamin D metabolism. In chronic pancreatitis, structural atrophy and ductal-related characteristics were correlated with vitamin D insufficiency. The ramifications of exocrine insufficiency, primarily signified by fecal elastase 1 levels, may be pertinent to serum vitamin D3 concentrations (Cai et al., 2022). Reduced vitamin D levels are documented to vary from 22.0% to 86.5% (Jøker-Jensen et al., 2020). Zhang and Gao observed a statistically significant decrease in vitamin D levels, particularly among patients with the alcoholic variant of chronic pancreatitis (Zheng & Gao, 2022). A comparison of vitamin D levels in patients with definitive chronic pancreatitis and those with early chronic pancreatitis revealed that vitamin D levels are diminished in the early form; however, this reduction is significantly less pronounced in the definitive form of the disease compared to the advanced form (Zheng & Gao, 2022).

14.17 Challenges and controversies

Vitamin D's role in diabetes management remains controversial due to inconsistencies in study outcomes. Variations in baseline vitamin D levels significantly influence results, with the most pronounced benefits observed in patients with severe deficiency. Conversely, studies involving participants with sufficient or mildly deficient vitamin D levels often report negligible improvements in glycemic control, suggesting a threshold effect. Participant demographics such as ethnicity further complicate findings, as differences in skin pigmentation, genetic polymorphisms in VDR genes, and lifestyle factors influence serum vitamin D levels and metabolic outcomes. Moreover, study design variability—ranging from differences in supplementation duration, dosing regimens, and control groups—adds to the heterogeneity of results.

Concerns about oversupplementation and vitamin D toxicity are growing, especially with high-dose regimens. While doses of up to 4000 IU/day are generally considered safe, chronic intake exceeding this threshold may lead to hypercalcemia, kidney stones, and vascular calcification. Defining the upper limit of safety is particularly challenging in populations with comorbidities or altered vitamin D metabolism, such as those with obesity or chronic kidney disease. Despite these risks, no consensus on standardized dosing protocols complicates clinical practice. For instance, some studies may advocate for individualized dosing based on baseline levels and genetic predispositions, while others recommend uniform doses, leading to inconsistent recommendations. Additionally, a meta-analysis carried out by Hu et al. showed benefits with short-term vitamin D supplementation but not long-term vitamin D supplementation, suggesting that the period of supplementation may also matter (Hu et al., 2019).

The lack of agreement on optimal vitamin D thresholds for supplementation—both for deficiency correction and therapeutic effects—further adds to the controversy. Recommendations vary widely between organizations, ranging from 20 to 30 ng/mL as the target serum 25(OH)D level, creating ambiguity in clinical guidelines. These discrepancies highlight the need for robust, large-scale trials that stratify participants by demographic and metabolic factors to establish evidence-based, standardized protocols (Cheng et al., 2024).

14.18 Future research directions

Future research on vitamin D and diabetes should prioritize long-term studies to evaluate its role in preventing diabetes onset and in diabetes treatment, particularly in at-risk populations such as individuals with prediabetes or metabolic syndrome. Large-scale, multicenter randomized controlled trials could provide clarity on optimal dosing regimens, timing, and baseline vitamin D thresholds necessary for maximum preventive effects. Additionally, studies should stratify participants by demographic and genetic factors, including ethnicity, skin pigmentation, and VDR polymorphisms, to better understand how these variables influence outcomes. Long-term longitudinal studies that track changes in glycemic markers, insulin resistance, and beta-cell function could also clarify vitamin D's potential to halt or reverse disease progression.

The development and study of vitamin D analogs represent another promising avenue for research. These analogs, designed to retain the therapeutic benefits of vitamin D while minimizing risks like hypercalcemia, could revolutionize treatment strategies. For example, certain analogs might selectively target VDR pathways involved in insulin sensitivity and immune modulation without affecting calcium metabolism. Investigating these compounds' pharmacodynamics and safety profiles, both in vitro and in vivo, will be critical. Preclinical studies in animal models, followed by human trials, could assess their efficacy in reducing glycemic variability, improving beta-cell survival, and modulating inflammatory pathways with fewer side effects.

Finally, integrating vitamin D supplementation with other therapies, such as metformin, dietary interventions, or microbiome-modulating strategies, warrants exploration. Research could assess synergistic effects that optimize metabolic outcomes while reducing reliance on pharmacological treatments. By leveraging genomic and metabolomic data, precision medicine approaches might help tailor vitamin D interventions to individual needs, enhancing their effectiveness and safety. These directions collectively aim to address current research gaps and unlock vitamin D's full potential in diabetes prevention and management.

References

Abbas, M. A. (2017). Physiological functions of Vitamin D in adipose tissue. *Journal of Steroid Biochemistry and Molecular Biology, 165*, 369–381. https://doi.org/10.1016/j.jsbmb.2016.08.004, www.elsevier.com/locate/jsbmb.

Acharya, M., Singh, N., Gupta, G., Tambuwala, M. M., Aljabali, A. A. A., Chellappan, D. K., Dua, K., & Goyal, R. (2024). Vitamin D, Calbindin, and calcium signaling: Unraveling the Alzheimer's connection. *Cellular Signalling, 116*. https://doi.org/10.1016/j.cellsig.2024.111043, https://www.sciencedirect.com/science/journal/08986568.

Adeleye, J. O., Emuze, M. E., Esan, A., & Bamidele, O. T. (2023). Serum vitamin D status and its relationship with insulin resistance amongst a cohort of Nigerian patients with type 2 diabetes mellitus. *Journal of Diabetology, 14*(4), 220–225. https://doi.org/10.4103/jod.jod_12_23, https://journals.lww.com/JODB/pages/default.aspx.

Aier, I., Semwal, R., Sharma, A., & Varadwaj, P. K. (2019). A systematic assessment of statistics, risk factors, and underlying features involved in pancreatic cancer. *Cancer Epidemiology, 58*, 104–110. https://doi.org/10.1016/j.canep.2018.12.001, http://www.elsevier.com.

Alvina, S., Immanuel, D. S., Harbuwono, F. D., Suyatna, A., Harahap, J., & Prihartono, P. (2023). Effect of three and six months of vitamin D supplementation on glycemic control and insulin resistance in type 2 diabetes mellitus: Randomized placebo-controlled trial. *Indonesian Biomedical Journal, 15*(3), 287–295. https://doi.org/10.18585/inabj.v15i3.2370, http://inabj.org/index.php/ibj.

Argano, C., Mirarchi, L., Amodeo, S., Orlando, V., Torres, A., & Corrao, S. (2023). The role of vitamin D and its molecular bases in insulin resistance, diabetes, metabolic syndrome, and cardiovascular disease: State of the art. *International Journal of Molecular Sciences, 24*(20), 15485. https://doi.org/10.3390/ijms242015485.

Azzini, E., Furini, T., Polito, A., Scalfi, L., Pinto, A., Gasperi, V., & Savini, I. (2024). Vitamin nutritional status in patients with pancreatic cancer: A narrative review. *International Journal of Molecular Sciences, 25*(9), 4773. https://doi.org/10.3390/ijms25094773.

Barker, J. M., Barriga, K. J., Yu, L., Miao, D., Erlich, H. A., Norris, J. M., Eisenbarth, G. S., & Rewers, M. (2004). Prediction of autoantibody positivity and progression to type 1 diabetes: Diabetes Autoimmunity Study in the Young (DAISY). *Journal of Clinical Endocrinology and Metabolism, 89*(8), 3896–3902. https://doi.org/10.1210/jc.2003-031887.

Beyer, G., Hoffmeister, A., Lorenz, P., Lynen, P., Lerch, M. M., & Mayerle, J. (2022). Acute and chronic pancreatitis. *Deutsches Ärzteblatt international, 119*.

Bourlon, P. M., Billaudel, B., & Faure-Dussert, A. (1999). Influence of vitamin D3 deficiency and 1,25 dihydroxyvitamin D3 on de novo insulin biosynthesis in the islets of the rat endocrine pancreas. *Journal of Endocrinology, 160*(1), 87–95. https://doi.org/10.1677/joe.0.1600087.

Cai, F., Hu, C., Chen, C. J., Han, Y. P., Lin, Z. Q., Deng, L. H., & Xia, Q. (2022). Vitamin D and pancreatitis: A narrative review of current evidence. *Nutrients, 14*(10). https://doi.org/10.3390/nu14102113, https://www.mdpi.com/2072-6643/14/10/2113/pdf?version=1652887013.

Capurso, G., Traini, M., Piciucchi, M., Signoretti, M., & Arcidiacono, P. G. (2019). Exocrine pancreatic insufficiency: Prevalence, diagnosis, and management. *Clinical and Experimental Gastroenterology, 12*, 129–139. https://doi.org/10.2147/CEG.S168266, https://www.dovepress.com/exocrine-pancreatic-insufficiency-prevalence-diagnosis-and-management-peer-reviewed-article-CEG.

Chagas, C. E. A., Borges, M. C., Martini, L. A., & Rogero, M. M. (2012). Focus on vitamin D, inflammation and type 2 diabetes. *Nutrients, 4*(1), 52–67. https://doi.org/10.3390/nu4010052, http://www.mdpi.com/2072-6643/4/1/52/pdf.

Chang, E., Donkin, S. S., & Teegarden, D. (2009). Parathyroid hormone suppresses insulin signaling in adipocytes. *Molecular and Cellular Endocrinology, 307*(1-2), 77–82. https://doi.org/10.1016/j.mce.2009.03.024.

Cheng, L., Lv, C., Xue, L., Zhang, C., Wang, L., Wang, X., Chen, S., Li, X., Feng, W., Xie, H., & Zhao, H. (2024). The prevention and improvement effects of vitamin D on type 2 diabetes mellitus: evidence from an umbrella review on meta-analyses of cohort studies and randomized controlled trials. *Frontiers in Nutrition, 11*. https://doi.org/10.3389/fnut.2024.1462535.

Chiu, K. C., Chu, A., Go, V. L. W., & Saad, M. F. (2004). Hypovitaminosis D is associated with insulin resistance and β cell dysfunction. *Journal of Clinical Nutrition, 79*(5), 820–825. https://doi.org/10.1093/ajcn/79.5.820, http://www.ajcn.org/contents-by-date.2005.shtml.

Choi, M., Ozeki, J., Hashizume, M., Kato, S., Ishihara, H., & Makishima, M. (2012). Vitamin D receptor activation induces peptide YY transcription in pancreatic islets. *Endocrinology, 153*(11), 5188–5199. https://doi.org/10.1210/en.2012-1396.

Christakos, S., Dhawan, P., Verstuyf, A., Verlinden, L., & Carmeliet, G. (2016). Vitamin D: Metabolism, molecular mechanism of action, and pleiotropic effects. *Physiological Reviews, 96*(1), 365–408. https://doi.org/10.1152/physrev.00014.2015.

Cojic, M., Kocic, R., Klisic, A., Cvejanov-Kezunovic, L., Kavaric, N., & Kocic, G. (2020). A novel mechanism of vitamin D anti-inflammatory/antioxidative potential in type 2 diabetic patients on metformin therapy. *Archives of Medical Science, 16*(5), 1004–1012. https://doi.org/10.5114/aoms.2020.92832.

Doroudi, M., Schwartz, Z., & Boyan, B. D. (2015). Membrane-mediated actions of 1,25-dihydroxy vitamin D3: A review of the roles of phospholipase A2 activating protein and Ca2+/calmodulin-dependent protein kinase II. *Journal of Steroid Biochemistry and Molecular Biology, 147*, 81–84. https://doi.org/10.1016/j.jsbmb.2014.11.002, www.elsevier.com/locate/jsbmb.

El-Sharkawy, A., & Malki, A. (2020). Vitamin D signaling in inflammation and cancer: Molecular mechanisms and therapeutic implications. *Molecules (Basel, Switzerland), 25*(14), 3219. https://doi.org/10.3390/molecules25143219.

Ellison, T. I., Dowd, D. R., & MacDonald, P. N. (2005). Calmodulin-dependent kinase IV stimulates vitamin D receptor-mediated transcription. *Molecular Endocrinology, 19*(9), 2309–2319. https://doi.org/10.1210/me.2004-0382UnitedStates, http://mend.endojournals.org/cgi/reprint/19/9/2309.

Fenercioglu, A. K. (2024). The anti-inflammatory roles of vitamin D for improving human health. *Current Issues in Molecular Biology, 46*(12), 13514–13525. https://doi.org/10.3390/cimb46120807.

Fleet, J. C. (2004). Rapid, membrane-initiated actions of 1,25 dihydroxyvitamin D: What are they and what do they mean? *Journal of Nutrition, 134*(12), 3215–3218. https://doi.org/10.1093/jn/134.12.3215, http://jn.nutrition.org.

Frøkjær, J. B., Olesen, S. S., & Drewes, A. M. (2013). Fibrosis, atrophy, and ductal pathology in chronic pancreatitis are associated with pancreatic function but independent of symptoms. *Pancreas, 42*(7), 1182–1187. https://doi.org/10.1097/MPA.0b013e31829628f4.

Gorchs, L., Ahmed, S., Mayer, C., Knauf, A., Fernández Moro, C., Svensson, M., Heuchel, R., Rangelova, E., Bergman, P., & Kaipe, H. (2020). The vitamin D analogue calcipotriol promotes an anti-tumorigenic phenotype of human pancreatic CAFs but reduces T cell mediated immunity. *Scientific Reports, 10*(1). https://doi.org/10.1038/s41598-020-74368-3.

Hashim, Z. R., Qasim, Q. A., & ALabbood, M. H. (2022). The association of serum calcium and vitamin D with insulin resistance and beta-cell dysfunction among people with type 2 diabetes. *Archives of Razi Institute, 77*(5), 1567–1574. https://doi.org/10.22092/ARI.2022.357641.2081, https://archrazi.areeo.ac.ir/article_126619_8419a435608e20562ae51a897693d935.pdf.

He, L. P., Song, Y. X., Zhu, T., Gu, W., & Liu, C. W. (2022). Progress in the relationship between vitamin D deficiency and the incidence of type 1 diabetes mellitus in children. *Journal of Diabetes Research, 2022*. https://doi.org/10.1155/2022/5953562, http://www.hindawi.com/journals/jdr/.

Hernandez, M., Recalde, S., González-Zamora, J., Bilbao-Malavé, V., Sáenz de Viteri, M., Bezunartea, J., Moreno-Orduña, M., Belza, I., Barrio-Barrio, J., Fernandez-Robredo, P., & García-Layana, A. (2021). Anti-inflammatory and anti-oxidative synergistic effect of vitamin D and nutritional complex on retinal pigment epithelial and endothelial cell lines against age-related macular degeneration. *Nutrients, 13*(5), 1423. https://doi.org/10.3390/nu13051423.

Hu, Z., Chen, Jin'an, Sun, X., Wang, L., & Wang, A. (2019). Efficacy of vitamin D supplementation on glycemic control in type 2 diabetes patients. *Medicine, 98*(14), e14970. https://doi.org/10.1097/md.0000000000014970.

Huh, J. H., Kim, J. W., & Lee, K. J. (2019). Vitamin D deficiency predicts severe acute pancreatitis. *United European Gastroenterology Journal, 7*(1), 90–95. https://doi.org/10.1177/2050640618811489, http://ueg.sagepub.com/.

Idevall-Hagren, O., & Tengholm, A. (2020). Metabolic regulation of calcium signaling in beta cells. *Seminars in Cell & Developmental Biology, 103*, 20–30. https://doi.org/10.1016/j.semcdb.2020.01.008.

Jøker-Jensen, H., Mathiasen, A. S., Køhler, M., Rasmussen, H. H., Drewes, A. M., & Olesen, S. S. (2020). Micronutrient deficits in patients with chronic pancreatitis: Prevalence, risk factors and pitfalls. *Journal of Gastroenterology and Hepatology, 32*(10), 1328–1334. https://doi.org/10.1097/MEG.0000000000001866, http://journals.lww.com/eurojgh/pages/default.aspx.

Khammissa, R. A. G., Fourie, J., Motswaledi, M. H., Ballyram, R., Lemmer, J., & Feller, L. (2018). The biological activities of vitamin D and its receptor in relation to calcium and bone homeostasis, cancer, immune and cardiovascular systems, skin biology, and oral health. *BioMed Research International, 2018*, 1–9. https://doi.org/10.1155/2018/9276380.

Klec, C., Ziomek, G., Pichler, M., Malli, R., & Graier, W. F. (2019). Calcium signaling in ß-cell physiology and pathology: A revisit. *International Journal of Molecular Sciences, 20*(24). https://doi.org/10.3390/ijms20246110, https://www.mdpi.com/1422-0067/20/24/6110/pdf.

Klöppel, G., & Maillet, B. (1992). The morphological basis for the evolution of acute pancreatitis into chronic pancreatitis. *Virchows Archiv. A, Pathological Anatomy and Histopathology, 420*(1), 1–4. https://doi.org/10.1007/bf01605976.

Krajewska, M., Witkowska-Sędek, E., Rumińska, M., Stelmaszczyk-Emmel, A., Sobol, M., Majcher, A., & Pyrżak, B. (2022). Vitamin D effects on selected anti-inflammatory and pro-inflammatory markers of obesity-related chronic inflammation. *Frontiers in Endocrinology, 13*. https://doi.org/10.3389/fendo.2022.920340, https://www.frontiersin.org/journals/endocrinology#.

Krul-Poel, Y. H. M., ter Wee, M. M., Lips, P., & Simsek, S. (2017). MANAGEMENT OF ENDOCRINE DISEASE: The effect of vitamin D supplementation on glycaemic control in patients with type 2 diabetes mellitus: a systematic review and meta-analysis. *European Journal of Endocrinology, 176*(1), R1. https://doi.org/10.1530/eje-16-0391.

Lai, X., Liu, X., Cai, X., & Zou, F. (2022). Vitamin D supplementation induces CatG-mediated CD4 + T cell inactivation and restores pancreatic β-cell function in mice with type 1 diabetes. *American Journal of Physiology-Endocrinology and Metabolism, 322*(1), E74. https://doi.org/10.1152/ajpendo.00066.2021.

Lee, S., Clark, S. A., Gill, R. K., & Christakos, S. (1994). 1,25-Dihydroxyvitamin D3 and pancreatic beta-cell function: Vitamin D receptors, gene expression, and insulin secretion. *Endocrinology, 134*(4), 1602–1610. https://doi.org/10.1210/endo.134.4.8137721.

Lei, X., Zhou, Q., Wang, Y., Fu, S., Li, Z., & Chen, Q. (2023). Serum and supplemental vitamin D levels and insulin resistance in T2DM populations: A meta-analysis and systematic review. *Scientific Reports, 13*(1). https://doi.org/10.1038/s41598-023-39469-9.

Leung, P. S. (2016). The potential protective action of vitamin D in hepatic insulin resistance and pancreatic islet dysfunction in type 2 diabetes mellitus. *Nutrients, 8*(3). https://doi.org/10.3390/nu8030147, http://www.mdpi.com/2072-6643/8/3/147/pdf.

Li, X., Gan, X., Gong, J., Mou, T., Zhou, H., & Li, M. (2021). Association between vitamin D receptor polymorphisms and acute pancreatitis: A protocol for systematic review and meta analysis. *Medicine (United States), 100*(16), E25508. https://doi.org/10.1097/MD.0000000000025508, https://journals.lww.com/md-journal/pages/default.aspx.

Li, Z., Guo, J., Xie, K., & Zheng, S. (2015). Vitamin D receptor signaling and pancreatic cancer cell EMT. *Current Pharmaceutical Design, 21*(10), 1262–1267. https://doi.org/10.2174/1381612821666141211151138.

Luo, W., Tao, J., Zheng, L., & Zhang, T. (2020). Current epidemiology of pancreatic cancer: Challenges and opportunities. *Chinese Journal of Cancer Research, 32*(6), 705–719. https://doi.org/10.21147/j.issn.1000-9604.2020.06.04.

Martens, P. J., Centelles-Lodeiro, J., Ellis, D., Cook, D. P., Sassi, G., Verlinden, L., Verstuyf, A., Raes, J., Mathieu, C., & Gysemans, C. (2022). High serum vitamin D concentrations, induced via diet, trigger immune and intestinal microbiota alterations leading to type 1 diabetes protection in NOD mice. *Frontiers in Immunology, 13*. https://doi.org/10.3389/fimmu.2022.902678, https://www.frontiersin.org/journals/immunology#.

Meyer, M. B., Watanuki, M., Kim, S., Shevde, N. K., & Pike, J. W. (2006). The human transient receptor potential vanilloid type 6 distal promoter contains multiple vitamin D receptor binding sites that mediate activation by 1,25-dihydroxyvitamin D3 in intestinal cells. *Molecular Endocrinology, 20*(6), 1447–1461. https://doi.org/10.1210/me.2006-0031, http://mend.endojournals.org/cgi/reprint/20/6/1447, UnitedStates.

Miettinen, M. E., Niinistö, S., Erlund, I., Cuthbertson, D., Nucci, A. M., Honkanen, J., Vaarala, O., Hyöty, H., Krischer, J. P., Knip, M., & Virtanen, S. M. (2020). Serum 25-hydroxyvitamin D concentration in childhood and risk of islet autoimmunity and type 1 diabetes: the TRIGR nested case–control ancillary study. *Diabetologia, 63*(4), 780–787. https://doi.org/10.1007/s00125-019-05077-4, link.springer.de/link/service/journals/00125/index.htm.

Mohapatra, S., Aggarwal, G., & Chari, S. T. (2020). Chronic pancreatitis. *Geriatric Gastroenterology, 1–16.*

Morró, M., Vilà, L., Franckhauser, S., Mallol, C., Elias, G., Ferré, T., Molas, M., Casana, E., Rodó, J., Pujol, A., Téllez, N., Bosch, F., & Casellas, A. (2020). Vitamin D receptor overexpression in β-cells ameliorates diabetes in mice. *Diabetes, 69*(5), 927–939. https://doi.org/10.2337/db19-0757.

Moz, S., Contran, N., Facco, M., Trimarco, V., Plebani, M., & Basso, D. (2020). Vitamin D prevents pancreatic cancer-induced apoptosis signaling of inflammatory cells. *Biomolecules, 10*(7), 1055. https://doi.org/10.3390/biom10071055.

Muniraj, T., Aslanian, H. R., Farrell, J., & Jamidar, P. A. (2014). Chronic pancreatitis, a comprehensive review and update. Part I: Epidemiology, etiology, risk factors, genetics, pathophysiology, and clinical features. *Disease-a-Month. 60*(12), 530–550. https://doi.org/10.1016/j.disamonth.2014.11.002, http://www.elsevier.com/inca/publications/store/6/2/3/2/9/2/index.htt.

Munnelly, S., Mitra, V., & Mole, D. (2024). Setting the top 10 research priorities for pancreatitis. *Gastrointestinal Nursing, 22*(1), 12–15. https://doi.org/10.12968/gasn.2024.22.1.12.

Musazadeh, V., Kavyani, Z., Mirhosseini, N., Dehghan, P., & Vajdi, M. (2023). Effect of vitamin D supplementation on type 2 diabetes biomarkers: An umbrella of interventional meta-analyses. *Diabetology & Metabolic Syndrome, 15*(1). https://doi.org/10.1186/s13098-023-01010-3.

Ozcan, C., Corapcıoglu, D., & Cerit, E. T. (2023). Relationship between vitamin D levels and β cell function and insulin resistance. *Cureus, 15*(1). https://doi.org/10.7759/cureus.33970.

Park, C. Y., & Han, S. N. (2021). The role of vitamin D in adipose tissue biology: Adipocyte differentiation, energy metabolism, and inflammation. *Journal of Lipid and Atherosclerosis, 10*(2), 130–144. https://doi.org/10.12997/jla.2021.10.2.130, https://e-jla.org/pdf/10.12997/jla.2021.10.2.130.

Petrov, M. S., & Yadav, D. (2019). Global epidemiology and holistic prevention of pancreatitis. *Nature Reviews Gastroenterology and Hepatology, 16*(3), 175–184. https://doi.org/10.1038/s41575-018-0087-5, http://www.nature.com/nrgastro/index.html.

Pittas, A. G., Lau, J., Hu, F. B., & Dawson-Hughes, B. (2007). The role of vitamin D and calcium in type 2 diabetes. A systematic review and meta-analysis. *The Journal of Clinical Endocrinology & Metabolism, 92*(6), 2017–2029. https://doi.org/10.1210/jc.2007-0298.

Pittas, A. G., Dawson-Hughes, B., Sheehan, P., Ware, J. H., Knowler, W. C., Aroda, V. R., Brodsky, I., Ceglia, L., Chadha, C., Chatterjee, R., Desouza, C., Dolor, R., Foreyt, J., Fuss, P., Ghazi, A., Hsia, D. S., Johnson, K. C., Kashyap, S. R., Kim, S., ... Staten, M. (2019). Vitamin D supplementation and prevention of type 2 diabetes. *New England Journal of Medicine, 381*(6), 520–530. https://doi.org/10.1056/NEJMoa1900906, http://www.nejm.org/medical-index.

Pérez, A. G., Serrano, A. A., & Serrano Ruiz, F. J. (2024). Etiological diagnosis of recurrent acute pancreatitis. *Revista Espanola de Enfermedades Digestivas, 116*(8), 399–403. https://doi.org/10.17235/reed.2024.10404/2024, https://www.reed.es/revista_20241168135.

Ryan, Z. C., Craig, T. A., Folmes, C. D., Wang, X., Lanza, I. R., Schaible, N. S., Salisbury, J. L., Nair, K. S., Terzic, A., Sieck, G. C., & Kumar, R. (2016). 1α, 25-Dihydroxyvitamin D3 regulates mitochondrial oxygen consumption and dynamics in human skeletal muscle cells. *Journal of Biological Chemistry, 291*(3), 1514–1528.

Sakorafas, G. H., & Tsiotou, A. G. (2000). Etiology and pathogenesis of acute pancreatitis: Current concepts. *Journal of Clinical Gastroenterology, 30*(4), 343–356. https://doi.org/10.1097/00004836-200006000-00002.

Sherman, M. H., Yu, R. T., Engle, D. D., Ding, N., Atkins, A. R., Tiriac, H., Collisson, E. A., Connor, F., Van Dyke, T., Kozlov, S., Martin, P., Tseng, T. W., Dawson, D. W., Donahue, T. R., Masamune, A., Shimosegawa, T., Apte, M. V., Wilson, J. S., Ng, B., ... Evans, R. M. (2014). Vitamin D receptor-mediated stromal reprogramming suppresses pancreatitis and enhances pancreatic cancer therapy. *Cell, 159*(1), 80–93. https://doi.org/10.1016/j.cell.2014.08.007, https://www.sciencedirect.com/journal/cell.

Siegel, R. L., Miller, K. D., & Jemal, A. (2019). Cancer statistics, 2019. *CA Cancer Journal for Clinicians, 69*(1), 7–34. https://doi.org/10.3322/caac.21551, http://onlinelibrary.wiley.com/journal/10.3322/(ISSN)1542-4863.

Spagnolo, D. M., Greer, P. J., Ohlsen, C. S., Mance, S., Ellison, M., Breze, C., Busby, B., Whitcomb, D. C., & Haupt, M. (2022). Acute and chronic pancreatitis disease prevalence, classification, and comorbidities: A cohort study of the UK BioBank. *Clinical and Translational Gastroenterology, 13*(1), E00455. https://doi.org/10.14309/ctg.0000000000000455, https://journals.lww.com/ctg/pages/currenttoc.aspx.

Strate, T., Yekebas, E., Knoefel, W. T., Bloechle, C., & Izbicki, J. R. (2002). Pathogenesis and the natural course of chronic pancreatitis. *European Journal of Gastroenterology and Hepatology, 14*(9), 929–934. https://doi.org/10.1097/00042737-200209000-00002.

Sung, C. C., Liao, M. T., Lu, K. C., & Wu, C. C. (2012). Role of vitamin D in insulin resistance. *Journal of Biomedicine and Biotechnology, 2012*. https://doi.org/10.1155/2012/634195.

Szatmary, P., Grammatikopoulos, T., Cai, W., Huang, W., Mukherjee, R., Halloran, C., Beyer, G., & Sutton, R. (2022). Acute pancreatitis: Diagnosis and treatment. *Drugs, 82*(12), 1251–1276. https://doi.org/10.1007/s40265-022-01766-4.

Talaei, A., Mohamadi, M., & Adgi, Z. (2013). The effect of vitamin D on insulin resistance in patients with type 2 diabetes. *Diabetology & Metabolic Syndrome, 5*(1). https://doi.org/10.1186/1758-5996-5-8.

Thomas, D. M., Rogers, S. D., Sleeman, M. W., Pasquini, G. M., Bringhurst, F. R., Ng, K. W., Zajac, J. D., & Best, J. D. (1995). Modulation of glucose transport by parathyroid hormone and insulin in UMR 106-01, a clonal rat osteogenic sarcoma cell line. *Journal of Molecular Endocrinology, 14*(2), 263–275. https://doi.org/10.1677/jme.0.0140263, http://jme.endocrinology-journals.org/.

Tobias, D. K., Pradhan, A., Duran, E., Li, C., Song, Y., Buring, J., Cook, N., Mora, S., & Manson, J. E. (2024). 8564 vitamin D supplementation and incident type 2 diabetes in the vitamin D and omega-3 trial. *Journal of the Endocrine Society, 8*(Supplement_1). https://doi.org/10.1210/jendso/bvae163.1004.

Trexler, A. J., & Taraska, J. W. (2017). Regulation of insulin exocytosis by calcium-dependent protein kinase C in beta cells. *Cell Calcium, 67*, 1–10. https://doi.org/10.1016/j.ceca.2017.07.008, http://www.elsevier-international.com/journals/ceca/.

Vujasinovic, M., Dobrijevic, L. N., Asplund, E., Rutkowski, W., Dugic, A., Kahn, M., Dahlman, I., Sääf, M., Hagström, H., & Löhr, J.-M. (2021). Low bone mineral density and risk for osteoporotic fractures in patients with chronic pancreatitis. *Nutrients, 13*(7), 2386. https://doi.org/10.3390/nu13072386.

Wang, Z., Wang, W., & Liu (2019). Vitamin D deficiency enhances insulin resistance by promoting inflammation in type 2 diabetes. *International Journal of Clinical and Experimental Pathology, 12*(5), 1859–1867.

Wu, M., Lu, L., Guo, K., Lu, J., & Chen, H. (2022). Vitamin D protects against high glucose-induced pancreatic β-cell dysfunction via AMPK-NLRP3 inflammasome pathway. *Molecular and Cellular Endocrinology, 547*, 111596. https://doi.org/10.1016/j.mce.2022.111596.

Zbaar, S. A. (2023). Review: How vitamin D supplementation improve insulin sensitivity in patients with metabolic syndrome. *Journal for Research in Applied Sciences and Biotechnology, 2*(3), 163–167. https://doi.org/10.55544/jrasb.2.3.21.

Zhang, Y., Tan, H., Tang, J., Li, J., Chong, W., Hai, Y., Feng, Y., Lunsford, L. D., Xu, P., Jia, D., & Fang, F. (2020). Effects of vitamin D supplementation on prevention of type 2 diabetes in patients with prediabetes: A systematic review and meta-analysis. *Diabetes Care, 43*(7), 1650–1658. https://doi.org/10.2337/dc19-1708.

Zhao, H., Zheng, C., Zhang, M., & Chen, S. (2021). The relationship between vitamin D status and islet function in patients with type 2 diabetes mellitus. *BMC Endocrine Disorders, 21*(1). https://doi.org/10.1186/s12902-021-00862-y.

Zheng, M., & Gao, R. (2022). Vitamin D: A potential star for treating chronic pancreatitis. *Frontiers in Pharmacology, 13*. https://doi.org/10.3389/fphar.2022.902639.

CHAPTER 15

Vitamin D and metabolic syndrome-associated diseases: interconnections and implications

Salaar Ahmed[1], and Syeda Sadia Fatima[2]

[1]*Medical College, Aga Khan University, Karachi, Pakistan* [2]*Department of Biological & Biomedical Sciences, Aga Khan University, Karachi, Pakistan*

15.1 Background

Metabolic syndrome (MetS) is not a single disease entity but instead a constellation of many metabolic changes occurring in the body that predispose to the development of cardiovascular disease (Huang, 2009). This includes abdominal obesity, insulin resistance, abnormal atherogenic lipid profile, and hypertension. Individuals suffering from metabolic syndrome, due to the clustering of these risk factors, have an increased risk of developing type 2 diabetes mellitus and atherosclerotic cardiovascular disease (Alexander et al., 2003; Isomaa et al., 2001; Lakka, 2002).

The International Diabetes Federation (IDF) consensus statement includes central obesity (instead of evidence of insulin resistance) as an absolute requirement for a MetS diagnosis (Zimmet et al., 2005). In addition to central obesity, at least two or more of the four factors should be present. This includes raised triglycerides, fasting blood glucose levels, blood pressure, or reduced HDL levels. While criticized by some for its emphasis on obesity and not insulin resistance, recent studies have shown the IDF definition to be better suited at estimating the risk of diabetes, especially in high-risk ethics groups, and, therefore, it is more commonly used in literature (Reaven, 2006; Zhu et al., 2020).

15.1.1 Prevalence and global impact

The global impact of MetS is immense and stems from a multitude of chronic diseases and risk factors it predisposes the patients to. While the international data on the prevalence of MetS is difficult to measure, there has been a significant increase in MetS-related conditions. It is estimated that the prevalence of obesity alone has doubled or even tripled in many countries over the last four decades ("Health Effects of Overweight and Obesity in 195 Countries over 25 Years," 2017). This especially includes children and adolescents. Similarly, the global prevalence of diabetes is expected to reach 10.4% by 2040 (Ogurtsova et al., 2017).

Considering existing data about MetS being at least thrice as common as diabetes, it is estimated that almost one-quarter of the world's population is affected by MetS.

Depending on the definition, the estimated prevalence of MetS is anywhere between 12.5% (according to ATP-3 considering BMI) to 31.4% (according to JIS) (Noubiap et al., 2022). According to the IDF criterion, 28.2% of people globally suffer from metabolic syndrome. MetS prevalence also varies considerably by geographical distribution and country income level. The Eastern Mediterranean region has the highest (36.6%), and the African region has the lowest (23.1%) estimated prevalence. Similarly, low- and low-middle-income countries have a lower estimated MetS prevalence than upper-middle- and high-income countries. However, more recent trends predict an exponential rise in rates of obesity and diabetes prevalence in low-income countries, such as in sub-Saharan Africa.

15.1.1.1 Pathophysiology and risk factors

The pathophysiology of MetS is complex and involves a connection between genetic and environmental risk factors. Adiposity is considered a main pillar in the pathophysiology of MetS, with visceral adipose tissue (VAT) and its endocrine function tying in closely to other associated factors such as insulin resistance, hypertension, and dyslipidemia. More recently, inflammation has also been studied as a fundamental factor in the pathophysiology of the disease. This is due to the proposed role of oxidative stress, proinflammatory cytokines, and inflammatory vascular dysfunction, as seen in metabolic syndrome. Studies show significantly higher levels of proinflammatory cytokines, such as TNF-α, leptin, and IL-6, in MetS patients compared to healthy controls (Esser et al., 2014; Zafar et al., 2019), as well as dysregulation of the activity of reactive oxygen species (ROS) producing systems (Chattopadhyay et al., 2015; Spahis et al., 2017).

Literature suggests that Insulin resistance (IR) precedes obesity, hence visceral adiposity. Indeed, a considerable number of individuals with a normal BMI may still present with IR (Blüher, 2010; Ferrannini et al., 1997). This also depends on age, gender, and ethnicity, among other factors. For instance, African-Americans have higher rates of IR while having lower VAT percentages (Conway et al., 1995). IR in body tissues causes hyperinsulinemia, which starts a cascade of metabolic changes, including central fat deposition (Kim & Reaven, 2008). Visceral adiposity leads to elevated free fatty acid (FFA) levels in the blood, which, in turn, leads to lipid deposition in vessels throughout the body (Rodriguez et al., 2007), as well as dysfunction at the cellular level in vital organs including the liver and pancreas (Buzzetti et al., 2016; Tan et al., 2017). The liver's response to chronically high levels of FFA (as well as other lipids) leads to hepatic IR and dysregulated gluconeogenesis. Response of skeletal muscles to high levels of FFA is also similar, leading to intramyocellular lipid accumulation (Tumova et al., 2016). This results in impaired beta-oxidation, reduced glucose oxidation, and glycogen synthesis. Again, all these factors contribute to local IR. Therefore, a vicious cycle of positive feedback begins with increasing levels of insulin resistance, adiposity, and, eventually, unregulated inflammation.

Another important component of MetS is hypertension, seen as a sustained rise in blood pressure and affects as many as 85% of the people suffering from MetS (Duvnjak et al., 2008; Mulè, 2014; Yanai et al., 2008). Oxidative stress, endothelial dysfunction secondary to chronic inflammation, the release of inflammatory mediators such as TNF-α, and insulin resistance itself are all believed to play a role in elevated blood pressure (Grundy, 1998; Rahmouni et al., 2005; Schinzari et al., 2010).

15.1.1.2 Link of vitamin D deficiency to metabolic syndrome

While previously mostly studied for its role in calcium and phosphorus homeostasis, and therefore bone and skeletal health, recent literature has demonstrated the protective role of Vitamin D against a variety of different diseases, including cancer, autoimmune disorders, and cardiovascular disease (Illescas-Montes et al., 2019; Jeon & Shin, 2018; Mozos & Marginean, 2015). It is also implicated for its role in hormone regulation and endocrine function, antiinflammatory effect, and antifibrotic properties (Lai & Fang, 2013). This is important to consider as previously described, the foundation of MetS rests on endocrine dysfunction and inflammation. Numerous studies around the world have been conducted to investigate the role of vitamin D deficiency in MetS, the pathophysiology behind it, and clinical outcomes in such patients.

The evidence surrounding vitamin D levels and their association with MetS remains inconsistent. Schmitt et al., Mutt et al., Huang et al., and many others point toward an inverse relation between vitamin D levels and metabolic syndrome (Huang, 2009; Mutt et al., 2019; Schmitt et al., 2018). Not only is a deficiency of vitamin D associated with a significantly higher prevalence of vitamin D, but the same studies also show a lower incidence of MetS in people taking vitamin D supplementation. Similarly, high levels of 25(OH)D have been shown to improve the metabolic profile by optimizing serum levels of cholesterol and LDL (Zhu & Heil, 2018). On the other hand, many studies have shown no significant association between vitamin D and MetS (Al-Dabhani et al., 2017; Hjelmesæth et al., 2010; Rueda et al., 2008), with hypovitaminosis D at times linked to increased risk for individual components of MetS such as abdominal obesity, elevated blood pressures, or impaired glucose metabolism but not MetS itself (Barbalho et al., 2018; Mansouri et al., 2018). Fig. 15.1 illustrates the synthesis, metabolism, and diverse physiological roles of vitamin D in the human body. Its impact on bone health, cardiovascular function, immune response, insulin regulation, and more, highlighting its critical role in maintaining overall health.

15.1.1.2.1 Prevalence of vitamin D deficiency in populations with metabolic syndrome

Worldwide, the prevalence rates of severe Vitamin D deficiency range anywhere between around 6% in the United States (Schleicher et al., 2016) to over 20% in countries like India and Pakistan (Arif et al., 2023; G & Gupta, 2014). Estimating the worldwide prevalence of hypovitaminosis D in MetS patients has been challenging due to a lack of global literature, varied diagnostic criteria of MetS used in studies, and slightly different vitamin D cutoffs for

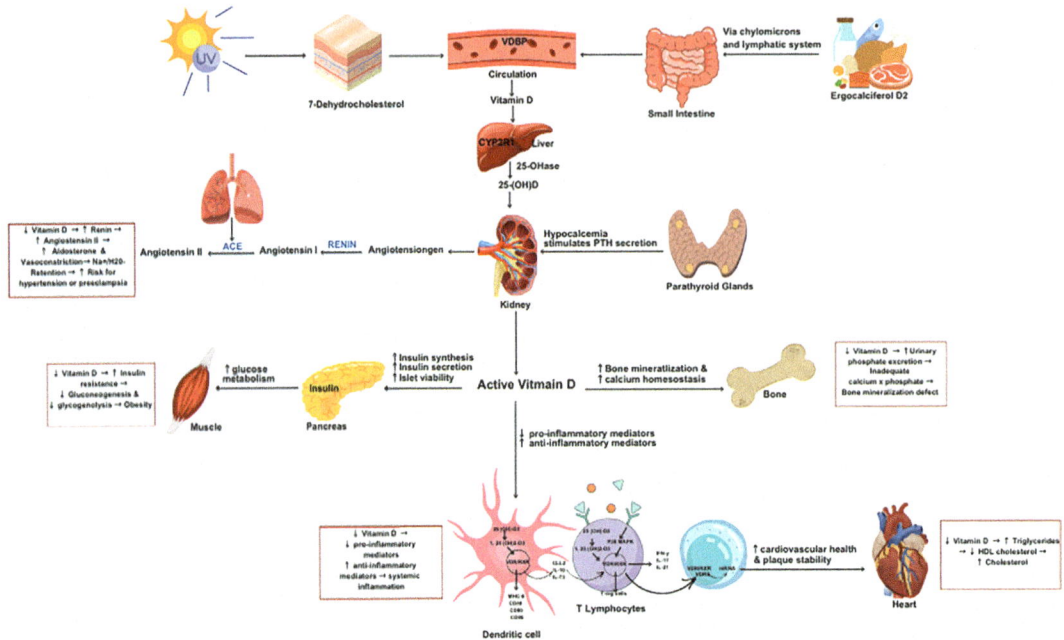

Figure 15.1

Overview of vitamin D metabolism and its systemic effects.

Figure illustrates the synthesis, metabolism, and diverse physiological roles of vitamin D in the human body. Its impact on bone health, cardiovascular function, immune response, insulin regulation, and more, highlighting its critical role in maintaining overall health.

Source: *Figure created by Hania Fatima, Medical Student. Aga Khan University.*

different populations. Studies show the estimated prevalence of MetS in vitamin D-deficient patients to be around 32%–60% (Ganji et al., 2020; Lee et al., 2019; Pott-Junior et al., 2020).

While these may be exaggerated numbers and not representative of the population globally (considering that most of these studies include elderly patients or patients from one gender), more convincing evidence of increased prevalence of MetS in vitamin D deficiency comes from successive increases in MetS prevalence moving down quartiles of vitamin D (Lee et al., 2019). For instance, MetS prevalence was seen to be 31.9% in the lowest 25(OH)D quartile but only 17.5% in the highest 25(OH)D quartile (Ganji et al., 2020). These risks are independent of age and sex and replicated in many modestly sized cross-sectional and observational studies throughout the world (Ganji et al., 2020; Huang et al., 2015).

15.1.1.2.2 Obesity and vitamin D

Vitamin D is a fat solute molecule, and adipose tissue is the primary site of storage for vitamin D (Heaney et al., 2011). While contradicting literature exists on the exact role of vitamin D in adipogenesis, its regulatory effects at different stages of adipogenesis are widely documented in the literature (Blumberg et al., 2006; Kong & Li, 2006; Nimitphong et al., 2012). Multiple large observational studies (Cheng et al., 2010; Yetley, 2008) have supported the association between obesity and low vitamin D status, with a meta-analysis of 34 cross-sectional studies in 2013 proving a significant inverse association between vitamin D levels and body mass index (BMI) (Saneei et al., 2013).

One proposed mechanism of how vitamin D deficiency can contribute to obesity is via higher serum levels of parathyroid hormone (PTH). This chronic elevation in PTH levels leads to calcium resorption from bones, resulting in high serum calcium levels. The influx of calcium into adipocytes can stimulate lipogenesis and, therefore, increase adiposity (Pereira-Santos et al., 2015). However, a bi-directional Mendelian randomization analysis of large cohort studies showed that it is obesity that predisposes patients to hypovitaminosis D, not vice versa, with an increase in one unit of BMI associated with a decrease in 25(OH)D by 1.15% (Vimaleswaran et al., 2013). These findings have subsequently been supported by many recent studies, reiterating that obesity (BMI > 30 kg/m^2) is an independent risk factor for vitamin D insufficiency, and any reverse relation, even if present, is small (Pereira-Santos et al., 2015; Shanmugalingam et al., 2014). The underlying pathophysiology, while debatable, is believed to be the dilution effect of circulating vitamin D in obese patients with larger body volumes and metabolic requirements (Drincic et al., 2012). Visceral adiposity, in particular, leads to insignificant changes in body surface area while resulting in a considerable change in body volume. This is also believed to reduce the relative sun exposure per unit volume, resulting in a deficiency of activated circulating vitamin D. Others believe that the skin of obese and older individuals may have impaired absorption of UV light and vitamin D synthesis, but the scientific evidence remains scarce.

Interestingly, the strength of association between obesity and hypovitaminosis D is considerably stronger in patients with type 2 diabetes (Rafiq & Jeppesen, 2018). This is important to understand as obesity may be one of the factors involved when considering the association of MetS with hypovitaminosis D, but a complex interplay of inflammation, oxidative stress, dyslipidemia, and vascular dysfunction alongside obesity may explain why it is difficult to establish linear relationships between vitamin D levels and MetS.

15.1.1.2.3 Insulin resistance, type 2 diabetes, and vitamin D

The role of vitamin D in maintaining glucose homeostasis is well-established in both basic and clinical literature (Lim et al., 2013; Maestro et al., 2000; Mitri et al., 2011). It does this by acting as a genomic stimulator for the expression of the insulin receptor gene and by increasing the insulin-induced responsiveness to glucose transport across cells (Maestro et al., 2000). High levels of 1,25 (OH)$_2$D3 also stimulate increased absorption of calcium in the gut, leading to increased levels of serum calcium. This is directly linked to increased insulin release from pancreatic beta cells. These beta cells also express receptors for 1,25 $(OH)_2D3$, the active form of vitamin D. In vitro trials on rat islets show that application of $1\alpha,25(OH)_2D_3$ to these cells results in a marked increase in cytosolic calcium levels and insulin secretion (Bland et al., 2004). Therefore, genetic polymorphisms of genes such as VDR (vitamin-D receptor) and DBP vitamin-D binding proteins can contribute to insulin resistance (Baier et al., 1998; Blanton et al., 2011; Faraco et al., 1989; McDermott et al., 1997). VDR is also expressed by immune cells, including macrophages, and is shown to play a role in immunomodulation (Chagas et al., 2012). Vitamin D exerts its antiinflammatory effect by inhibiting NF-κB and, therefore, reducing TNFα levels (as NF-κB is a transcription activator for TNF) (Cohen-Lahav et al., 2006), as well as suppressing TLR2 and TLR4 proteins (Sadeghi et al., 2006). As previously discussed, inflammation is a cornerstone for the development of MetS and T2DM through insulin resistance among other factors. Therefore, vitamin D acts to reduce insulin resistance by reducing inflammation.

Some studies have shown improvement in glucose control with the use of vitamin D supplementation alone or in combination with calcium (Pittas, Harris, et al., 2007), but there are no large trials or studies to support these claims. However, in cases of patients suffering from T1DM, the literature is more favorable, pointing toward the use of Vitamin D supplementation in patients suffering from hypovitaminosis D (Jorde & Figenschau, 2009; Nikooyeh et al., 2011). This has been shown to improve glucose homeostasis and optimize HBA1C levels in the short term; however, an RCT in 2014 concluded that it did not affect long-term glycemic control in patients with T2DM (Ryu et al., 2014). A meta-analysis of observational studies and trials revealed a significant inverse association between total vitamin D intake (in the form of diet and supplementation) and risk of developing type 2 DM (Pittas, Lau, et al., 2007). It is interesting to note, however, that the association was weakened after adjusting for dietary factors, such as calcium and magnesium. Therefore the question as to how much vitamin D supplementation may help in reducing insulin resistance and MetS remains unanswered.

15.1.1.2.4 Hypertension and vitamin D

Vitamin D has a well-known role in the regulation of the renin–angiotensin–aldosterone system (RAAS) through the inhibition of renin secretion (Li et al., 2004). This reduction in renin secretion is attributed to the blocking of the activity of cyclic AMP response element in the renin gene promoter region (Yuan et al., 2007). This results in reduced transcription and, therefore, inhibited secretion of renin throughout the body. This, in turn, leads to reduced levels of Angiotensin 1 and Angiotensin 2 and subsequent reduction in blood pressure. In contrast, vitamin D deficiency results in reduced binding to VDR, which allows for active transcription (and therefore translation) of renin mRNA. Thus, low levels of 25(OH)D relate to RAAS hyperactivation, the primary known mechanism in the development of hypertension (Canale et al., 2014).

Hypertension occurs as a result of increased water and sodium retention, sympathetic activation, and peripheral vasoconstriction. All these events are implicated with an increased risk of developing vascular endothelial dysfunction and inflammatory changes, therefore, an aggravated risk of chronic hypertension and arteriosclerosis. Moreover, PTH is another activator of the RAAS system (Zheng et al., 2020). Elevated levels of PTH cause hypercalcemia, and significant hypercalcemia is linked to elevated blood pressure (Iseki et al., 1986). Vitamin D can inhibit PTH secretion through a negative feedback mechanism, which, in turn, reduces blood pressure. In fact, some studies report that the association between vitamin D and blood pressure is mediated primarily through changes in the level of PTH and not the direct effect of vitamin D on the RAAS system (He & Scragg, 2011).

Multiple large trials have looked at vitamin D, either used alone or alongside another antihypertensive medication as a supplement to evaluate blood pressure control. While most such trials have found no significant association between vitamin D and blood pressure in hypertensive or prehypertensive patients, a few have shown modest cardioprotective benefits of vitamin D supplementation (Arora et al., 2015; Grübler et al., 2016; Zaheer et al., 2018).

For instance, supplementation with dietary vitamin D3 is shown to result in decreased plasma renin concentration and activity in congestive heart failure (CGF) patients (Schroten et al., 2013). Nganou-Gnindjio et al. is the one clinical trial that showed not only a reduction in diurnal blood pressure but also a decrease in inflammatory markers associated with supplementation with calcium and vitamin D in postmenopausal hypertensive women (Nadège Nganou-Gnindjio et al., 2021). However, it is interesting to consider that in this trial, a significant reduction in diurnal blood pressure was noted, even with calcium supplementation alone, and therefore, raises the question of the role of vitamin D in such cases where all evidence points otherwise.

15.2   Dyslipidemia and vitamin D

Like its role in other biochemical processes, vitamin D influences lipid metabolism through mechanisms mediated via VDR. Indeed certain polymorphisms of VDR are associated with elevated levels of lipids in blood (He & Wang, 2015; Xia et al., 2017). One such lipid is cholesterol, whose concentration in blood is regulated by vitamin D via inhibition of liver X receptor alpha (LXR-alpha) signaling (Gonzalez & Moschetta, 2014; Jiang et al., 2006). This is important in the pathway for bile acid synthesis and, therefore, bodily excretion of excess cholesterol.

Vitamin D can also have an indirect effect on lipid uptake and metabolism through its effect on serum calcium levels. For instance, increased calcium absorption in the gut modulates microsomal triglyceride transfer protein (MTP), which results in reduced synthesis of triglycerides (Hussain et al., 2011). Reduced absorbed calcium levels in the intestines (as seen in vitamin D deficiency) can result in increased FFA uptake, as less calcium is available to bind FFAs and form insoluble complexes. This is interesting as FFAs play an important role in inflammatory and atherosclerotic changes, which are a hallmark of MetS (Malekmohammad et al., 2021).

A recent meta-analysis of 17 studies found vitamin D to optimize serum triglyceride, total cholesterol, and LDL levels without improving HDL levels (Jafari et al., 2016). Another study, including a sample of over 4.06 million laboratory tests, found optimal vitamin D levels to be significantly associated with a better lipid profile, including reduced serum cholesterol, LDL, and triglycerides, as well as higher HDL (Ponda et al., 2012). However, when retrospectively analyzed, it was found that optimizing vitamin D levels through supplementation in patients with hypovitaminosis D did not translate into clinically meaningful changes in the lipid profile. Similar results have been seen in multiple studies with higher quartiles of vitamin D associated with lower levels of cholesterol, LDL, and triglycerides, but more importantly, with improvement in HDL levels (Auwerx et al., 1992; Chaudhuri et al., 2013; Jiang et al., 2006; Karhapää et al., 2010). Interestingly, a vast majority of interventional studies where vitamin D supplementation is used in patients with hypovitaminosis D report either no significant improvement in lipid parameters or modest changes in some parameters (Andersen et al., 2009; Chai et al., 2013; Makariou et al., 2017; Muldowney et al., 2012; Witham et al., 2013; Wongwiwatthananukit et al., 2013; Wood et al., 2012; Xiao, no date; Yin et al., 2016). Therefore discussion around the prospects of mitigating the cardiovascular risks of dyslipidemia with vitamin D supplementation should be met with caution at best.

15.3   Future directions and research gaps in vitamin D and metabolic health

15.3.1   Optimal levels of vitamin D for metabolic health

Despite substantial evidence linking vitamin D deficiency to metabolic disorders, there is still no consensus on the optimal levels of vitamin D for metabolic health. Most studies suggest a serum level of 25(OH)D between 20 and 40 ng/mL, but these ranges may not be ideal for all populations, particularly those with metabolic syndrome or diabetes. Future research should focus on determining the precise vitamin D thresholds that maximize metabolic health outcomes, including insulin sensitivity, lipid profiles, and inflammatory markers.

15.3.2   Long-term effects of supplementation

While short-term supplementation with vitamin D has shown promising results in improving metabolic health markers, the long-term effects are less clear. There is a need for large-scale, long-duration studies to assess the sustained benefits and potential risks of high-dose supplementation. This includes understanding the impact of vitamin D on bone health, cardiovascular risk, and other chronic conditions that commonly co-occur with metabolic syndrome.

15.3.3 Genetic factors influencing vitamin D metabolism

Genetic variations, such as those in the VDR (vitamin D receptor) gene, CYP2R1, and CYP27B1, influence how individuals metabolize vitamin D. Understanding these genetic differences can help tailor personalized approaches to vitamin D supplementation, ensuring that individuals with certain genetic profiles receive optimal benefits. Further research into pharmacogenetics related to vitamin D could allow for more precise recommendations for individuals with metabolic syndrome or diabetes.

15.3.4 Interaction between vitamin D and other nutrients

The complex interactions between vitamin D and other nutrients, such as calcium, magnesium, and omega-3 fatty acids, are under-explored in the context of metabolic health. Vitamin D's role in calcium metabolism and its potential synergy with other micronutrients could play a critical role in modulating insulin resistance, inflammation, and cardiovascular risk. Research should focus on understanding these nutrient interactions and their combined effects on metabolic syndrome and its related disorders.

15.4 Clinical and public health recommendations

15.4.1 Strategies for improving vitamin D status in at-risk populations

Certain populations, such as individuals with obesity, older adults, and those living in regions with limited sunlight, are at increased risk for vitamin D deficiency. Public health strategies should prioritize identifying these at-risk groups through screening and targeted interventions. For example, community-based programs offering affordable vitamin D supplementation, education on sun exposure, and dietary modifications could help address this gap. Special attention should also be given to vulnerable groups, such as pregnant women and ethnic minorities, who may have a higher risk of deficiency.

15.4.2 Integrating vitamin D management into metabolic syndrome treatment plans

Given the strong association between low vitamin D levels and metabolic syndrome, it is crucial to integrate vitamin D assessment and management into clinical guidelines for treating metabolic disorders. This could include routine screening for vitamin D deficiency in patients with metabolic syndrome, diabetes, or cardiovascular risk factors. In clinical practice, this could mean incorporating vitamin D supplementation as a complementary approach to traditional treatments, such as lifestyle changes and pharmacological interventions. Multidisciplinary care teams, including endocrinologists, nutritionists, and public health experts, should collaborate to optimize patient outcomes through comprehensive vitamin D management in the context of metabolic syndrome.

References

Al-Dabhani, K., Tsilidis, K. K., Murphy, N., Ward, H. A., Elliott, P., Riboli, E., Gunter, M., & Tzoulaki, I. (2017). Prevalence of vitamin D deficiency and association with metabolic syndrome in a Qatari population. *Nutrition & Diabetes, 7*(4), e263. https://doi.org/10.1038/nutd.2017.14.

Alexander, C. M., Landsman, P. B., Teutsch, S. M., & Haffner, S. M. (2003). NCEP-defined metabolic syndrome, diabetes, and prevalence of coronary heart disease among NHANES III participants age 50 years and older. *Diabetes, 52*(5), 1210–1214. https://doi.org/10.2337/diabetes.52.5.1210.

Andersen, R., Brot, C., Mejborn, H., Mølgaard, C., Skovgaard, L. T., Trolle, E., & Ovesen, L. (2009). Vitamin D supplementation does not affect serum lipids and lipoproteins in Pakistani immigrants. *European Journal of Clinical Nutrition, 63*(9), 1150–1153. https://doi.org/10.1038/ejcn.2009.18.

Arif, A., Mohan Lal, P., Shaikh, O. A., & Mohan, A. (2023). High prevalence of vitamin D deficiency in Pakistan and its relation to uterine fibroids development and progression. *International Journal of Surgery: Global Health, 6*(2), e124. https://doi.org/10.1097/gh9.0000000000000124.

Arora, P., Song, Y., Dusek, J., Plotnikoff, G., Sabatine, M. S., Cheng, S., Valcour, A., Swales, H., Taylor, B., Carney, E., Guanaga, D., Young, J. R., Karol, C., Torre, M., Azzahir, A., Strachan, S. M., O'Neill, D. C., Wolf, M., Harrell, F., ... Wang, T. J. (2015). Vitamin D therapy in individuals with prehypertension or hypertension the DAYLIGHT trial. *Circulation, 131*(3), 254–262. https://doi.org/10.1161/CIRCULATIONAHA.114.011732, http://circ.ahajournals.org.

Auwerx, J., Bouillon, R., & Kesteloot, H. (1992). Relation between 25-hydroxyvitamin D3, apolipoprotein A-I, and high density lipoprotein cholesterol. *Arteriosclerosis and Thrombosis: A Journal of Vascular Biology, 12*(6), 671–674. https://doi.org/10.1161/01.atv.12.6.671.

Baier, L. J., Dobberfuhl, A. M., Pratley, R. E., Hanson, R. L., & Bogardus, C. (1998). Variations in the vitamin D-binding protein (Gc locus) are associated with oral glucose tolerance in nondiabetic Pima Indians. *Journal of Clinical Endocrinology and Metabolism, 83*(8), 2993–2996. https://doi.org/10.1210/jcem.83.8.5043, http://jcem.endojournals.org.

Barbalho, S. M., Tofano, R. J., de Campos, A. L., Rodrigues, A. S., Quesada, K., Bechara, M. D., de Alvares Goulart, R., & Oshiiwa, M. (2018). Association between vitamin D status and metabolic syndrome risk factors. *Diabetes and Metabolic Syndrome: Clinical Research and Reviews, 12*(4), 501–507. https://doi.org/10.1016/j.dsx.2018.03.011, http://www.journals.elsevier.com/diabetes-and-metabolic-syndrome-clinical-research-and-reviews/.

Bland, R., Markovic, D., Hills, C. E., Hughes, S. V., Chan, S. L. F., Squires, P. E., & Hewison, M. (2004). Expression of 25-hydroxyvitamin D3-1α-hydroxylase in pancreatic islets. *Journal of Steroid Biochemistry and Molecular Biology, 89-90*, 121–125. https://doi.org/10.1016/j.jsbmb.2004.03.115.

Blanton, D., Han, Z., Bierschenk, L., Linga-Reddy, M. V. P., Wang, H., Clare-Salzler, M., Haller, M., Schatz, D., Myhr, C., She, J. X., Wasserfall, C., & Atkinson, M. (2011). Reduced serum vitamin D-binding protein levels are associated with type 1 diabetes. *Diabetes, 60*(10), 2566–2570. https://doi.org/10.2337/db11-0576, http://diabetes.diabetesjournals.org/content/60/10/2566.full.pdf+html. United States.

Blüher, M. (2010). The distinction of metabolically 'healthy' from 'unhealthy' obese individuals. *Current Opinion in Lipidology, 21*(1), 38–43. https://doi.org/10.1097/mol.0b013e3283346ccc.

Blumberg, J. M., Tzameli, I., Astapova, I., Lam, F. S., Flier, J. S., & Hollenberg, A. N. (2006). Complex role of the vitamin D receptor and its ligand in adipogenesis in 3T3-L1 cells. *Journal of Biological Chemistry, 281*(16), 11205–11213. https://doi.org/10.1074/jbc.M510343200, http://www.jbc.org/cgi/reprint/281/16/11205. United States.

Buzzetti, E., Pinzani, M., & Tsochatzis, E. A. (2016). The multiple-hit pathogenesis of non-alcoholic fatty liver disease (NAFLD). *Metabolism: Clinical and Experimental, 65*(8), 1038–1048. https://doi.org/10.1016/j.metabol.2015.12.012.

Canale, D., De Bragança, A. C., Gonçalves, J. G., Shimizu, M. H. M., Sanches, T. R., Andrade, L., Volpini, R. A., & Seguro, A. C. (2014). Vitamin D deficiency aggravates nephrotoxicity, hypertension and dyslipidemia caused by tenofovir: Role of oxidative stress and renin-angiotensin system. *PLoS ONE, 9*(7). https://doi.org/10.1371/journal.pone.0103055, http://www.plosone.org/article/fetchObject.action?uri=info%3Adoi%2F10.1371%2Fjournal.pone.0103055&representation=PDF.

Chagas, C. E. A., Borges, M. C., Martini, L. A., & Rogero, M. M. (2012). Focus on vitamin D, inflammation and type 2 diabetes. *Nutrients, 4*(1), 52–67. https://doi.org/10.3390/nu4010052, http://www.mdpi.com/2072-6643/4/1/52/pdf.

Chai, W., Cooney, R. V., Franke, A. A., & Bostick, R. M. (2013). Effects of calcium and vitamin D supplementation on blood pressure and serumlipids and carotenoids: A randomized, double-blind, placebo-controlled, clinicaltrial. *Annals of Epidemiology, 23*(9), 564–570. https://doi.org/10.1016/j.annepidem.2013.07.003.

Chattopadhyay, M., Khemka, V. K., Chatterjee, G., Ganguly, A., Mukhopadhyay, S., & Chakrabarti, S. (2015). Enhanced ROS production and oxidative damage in subcutaneous white adipose tissue mitochondria in obese and type 2 diabetes subjects. *Molecular and Cellular Biochemistry, 399*(1-2), 95–103. https://doi.org/10.1007/s11010-014-2236-7, http://www.kluweronline.com/issn/0300-8177/.

Chaudhuri, J. R., Mridula, K. R., Anamika, A., Boddu, D. B., Misra, P. K., Lingaiah, A., Balaraju, B., & Bandaru, V. S. (2013). Deficiency of 25-hydroxyvitamin D and dyslipidemia in Indian subjects. *Journal of Lipids, 2013*, 1–7. https://doi.org/10.1155/2013/623420.

Cheng, S., Massaro, J. M., Fox, C. S., Larson, M. G., Keyes, M. J., McCabe, E. L., Robins, S. J., Donnell, C. J. O., Hoffmann, U., Jacques, P. F., Booth, S. L., Vasan, R. S., Wolf, M., & Wang, T. J. (2010). Adiposity, cardiometabolic risk, and vitamin D status: The framingham heart study. *Diabetes, 59*(1), 242–248. https://doi.org/10.2337/db09-1011, http://diabetes.diabetesjournals.org/content/59/1/242.full.pdf+html. United States.

Cohen-Lahav, M., Shany, S., Tobvin, D., Chaimovitz, C., & Douvdevani, A. (2006). Vitamin D decreases NFκB activity by increasing IκBα levels. *Nephrology Dialysis Transplantation, 21*(4), 889–897. https://doi.org/10.1093/ndt/gfi254.

Conway, J. M., Yanovski, S. Z., Avila, N. A., & Hubbard, V. S. (1995). Visceral adipose tissue differences in black and white women. *The American Journal of Clinical Nutrition, 61*(4), 765–771. https://doi.org/10.1093/ajcn/61.4.765.

Drincic, A. T., Armas, L. A. G., Van Diest, E. E., & Heaney, R. P. (2012). Volumetric dilution, rather than sequestration best explains the low vitamin D status of obesity. *Obesity, 20*(7), 1444–1448. https://doi.org/10.1038/oby.2011.404.

Duvnjak, L., Bulum, T., & Metelko, Z. (2008). Hypertension and the metabolic syndrome. *Diabetologia Croatica, 37*(4), 83–89.

Esser, N., Legrand-Poels, S., Piette, J., Scheen, A. J., & Paquot, N. (2014). Inflammation as a link between obesity, metabolic syndrome and type 2 diabetes. *Diabetes Research and Clinical Practice, 105*(2), 141–150. https://doi.org/10.1016/j.diabres.2014.04.006, www.elsevier.com/locate/diabres.

Faraco, J. H., Morrison, N. A., Baker, A., Shine, J., & Frossard, P. M. (1989). ApaI dimorphism at the human vitamin D receptor gene locus. *Nucleic Acids Research, 17*(5), 2150. https://doi.org/10.1093/nar/17.5.2150.

Ferrannini, E., Natali, A., Bell, P., Cavallo-Perin, P., Lalic, N., & Mingrone, G. (1997). Insulin resistance and hypersecretion in obesity. European Group for the Study of Insulin Resistance (EGIR). *Journal of Clinical Investigation, 100*(5), 1166–1173. https://doi.org/10.1172/JCI119628.

G, R., & Gupta, A. (2014). Vitamin D Deficiency in India: Prevalence, Causalities and Interventions. *Nutrients, 6*(2), 729–775. https://doi.org/10.3390/nu6020729.

Ganji, V., Sukik, A., Alaayesh, H., Rasoulinejad, H., & Shraim, M. (2020). Serum vitamin D concentrations are inversely related to prevalence of metabolic syndrome in Qatari women. *BioFactors (Oxford, England), 46*(1), 180–186. https://doi.org/10.1002/biof.1572.

Gonzalez, F. J., & Moschetta, A. (2014). Potential role of the vitamin D receptor in control of cholesterol levels. *Gastroenterology, 146*(4), 899–902. https://doi.org/10.1053/j.gastro.2014.02.022, http://www.journals.elsevier.com/gastroenterology/.

Grübler, M. R., Gaksch, M., Kienreich, K., Verheyen, N., Schmid, J., Ó Hartaigh, B. W. J., Richtig, G., Scharnagl, H., Meinitzer, A., Pieske, B., Fahrleitner-Pammer, A., März, W., Tomaschitz, A., & Pilz, S. (2016). Effects of vitamin D supplementation on plasma aldosterone and renin—A randomized placebo-controlled trial. *Journal of Clinical Hypertension, 18*(7), 608–613. https://doi.org/10.1111/jch.12825, http://onlinelibrary.wiley.com/journal/10.1111/(ISSN)1751-7176.

Grundy, S. M. (1998). Hypertriglyceridemia, atherogenic dyslipidemia, and the metabolic syndrome. *The American Journal of Cardiology, 81*(4), 18B. https://doi.org/10.1016/s0002-9149(98)00033-2.

He, J. L., & Scragg, R. K. (2011). Vitamin D, parathyroid hormone, and blood pressure in the national health and nutrition examination surveys. *American Journal of Hypertension, 24*(8), 911–917. https://doi.org/10.1038/ajh.2011.73.

He, L., & Wang, M. (2015). Association of vitamin d receptor-a gene polymorphisms with coronary heart disease in Han Chinese. *International Journal of Clinical and Experimental Medicine, 8*(4), 6224–6229. http://www.ijcem.com/files/ijcem0006672.pdf.

Health effects of overweight and obesity in 195 countries over 25 years. (2017). *New England Journal of Medicine, 377*(1), 13–27. https://doi.org/10.1056/NEJMoa1614362.

Heaney, R. P., Recker, R. R., Grote, J., Horst, R. L., & Armas, L. A. G. (2011). Vitamin D3 is more potent than vitamin D2in humans. *Journal of Clinical Endocrinology and Metabolism, 96*(3), E447. https://doi.org/10.1210/jc.2010-2230, http://jcem.endojournals.org/cgi/reprint/96/3/E447. United States.

Hjelmesæth, J., Røislien, J., Hofsø, D., & Bollerslev, J. (2010). Plasma 25-hydroxyvitamin D concentration and metabolic syndrome among middle-aged and elderly Chinese individuals. *Diabetes Care, 33*(1), e13. https://doi.org/10.2337/dc09-1568.

Huang, C. Y., Chang, H. H., Lu, C. W., Tseng, F. Y., Lee, L. T., & Huang, K. C. (2015). Vitamin D status and risk of metabolic syndrome among non-diabetic young adults. *Clinical Nutrition, 34*(3), 484–489. https://doi.org/10.1016/j.clnu.2014.05.010, http://www.elsevier-international.com/journals/clnu/.

Huang, P. L. (2009). A comprehensive definition for metabolic syndrome. *Disease Models & Mechanisms, 2*(5-6), 231–237. https://doi.org/10.1242/dmm.001180.

Hussain, M. M., Nijstad, N., & Franceschini, L. (2011). Regulation of microsomal triglyceride transfer protein. *Clinical Lipidology, 6*(3), 293–303. https://doi.org/10.2217/clp.11.21.

Illescas-Montes, R., Melguizo-Rodríguez, L., Ruiz, C., & Costela-Ruiz, V. J. (2019). Vitamin D and autoimmune diseases. *Life Sciences, 233*, 116744. https://doi.org/10.1016/j.lfs.2019.116744.

Iseki, K., Massry, S. G., & Campese, V. M. (1986). Effects of hypercalcemia and parathyroid hormone on blood pressure in normal and renal-failure rats. *American Journal of Physiology-Renal Physiology, 250*(5), F924. https://doi.org/10.1152/ajprenal.1986.250.5.f924.

Isomaa, B., Almgren, P., Tuomi, T., Forsén, B., Lahti, K., Nissén, M., Taskinen, M. R., & Groop, L. (2001). Cardiovascular morbidity and mortality associated with the metabolic syndrome. *Diabetes Care, 24*(4), 683–689. https://doi.org/10.2337/diacare.24.4.683, http://care.diabetesjournals.org/.

Jafari, T., Fallah, A. A., & Barani, A. (2016). Effects of vitamin D on serum lipid profile in patients with type 2 diabetes: A meta-analysis of randomized controlled trials. *Clinical Nutrition, 35*(6), 1259–1268. https://doi.org/10.1016/j.clnu.2016.03.001, http://www.elsevier-international.com/journals/clnu/.

Jeon, S. M., & Shin, E. A. (2018). Exploring vitamin D metabolism and function in cancer. *Experimental and Molecular Medicine, 50*(4). https://doi.org/10.1038/s12276-018-0038-9, https://www.nature.com/emm/.

Jiang, W., Miyamoto, T., Kakizawa, T., Nishio, S.-ich, Oiwa, A., Takeda, T., Suzuki, S., & Hashizume, K. (2006). Inhibition of LXRα signaling by vitamin D receptor: Possible role of VDR in bile acid synthesis. *Biochemical and Biophysical Research Communications, 351*(1), 176–184. https://doi.org/10.1016/j.bbrc.2006.10.027.

Jorde, R., & Figenschau, Y. (2009). Supplementation with cholecalciferol does not improve glycaemic control in diabetic subjects with normal serum 25-hydroxyvitamin D levels. *European Journal of Nutrition, 48*(6), 349–354. https://doi.org/10.1007/s00394-009-0020-3.

Karhapää, P., Pihlajamäki, J., Pörsti, I., Kastarinen, M., Mustonen, J., Niemelä, O., & Kuusisto, J. (2010). Diverse associations of 25-hydroxyvitamin D and 1,25-dihydroxy-vitamin D with dyslipidaemias. *Journal of Internal Medicine, 268*(6), 604–610. https://doi.org/10.1111/j.1365-2796.2010.02279.x.

Kim, S. H., & Reaven, G. M. (2008). Insulin resistance and hyperinsulinemia. *Diabetes Care, 31*(7), 1433–1438. https://doi.org/10.2337/dc08-0045, http://care.diabetesjournals.org/cgi/reprint/31/7/1433. United States.

Kong, J., & Li, Y. C. (2006). Molecular mechanism of 1,25-dihydroxyvitamin D3 inhibition of adipogenesis in 3T3-L1 cells. *American Journal of Physiology - Endocrinology and Metabolism, 290*(5), E916. https://doi.org/10.1152/ajpendo.00410.2005, http://ajpendo.physiology.org/cgi/reprint/290/5/E916. United States.

Lai, Y.-H., & Fang, T.-C. (2013). The pleiotropic effect of vitamin D. *ISRN Nephrology, 2013*(4), 1–6. https://doi.org/10.5402/2013/898125.

Lakka, H.-M. (2002). The metabolic syndrome and total and cardiovascular disease mortality in middle-aged men. *The Journal of the American Medical Association, 288*(21), 2709. https://doi.org/10.1001/jama.288.21.2709.

Lee, S. J., Lee, E. Y., Lee, J. H., Kim, J. E., Kim, K. J., Rhee, Y., Kim, H. C., Youm, Y., & Kim, C. O. (2019). Associations of serum 25-hydroxyvitamin D with metabolic syndrome and its components in elderly men and women: The Korean Urban Rural Elderly cohort study. *BMC Geriatrics, 19*(1). https://doi.org/10.1186/s12877-019-1118-y, http://www.biomedcentral.com/bmcgeriatr/.

Li, Y. C., Qiao, G., Uskokovic, M., Xiang, W., Zheng, W., & Kong, J. (2004). Vitamin D: A negative endocrine regulator of the renin-angiotensin system and blood pressure. *Journal of Steroid Biochemistry and Molecular Biology, 89-90*, 387–392. https://doi.org/10.1016/j.jsbmb.2004.03.004.

Lim, S., Kim, M. J., Lim, S., Kim, M. J., Choi, S. H., Shin, C. S., Park, K. S., Jang, H. C., Billings, L. K., Meigs, J. B., Choi, S. H., Shin, C. S., Park, K. S., Jang, H. C., Billings, L. K., & Meigs, J. B. (2013). Association of vitamin D deficiency with incidence of type 2 diabetes in high-risk Asian subjects. *The American Journal of Clinical Nutrition, 97*(3), 524–530. https://doi.org/10.3945/ajcn.112.048496.

Maestro, B., Campión, J., Dávila, N., & Calle, C. (2000). Stimulation by 1,25-dihydroxyvitamin D3 of insulin receptor expression and insulin responsiveness for glucose transport in U-937 human promonocytic cells. *Endocrine Journal, 47*(4), 383–391. https://doi.org/10.1507/endocrj.47.383.

Makariou, S. E., Elisaf, M., Challa, A., Tentolouris, N., & Liberopoulos, E. N. (2017). No effect of vitamin D supplementation on cardiovascular risk factors in subjects with metabolic syndrome: a pilot randomised study. *Archives of Medical Science – Atherosclerotic Diseases, 2*(1), 52–60. https://doi.org/10.5114/amsad.2017.70504.

Malekmohammad, K., Bezsonov, E. E., & Rafieian-Kopaei, M. (2021). Role of lipid accumulation and inflammation in atherosclerosis: Focus on molecular and cellular mechanisms. *Frontiers in Cardiovascular Medicine, 8*. https://doi.org/10.3389/fcvm.2021.707529, http://www.frontiersin.org/journals/cardiovascular-medicine.

Mansouri, M., Abasi, R., Nasiri, M., Sharifi, F., Vesaly, S., Sadeghi, O., Rahimi, N., & Sharif, N. A. (2018). Association of vitamin D status with metabolic syndrome and its components: A cross-sectional study in a population of high educated Iranian adults. *Diabetes and Metabolic Syndrome: Clinical Research and Reviews, 12*(3), 393–398. https://doi.org/10.1016/j.dsx.2018.01.007, http://www.journals.elsevier.com/diabetes-and-metabolic-syndrome-clinical-research-and-reviews/.

McDermott, M. F., Ramachandran, A., Ogunkolade, B. W., Aganna, E., Curtis, D., Boucher, B. J., Snehalatha, C., & Hitman, G. A. (1997). Allelic variation in the vitamin D receptor influences susceptibility to IDDM in Indian Asians. *Diabetologia, 40*(8), 971–975. https://doi.org/10.1007/s001250050776.

Mitri, J., Dawson-Hughes, B., Hu, F. B., & Pittas, A. G. (2011). Effects of vitamin D and calcium supplementation on pancreatic β cell function, insulin sensitivity, and glycemia in adults at high risk of diabetes: The Calcium and Vitamin D for Diabetes Mellitus (CaDDM) randomized controlled trial. *American Journal of Clinical Nutrition, 94*(2), 486–494. https://doi.org/10.3945/ajcn.111.011684, http://www.ajcn.org/content/94/2/486.full.pdf+html. United States.

Mozos, I., & Marginean, O. (2015). Links between Vitamin D deficiency and cardiovascular diseases. *BioMed Research International, 2015*, 1–12. https://doi.org/10.1155/2015/109275.

Muldowney, S., Lucey, A. J., Hill, T. R., Seamans, K. M., Taylor, N., Wallace, J. M. W., Horigan, G., Barnes, M. S., Bonham, M. P., Duffy, E. M., Strain, J. J., Cashman, K. D., & Kiely, M. (2012). Incremental cholecalciferol supplementation up to 15 μg/d throughout winter at 51-55° N has no effect on biomarkers of cardiovascular risk in healthy young and older adults. *Journal of Nutrition, 142*(8), 1519–1525. https://doi.org/10.3945/jn.111.154005, http://jn.nutrition.org/content/142/8/1519.full.pdf.

Mulè, G. (2014). Metabolic syndrome in hypertensive patients: An unholy alliance. *World Journal of Cardiology, 6*(9), 890. https://doi.org/10.4330/wjc.v6.i9.890.

Mutt, S. J., Jokelainen, J., Sebert, S., Auvinen, J., Järvelin, M. R., Keinänen-Kiukaanniemi, S., & Herzig, K. H. (2019). Vitamin D status and components of metabolic syndrome in older subjects from Northern Finland (Latitude 65∘North). *Nutrients, 11*(6). https://doi.org/10.3390/nu11061229, https://www.mdpi.com/2072-6643/11/6/1229/pdf.

Nadège Nganou-Gnindjio, C., Jocelyne Ama Moor, V., Anatole Pieme, C., Sadeu Wafeu, G., Ngandjeu Kamtchoum, I., Yerema, R., & Patrick Menanga, A. (2021). Short-term effects of calcium and vitamin D supplementation in postmenopausal hypertensive patients in sub-Saharan Africa: A double blinded randomized controlled trial. *Acta Scientific Women's Health, 1*(3), 59–64. https://doi.org/10.31080/aswh.2021.si.03.0010.

Nikooyeh, B., Neyestani, T. R., Farvid, M., Alavi-Majd, H., Houshiarrad, A., Kalayi, A., Shariatzadeh, N., Gharavi, A., Heravifard, S., Tayebinejad, N., Salekzamani, S., & Zahedirad, M. (2011). Daily consumption of vitamin D- or vitamin D + calcium-fortified yogurt drink improved glycemic control in patients with type 2 diabetes: A randomized clinical trial. *American Journal of Clinical Nutrition, 93*(4), 764–771. https://doi.org/10.3945/ajcn.110.007336, http://www.ajcn.org/content/93/4/764.full.pdf+html. Iran.

Nimitphong, H., Holick, M. F., Fried, S. K., & Lee, M. J. (2012). 25-Hydroxyvitamin D3 and 1,25-dihydroxyvitamin D3 promote the differentiation of human subcutaneous preadipocytes. *PLoS ONE, 7*(12). https://doi.org/10.1371/journal.pone.0052171, http://www.plosone.org/article/fetchObjectAttachment.action?uri=info%3Adoi%2F10.1371%2Fjournal.pone.0052171&representation=PDF. Thailand.

Noubiap, J. J., Nansseu, J. R., Lontchi-Yimagou, E., Nkeck, J. R., Nyaga, U. F., Ngouo, A. T., Tounouga, D. N., Tianyi, F. L., Foka, A. J., Ndoadoumgue, A. L., & Bigna, J. J. (2022). Geographic distribution of metabolic syndrome and its components in the general adult population: A meta-analysis of global data from 28 million individuals. *Diabetes Research and Clinical Practice, 188.* https://doi.org/10.1016/j.diabres.2022.109924, www.elsevier.com/locate/diabres.

Ogurtsova, K., da Rocha Fernandes, J. D., Huang, Y., Linnenkamp, U., Guariguata, L., Cho, N. H., Cavan, D., Shaw, J. E., & Makaroff, L. E. (2017). IDF Diabetes Atlas: Global estimates for the prevalence of diabetes for 2015 and 2040. *Diabetes Research and Clinical Practice, 128*, 40–50. https://doi.org/10.1016/j.diabres.2017.03.024.

Pereira-Santos, M., Costa, P. R. F., Assis, A. M. O., Santos, C. A. S. T., & Santos, D. B. (2015). Obesity and vitamin D deficiency: A systematic review and meta-analysis. *Obesity Reviews, 16*(4), 341–349. https://doi.org/10.1111/obr.12239.

Pittas, A. G., Lau, J., Hu, F. B., & Dawson-Hughes, B. (2007). Review: The role of vitamin D and calcium in type 2 diabetes. A systematic review and meta-analysis. *Journal of Clinical Endocrinology and Metabolism, 92*(6), 2017–2029. https://doi.org/10.1210/jc.2007-0298, http://jcem.endojournals.org/cgi/reprint/92/6/2017.pdf.

Pittas, A. G., Harris, S. S., Stark, P. C., & Dawson-Hughes, B. (2007). The effects of calcium and vitamin D supplementation on blood glucose and markers of inflammation in nondiabetic adults. *Diabetes Care, 30*(4), 980–986. https://doi.org/10.2337/dc06-1994, http://care.diabetesjournals.org/cgi/reprint/30/4/980. United States.

Ponda, M. P., Huang, X., Odeh, M. A., Breslow, J. L., & Kaufman, H. W. (2012). Vitamin D may not improve lipid levels: A serial clinical laboratory data study. *Circulation, 126*(3), 270–277. https://doi.org/10.1161/CIRCULATIONAHA.111.077875.

Pott-Junior, H., Nascimento, C. M. C., Costa-Guarisco, L. P., Gomes, G. Ad. O., Gramani-Say, K., Orlandi, Fd. S., Gratão, A. C. M., Orlandi, A. A. D. S., Pavarini, S. C. I., Vasilceac, F. A., Zazzetta, M. S., & Cominetti, M. R.

(2020). Vitamin D deficient older adults are more prone to have metabolic syndrome, but not to a greater number of metabolic syndrome parameters. *Nutrients, 12*(3). https://doi.org/10.3390/nu12030748, https://www.mdpi.com/2072-6643/12/3/748/pdf.

Rafiq, S., & Jeppesen, P. B. (2018). Body mass index, vitamin D, and type 2 diabetes: A systematic review and meta-analysis. *Nutrients, 10*(9), 1182. https://doi.org/10.3390/nu10091182.

Rahmouni, K., Correia, M. L. G., Haynes, W. G., & Mark, A. L. (2005). Obesity-associated hypertension: New insights into mechanisms. *Hypertension, 45*(1), 9–14. https://doi.org/10.1161/01.HYP.0000151325.83008.b4.

Reaven, G. M. (2006). The metabolic syndrome: Is this diagnosis necessary?[1,2]. *The American Journal of Clinical Nutrition, 83*(6), 1237–1247. https://doi.org/10.1093/ajcn/83.6.1237.

Rodriguez, A., Catalan, V., Gomez-Ambrosi, J., & Fruhbeck, G. (2007). Visceral and subcutaneous adiposity: Are both potential therapeutic targets for tackling the metabolic syndrome? *Current Pharmaceutical Design, 13*(21), 2169–2175. https://doi.org/10.2174/138161207781039599.

Rueda, S., Fernández-Fernández, C., Romero, F., Martínez de Osaba, M. J., & Vidal, J. (2008). Vitamin D, PTH, and the metabolic syndrome in severely obese subjects. *Obesity Surgery, 18*(2), 151–154. https://doi.org/10.1007/s11695-007-9352-3.

Ryu, O. H., Lee, S., Yu, J., Choi, M. G., Yoo, H. J., & Mantero, F. (2014). A prospective randomized controlled trial of the effects of vitamin D supplementation on long-term glycemic control in type 2 diabetes mellitus of Korea. *Endocrine Journal, 61*(2), 167–176. https://doi.org/10.1507/endocrj.EJ13-0356, https://www.jstage.jst.go.jp/article/endocrj/61/2/61_EJ13-0356/_pdf. South Korea.

Sadeghi, K., Wessner, B., Laggner, U., Ploder, M., Tamandl, D., Friedl, J., Zügel, U., Steinmeyer, A., Pollak, A., Roth, E., Boltz-Nitulescu, G., & Spittler, A. (2006). Vitamin D3 down-regulates monocyte TLR expression and triggers hyporesponsiveness to pathogen-associated molecular patterns. *European Journal of Immunology, 36*(2), 361–370. https://doi.org/10.1002/eji.200425995.

Saneei, P., Salehi-Abargouei, A., & Esmaillzadeh, A. (2013). Serum 25-hydroxy vitamin D levels in relation to body mass index: A systematic review and meta-analysis. *Obesity Reviews, 14*(5), 393–404. https://doi.org/10.1111/obr.12016.

Schinzari, F., Tesauro, M., Rovella, V., Galli, A., Mores, N., Porzio, O., Lauro, D., & Cardillo, C. (2010). Generalized impairment of vasodilator reactivity during hyperinsulinemia in patients with obesity-related metabolic syndrome. *American Journal of Physiology-Endocrinology and Metabolism, 299*(6), E947. https://doi.org/10.1152/ajpendo.00426.2010.

Schleicher, R. L., Sternberg, M. R., Looker, A. C., Yetley, E. A., Lacher, D. A., Sempos, C. T., Taylor, C. L., Durazo-Arvizu, R. A., Maw, K. L., Chaudhary-Webb, M., Johnson, C. L., & Pfeiffer, C. M. (2016). National estimates of serum total 25-hydroxyvitamin D and metabolite concentrations measured by liquid chromatography-tandem mass spectrometry in the US population during 2007-2010. *Journal of Nutrition, 146*(5), 1051–1061. https://doi.org/10.3945/jn.115.227728, http://jn.nutrition.org/content/146/5/1051.full.pdf.

Schmitt, E. B., Nahas-Neto, J., Bueloni-Dias, F., Poloni, P. F., Orsatti, C. L., & Petri Nahas, E. A. (2018). Vitamin D deficiency is associated with metabolic syndrome in postmenopausal women. *Maturitas, 107*, 97–102. https://doi.org/10.1016/j.maturitas.2017.10.011, www.elsevier.com/locate/maturitas.

Schroten, N. F., Ruifrok, W. P. T., Kleijn, L., Dokter, M. M., Silljé, H. H., Lambers Heerspink, H. J., Bakker, S. J. L., Kema, I. P., Van Gilst, W. H., Van Veldhuisen, D. J., Hillege, H. L., & De Boer, R. A. (2013). Short-term vitamin D3 supplementation lowers plasma renin activity in patients with stable chronic heart failure: An open-label, blinded end point, randomized prospective trial (VitD-CHF trial). *American Heart Journal, 166*(2), 357. https://doi.org/10.1016/j.ahj.2013.05.009, http://www.elsevier.com/inca/publications/store/6/2/3/2/7/2/index.htt.

Shanmugalingam, T., Crawley, D., Bosco, C., Melvin, J., Rohrmann, S., Chowdhury, S., Holmberg, L., & Van Hemelrijck, M. (2014). Obesity and cancer: The role of vitamin D. *BMC Cancer, 14*(1). https://doi.org/10.1186/1471-2407-14-712.

Spahis, S., Borys, J. M., & Levy, E. (2017). Metabolic syndrome as a multifaceted risk factor for oxidative stress. *Antioxidants and Redox Signaling, 26*(9), 445–461. https://doi.org/10.1089/ars.2016.6756, www.liebertonline.com/ars.

Tan, H. W., Zhao, N. Q., Yu, Y. R., Han, L. N., & Zhang, X. X. (2017). Pancreatic β-cell dysfunction and apoptosis induced by klevated free fatty acids synergize with hyperglycemia. *Journal of Sichuan University (Medical Science Edition), 48*(1), 71–75. http://hxykdxxb.periodicals.net.cn/default.html.

Tumova, J., Andel, M., & Trnka, J. (2016). Excess of free fatty acids as a cause of metabolic dysfunction in skeletal muscle. *Physiological Research, 65*(2), 193–207. https://doi.org/10.33549/physiolres.932993.

Vimaleswaran, K. S., Berry, D. J., Lu, C., Tikkanen, E., Pilz, S., Hiraki, L. T., Cooper, J. D., Dastani, Z., Li, R., Houston, D. K., Wood, A. R., Michaëlsson, K., Vandenput, L., Zgaga, L., Yerges-Armstrong, L. M., McCarthy, M. I., Dupuis, J., Kaakinen, M., Kleber, M. E., ... Hirschhorn, J. N. (2013). Causal relationship between obesity and vitamin D status: Bi-directional mendelian randomization analysis of multiple cohorts. *PLoS Medicine, 10*(2). https://doi.org/10.1371/journal.pmed.1001383, http://www.plosmedicine.org/article/fetchObjectAttachment.action?uri=info%3Adoi%2F10.1371%2Fjournal.pmed.1001383&representation=PDF.

Witham, M. D., Adams, F., Kabir, G., Kennedy, G., Belch, J. J. F., & Khan, F. (2013). Effect of short-term vitamin D supplementation on markers of vascular health in South Asian women living in the UK - A randomised controlled trial. *Atherosclerosis, 230*(2), 293–299. https://doi.org/10.1016/j.atherosclerosis.2013.08.005.

Wongwiwatthananukit, S., Sansanayudh, N., Phetkrajaysang, N., & Krittiyanunt, S. (2013). Effects of vitamin D2 supplementation on insulin sensitivity and metabolic parameters inmetabolic syndrome patients. *Journal of Endocrinological Investigation, 36*(8), 558–563. https://doi.org/10.3275/8817, www.jendocrinolinvest.it/jei/en. United States.

Wood, A. D., Secombes, K. R., Thies, F., Aucott, L., Black, A. J., Mavroeidi, A., Simpson, W. G., Fraser, W. D., Reid, D. M., & Macdonald, H. M. (2012). Vitamin D 3 supplementation has no effect on conventional cardiovascular risk factors: A parallel-group, double-blind, placebo-controlled RCT. *Journal of Clinical Endocrinology and Metabolism, 97*(10), 3557–3567. https://doi.org/10.1210/jc.2012-2126, http://jcem.endojournals.org/content/97/10/3557.full.pdf+html. United Kingdom.

Xia, Z., Hu, Y., Han, Z., Gao, Y., Bai, J., He, Y., Zhao, H., & Zhang, H. (2017). Association of vitamin D receptor gene polymorphisms with diabetic dyslipidemia in the elderly male population in North China. *Clinical interventions in aging, 12*, 1673–1679. https://doi.org/10.2147/cia.s145700.

Yanai, H., Tomono, Y., Ito, K., Furutani, N., Yoshida, H., & Tada, N. (2008). The underlying mechanisms for development of hypertension in the metabolic syndrome. *Nutrition Journal, 7*(1). https://doi.org/10.1186/1475-2891-7-10.

Yetley, E. A. (2008). Assessing the vitamin D status of the US population. *The American Journal of Clinical Nutrition, 88*(2), 558S. https://doi.org/10.1093/ajcn/88.2.558s.

Yin, X., Yan, L., Lu, Y., Jiang, Q., Pu, Y., & Sun, Q. (2016). Correction of hypovitaminosis D does not improve the metabolic syndrome risk profile in a Chinese population: A randomized controlled trial for 1 year. *Asia Pacific Journal of Clinical Nutrition, 25*(1), 71–77. https://doi.org/10.6133/apjcn.2016.25.1.06, http://apjcn.nhri.org.tw/server/APJCN/25/1/71.pdf.

Yuan, W., Pan, W., Kong, J., Zheng, W., Szeto, F. L., Wong, K. E., Cohen, R., Klopot, A., Zhang, Z., & Yan, C. L. (2007). 1,25-Dihydroxyvitamin D3 suppresses renin gene transcription by blocking the activity of the cyclic AMP response element in the renin gene promoter. *Journal of Biological Chemistry, 282*(41), 29821–29830. https://doi.org/10.1074/jbc.M705495200, http://www.jbc.org/cgi/reprint/282/41/29821. United States.

Zafar, U., Khaliq, S., Ahmad, H. U., & Lone, K. P. (2019). Serum profile of cytokines and their genetic variants in metabolic syndrome and healthy subjects: A comparative study. *Bioscience Reports, 39*(2). https://doi.org/10.1042/BSR20181202, http://www.bioscirep.org/content/39/2/BSR20181202.full-text.pdf.

Zaheer, S., Taquechel, K., Brown, J. M., Adler, G. K., Williams, J. S., & Vaidya, A. (2018). A randomized intervention study to evaluate the effect of calcitriol therapy on the renin-angiotensin system in diabetes. *Journal of the Renin-Angiotensin-Aldosterone System, 19*(1). https://doi.org/10.1177/1470320317754178.

Zheng, M. H., Li, F. X. Z., Xu, F., Lin, X., Wang, Y., Xu, Q. S., Guo, B., & Yuan, L. Q. (2020). The interplay between the renin-angiotensin-aldosterone system and parathyroid hormone. *Frontiers in Endocrinology, 11*. https://doi.org/10.3389/fendo.2020.00539, https://www.frontiersin.org/journals/endocrinology#.

Zhu, L., Spence, C., Yang, W. J., & Ma, G. X. (2020). The idf definition is better suited for screening metabolic syndrome and estimating risks of diabetes in asian american adults: Evidence from nhanes 2011–2016. *Journal of Clinical Medicine, 9*(12), 1–13. https://doi.org/10.3390/jcm9123871, https://www.mdpi.com/2077-0383/9/12/3871/pdf.

Zhu, W., & Heil, D. P. (2018). Associations of vitamin D status with markers of metabolic health: A community-based study in Shanghai, China. *Diabetes and Metabolic Syndrome: Clinical Research and Reviews, 12*(5), 727–732. https://doi.org/10.1016/j.dsx.2018.04.010, http://www.journals.elsevier.com/diabetes-and-metabolic-syndrome-clinical-research-and-reviews/.

Zimmet, P., Magliano, D., Matsuzawa, Y., Alberti, G., & Shaw, J. (2005). The metabolic syndrome: A global public health problem and a new definition. *Journal of Atherosclerosis and Thrombosis, 12*(6), 295–300. https://doi.org/10.5551/jat.12.295.

CHAPTER 16

Vitamin D and Reproductive health: a critical link of vitamin D deficiency with subfertility

Arfa Azhar[1], Rehana Rehman[2], and Chaman Nasrullah[1]

[1]University College of Medicine & Dentistry, The University of Lahore, Lahore, Pakistan [2]Department of Biological & Biomedical Sciences, Aga Khan University, Karachi, Pakistan

16.1 Subfertility

16.1.1 Definition and prevalence

Subfertility is defined as a lower likelihood of becoming pregnant after a year of persistent, unprotected relationship, as opposed to infertility, which is expressed as the inability to conceive (Malhotra et al., 2024). It poses a major health issue for numerous young females in Pakistan, with 22% females of reproductive age experiencing this condition (Deshpande & Gupta, 2019). The World Health Organization (WHO) estimates that around 48.5 million couples universally face challenges in conceiving (Kayani et al., 2024). The total fertility rate (TFR) has also decreased from 4.2 in 1990 to 2.6 in 2012 in South Asia (Gajanayake et al., 2024).

Primary subfertility pertains to challenges in achieving pregnancy in couples without any previous pregnancies (Farquhar et al., 2019). Studies show that 1.9% of women who are 20 years old face primary subfertility (Gunawardhana et al., 2024), which impacts 10%–15% of couples of reproductive age worldwide (Dewau et al., 2021). Additionally, 10.5% of women who have given birth before encounter difficulties in getting pregnant again, a situation referred to as secondary subfertility(Alam, 2020; Barrera et al., 2022).

16.1.2 Causes and risk factors

This condition may result from different factors, such as hormonal inequalities, structural irregularities, lifestyle impacts, and nutritional deficits (Feskens et al., 2022). Subfertility is a complex condition that necessitates comprehensive examination, especially in our nation, where tuberculosis significantly leads to tubal obstruction from strictures (Mondal et al., 2024).

The Impact of Vitamin D on Health and Disease. DOI: https://doi.org/10.1016/B978-0-443-34037-6.00017-0

Over 70% of female subfertility cases are associated with factors such as low ovarian reserve or dysfunction, uterine and cervical issues, problems with the tubes, endometriosis, and pelvic adhesions. However, approximately 30% of instances remain unexplained (Barbieri, 2019).

Key elements leading to subfertility include sexually transmitted diseases, tuberculosis, uterine abnormalities, stress, male subfertility, and unexplained infertility (Alam, 2020). Furthermore, the rising prevalence of conditions such as hypothyroidism, diabetes, auto-immune disorders, hypertension, obesity, and substance dependence among youth has exacerbated the issue (Ciężki et al., 2024).

Nutrition also plays a vital part in sustaining general health, encompassing reproductive health. Sufficient nutrition is required to perform vital reproductive functions equally in males and females (Shukla & Shrivastava, 2024). Essential vitamins, minerals, and nutrients are therefore vital for reproductive processes like hormone regulation, ovulation, and sperm mobility (Ma et al., 2022).

Hormonal imbalances and ovulation issues, for example, polycystic ovarian syndrome (PCOS), can disturb normal ovulation, hindering conception. Fertilization and embryo implantation may be hindered by structural issues like endometriosis, fibroids, or blocked fallopian tubes, often resulting from infections (Shukla & Shrivastava, 2024). Another significant factor is age, as women's fertility decreases with advancing years, particularly after 35, due to decreased quantity and quality of eggs (Monaghan et al., 2020). Inflammation and scarring caused by endometriosis change the reproductive structures and may further complicate fertility (Coccia et al., 2022). Genetic compatibility is essential since one partner's genetic traits can affect the other's capacity to conceive, complicating the process of conception (Kimmins et al., 2024)

16.1.3   Impact of subfertility on individuals and couples

Subfertility can have considerable importance on the emotional, psychological, and social health of individuals and couples (Sharma & Shrivastava, 2022). It often leads to anxiety, sadness, irritability, and a diminished sense of self-worth (Azhar et al., 2024).

Many feel a loss of control over their lives and futures, with some experiencing emotional detachment or isolation during treatment, especially when partners struggle to communicate their emotions (Sharma & Shrivastava, 2022). It might be beneficial to find assistance from individuals who relate to the challenges faced by such couples, possibly via support groups or therapy. Transparent discussions regarding their experience of subfertility, how they coped with that, can enhance connections and lessen feelings of loneliness (Shukla & Shrivastava, 2024). Cultural pressures also add to the burden, with subfertility often linked to shame or inadequacy, particularly for women in societies that place a high value on parenthood (Xie et al., 2023). Additionally, the financial strain of expensive fertility treatments creates further stress and anxiety. Support and understanding are vital to addressing these challenges (Shukla & Shrivastava, 2024).

16.2   Vitamin D: reproductive health and subfertility

16.2.1   Vitamin D

Vitamin D is a steroid hormone needed for reproductive health in both sexes. Its metabolizing enzymes are found in reproductive tissues, including the ovaries, testes, uterus, and placenta, along with endocrine organs such as the pituitary gland and hypothalamus. Although sunlight is the main source of vitamin D, it can likewise be obtained from foods like fatty fish (including salmon and mackerel), fortified dairy items, egg yolks, and mushrooms (Azhar et al., 2022). Vitamin D further enhances the synthesis of essential reproductive hormones like estradiol and progesterone. Research in both animals and humans indicates that vitamin D takes part in folliculogenesis, steroidogenesis, and the maintenance of the endometrium in females (Azhar et al., 2024). Vitamin D can be attained from sunlight, fatty fish (including salmon and mackerel), fortified items (such as milk and orange juice), and dietary supplements (Benedik, 2022).

Polycystic ovary syndrome (PCOS), a primary factor in subfertility, particularly in South Asian women, is often linked to a deficiency in vitamin D. Although many Asian countries receive abundant sunlight, vitamin D deficiency is still widespread due to additional factors influencing vitamin D levels (Azhar et al., 2023).

16.3   Mechanisms linking vitamin D and reproduction

Vitamin D is recognized as an important pillar for follicular growth and oocyte maturation. Vitamin D, specifically, aids in improving modifiable reproductive hormones, such as estrogen and progesterone, and is crucial for ovulation and the uniformity of menstruation in females (Calcaterra et al., 2024). Furthermore, having adequate vitamin D levels throughout pregnancy can reduce the likelihood of issues such as gestational diabetes and preeclampsia (Shukla & Shrivastava, 2024). Results from early research of the 1980s and later studies need further elaboration due to the intricacy of Vitamin D metabolism and its extensive impact on the reproductive, endocrine, and neurological systems.

16.3.1   Vitamin D receptors and reproductive organs

Vitamin D mediates its role in fertility, conception, and embryogenesis through vitamin D receptors (VDR), which are nuclear receptors found in the ovary, primordial, primary follicles, and oocytes, endometrium, and placenta. Vitamin D supplementation increases VDR expression and signaling in a positive feedback loop, intensifying vitamin D's effects in the ovary (Makieva et al., 2021). VDR are found to be present in the ovaries of various birds as well as mammals (Pejovic et al., 2020). Other studies in fish, goat, and rhesus monkey showed the presence of VDR in oocytes of primordial follicles. VDR signaling is found to be dominant in theca cells (TCs) and granulosa cells (GCs) in the primary and secondary follicles of rats and goats (Xu et al., 2021).

VDR expression in ovarian follicles depends on the stage of follicular development, and it increases as the follicle grows (Li et al., 2024). In human ovarian surface epithelial cells that have been cultured, supplementation increases the expression of the VDR protein(Pejovic et al., 2020). Vitamin D's signaling system affects several important ovarian functions, including follicular growth, steroidogenesis, and oocyte maturation. VDR-null animals exhibit defective folliculogenesis, decreased aromatase activity, and uterine hypoplasia (Xu et al., 2021) (Fig. 16.1).

Primordial follicles represent the "ovarian reserve". Serum vitamin D levels and ovarian reserve indicators are not correlated in most clinical trials (Xu et al., 2021). There was no discernible effect of vitamin D insufficiency on ovarian reserve in studies conducted on oocyte donors and women receiving infertility therapy. Nonetheless, a negative correlation has been noted in patients with uterine fibroids, and some research indicates that extremely low vitamin D levels may lower ovarian reserve. Clarifying the connection between the ovarian reserve and vitamin D status requires direct evaluation of primordial follicles; however, this is still challenging for human studies (Arefi et al., 2018).

16.3.2   Vitamin D and follicle maturation

Follicles, having follicular cells and oocytes, are the main functional part of the ovaries. Folliculogenesis is a dynamic process, and follicles undergo different phases of development,

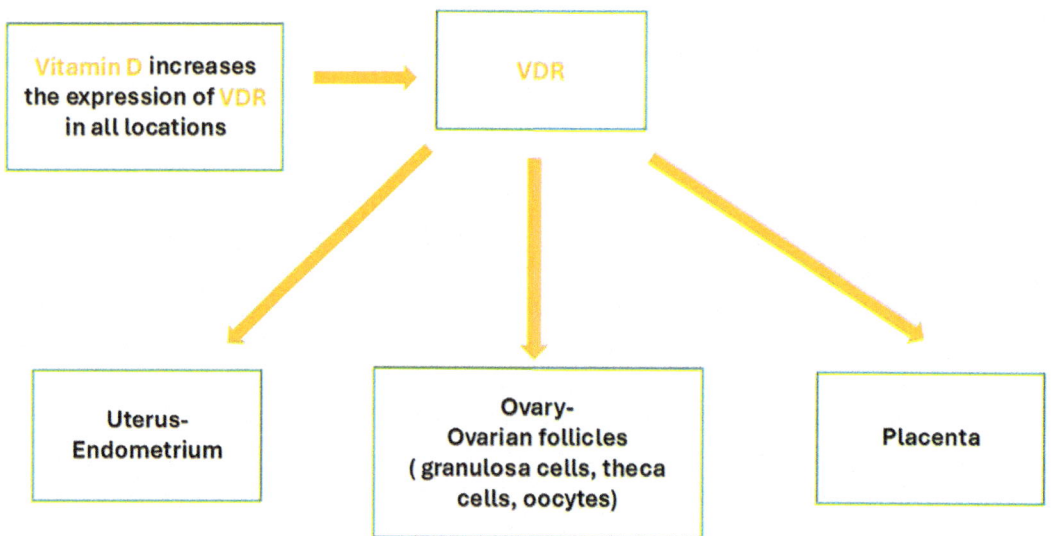

Figure 16.1
Location of VDR. *VDR*, Vitamin D receptors.

including primordial, primary, secondary, antral, and mature follicles. The developing follicle enters the hormone-dependent stage when pregranulosa cells of the primordial follicle undergo maturation and start to express the receptors for follicle-stimulating hormone (FSH), estrogen, and androgen hormones (Li et al., 2024) (Fig. 16.2).

By controlling endocrine and paracrine elements in the ovarian microenvironment, vitamin D aids in this process. Studies in animals show that a vitamin D shortage impairs follicular development, resulting in lower ovarian weight, extended estrous cycles, and arrested growth. On the other hand, Vitamin D supplementation improves follicular shape, increases steroid hormone production (progesterone and estradiol), and improves follicular vitality, especially in models of polycystic ovarian syndrome (PCOS). (Grzeczka et al., 2022; Xu et al., 2021).

Follicular vitamin D may have an intraovarian or systemic origin. The CYP2R1 and CYP27B1 genes encode the essential enzymes for the synthesis of calcitriol, 25-hydroxylase,

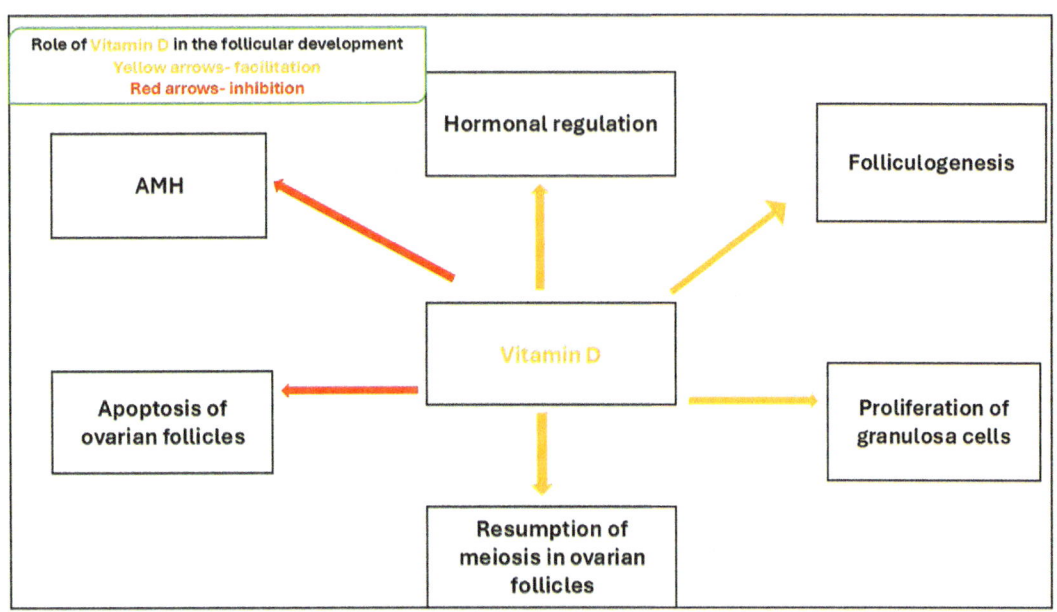

Figure 16.2
Vitamin D and ovarian reserve. Role of vitamin D in the follicular development.

and 1-α-hydroxylase, respectively (Bièche et al., 2007). Human ovaries, as well as the growing follicles of nonhuman primates, express the mRNA of these enzymes. Vitamin D supplementation leads to an increased proportion of growing follicles as well as an increased diameter of oocytes of antral follicles in an in vitro study in primates.

Vitamin D is essential for granulosa cell (GC) proliferation. Research has demonstrated that GC proliferation is stimulated in a dose-dependent manner by modest concentrations of vitamin D, as seen in the follicles of goats and hens. Vitamin D achieves this target by controlling the cell cycle and upregulating the expression of cyclin-dependent kinase 4 (CDK4) and Cyclin D1 while downregulating the expression of cell cycle inhibitors such as P21. This facilitates cell cycle progression and GC proliferation by encouraging GCs to move from the G0/G1 phase to the S phase (Cong et al., 2017). The effects of high vitamin D on GC proliferation and the mechanism behind it require more investigation.

Vitamin D levels are positively correlated with improved follicular fluid composition, which promotes oocyte development. On the other hand, vitamin D deficiency hinders follicular growth, which may be responsible for decreased ovarian reserve and polycystic ovary syndrome (PCOS) (Grzeczka et al., 2022). Vitamin D significantly affects folliculogenesis by regulating hormone synthesis and receptor activity in granulosa and theca cells. The anti-Müllerian hormone (AMH), a crucial regulator of ovarian reserve, interacts with vitamin D through its receptors. Vitamin D balances follicular recruitment by improving AMH control (Grzeczka et al., 2022). Hormone receptors start to express as secondary follicles change into antral follicles, marking the start of the gonadotropin-dependent stage. Vitamin D supports follicular development by aiding in oocyte meiosis, promoting granulosa cell proliferation, increasing follicular cell secretion of progesterone and estrogen, blocking AMH inhibitory impact on FSH, and lowering cellular apoptosis (Li et al., 2024).

16.3.3   Vitamin D and oocyte maturation

The oocyte is kept arrested in the prophase of the first meiosis for a few hours before ovulation. Oocyte accumulates various proteins for embryogenesis during this period. The C-type natriuretic peptide pathway (NPCC) is responsible for this process. Mural granulosa cells secrete NPPC when it binds to its receptors, NPR2, and leads to the synthesis of cGMP, which enters oocytes by passing through gap junctions.

When transforming growth factor-beta (TGF-β) binds to its receptor TGFR, transcription protein Smad-2/3 is activated. Activated Smads2/3 form heteromeric complexes with Smad4 attach to the promoter region of NPPC after translocating to the nucleus and dramatically raise the levels of NPPC in the cultured MGCs (Li et al., 2024). Vitamin D may encourage oocyte growth by lowering TGF-β1 levels and restoring the meiotic condition of oocytes. Vitamin D supplementation decreased the expression of the gene for TGF-β1 and also phosphorylated the Smad-2/3 in the lungs using the TGF-β1 transgenic mouse model. By increasing VDR expression and blocking the signaling pathway for TGF-β1/Smad3, vitamin D is found to be beneficial in reducing renal fibrosis in the rat model of chronic kidney disease (CKD) (Li et al., 2024).

NPPC leads to the production of cGPM. cGMP needs connexins 43,37 to enter the oocytes and to arrest the meiosis. Vitamin D can lower NPPC levels, overcome oocyte meiotic arrest, and encourage follicular growth via blocking the TGF-β1/Smad3 signaling pathways. Vitamin D increases the expression of connexin mimetic peptides CX43 to break the gap junctions so that cGMP is not able to penetrate the oocytes, leading to the resumption of meiosis (Li et al., 2024) (Fig. 16.3).

16.3.3.1   Vitamin D and hormonal regulation

16.3.3.1.1   Anti-Mullerian hormone

AMH is the "guardian" of ovarian reserve, preventing the overactivation of primary follicles and the growth of an excessive number of antral follicles by decreasing their receptor sensitivity to follicle-stimulating hormone (FSH). The AMH coding sequence was shown to contain VD-

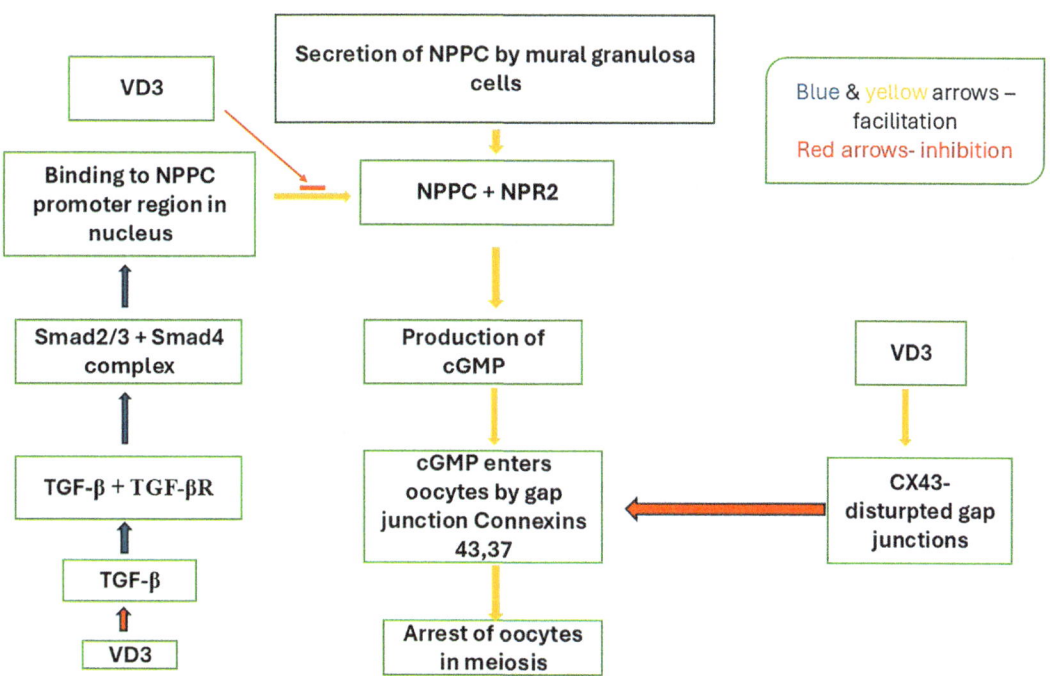

Figure 16.3

Vitamin D and oocyte maturation. *cGMP*, Cyclic GMP; *NPR2*, C-type natriuretic peptide receptors; *TGF-β*, transforming growth factor-beta.

responsive sites. VDR causes AMH to be downregulated, but it is also likely that AMH and VDR work in concert because AMH, a measure of ovarian reserve, prevents primordial follicles from being recruited into active folliculogenesis. The AMH gene's promoter region has a functional VD response element (VDRE) for vitamin D, which connects its modulation to AMH levels. According to human studies, vitamin D and AMH levels are positively correlated, and taking vitamin D supplements can reverse seasonal declines in AMH. In a study, GCs from women who were undergoing in vitro fertilization were used to investigate the function of vitamin D on follicular development as well as steroidogenesis (Merhi, 2019).

The results showed that in cumulus GCs of small follicles, higher expression of AMH receptor (AMHR-II) mRNA was linked to lower levels of vitamin D in follicular fluid. Vitamin D treatment increased 3β-hydroxysteroid dehydrogenase (3β-HSD) mRNA and enzyme activity while decreasing mRNA levels of AMHR-II and FSH receptors, which led to increased progesterone synthesis. Vitamin D decreased the phosphorylation of Smad 1/5/8, a crucial element of AMH signaling, but did not affect the generation of estradiol (E2) triggered by FSH. These findings show that vitamin D may play a crucial role in fertility by modulating AMH signaling and promoting GC luteinization (Merhi et al., 2014)

An analysis of previous research studies showed that vitamin D supplementation affected blood AMH levels differentially depending on ovulation state. After taking supplements, AMH levels dramatically dropped in anovulatory PCOS patients while rising in ovulatory non-PCOS women. This implies that vitamin D regulates AMH bidirectionally (Moridi et al., 2020).

16.3.3.1.2   Estradiol and vitamin D

Vitamin D directly affects ovarian steroidogenesis by regulating the generation of progesterone, estradiol, and oestrone in human ovarian cells by affecting the manifestation of steroidogenic enzymes such as aromatase and 3β-hydroxysteroid dehydrogenase (Harmon et al., 2020). Vitamin D regulates estrogen production by controlling calcium balance and potentially exhibits direct effects on the aromatase gene (Parikh et al., 2010).

A retrospective research study, including 89 women of reproductive age, indicated that low levels of vitamin D (< 30 ng/mL) were related to reduced estradiol (E2) concentrations throughout the menstrual cycle (Hong et al., 2017). Adding vitamin D to cultured human ovarian tissue boosted estradiol synthesis by 9%, and when paired with insulin, the rise was 60%, indicating a synergistic impact.

16.3.3.1.3   Progesterone and vitamin D

Vitamin D supplementation increases the production of progesterone (P4) in human granulosa cells by increasing the activity and expression of 3β-hydroxysteroid dehydrogenase, the regulating enzyme for progesterone synthesis (Merhi et al., 2014).

Progesterone and vitamin D have comparable effects and share structural and functional traits. Vitamin D3 deficiency may impair the production of P4. 25-Hydroxyvitamin D1α-hydroxylase null mice showed lower serum levels of progesterone and estrogen. The production of P4 is controlled by the protein, steroidogenic acute regulatory protein (StAR), and the enzyme 3β-hydroxysteroid dehydrogenase (3β-HSD) (Stensen et al., 2014). Vitamin D also increased the expression of StAR mRNA and 3β-HSD, indicating that it increases the expression of steroidogenic genes, which in turn stimulates P4 production. Supplementing egg-laying hens' diets with vitamin D dramatically raised their serum P4 levels while lowering their overall cholesterol levels. Vitamin D3 dramatically increased CYP11A1 mRNA levels, which encode an enzyme that converts cholesterol into P4, enhancing follicular growth and promoting progesterone synthesis (Cheng et al., 2023) (Fig.16.4).

Vitamin D (1,25-dihydroxyvitamin D3) protects ovarian granulosa cells by reducing the oxidative and mitochondrial damage induced by endocrine disruptors such as bisphenol A (BPA). It restores mitochondrial function by lowering BPA-induced mitochondrial DNA deletion, raising total superoxide dismutase (SOD) activity, and boosting mitochondrial biogenesis-related protein expression through the PI3K-Akt pathway. Furthermore, vitamin D restores hormonal balance and cellular energy production by counteracting BPA's induced decrease in the cytochrome c oxidase subunit I levels and 17β-estradiol secretion (Lee et al., 2019). In GCs from a PCOS mouse model, vitamin D supplementation in the culture media

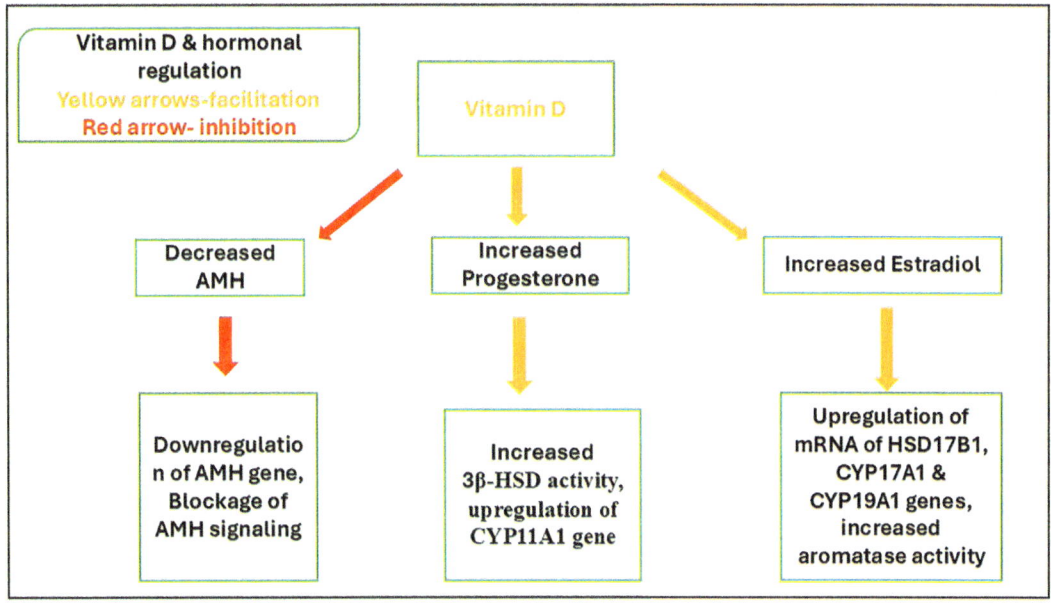

Figure 16.4
Vitamin D and hormonal regulation.

enhanced the number of mitochondrial DNA copies, biogenesis, and membrane integrity. It also raised the expression of genes related to antioxidant and antiapoptotic factors (Safaei et al., 2020). Vitamin D–controlled biogenesis of mitochondria and its functions in the oocyte are not well understood, but this data lay the ground for future in vivo research as well as investigations in humans or other animal models to better understand vitamin D–controlled mitochondrial functions during the process of folliculogenesis and oocyte maturation.

16.3.3.2   Vitamin D and inflammation

Vitamin D reduces various harmful elements like reactive oxygen species (ROS) as well as advanced glycation end products (AGEs). Follicular development is affected by oxidative stress as it induces oocyte aging. Vitamin D itself reduced the levels of reactive oxygen species (ROS) in goat granulosa cells and increased the genes for antioxidant enzymes like [superoxide dismutase 2 (SOD2) and catalase (CAT)], which in turn encourages the proliferation of GC (Merhi, 2019).

AGEs can also have a detrimental effect on follicular growth by binding to receptors on granulosa and theca cells, called RAGE (Stensen et al., 2014). Soluble RAGE (sRAGE) binds with free AGEs and thus blocks its actions (Merhi, 2019). Vitamin D raises Soluble RAGE (sRAGE) levels in ovaries and decreases the negative effects of AGEs on follicle development. Studies reveal that vitamin D decreases the overexpression of steroidogenesis-related genes, including CYP11A1, StAR, and CYP17A1, in luteinized human GCs and prevents AGE-induced inflammation. Furthermore, AGEs increase the phosphorylation of SMAD 1/5/8 by recombinant AMH, whereas adding vitamin D could reverse these changes and decrease the expression of mRNA of AMHR-II, which was brought about by AGEs (Merhi, 2019).

16.4   Vitamin D and female subfertility

Lack of vitamin D is associated with abnormal menstrual cycles and diseases such as PCOS, which may interfere with ovulation. Acceptable levels of vitamin D augment ovarian function and boost the probability of successful implantation (Azhar et al., 2023).

Menstruation returned to normal for PCOS individuals who took calcium and vitamin D supplements. A diet lacking vitamin D caused mice to have longer estrous cycles and delayed ovarian development in a study employing CYP27B1 knockout animals. However, the estrous cycles restored to normal when vitamin D was incorporated into the diet (Mohan et al., 2023; Wu et al., 2018). Vitamin D insufficiency and PCOS, a major cause of female subfertility, are frequently linked. In women with PCOS, clinical studies show that using VD supplements enhances ovulation, hormonal balance, and monthly regularity. Calcitriol supplementation has been demonstrated to enhance IVF results and encourage spontaneous ovulation in PCOS patients with VD deficiency (Xu et al., 2021).

16.5   Conclusion

Vitamin D is important for numerous body functions, such as immune system response and bone health, being vital for reproductive health. Vitamin D is recognized as an important pillar for female reproductive health. It plays a vital role in follicular growth and oocyte maturation. Well-controlled animal models are necessary to investigate the molecular processes of vitamin D in the ovary. Furthermore, clinical research employing uniform patient groups and standardized experimental setups can more accurately assess vitamin D's role in the maintenance of female reproductive health.

AI disclosure

During the preparation of this work, the author(s) used an AI Chat Bot to use for grammatical correction. After using this tool/service, the author(s) reviewed and edited the content as needed and take(s) full responsibility for the content of the publication.

References

Alam, F. (2020). *Introduction to subfertility subfertility: Recent advances in management and prevention.* Brunei Darussalam: Elsevier, 97–106. http://doi.org/10.1016/B978-0-323-75945-8.00005-0, https://www.elsevier.com/books/subfertility/978-0-323-75945-8.

Arefi, S., Khalili, G., Iranmanesh, H., Farifteh, F., Hosseini, A., Fatemi, H. M., & Lawrenz, B. (2018). Is the ovarian reserve influenced by Vitamin D deficiency and the dress code in an infertile Iranian population? *Journal of Ovarian Research, 11*(1). http://doi.org/10.1186/s13048-018-0435-7, http://www.ovarianresearch.com/.

Azhar, A., Alam, S. M., Ashraf, M., Malick, A., Riffat, S., & Rehman, R. (2023). Vitamin D status and its relationship with oxidative stress markers in infertile women with polycystic ovary syndrome. *Pakistan Journal of Pharmaceutical Sciences, 36*(2), 331–335. https://doi.org/10.36721/PJPS.2023.36.1.SP.331-335.1, https://www.pjps.pk/uploads/pdfs/36/1/Special/16-11315-SP.pdf.

Azhar, A., Alam, S. M., & Rehman, R. (2024). Vitamin D and lipid profiles in infertile PCOS and Non-PCOS females. *Journal of the College of Physicians and Surgeons Pakistan. 34*(7), 767–770. https://doi.org/10.29271/jcpsp.2024.07.767, https://www.jcpsp.pk/article-detail/pvitamin-d-and-lipid-profiles-in-infertile-pcos-and-nonpcos-femalesorp.

Azhar, A., Naseem, Z., Haider, G., Farooqui, N., Farhat, S., & Rehman, R. (2022). PCOS model: Apoptotic changes and role of vitamin D. *Electronic Journal of General Medicine, 19*(5), em398. https://doi.org/10.29333/ejgm/12275.

Barbieri, R. L. (2019). *Female infertility yen & Jaffe's reproductive endocrinology: Physiology, pathophysiology, and clinical management: Eighth Edition.* United States: Elsevier Inc, 556. http://doi.org/10.1016/B978-0-323-47912-7.00022-6, http://www.sciencedirect.com/science/book/9780323479127.

Barrera, N., Omolaoye, T. S., & Du Plessis, S. S. (2022). A contemporary view on global fertility, infertility, and assisted reproductive techniques. In *Fertility, Pregnancy, and Wellness.* Uruguay: Elsevier, 93–120. http://doi.org/10.1016/B978-0-12-818309-0.00009-5, https://www.sciencedirect.com/book/9780128183090.

Benedik, E. (2022). Sources of vitamin D for humans. *International Journal for Vitamin and Nutrition Research, 92*(2), 118–125. https://doi.org/10.1024/0300-9831/a000733, https://econtent.hogrefe.com/loi/vit.

Bièche, I., Narjoz, C., Asselah, T., Vacher, S., Marcellin, P., Lidereau, R., Beaune, P., & De Waziers, I. (2007). Reverse transcriptase-PCR quantification of mRNA levels from cytochrome (CYP)1, CYP2 and CYP3 families in 22 different human tissues. *Pharmacogenetics and Genomics, 17*(9), 731–742. https://doi.org/10.1097/FPC.0b013e32810f2e58, http://journals.lww.com/jpharmacogenetics.

Calcaterra, V., Magenes, V. C., Massini, G., De Sanctis, L., Fabiano, V., & Zuccotti, G. (2024). High fat diet and polycystic ovary syndrome (PCOS) in adolescence: An overview of nutritional strategies. *Nutrients, 16*(7), 938. https://doi.org/10.3390/nu16070938.

Cheng, M., Song, Z., Guo, Y., Luo, X., Li, X., Wu, X., & Gong, Y. (2023). 1α,25-Dihydroxyvitamin D3 improves follicular development and steroid hormone biosynthesis by regulating vitamin D receptor in the layers model. *Current Issues in Molecular Biology, 45*(5), 4017–4034. https://doi.org/10.3390/cimb45050256.

Ciężki, S., Odyjewska, E., Bossowski, A., & Głowińska-Olszewska, B. (2024). Not only metabolic complications of childhood obesity. *Nutrients, 16*(4), 539. https://doi.org/10.3390/nu16040539.

Coccia, M. E., Nardone, L., & Rizzello, F. (2022). Endometriosis and infertility: A long-life approach to preserve reproductive integrity. *International Journal of Environmental Research and Public Health, 19*(10), 6162. https://doi.org/10.3390/ijerph19106162.

Cong, M., Wen, L., Han, F., Xu, Y., & Shi, Y. (2017). Alterations in cyclin D1 and cyclin-dependent kinase 4 expression in the amygdalae of post-traumatic stress disorder rats. *Molecular Medicine Reports, 16*(6), 8351–8358. https://doi.org/10.3892/mmr.2017.7613.

Deshpande, P., & Gupta, A. (2019). Causes and prevalence of factors causing infertility in a public health facility. *Journal of Human Reproductive Sciences, 12*(4), 287–293. https://doi.org/10.4103/jhrs.JHRS_140_18, http://www.jhrsonline.org.

Dewau, R., Mekonnen, F. A., & Seretew, W. S. (2021). Time to first birth and its predictors among reproductive-age women in Ethiopia: Inverse Weibull gamma shared frailty model. *BMC Women's Health, 21*(1). https://doi.org/10.1186/s12905-021-01254-z, http://www.biomedcentral.com/bmcwomenshealth/.

Farquhar, C. M., Bhattacharya, S., Repping, S., Mastenbroek, S., Kamath, M. S., Marjoribanks, J., & Boivin, J. (2019). Female subfertility. *Nature Reviews Disease Primers, 5*(1). https://doi.org/10.1038/s41572-018-0058-8, http://www.nature.com/nrdp/.

Feskens, E. J. M., Bailey, R., Bhutta, Z., Biesalski, H. K., Eicher-Miller, H., Krämer, K., Pan, W. H., & Griffiths, J. C. (2022). Women's health: Optimal nutrition throughout the lifecycle. *European Journal of Nutrition, 61*, 1–23. https://doi.org/10.1007/s00394-022-02915-x, https://www.springer.com/journal/394.

Gajanayake, C., Munasinghe, P. M., Kalubowila, K. C., Gunathilake, J., Denawaka, C., & Kahangamage, D. (2024). Sub-fertility and life style factors which affecting sub-fertility among women in Regional Director of Health Service area, Colombo. *Sri Lankan Journal of Medical Administration, 24*(2), 91–98. https://doi.org/10.4038/sljma.v24i2.5431.

Grzeczka, A., Graczyk, S., Skowronska, A., Skowronski, M. T., & Kordowitzki, P. (2022). Relevance of vitamin D and its deficiency for the ovarian follicle and the oocyte: An update. *Nutrients, 14*(18). https://doi.org/10.3390/nu14183712, http://www.mdpi.com/journal/nutrients/.

Gunawardhana, G. K., Godakandage, S., & Weerasinghe, M. (2024). Prevalence of primary and secondary subfertility and its associated factors in Regional Director of Health Services area in Colombo district Sri Lanka: A community-based cross-sectional study. *Ceylon Medical Journal, 68*(2), 52–60. https://doi.org/10.4038/cmj.v68i2.9732.

Harmon, Q. E., Kissell, K., Jukic, A. M. Z., Kim, K., Sjaarda, L., Perkins, N. J., Umbach, D. M., Schisterman, E. F., Baird, D. D., & Mumford, S. L. (2020). Vitamin D and reproductive hormones across the menstrual cycle. *Human Reproduction, 35*(2), 413–423. https://doi.org/10.1093/humrep/dez283.

Hong, S. H., Lee, J. E., An, S. M., Shin, Y. Y., Hwang, D. Y., Yang, S. Y., Cho, S. K., & An, B. S. (2017). Effect of vitamin d3 on biosynthesis of estrogen in porcine granulosa cells via modulation of steroidogenic enzymes. *Toxicological Research, 33*(1), 49–54. https://doi.org/10.5487/TR.2017.33.1.049, http://society.kisti.re.kr/sv/SV_svpsbs03V.do?method=download&cn1=JAKO201710758144178.

Kayani, A., Khan, R., Siddiqui, T. S., Rehman, A. U., Ahmed, R., & Khan, Y. (2024). Hysterosalpingographic pattern of primary sub-fertility and secondary sub-fertility in women of reproductive age. *Pakistan Armed Forces Medical Journal, 74*(5), 1251–1254. https://doi.org/10.51253/pafmj.v74i5.5394, https://www.pafmj.org/PAFMJ/article/download/5394/6484.

Kimmins, S., Anderson, R. A., Barratt, C. L. R., Behre, H. M., Catford, S. R., De Jonge, C. J., Delbes, G., Eisenberg, M. L., Garrido, N., Houston, B. J., Jørgensen, N., Krausz, C., Lismer, A., McLachlan, R. I., Minhas, S., Moss, T., Pacey, A., Priskorn, L., Schlatt, S., ... O'Bryan, M. K. (2024). Frequency, morbidity and equity—the case for increased research on male fertility. *Nature Reviews Urology, 21*(2), 102–124. https://doi.org/10.1038/s41585-023-00820-4, https://www.nature.com/nrurol/.

Lee, C. T., Wang, J. Y., Chou, K. Y., & Hsu, M. I. (2019). 1,25-Dihydroxyvitamin D 3 modulates the effects of sublethal BPA on mitochondrial function via activating PI3K-Akt pathway and 17β-estradiol secretion in rat granulosa cells. *Journal of Steroid Biochemistry and Molecular Biology, 185*, 200–211. https://doi.org/10.1016/j.jsbmb.2018.09.002, http://www.elsevier.com/locate/jsbmb.

Li, M., Hu, S., Sun, J., & Zhang, Y. (2024). The role of vitamin D3 in follicle development. *Journal of Ovarian Research, 17*(1). https://doi.org/10.1186/s13048-024-01454-9.

Ma, X., Wu, L., Wang, Y., Han, S., El-Dalatony, M. M., Feng, F., Tao, Z., Yu, L., & Wang, Y. (2022). Diet and human reproductive system: Insight of omics approaches. *Food Science and Nutrition, 10*(5), 1368–1384. https://doi.org/10.1002/fsn3.2708, onlinelibrary.wiley.com/journal/10.1002/%28ISSN%292048-7177.

Makieva, S., Reschini, M., Ferrari, S., Bonesi, F., Polledri, E., Fustinoni, S., Restelli, L., Sarais, V., Somigliana, E., & Viganò, P. (2021). Oral Vitamin D supplementation impacts gene expression in granulosa cells in women undergoing IVF. *Human Reproduction, 36*(1), 130–144. https://doi.org/10.1093/humrep/deaa262, http://humrep.oxfordjournals.org/.

Malhotra, J., Gouri Devi, M., & Patil, M. (2024). Best practice recommendations for infertility management. *Journal of Human Reproductive Sciences, 17*(1), S1. https://doi.org/10.4103/jhrs.JHRS_ISAR_IFS, http://www.jhrsonline.org.

Merhi, Z. (2019). Vitamin D attenuates the effect of advanced glycation end products on anti-Mullerian hormone signaling. *Molecular and Cellular Endocrinology, 479*, 87–92. https://doi.org/10.1016/j.mce.2018.09.004.

Merhi, Z., Doswell, A., Krebs, K., & Cipolla, M. (2014). Vitamin D alters genes involved in follicular development and steroidogenesis in human cumulus granulosa cells. *The Journal of Clinical Endocrinology & Metabolism, 99*(6), E1137. https://doi.org/10.1210/jc.2013-4161.

Mohan, A., Haider, R., Fakhor, H., Hina, F., Kumar, V., Jawed, A., Majumder, K., Ayaz, A., Mohan Lal, P., Tejwaney, U., Ram, N., & Kazeem, S. (2023). Vitamin D and polycystic ovary syndrome (PCOS): A review. *Annals of Medicine & Surgery, 85*(7), 3506–3511. https://doi.org/10.1097/ms9.0000000000000879.

Monaghan, P., Maklakov, A. A., & Metcalfe, N. B. (2020). Intergenerational transfer of ageing: Parental age and offspring lifespan. *Trends in Ecology and Evolution, 35*(10), 927–937. https://doi.org/10.1016/j.tree.2020.07.005, https://www.sciencedirect.com/journal/trends-in-ecology-and-evolution.

Mondal, R., Jaiswal, N., Bhave, P., & Mandal, P. (2024). Laparoscopic and hysteroscopic findings in women with sub-fertility and tuberculosis: A case series. *BJOG: An International Journal of Obstetrics & Gynaecology, 131*(7), 929–940. https://doi.org/10.1111/1471-0528.17701.

Moridi, I., Chen, A., Tal, O., & Tal, R. (2020). The association between vitamin D and Anti-Müllerian hormone: A systematic review and meta-analysis. *Nutrients, 12*(6), 1567. https://doi.org/10.3390/nu12061567.

Parikh, G., Varadinova, M., Suwandhi, P., Araki, T., Rosenwaks, Z., Poretsky, L., & Seto-Young, D. (2010). Vitamin D regulates steroidogenesis and insulin-like growth factor binding protein-1 (IGFBP-1) production in human ovarian cells. *Hormone and Metabolic Research, 42*(10), 754–757. https://doi.org/10.1055/s-0030-1262837.

Pejovic, T., Joshi, S., Campbell, S., Thisted, S., Xu, F., & Xu, J. (2020). Association between vitamin D and ovarian cancer development in BRCA1 mutation carriers. *Oncotarget, 11*(45), 4104–4114. https://doi.org/10.18632/oncotarget.27803.

Safaei, Z., Bakhshalizadeh, S., Nasr-Esfahani, M. H., Akbari Sene, A., Najafzadeh, V., Soleimani, M., & Shirazi, R. (2020). Vitamin D3 affects mitochondrial biogenesis through mitogen-activated protein kinase in polycystic ovary syndrome mouse model. *Journal of Cellular Physiology, 235*(9), 6113–6126. https://doi.org/10.1002/jcp.29540, http://onlinelibrary.wiley.com/journal/10.1002/(ISSN)1097-4652.

Sharma, A., & Shrivastava, D. (2022). Psychological problems related to infertility. *Cureus, 14*(10). https://doi.org/10.7759/cureus.30320.

Shukla, S., & Shrivastava, D. (2024). Nutritional deficiencies and subfertility: A comprehensive review of current evidence. *Cureus, 16*(8). https://doi.org/10.7759/cureus.66477.

Stensen, M. H., Tanbo, T., Storeng, R., & Fedorcsak, P. (2014). Advanced glycation end products and their receptor contribute to ovarian ageing. *Human Reproduction, 29*(1), 125–134. https://doi.org/10.1093/humrep/det419, http://humrep.oxfordjournals.org/.

Wu, L., Kwak-Kim, J., Zhang, R., Li, Q., Lu, F. T., Zhang, Y., Wang, H. Y., Zhong, L. W., & Liu, Y. S. (2018). Vitamin D level affects IVF outcome partially mediated via Th/Tc cell ratio. *American Journal of Reproductive Immunology, 80*(6). http://doi.org/10.1111/aji.13050, http://onlinelibrary.wiley.com/journal/10.1111/(ISSN)1600-0897.

Xie, Y., Ren, Y., Niu, C., Zheng, Y., Yu, P., & Li, L. (2023). The impact of stigma on mental health and quality of life of infertile women: A systematic review. *Frontiers in Psychology, 13*. https://doi.org/10.3389/fpsyg.2022.1093459.

Xu, F., Wolf, S., Green, O., & Xu, J. (2021). Vitamin D in follicular development and oocyte maturation. *Reproduction (Cambridge, England), 161*(6), R129. https://doi.org/10.1530/rep-20-0608.

CHAPTER 17

Vitamin D and male reproductive health: complex interplay in male fertility

Rashida Sultana[1], and Sofia Amjad[2]

[1]*Department of Obstetrics and Gynaecology, Azra Naheed Medical College, Faculty of Medical Sciences, The Superior University, Lahore, Punjab, Pakistan* [2]*Department of Physiology, Faculty of Medical Sciences, Azra Naheed Medical College, The Superior University, Lahore, Pakistan*

17.1 Introduction

Male infertility accounts for 50% of cases of infertility, which affects 8%–12% of noncontracepting couples globally (Agarwal et al., 2021). Its etiology includes disorders of the "hypothalamic–pituitary–gonadal axis" (HPG), genetic, environmental, psychological, lifestyle factors, and structural abnormalities of the "male reproductive tract." Even in the era of modern reproductive medicine, a significant percentage of male infertility remains idiopathic. So, structural and functional optimization of the "male reproductive system" provides the basis for fertility outcomes (Balen, 2022). Research has suggested that adequate vitamin D (Vit.D) levels are essential for male fertility, as a deficiency in Vit.D negatively affects semen quality and hormone function in animals and humans (Cito et al., 2020).

17.2 Physiology of spermatogenesis

"Spermatogenesis" is the process that produces male gametes in the seminiferous tubules. This process occurs in a specialized testicular environment, where developing sperm closely interact with accessory cells to support their maturation. It includes spermatogonial mitosis, spermatocyte meiosis, and spermiogenesis (Wang et al., 2019). Stem cells form spermatogonia, which increase in number during puberty and develop into primary spermatocytes. Primary spermatocytes form spermatids through meiosis. Spermatids undergo spermiogenesis and form "mature spermatozoa" (Moore et al., 2018). Spermatogenesis takes 64–72 days. "Mature spermatozoa are released into the seminiferous tubules by the process of Spermiation" (Griswold, 2016).

The Impact of Vitamin D on Health and Disease. DOI: https://doi.org/10.1016/B978-0-443-34037-6.00021-2

"Follicle-stimulating hormone" (FSH), "luteinizing hormone" (LH), and "testosterone" play a vital role in sperm production. This process is regulated by the HPG axis. The hypothalamus produces gonadotropin-releasing hormone that stimulates the anterior pituitary gland to release FSH and LH. FSH accelerates sperm development, while LH increases testosterone to facilitate sperm production. Additionally, testosterone promotes the growth of male secondary sexual characteristics (Nishimura & Hernault, 2017). Thus, the "male reproductive system" is an integrated pathway for sperm production, maturation, and transport (Dwyer & Quinton, 2019).

17.3   Role of vitamin D in male reproductive system

17.3.1   Vitamin D and male reproductive cell biology

Several factors, such as age, hormone levels, nutrition, and lifestyle choices, including stimulants and medications, affect male reproductive function (Sharma et al., 2013). Maintaining a balance of hormones and vitamins is essential for supporting reproductive health. Vit.D significantly contributes to the male reproductive system with endocrine, autocrine, and paracrine functions. Vit.D mediates these functions through both genomic and nongenomic actions (Kochupillai, 2008). Receptors for Vit.D and enzymes for its metabolism are present in the "male reproductive system," with the highest expression in the seminal vesicle and epididymis (Boisen et al., 2018). The biologically active form of Vit.D, "125 dihydroxy vitamin D" (calcitriol), binds to "vitamin D receptors" (VDR). VDR, a nuclear receptor, forms a "heterodimer with the retinoid X receptor," which then binds to "Vitamin D response elements" (VDRE) in DNA, thereby modulating the transcription of target genes (Rochel, 2022). This modulation regulates gene expression in cellular proliferation, differentiation, programmed cell death, and inflammatory responses in the male reproductive tract (Dutta et al., 2021).

17.3.2   Vitamin D and metabolizing enzymes

The male reproductive system shows a diverse expression of Vit.D messenger RNA and metabolizing enzymes. Significant expression of Vit.D activating enzymes such as "CYP2R1" and "CYP27B1" and minor expressions of Vit.D inactivating enzymes like "CYP24A1" have been identified in testes, seminal vesicles, and prostate (Blomberg Jensen et al., 2010).

17.3.3   Vitamin D and immunity

Vit.D maintains a balanced immune response by downregulating "proinflammatory cytokines" and upregulating "antiinflammatory cytokines" for germ cell protection (Keane et al., 2017). It also helps maintain the integrity of the blood-testis barrier through tight cellular junctions. Vit.D reduces the expression of inflammatory cytokines and promotes interleukin 10 (1L-10) in the prostate, leading to a balanced immune response. Vit.D also enhances the gene expression for antimicrobial peptides such as "cathelicidin," leading to a strengthened defense system against infection (Chung et al., 2020). Vit.D is also essential in controlling cell proliferation and programmed cell death to maintain tissue growth and eliminate damaged cells (Uberti et al., 2014).

17.3.4 Vitamin D and spermatogenesis

Blomberg Jensen et al. (2010) found VDR expression at the postacrosomal part, neck, and mid-piece of spermatozoa, suggesting a probable role of Vit.D in sperm production and maturation. In adult testes, germ cells like spermatogonia, spermatocytes, and spermatids exhibit VDRs and metabolizing enzymes, indicating the necessity of Vit.D in sperm production and function. The VDR expression in Sertoli cells indicates its role in spermatogenesis as Sertoli cells nourish and support the development of sperm (Adamczewska et al., 2023).

17.3.5 Vitamin D and sperm quality

Sperm quality is a crucial indicator of fertility potential. Sperm quality refers to its motility and morphology, both essential for fertilization (García-Vázquez et al., 2016). Vit.D is vital in calcium homeostasis, regulating intracellular signaling in Sertoli and sperm cells. "Calcium signaling pathways" facilitate sperm motility (Yahyavi et al., 2024). Calcium influx promotes an acrosomal reaction, which is necessary for ovum penetration during the process of fertilization (Beigi Harchegani et al., 2019). Vit.D influences sperm motility and metabolism, affecting their ability to undergo the acrosome reaction and fertilize the ovum (Keane et al., 2017). Vit.D facilitates capacitation and enhances acrosome reaction by regulating "tyrosine kinase" and "protein phosphorylation," which are responsible for high-amplitude and asymmetrical flagellar movements (Morris, 2014).

Jueraitetibaike et al. evaluated the impact of Vit.D on the kinetic characteristics of sperm and found that it increases ATP production and sperm motility. Increased ATP production raises the level of intracellular calcium ions, resulting in improved sperm motility. Thus, activated Vit.D augments the motility parameters by enhancing ATP production and promoting better utilization of these energy resources (Jueraitetibaike et al., 2019). Moreover, Vit.D regulates cell cycle progression by balancing proapoptotic and antiapoptotic factors, which is beneficial for healthy spermatozoa (Dwivedi et al., 2024).

17.3.6 Vitamin D and testosterone synthesis

Vit.D participates in testosterone production directly and indirectly, improving sperm quality. When it binds with VDR in the Leydig cell, the biologically active form of Vit.D affects gene transcription and increases testosterone production. Vit.D regulates the expression of "Steroidogenic Acute Regulatory Protein" (StARP), "3β-hydroxysteroid dehydrogenase," and "cytochrome p450 enzymes" in Leydig cells, indirectly increasing testosterone biosynthesis (Manna et al., 2016). Vit.D plays a role in androgen receptor signaling, enhances their expression, and positively impacts testosterone-mediated responses. The role of Vit.D in calcium homeostasis also activates enzymes necessary for testosterone synthesis (Blomberg Jensen, 2012).

17.3.7 Vitamin D and oxidative stress

Spermatozoa are susceptible to oxidative stress due to their naturally limited antioxidant defense and DNA repair mechanisms (Shahid et al., 2021). Vit.D possesses antioxidant properties that reduce oxidative stress (OS) in sperm cells by enhancing oxidative stress management. Vit.D thereby safeguards macromolecules like deoxyribonucleic acid (DNA) from oxidative damage, prevents fatty acid peroxidation in cell membranes, and upholds the stability and integrity of plasma membranes. By enhancing the stability of sperm cell membranes, Vit.D improves sperm motility and the acrosomal reaction. Thus, Vit.D deficiency impairs the motility and fertilizing potential of sperm, contributing to male factor infertility (Maghsoumi-Norouzabad et al., 2022). Additionally, Vit.D boosts the expression of antioxidant enzymes such as "superoxide dismutase" and "glutathione peroxidase" while also reducing levels of reactive oxygen species (ROS) (Mokhtari et al., 2016).

17.4 Vitamin D deficiency and male factor infertility

Vit.D plays both direct and indirect roles in male reproductive health. It directly influences sperm production and maturation, and indirectly regulates testosterone levels, while also reducing oxidative stress. Thus, maintaining adequate Vit.D levels may enhance male reproductive health and support fertility by regulating testicular function. Vit.D has significant participation in initiating "spermatozoa maturation" and the "acrosomal reaction" (Wadhwa et al., 2020). Vit.D also has a role in the HPG axis as VDR and Vit.D metabolizing enzymes are found in the hypothalamus and pituitary gland (Ajdžanović et al., 2024).

Vit.D deficiency negatively affects sperm quality, thus impairing fertilizing capacity. Furthermore, animal studies have shown DNA fragmentation (Shahreza et al., 2020). Structural alterations of the epididymis have been reported in moderate to severe Vit.D deficiency, which adversely affects sperm maturation and motility. Males with Vit,D deficiency exhibit reduced sperm counts, impaired Sertoli cells, few Leydig cells, and degeneration in the reproductive tissues (Adamczewska et al., 2023). Spermatogenesis in rats with Vit.D deficiency exhibited lower "testicular glutamyl transpeptidase activity," indicating reduced Sertoli cell function. The histological analysis of testicular tissue of rats revealed a profound decrease in Leydig cells and "degenerative changes" in the germinal epithelium, highlighting its role in testicular functioning (Wadhwa et al., 2020). This modulation of serum testosterone in moderate to severe Vit.D deficiency leads to impaired spermatogenesis and loss of libido (Karim et al., 2021). Even infertile men with Vit.D deficiency have also experienced a higher rate of pregnancy loss (Banks et al., 2021).

17.5 Role of vitamin D in the treatment of male infertility

Male infertility is a global issue affecting the quality of life for both members of the infertile couple. It needs to be addressed in terms of prevention and treatment. Considering Vit.D as a significant cause of male infertility, we can proceed with targeted medical therapy in terms of Vit.D supplementation. Even the patients opting for the alternative plan of assisted reproductive technology (ART) as a treatment option can be facilitated (Amjad & Rehman, 2021). Literature reveals Vit.D supplementation is a targeted medical therapy that leads to measurable improvement in semen volume, sperm concentration, sperm motility, and spontaneous pregnancy rates (Blomberg Jensen et al., 2018; Cito et al., 2020). Vit.D supplements have shown improvement in sperm motility, particularly progressive motility in infertile men with vitamin D deficiency, with no significant effect on testosterone levels (Calagna et al., 2022; Maghsoumi-Norouzabad et al., 2022) (Fig. 17.1). Overall, improvements in sperm quality may result in better outcomes in ART (Amjad et al., 2021).Thus this reveals that adequate Vit.D levels have enhanced fertility outcomes in infertile male candidates for "Intra-Cytoplasmic Sperm Insemination" (Chen & Zhi, 2020).

17.6 Future recommendations

Vit.D functions as a regulator in men's reproductive health, as evidenced by "VDR gene expression" and "Vit.D metabolizing enzymes" in the male reproductive system. However, heterogeneity in Vit.D deficiency and fertility outcomes indicates potential genetic variations. This complex interplay between Vit.D and male reproductive health provides grounds for further research addressing all aspects in detail for an integrated understanding of its impact on male fertility regarding clinical significance and therapeutic potential. Limitations of the available data include the observational research design, the small sample size, and short follow-up. Conducting large triple-blinded randomized controlled trials to evaluate the multilayered role of Vit.D in male infertility, particularly addressing its genetic variation and interaction with other causes of fertility, may support existing data.

As Vit.D directly and indirectly influences male reproductive health, investigating serum 25 (OH) D levels can give insight into male fertility status and reproductive health. Early identification, monitoring, and optimization of Vit.D levels may improve overall reproductive health for men with Vit.D deficiency (Fig.17.1).

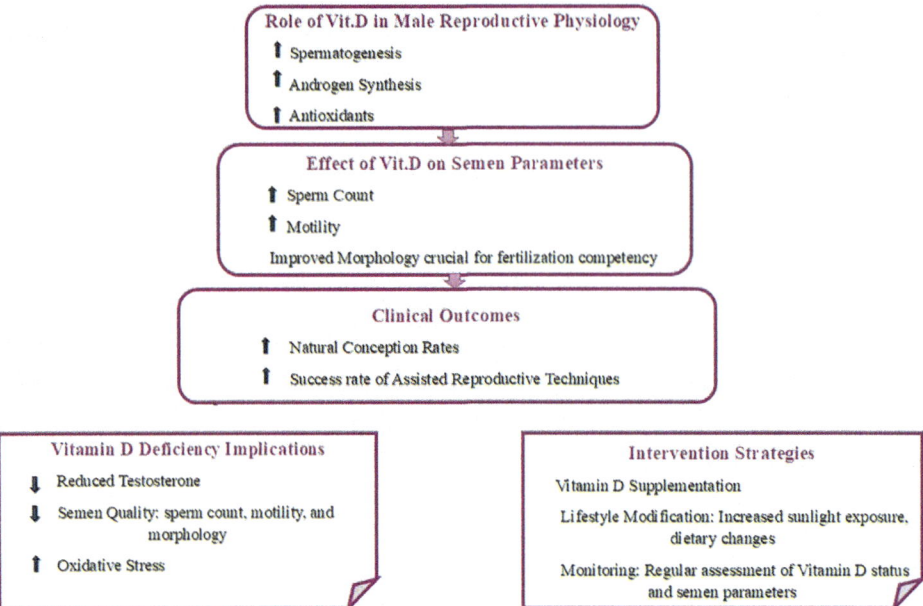

Figure 17.1
Mechanistic role of vitamin D in male infertility.

17.7   Conclusion

Recognizing "VDR expression" and "Vit.D metabolizing enzymes" in male reproductive organs suggests their potential role in reproductive health. Vit.D influences semen quality through both genomic and non-genomic mechanisms. Its comprehensive role in male reproductive health includes effects on hormonal regulation, spermatogenesis, sperm molecular and kinetic parameters, and modulation of reactive oxygen species (Fig. 17.1). This physiological and biological significance highlights the need for research into the various aspects of male reproduction. The heterogeneity in the results of multiple studies on the role of Vit.D in male reproductive health is challenging. Researchers need to consider the dose and duration of Vit.D Supplementation.

AI disclosure

During the preparation of this work, the authors used Grammarly Premium in order to get help in the grammar. After using this tool/service, the authors reviewed and edited the content as needed and take full responsibility for the content of the publication.

References

Adamczewska, D., Słowikowska-Hilczer, J., & Walczak-Jędrzejowska, R. (2023). The association between vitamin D and the components of male fertility: A systematic review. *Biomedicines, 11*(1), 90. https://doi.org/10.3390/biomedicines11010090.

Agarwal, A., Baskaran, S., Parekh, N., Cho, C. L., Henkel, R., Vij, S., Arafa, M., Panner Selvam, M. K., & Shah, R. (2021). Male infertility. *The Lancet, 397*(10271), 319–333. https://doi.org/10.1016/S0140-6736(20)32667-2, http://www.journals.elsevier.com/the-lancet/.

Ajdžanović, V., Šošić-Jurjević, B., Živanović, J., Miler, M., Stanković, S., Ranin, J., & Filipović, B. (2024). Vitamin D3 application and factors of its activity in the adrenal cortex of andropausal rats: A functionally-histological study. *Annals of Anatomy - Anatomischer Anzeiger, 256*, 152322. https://doi.org/10.1016/j.aanat.2024.152322.

Amjad, S., Mushtaq, S., Rehman, R., Munir, A., Zahid, N., & Siddique, P. Q. R. (2021). Protamine 1/Protamine 2 mRNA ratio in nonobstructive azoospermic patients. *Andrologia, 53*(3). https://doi.org/10.1111/and.13936, http://onlinelibrary.wiley.com/journal/10.1111/(ISSN)1439-0272.

Amjad, S., & Rehman, R. (2021). Assisted reproductive techniques. *Subfertility,* 185–197.

Balen, A. (2022). *Infertility in practice.* CRC Press. http://doi.org/10.1201/9781003094951.

Banks, N., Sun, F., Krawetz, S. A., Coward, R. M., Masson, P., Smith, J. F., Trussell, J. C., Santoro, N., Zhang, H., & Steiner, A. Z. (2021). Male vitamin D status and male factor infertility. *Fertility and Sterility, 116*(4), 973–979. https://doi.org/10.1016/j.fertnstert.2021.06.035, www.elsevier.com/locate/fertnstert.

Beigi Harchegani, A., Irandoost, A., Mirnamniha, M., Rahmani, H., Tahmasbpour, E., & Shahriary, A. (2019). Possible mechanisms for the effects of calcium deficiency on male infertility. *International Journal of Fertility and Sterility, 12*(4), 267–272. https://doi.org/10.22074/ijfs.2019.5420, http://ijfs.ir/journal/article/12894/download.

Blomberg Jensen, M. (2012). Vitamin D metabolism, sex hormones, and male reproductive function. *Reproduction (Cambridge, England), 144*(2), 135–152. https://doi.org/10.1530/rep-12-0064.

Blomberg Jensen, M., Lawaetz, J. G., Petersen, J. H., Juul, A., & Jørgensen, N. (2018). Effects of Vitamin D supplementation on semen quality, reproductive hormones, and live birth rate: A randomized clinical trial. *The Journal of Clinical Endocrinology & Metabolism, 103*(3), 870–881. https://doi.org/10.1210/jc.2017-01656.

Blomberg Jensen, M., Nielsen, J. E., Jørgensen, A., Rajpert-De Meyts, E., Kristensen, D. M., Jørgensen, N., Skakkebaek, N. E., Juul, A., & Leffers, H. (2010). Vitamin D receptor and vitamin D metabolizing enzymes are expressed in the human male reproductive tract. *Human Reproduction, 25*(5), 1303–1311. https://doi.org/10.1093/humrep/deq024, http://humrep.oxfordjournals.org/.

Boisen, I. M., Hansen, L. B., Mortensen, L. J., & Jensen, M. B. (2018). Vitamin D, reproductive biology, and dysfunction in men. *Vitamin D: Fourth Edition. 1*, 797–824. https://doi.org/10.1016/B978-0-12-809965-0.00044-6, http://www.sciencedirect.com/science/book/9780128099650.

Calagna, G., Catinella, V., Polito, S., Schiattarella, A., De Franciscis, P., D'Antonio, F., Calì, G., Perino, A., & Cucinella, G. (2022). Vitamin D and male reproduction: Updated evidence based on literature review. *Nutrients, 14*(16), 3278. https://doi.org/10.3390/nu14163278.

Chen, Y., & Zhi, X. (2020). Roles of vitamin D in reproductive systems and assisted reproductive technology. *Endocrinology, 161*(4). https://doi.org/10.1210/endocr/bqaa023.

Chung, C., Silwal, P., Kim, I., Modlin, R. L., & Jo, E. K. (2020). Vitamin D-cathelicidin axis: At the crossroads between protective immunity and pathological inflammation during infection. *Immune Network, 20*(2). https://doi.org/10.4110/in.2020.20.e12, http://www.immunenetwork.org/Synapse/Data/PDFData/0078IN/in-20-e12.pdf.

Cito, G., Cocci, A., Micelli, E., Gabutti, A., Russo, G. I., Coccia, M. E., Franco, G., Serni, S., Carini, M., & Natali, A. (2020). Vitamin D and male fertility: An updated review. *World Journal of Men's Health, 38*(2), 164–177. https://doi.org/10.5534/wjmh.190057, https://wjmh.org/Synapse/Data/PDFData/2074WJMH/wjmh-38-164.pdf.

Dutta, S., Sengupta, P., Slama, P., & Roychoudhury, S. (2021). Oxidative stress, testicular inflammatory pathways, and male reproduction. *International Journal of Molecular Sciences, 22*(18), 10043. https://doi.org/10.3390/ijms221810043.

Dwivedi, S., Singh, V., Sen, A., Yadav, D., Agrawal, R., Kishore, S., Misra, S., & Sharma, P. (2024). Vitamin D in disease prevention and cure-part I: An update on molecular mechanism and significance on human health. *Indian Journal of Clinical Biochemistry.* https://doi.org/10.1007/s12291-024-01251-7, https://www.springer.com/journal/12291.

Dwyer, A. A., & Quinton, R. (2019). Anatomy and physiology of the hypothalamic-pituitary-gonadal (HPG) axis. In *Advanced practice in endocrinology nursing.* United States: Springer International Publishing, 839–852. http://doi.org/10.1007/978-3-319-99817-6_43, https://link.springer.com/book/10.1007/978-3-319-99817-6.

García-Vázquez, F., Gadea, J., Matás, C., & Holt, W. (2016). Importance of sperm morphology during sperm transport and fertilization in mammals. *Asian Journal of Andrology, 18*(6), 844–850. https://doi.org/10.4103/1008-682X.186880, http://www.ajandrology.com/backissues.asp.

Griswold, M. D. (2016). Spermatogenesis: The commitment to Meiosis. *Physiological Reviews, 96*(1), 1–17. https://doi.org/10.1152/physrev.00013.2015, http://physrev.physiology.org/content/96/1/1.full.pdf.

Jueraitetibaike, K., Ding, Z., Wang, D. D., Peng, L. P., Jing, J., Chen, L., Ge, X., Qiu, X. H., & Yao, B. (2019). The effect of Vitamin D on sperm motility and the underlying mechanism. *Asian Journal of Andrology, 21*(4), 400–407. https://doi.org/10.4103/aja.aja_105_18, http://www.ajandrology.com/backissues.asp.

Karim, D. H., Mohammed, S. M., & Azeez, H. A. (2021). Impact of vitamin D3 Nanoemulsion on spermatogenesis and antioxidant enzymes in Vitamin D deficient induced albino male rats. *Zanco Journal of Pure and Applied Sciences, 33*(1), 55–67. https://doi.org/10.21271/ZJPAS.33.1.7, https://zancojournal.su.edu.krd/index.php/JPAS/article/download/1847/799.

Keane, K. N., Cruzat, V. F., Calton, E. K., Hart, P. H., Soares, M. J., Newsholme, P., & Yovich, J. L. (2017). Molecular actions of Vitamin D in reproductive cell biology. *Reproduction (Cambridge, England), 153*(1), R29. https://doi.org/10.1530/REP-16-0386, http://www.reproduction-online.org/content/153/1/R29.full.pdf+html.

Kochupillai, N. (2008). The physiology of vitamin D: Current concepts. *Indian Journal of Medical Research, 127*(3), 256–262. http://icmr.nic.in/ijmr/2008/march/0307.pdf.

Maghsoumi-Norouzabad, L., Javid, A. Z., Mansoori, A., Dadfar, M., & Serajian, A. (2022). Vitamin D3 supplementation effects on spermatogram and oxidative stress biomarkers in asthenozoospermia infertile men: A Randomized, triple-blind, placebo-controlled clinical trial. *Reproductive Sciences, 29*(3), 823–835. https://doi.org/10.1007/s43032-021-00769-y.

Manna, P. R., Stetson, C. L., Slominski, A. T., & Pruitt, K. (2016). Role of the steroidogenic acute regulatory protein in health and disease. *Endocrine, 51*(1), 7–21. https://doi.org/10.1007/s12020-015-0715-6, http://www.springer.com/humana+press/journal/12020.

Mokhtari, Z., Hekmatdoost, A., & Nourian, M. (2016). Antioxidant efficacy of vitamin D. *Journal of Parathyroid Disease. 5,* 11–16.

Moore, K. L., Persaud, T. V. N., & Torchia, M. G. (2018). *The developing human-E-book: The developing human-E-book.* Elsevier Health Sciences.

Morris, J. T. (2014). *The role of calcium stores in calcium signalling in human sperm.*

Nishimura, H., & Hernault, S. W. (2017). Spermatogenesis. *Current Biology, 27*(18).

Rochel, N. (2022). Vitamin D and its receptor from a structural perspective. *Nutrients, 14*(14), 2847. https://doi.org/10.3390/nu14142847.

Shahid, M., Khan, S., Ashraf, M., Mudassir, H. A., & Rehman, R. (2021). Male infertility: Role of vitamin D and oxidative stress markers. *Andrologia, 53*(8). https://doi.org/10.1111/and.14147.

Shahreza, F. D., Hajian, M., Gharagozloo, P., Drevet, J. R., & Nasr-Esfahani, M. H. (2020). Impact of vitamin D deficiency on mouse sperm structure and function. *Andrology, 8*(5), 1442–1455. https://doi.org/10.1111/andr.12820, http://onlinelibrary.wiley.com/journal/10.1111/(ISSN)2047-2927.

Sharma, R., Biedenharn, K. R., Fedor, J. M., & Agarwal, A. (2013). Lifestyle factors and reproductive health: Taking control of your fertility. *Reproductive Biology and Endocrinology, 11*(1). https://doi.org/10.1186/1477-7827-11-66, http://www.rbej.com/content/11/1/66.

Uberti, F., Lattuada, D., Morsanuto, V., Nava, U., Bolis, G., Vacca, G., Squarzanti, D. F., Cisari, C., & Molinari, C. (2014). Vitamin D protects human endothelial cells from oxidative stress through the autophagic and survival pathways. *The Journal of Clinical Endocrinology & Metabolism, 99*(4), 1367–1374. https://doi.org/10.1210/jc.2013-2103.

Wadhwa, L., Priyadarshini, S., Fauzdar, A., Wadhwa, S. N., & Arora, S. (2020). Impact of vitamin D supplementation on semen quality in vitamin D-deficient infertile males with oligoasthenozoospermia. *Journal of Obstetrics and Gynecology of India, 70*(1), 44–49. https://doi.org/10.1007/s13224-019-01251-1, http://medind.nic.in/jaq/jaqm.shtml.

Wang, T., Gao, H., Li, W., & Liu, C. (2019). Essential role of histone replacement and modifications in male fertility. *Frontiers in Genetics, 10.* https://doi.org/10.3389/fgene.2019.00962.

Yahyavi, S. K., Boisen, I. M., Cui, Z., Jorsal, M. J., Kooij, I., Holt, R., Juul, A., & Blomberg Jensen, M. (2024). Calcium and vitamin D homoeostasis in male fertility. *Proceedings of the Nutrition Society, 83*(2), 95–108. https://doi.org/10.1017/S002966512300486X, http://journals.cambridge.org/PNS.

CHAPTER 18

Vitamin D and cancer

Ya Chee Lim[1], Khalid Ahmed[2], and Siti Rohaiza Ahmad[1]

[1]PAPRSB Institute of Health Sciences, Universiti Brunei Darussalam, Bandar Seri Begawan, Brunei-Muara, Brunei [2]Department of Biological & Biomedical Sciences, Aga Khan University, Karachi, Pakistan

18.1 Vitamin D and cancers

In 2024, around 2 million cancer cases and 600,000 cancer related deaths were projected (Siegel et al., 2024). Lifestyle factors, such as diet, physical activity, and smoking habits, affect cancer risk. Low vitamin D levels are associated with breast, colon, and prostate cancer risk (Carlberg & Muñoz, 2022). The relationship between vitamin D and breast cancer has been extensively explored in recent years. The role of vitamin D in influencing the risk, progression, and prognosis of breast cancer is being explored. Many studies aimed to elucidate the role of vitamin D in both the prevention of breast cancer and in the potential treatment of the disease have been conducted. In this chapter, we will look into the relationship between vitamin D levels and various cancers.

18.2 Breast cancer risk and its association to vitamin D

Breast cancer affects millions of women per year, making it one of the most prevalent cancers globally. Although there have been significant improvements in early detection, prevention, and treatment, incidences of breast cancer continue to rise. Recently, there has been evidence that vitamin D decreases the risk of breast cancer, slows down tumor growth, and improves patients' outcomes.

A meta analysis of five studies concluded that higher vitamin D levels in blood at the time of diagnosis are correlated with better survival outcomes of breast cancer patients. Approximately 50% lower death rate from breast cancer for those in the highest quartile of vitamin D levels compared to those in the lowest quartile was observed (Mohr et al., 2014). Mohr et al. (2014) suggest that vitamin D levels in the blood of breast cancer patients to be raised to the normal range of 30 to 80 ng/mL. This study therefore supported the hypothesis that vitamin D deficiency may contribute to breast cancer development.

The Impact of Vitamin D on Health and Disease. DOI: https://doi.org/10.1016/B978-0-443-34037-6.00029-7

In a dose response meta analysis of 50 studies on vitamin D levels in blood and 20 studies of vitamin D intake, a 5 nmol/L rise in serum vitamin D level equates 6% drop in breast cancer risk. Within the same research initiative, the team found that this association is limited only to breast cancer risk and vitamin D level in serum. There was no significant association between vitamin D intake and breast cancer risk.

An umbrella review of 17 meta-analyses investigated the BsmI, Cdx2, and poly(A) polymorphisms of the vitamin D receptor (VDR) gene among 119 datasets. The results were mixed, garnering the conclusion that these VDR polymorphisms are not strongly associated with breast cancer risk in general. An earlier study conducted in Taiwan, nevertheless, studied ApaI, TaqI, and BsmI polymorphisms in the 3' end of the VDR gene and their associations with breast cancer risk. The findings were that there was an increasing risk for increased numbers of BsmI B alleles and ApaI AA genotypes, while there was no association observed for TaqI polymorphism. In another study by Huss et al. (2024), whereby immunohistochemistry of 878 Swedish breast cancer tumor samples was analyzed, reported increased VDR staining was observed with better cancer free interval and more positive tumor features. This report suggested that VDR may be a prognostic marker for breast cancer diagnosis.

Five year integrative literature review by Torres et al. (2024) with statistical analyses deduced that serum levels of vitamin D ≥ 40.26 ng/mL ± 14.19 ng/mL may have a protective effect against breast cancer. In a systematic review and meta-analysis of 25 studies by calculated the mean level of vitamin D in patients with breast cancer to be 26.88 ng/mL, while the mean level of vitamin D in controls was 31.41 ng/mL. 67% of breast cancer patients had serum vitamin D levels less than 30 ng/mL, while this only occurred in 34% of controls, illustrating the plausible pathophysiological causative association of vitamin D insufficiency and breast cancer (Voutsadakis, 2021).

A 2021 research article by Li et al. reported that vitamin D affects the epithelial to mesenchymal transition of cancer cells via interacting with chemokine CXC motif chemokine 12 (CXCL12) and its receptor CXC chemokine receptor type 4 (CXCR4). Replenishment of vitamin D reduces the invasiveness of tumor cells and increases CXCL12/CXCR4 colocalization by two and a half times. Therefore, this suggests supplementing cancer patients' diet with vitamin D to slow down the invasiveness of cancer cells and the growth of tumor cells. The presence of VDR is needed for the correct functioning of vitamin D to hinder the migration of cancer cells. This is supported by the work of Horas et al. (2019), which demonstrated that VDR knockdown increases the metastatic potential of MDA-MB-231 human breast cancer cells to bone.

18.3   Colorectal cancer risk and its association with vitamin D

Hypovitaminosis D is associated with various illnesses, as vitamin D plays antiinflammatory, antiangiogenic, and immunomodulatory roles in the human body. Colorectal cancer (CRC) is the third leading cause of cancer deaths in the United States and the second leading cancer-related death globally. Although advancements in treatment and screening in colorectal cancer have improved survival rates, there has been a rise in incidences of early onset CRC (Peixoto et al., 2022). The serum vitamin D levels of 257 colorectal cancer patients in Japan were measured at the time of surgery. Better survival rates were observed among colorectal cancer patients with higher serum vitamin D levels (Mezawa et al., 2010). In a further study, the blood plasma vitamin D levels of 515 stage IV colorectal cancer patients were quantified. Overall, 82% of the patients had vitamin D insufficiency, with 50% of them being vitamin D deficient, further emphasizing that vitamin D deficiency is actually prevalent within stage IV colorectal cancer patients. A meta-analysis of 11 original studies consisting of 7718 CRC patients from both PubMed and Web of Science databases illustrated that a linear correlation between vitamin D level in blood plasma and better CRC specific and overall survival outcomes for CRC patients, emphasizing the need for vitamin D supplementation for CRC (Maalmi et al., 2018). A recent systematic review investigated the impact of prechemotherapy plasma vitamin D level exert on the time to outcome of metastatic colorectal cancer patients. The overall survival shows 47% increased mortality risk for 1712 patients, while progression-free survival accounts for 38% increased risk of progression for 1264 patients with lower vitamin D levels (Ottaiano et al., 2024). In a publication by the Journal of the National Cancer Institute, McCullough et al. (2019) pooled 17 international cohorts involving 5706 colorectal cancer patients and 7107 control participants. The investigations demonstrated that individual with less than 30 nmol/L vitamin D blood level was associated with 31% higher colorectal cancer risk, while individuals with vitamin D levels between 75 and 87.5 nmol/L and between 87.5 and 100 nmol/L were associated with 19% and 27% lower risks of CRC, respectively. There is, however, no statistical significance in colorectal cancer risk reduction with blood vitamin D levels of 100 nmol/L and higher (McCullough et al., 2019).

In an evaluation of the association between vitamin D serum levels and CRC risks from 403 170 UK Biobank Project participants, there has been no significant association between the polymorphisms rs4588 or rs7041of vitamin D binding protein, as well as rs11568820, rs2228570 and rs1544410 of vitamin D receptor, and vitamin D circulating levels in blood. An earlier study showed the association of better absorption of vitamin D with the mutant ApaI A allele as compared to ApaI aa carriers with lower vitamin D intake and so, lower colorectal cancer risk. Other polymorphisms, such as FokI, BsmI, and Taq1 of VDR, did not indicate any association with calcium or vitamin D intake, and therefore, no association with colorectal cancer risk was found.

Recently, *Carnobacterium maltaromaticum* has been found to disminished intestinal tumor formation in two female CRC mice models. The action of this bacterium is gender specific as it requires estrogen to enable the bacterium to attach and colonise. Female mice being fed with *C. maltaromaticum* illustrated abundant vitamin D related metabolites. It is therefore hypothesized that *C. maltaromaticum* interacts with other microbes to enhance vitamin D production via activation of VDR, resulting in curbing of CRC tumors (Li et al., 2023).

18.4 Mechanisms influencing cancer development

Epidemiological studies and experimental investigations have reported that the risk of cancer development is affected by vitamin D, for instance, it has been shown that vitamin D may be associated with the prevention of cancer development as it decreases tumor progression and metastasis, reduces formation of new blood vessels, increases apoptosis, decreases cancer cell growth, promotes cellular differentiation and tend to enhance antitumor immunity (Muñoz & Grant, 2022). 1,25D is an active metabolite of vitamin D that binds with VDR, which then interacts with RXR to form a heterodimer, and ligand activated VDR-RXR initiates biological responses that are primarily related to calcium homeostasis involving phosphate and calcium intestinal absorption. 1,25D may have pleiotropic effects that can modulate apoptosis, cell proliferation, and cell differentiation via genomic and nongenomic pathways. These pathways involve mechanisms that primarily involve VDR mediated changes in the transcriptional regulation and its interaction with other key cell signaling pathways. Among the major involved mechanisms involve cell cycle arrest, induction of apoptosis, and enhancement of differentiation (Carlberg & Muñoz, 2022). 1,25D can induce G1 phase cell cycle arrest by upregulation of CDK inhibitors such as p27 and p21, which lead to the reduction in the phosphorylation of the Rb protein; therefore, suppressing cyclin D1 results in disruption of CDK4/6 activity, thereby preventing G1 to S phase progression (Bhoora & Punchoo, 2020). Related to apoptosis, vitamin D causes modulation of proteins of Bcl-2 family, and it increased apoptosis by increased prop-apoptotic proteins such as Bak, Bax, etc. and reduces expression of antiapoptotic Bcl-2 protein (Starska-Kowarska, 2023). The increased apoptosis is carried out by activating caspase pathways related to caspases 9,8, which are initiator caspases, and caspase 3, which is an effector caspase. In addition, an increase in cellular concentration of calcium results in activation of proteases, such as microcalpain and caspase 12, leading to cellular death. 1,25D increased differentiation of epithelial cells by increased expression of E-cadherin, activation of AP1 transcription factors, and reduction of β-catenin/ TCF signaling. For instance, in keratinocytes, the differentiation is caused by increased cellular calcium level that is related to the involvement of calcium sensing receptors (CaSR), phospholipase C. In addition, there are other underlying mechanisms involved in modulation of VDR mediated transcription, where by vitamin D response elements in target genes can regulate cell differentiation and the cell cycle. Vitamin D cell signaling pathway and its cross-talk with the growth factors, such as inhibition of EGFR, can result in the activation of TGF-β pathway, thereby contributing toward growth suppression. Vitamin D can also inhibit Wnt/β-Catenin pathways, which results in reduced levels of nuclear β-catenin; therefore, it can reduce transcription of oncogenic pathways. These mechanisms illustrate the role of vitamin D as a potential antiproliferative agent with a role in the modulation of cellular differentiation.

Vitamin D and its main active form 1,25D have a critical role in many cellular processing that involves the interaction between VDR and the regulation of gene expression, and the corresponding biological effects can be divided into two categories, for example, nongenomic and genomic effects. Among genomic mechanisms, it involves the regulation of VDR activation and the regulation of gene expression, which involves the binding of 1,25D with VDR that forms a heterodimer with RXR, and the complex binds to Vitamin D Response Elements (VDREs) in the promoter region of target genes. In addition, 1,25D-VDR signaling pathways regulate phosphate and calcium absorption by upregulation of PMCA1b, calbindin, and TRPV6 that increase intestinal absorption of calcium. In the kidneys, it regulated calcium transport through TRPV5 and increases reabsorption of phosphate via Npt2c regulation. In bone, 1,25D balances bone formation and reabsorption by regulating osteocalcin and RANKL in osteoclasts and osteoblast cells (van Driel & van Leeuwen, 2023). 1,25D also regulates innate immune response where in increase antimicrobial defense in macrophages by regulating the expression of defensins and cathelicidins (Ismailova & White, 2022). In addition, it can modulate the adaptive part of the immunity and suppresses inflammatory-associated pathways by modulating NF-κB and regulation of T-cell differentiation. The reported mechanisms related to nongenomic effects show that 1,25D can have membrane-initiated rapid signaling effects that can be independent of the changes in the gene transcription (Żmijewski, 2022). Furthermore, vitamin D can change cellular responses in immune, muscle, and bone cells by its interaction with ion transporters and calcium channels. These mechanisms illustrate that 1,25D can have multiple roles in the cell, ranging from prevention of cancer to immune response modulation to mineral metabolism.

In addition, vitamin D can have a role in reduced angiogenesis in tumor tissues by reducing the expression of vascular endothelial growth factor (VEGF), which may result in reduced formation of new blood vessels (Fleet et al., 2012). In addition, it may reduce the formation of new vessels and may limit the supply of nutrients to tumor tissues. 1,25D can modulate antitumor response of the immune system by inducing the immunomodulatory effect, where it changes the immune response to enhance antitumor response, for instance, it can increase the activity of cytotoxic T lymphocytes and natural killer cells, while at the same time it suppressed pro-inflammatory cytokines (Kim et al., 2022). Vitamin D can have a role in DNA repair and oxidative stress, for instance, it increases the expression of thioredoxin reductase and superoxide dismutase, which are antioxidant enzymes and can reduce the oxidative stress associated DNA damage. Furthermore, it can enhance DNA repair mechanisms, which may have a protective effect against carcinogenesis. Autophagy has an important role in cancer biology of various cancers, and it has been reported that vitamin D can enhance autophagy in cells, whereby it can enhance cellular degradation pathways that may reduce tumor growth by increased expression of Beclin1 which is a key regulator of autophagy and may result in the reduce activity in mTOR signaling pathway (Bhutia, 2022). Furthermore, vitamin D can modulate histone modification and DNA methylation, which are two major epigenetic mechanisms that may lead to the increased expression of tumor suppressor genes and may negatively affect the tumor growth. In addition, it has been reported that some cancers can develop resistant to vitamin D due to VDR mutations or due to increased expression of enzymes that cause degradation of vitamin D metabolites, such as CYP24A1. The above discussion illustrates that the role of vitamin D in the cancer treatment and prevention may depend on tissue type and may require further research to develop vitamin D-targeted analogs with increase anticancer properties. However, vitamin D shows a good promise to be used as a cancer prevention strategy and may be further investigated as a targeted potential therapeutic target in cancer therapy.

18.5   Clinical trials on vitamin D and cancer

Over the years, numerous clinical trials have studied the impact of vitamin D on cancer prognosis, either as a standalone supplement or in combination with other minerals, nutrients, or dietary interventions. Research has sought to understand the relationship between circulating vitamin D levels and cancer incidence, with findings suggesting that potential benefits might be limited to specific populations. Various studies have explored the role of vitamin D in different age groups including adults, the elderly, and adolescents while also evaluating the influence of vitamin D condition (whether deficient or sufficient) on cancer outcomes. In particular, the potential role of vitamin D in individuals with P53 immunoreceptivity has been a focus of recent research, as it could indicate a subgroup of patients who may respond more favorably to supplementation.

18.6   Vitamin D and cancer prevention

The contribution of vitamin D in cancer prevention has been widely debated, with mixed findings from clinical trials. Some studies have shown promising results, while others have found no significant protective effects. For instance, a study investigating the effects of calcium and vitamin D supplementation on CRC incidence found no significant decline in cancer occurrence. Similarly, a large study examining postmenopausal women concluded that calcium and vitamin D intake did not lower the incidence of invasive breast cancer, nor was there any significant association between 25 hydroxyvitamin D levels and risk of breast cancer. These results suggest that vitamin D supplementation singly may not be enough to prevent the development of certain cancers.

However, evidence supporting the potential protective effects of vitamin D in melanoma has been more encouraging. A randomized, double blind, placebo controlled trial found that vitamin D intake helped prevent melanoma recurrence, leading to better clinical outcomes and an overall improved quality of life for patients. In contrast, another study observed that while vitamin D and calcium supplementation did not significantly reduce the overall incidence of melanoma or non-melanoma skin cancer (NMSC), it did appear to lower melanoma risk in women with a history of NMSC. This suggests that high-risk populations may benefit from vitamin D supplementation, though further investigation is required to confirm these findings.

18.7   Vitamin D and cancer prognosis

Several studies have explored the correlation between vitamin D status and cancer prognosis, with many findings pointing to its potential role in disease progression and survival outcomes.

In follicular lymphoma (FL), for example, deficient vitamin D has been linked to worse progression free and overall survival, indicating that maintaining sufficient vitamin D levels could play a role in improving prognosis for FL patients.

Similarly, in CRC, research has found that patients with elevated levels of the soluble CD40 ligand (sCD40L) had better recurrence free survival (RFS) when taking vitamin D supplements. However, high sCD40L levels were also identified as a poor prognostic marker, suggesting that vitamin D supplementation may be more beneficial for patients with elevated sCD40L.

One of the largest and most comprehensive clinical trials exploring vitamin D and cancer was the VITamin D and OmegA3 TriaL (VITAL). This large scale, nationwide, randomized, placebo-controlled study evaluated the impact of daily vitamin D3 (2000 IU) and marine omega-3 fatty acids (1 g) on the prevention of cancer and cardiovascular disease (CVD). The trial included 25,871 participants in the U.S., spanning various demographic groups, including men aged 50 and older, women aged 55 and older, and a significant proportion of African American participants. While daily vitamin D3 supplementation was associated with a significant reduction in cancer mortality, it did not have a measurable impact on cancer incidence or cardiovascular disease outcomes, indicating that vitamin D might be more beneficial for survival rather than prevention.

Another trial, the Finnish Vitamin Trial, found that vitamin D3 supplementation did not decrease the frequency of major cardiac events or invasive cancer among older adults. Researchers suggested that this could be due to most participants already having sufficient vitamin D levels at baseline, making additional supplementation unnecessary.

Long term follow up data have also suggested mixed effects. In postmenopausal women, long-term calcium and vitamin D supplementation appeared to reduce cancer-related mortality; however, it was linked with an rise in cardiovascular disease-related mortality, with no overall effect on all-cause mortality.

18.8 Vitamin D in cancer treatment and supportive care

Beyond prevention and prognosis, vitamin D has also been studied in the context of cancer treatment and supportive care, particularly in its potential role in improving patient well being and reducing treatment related side effects. For example, among breast cancer patients receiving active therapy, those who took weekly vitamin D supplements and omega3 showed better nutritional status, including higher blood albumin levels, improved dietary energy and protein intake, and better PG-SGA scores.

A study investigating the impact of yoga combined with high dose vitamin D supplementation in breast cancer survivors found that this approach improved mental and physical well being while also enhancing systemic levels of inflammatory cytokines, suggesting a potential role in managing cancer related side effects.

Similarly, the DEDiCa trial, which included 227 breast cancer survivors, examined the effects of a lifestyle modification program incorporating vitamin D, exercise, and a Mediterranean diet. The results indicated that while a healthy lifestyle positively influenced health related quality of life (HRQoL) by reducing body weight, vitamin D deficiency may worsen symptoms associated with breast cancer, emphasizing the importance of maintaining adequate vitamin D levels in survivors.

However, research regarding vitamin D's role in chemotherapy induced infertility has been less conclusive. A study assessing vitamin D's potential in protecting ovarian reserve in young women undergoing chemotherapy found no significant protective effect, despite a slight increase in AMH levels after six months.

18.9 Vitamin D and prostate cancer

In prostate cancer, particularly for patients undergoing androgen deprivation therapy (ADT), vitamin D has been studied for its potential bone protective effects. ADT is known to cause bone mineral density (BMD) loss, increasing the risk of fractures. High dose vitamin D (HDVD) supplementation was found to be a safe and effective intervention, significantly reducing BMD loss in the hip and femoral neck, especially in patients with low baseline 25 hydroxyvitamin D levels.

However, a separate study investigating the outcome of a multicomponent resistance based workout program combined with protein, vitamin D, and calcium supplements on cognitive function in men with prostate cancer on ADT found no significant cognitive benefits.

18.10 Emerging research and future directions

Recent meta analyses of randomized clinical trials suggest that daily vitamin D3 supplementation may reduce cancer mortality, though further research is needed. One study found that vitamin D supplementation significantly lowered death risk or recurrence in a subcategory of digestive tract cancer patients who were p53 immune reactive, indicating the potential for personalized vitamin D-based treatments.

Additionally, vitamin D has been found to influence gut microbiota, with observed sex differences, suggesting the need for more research on gender specific responses. Furthermore, combining vitamin D with synbiotic supplements showed synergistic anti inflammatory effects, highlighting a new potential therapeutic approach.

AI disclosure

During the preparation of this work the author(s) used ChatGPT in order to assist with outline and referencing format. After using this tool/service, the author(s) reviewed and edited the content as needed and take(s) full responsibility for the content of the publication.

References

Bhoora, S., & Punchoo, R. (2020). Policing cancer: Vitamin D arrests the cell cycle. *International Journal of Molecular Sciences, 21*(23), 9296. https://doi.org/10.3390/ijms21239296.

Bhutia, S. K. (2022). Vitamin D in autophagy signaling for health and diseases: Insights on potential mechanisms and future perspectives. *The Journal of Nutritional Biochemistry, 99*, 108841. https://doi.org/10.1016/j.jnutbio.2021.108841.

Carlberg, C., & Muñoz, A. (2022). An update on vitamin D signaling and cancer. *Seminars in Cancer Biology, 79*, 217–230. https://doi.org/10.1016/j.semcancer.2020.05.018.

Fleet, J. C., DeSmet, M., Johnson, R., & Li, Y. (2012). Vitamin D and Cancer: A review of molecular mechanisms. *Biochemical Journal, 441*(1), 61. https://doi.org/10.1042/BJ20110744.

Horas, K., Zheng, Y., Fong-Yee, C., Macfarlane, E., Manibo, J., Chen, Y., Qiao, J., Gao, M., Haydar, N., M McDonald, M., I Croucher, P., Hong, Z., & J Seibel, M. (2019). Loss of the vitamin D receptor in human breast cancer cells promotes epithelial to mesenchymal cell transition and skeletal colonization. *Journal of Bone and Mineral Research, 34*(9), 1721. https://doi.org/10.1002/jbmr.3744.

Huss, L., Gulz-Haake, I., Nilsson, E., Tryggvadottir, H., Linn, N., Nodin, B., Jirström, K., Isaksson, K., & Jernström, H. (2024). The vitamin D receptor as a prognostic marker in breast cancer-a cohort study. *Nutrients, 16*(7), 931. https://doi.org/10.3390/nu16070931.

Ismailova, A., & White, J. H. (2022). Vitamin D, infections and immunity. *Reviews in Endocrine and Metabolic Disorders, 23*(2), 265–277. https://doi.org/10.1007/s11154-021-09679-5, https://www.springer.com/journal/11154.

Kim, H., Kim, J., Sa, J. K., Ryu, B. K., Park, K. J., Kim, J., Ha, H., Park, Y., Shin, M. H., Kim, J., Lee, H., Kim, D., Lee, K., Jang, B., Lee, K. M., & Kang, S. H. (2022). Calcipotriol, a synthetic Vitamin D analog, promotes antitumor immunity via CD^4+T-dependent CTL/NK cell activation. *Biomedicine and Pharmacotherapy, 154*. https://doi.org/10.1016/j.biopha.2022.113553, https://www.journals.elsevier.com/biomedicine-and-pharmacotherapy.

Li, Q., Chan, H., Liu, W. X., Liu, C. A., Zhou, Y., Huang, D., Wang, X., Li, X., Xie, C., Liu, W. Y. Z., Wang, X. S., Ng, S. K., Gou, H., Zhao, L. Y., Fong, W., Jiang, L., Lin, Y., Zhao, G., Bai, F., ... Yu, J. (2023). Carnobacterium maltaromaticum boosts intestinal vitamin D production to suppress colorectal cancer in female mice. *Cancer cell, 41*(8), 1450. https://doi.org/10.1016/j.ccell.2023.06.011, https://www.journals.elsevier.com/cancer-cell.

Maalmi, H., Walter, V., Jansen, L., Boakye, D., Schöttker, B., Hoffmeister, M., & Brenner, H. (2018). Association between blood 25-hydroxyvitamin D levels and survival in colorectal cancer patients: An updated systematic review and meta-analysis. *Nutrients, 10*(7), 896. https://doi.org/10.3390/nu10070896.

McCullough, P. J., Lehrer, D. S., & Amend, J. (2019). Daily oral dosing of vitamin D3 using 5000 TO 50,000 international units a day in long-term hospitalized patients: Insights from a seven year experience. *Journal of Steroid Biochemistry and Molecular Biology, 189*, 228–239. https://doi.org/10.1016/j.jsbmb.2018.12.010.

McCullough, M. L., Zoltick, E. S., Weinstein, S. J., Fedirko, V., Wang, M., Cook, N. R., Eliassen, A. H., Zeleniuch-Jacquotte, A., Agnoli, C., Albanes, D., Barnett, M. J., Buring, J. E., Campbell, P. T., Clendenen, T. V., Freedman, N. D., Gapstur, S. M., Giovannucci, E. L., Goodman, G. G., Haiman, C. A., ... Smith-Warner, S. A. (2019). Circulating Vitamin D and colorectal cancer risk: An international pooling project of 17 cohorts. *Journal of the National Cancer Institute, 111*(2), 158–169. https://doi.org/10.1093/jnci/djy087, http://jnci.oxfordjournals.org/.

Mezawa, H., Sugiura, T., Watanabe, M., Norizoe, C., Takahashi, D., Shimojima, A., Tamez, S., Tsutsumi, Y., Yanaga, K., & Urashima, M. (2010). Serum vitamin D levels and survival of patients with colorectal cancer: Post-hoc analysis of a prospective cohort study. *BMC Cancer, 10*. https://doi.org/10.1186/1471-2407-10-347Japan, http://www.biomedcentral.com/1471-2407/10/347.

Mohr, S. B., Gorham, E. D., Kim, J., Hofflich, H., & Garland, C. F. (2014). Meta-analysis of vitamin D sufficiency for improving survival of patients with breast cancer. *Anticancer Research, 34*(3), 1163–1166. http://ar.iiarjournals.org/content/34/3/1163.full.pdf+html.

Muñoz, A., & Grant, W. B. (2022). Vitamin D and cancer: An historical overview of the epidemiology and mechanisms. *Nutrients, 14*(7). https://doi.org/10.3390/nu14071448, https://www.mdpi.com/2072-6643/14/7/1448/pdf.

Ottaiano, A., Iacovino, M. L., Santorsola, M., Facchini, S., Iervolino, D., Perri, F., Nasti, G., Quagliariello, V., Maurea, N., Ronchi, A., Facchini, B. A., Bignucolo, A., & Berretta, M. (2024). Circulating vitamin D level before initiating chemotherapy impacts on the time-to-outcome in metastatic colorectal cancer patients: Systematic review and meta-analysis. *Journal of translational medicine, 22*(1). https://doi.org/10.1186/s12967-024-04889-2, https://translational-medicine.biomedcentral.com.

Peixoto, R. D. A., Oliveira, L. Jd. C., Passarini, Td. M., Andrade, A. C., Diniz, P. H., Prolla, G., Amorim, L. C., Gil, M., Lino, F., Garicochea, B., Jácome, A., & Ng, K. (2022). Vitamin D and colorectal cancer – A practical review of the literature. *Cancer Treatment and Research Communications. 32*. https://doi.org/10.1016/j.ctarc.2022.100616, https://www.journals.elsevier.com/cancer-treatment-and-research-communications/.

Siegel, R. L., Giaquinto, A. N., & Jemal, A. (2024). Cancer statistics, 2024. *CA Cancer Journal for Clinicians, 74*(1), 12–49. https://doi.org/10.3322/caac.21820, http://onlinelibrary.wiley.com/journal/10.3322/.

Starska-Kowarska, K. (2023). Role of vitamin D in head and neck cancer—Immune function, anti-tumour effect, and its impact on patient prognosis. *Nutrients, 15*(11), 2592. https://doi.org/10.3390/nu15112592.

Torres, A., Cameselle, C., Otero, P., & Simal-Gandara, J. (2024). The impact of vitamin D and its dietary supplementation in breast cancer prevention: an integrative review. *Nutrients, 16*(5), 573. https://doi.org/10.3390/nu16050573.

van Driel, M., & van Leeuwen, J. (2023). Vitamin D and bone: a story of endocrine and auto/paracrine action in osteoblasts. *Nutrients, 15*(3), 480. https://doi.org/10.3390/nu15030480.

Voutsadakis, I. A. (2021). Vitamin D baseline levels at diagnosis of breast cancer: A systematic review and meta-analysis. *Hematology/ Oncology and Stem Cell Therapy, 14*(1), 16–26. https://doi.org/10.1016/j.hemonc.2020.08.005, http://www.elsevier.com/journals/hematology-oncology-and-stem-cell-therapy/1658-3876.

Żmijewski, M. A. (2022). Nongenomic activities of vitamin D. *Nutrients, 14*(23), 5104. https://doi.org/10.3390/nu14235104.

CHAPTER 19

Vitamin D, paarthyroid function and renal bone disease: interplay with FGF23

Lena Jafri

Section of Chemical Pathology, Department of Pathology and Laboratory Medicine, Aga Khan University, Karachi, Sindh, Pakistan

19.1 Introduction

Chronic kidney disease (CKD) is a global health concern affecting over 10% of the population worldwide (Rovin et al., 2024). A typical consequence of CKD and a major contributor to higher morbidity and a lower quality of life is disturbances in bone and mineral metabolism (Aljawadi et al., 2024). Patients with CKD are at a higher risk of osteoporosis, fragility fractures, and even extra-skeletal calcification (Pimentel et al., 2021; Simic, 2024). Metabolic bone diseases in patients with CKD are often referred to as CKD–mineral and bone disorder (CKD–MBD). One part of the CKD–MBD, renal osteodystrophy, is identified by bone biopsy and characterizes the pathological alteration of bone morphology in CKD patients (Moe et al., 2006). However, CKD–MBD refers to a broader clinical entity that encompasses CKD-related diseases of mineral and bone metabolism (Ketteler et al., 2017).

According to the Kidney Disease Improving Global Outcomes (KDIGO) position statement, CKD–MBD is a systemic condition and is characterized by aberrant bone turnover, mineralization, volume, linear growth, strength, and/or extra skeletal (vascular or soft tissue) calcification, as well as inappropriate metabolism of calcium (Ca), phosphorus (P), parathyroid hormone (PTH), or vitamin D (Moe et al., 2006). The metabolic bone disorder can be recognized to exist even in the early stages of CKD with the help of some biochemical markers and hormones. The biochemical signs of CKD–MBD are mainly evident in stages 3 and 4 of CKD. The glomerular filtration rate in stages 3 A and 3B of CKD is 45–59 and 30–44 mL/min, respectively. While the glomerular filtration rate is 15–29 mL/min in stage 4 of CKD (Levey et al., 2020). Derangement in the metabolism of PTH, Ca, P, and vitamin D is the characteristic of CKD–MBD (Lucca et al., 2021). In addition, there may be Ca accumulation in soft tissues like blood vessels and concerns with bone mineralization, bone development, and bone strength (Kaur & Singh, 2022). Low levels of active vitamin D, P accumulation, reduced intestinal absorption of Ca, inadequate synthesis of an alpha-klotho by the kidneys, and increased levels of fibroblast growth factor 23 (FGF23) all contribute to the development of

The Impact of Vitamin D on Health and Disease. DOI: https://doi.org/10.1016/B978-0-443-34037-6.00024-8

CKD-MBD (Mußmächer, 2024). All these factors contribute to secondary hyperparathyroidism and structural abnormalities in the bones, resulting in poor bone mineralization, lower bone mineral density (BMD), and a higher risk of fractures. Early diagnosis and management of CKD–MBD is paramount to prevent potential complications. The CKD–MBD is a complex syndrome characterized by disruptions in Ca, P, PTH, vitamin D, and FGF23 levels (Waziri et al., 2019). The focus of this chapter is on exploring the interplay between these metabolites and hormones in the pathophysiology of CKD–MBD.

19.2 Definition of chronic kidney disease–mineral and bone disorder

The National Kidney Foundation proposed in 2003 that renal osteodystrophy should be defined as a constellation of bone disorders present or exacerbated by CKD that lead to bone fragility and fractures, deranged mineral metabolism, and extra-skeletal manifestations. Although this definition included a triad of abnormal mineral metabolism, skeletal, and extra-skeletal manifestations, it was not widely accepted, so the second KDIGO controversies conference in 2005 came up with a broader term, CKD–MBD (Moe et al., 2006). The conference participants agreed that the term "renal osteodystrophy" be limited to describing the bone pathology related with CKD and that CKD–MBD should be defined as a systemic disorder of bone and mineral metabolism due to CKD manifested by either one or a combination of the following: (1) abnormalities of Ca, P, PTH, or vitamin D metabolism; (2) abnormalities in bone turnover, mineralization, volume, linear growth, or strength; or (3) vascular or other soft tissue calcification. This globally recognized definition has made it easier to compare research in the CKD–MBD field. Having one universally recognized definition ensures consistency in how CKD–MBD is diagnosed, classified, and researched, and improving patient outcomes globally. The previous definition of renal osteodystrophy did not exactly incorporate this more diverse clinical spectrum, based on serum biomarkers, noninvasive imaging, and bone abnormalities on biopsy.

19.3 Vitamin D metabolism, parathyroid hormone, and chronic kidney disease–mineral and bone disorder

19.3.1 Vitamin D synthesis

The biggest source of vitamin D is the sun. Other sources include foods like fatty fish, cod liver oil, fortified foods like vitamin D fortified milk and dairy products, egg, beef liver, and vitamin D supplements. Vitamin is primarily formed in the skin by sunlight. The synthesis of Vitamin D begins in the skin when ultraviolet B rays convert 7-dehydrocholesterol to cholecalciferol. Next, hydroxylation of cholecalciferol occurs in the liver, and 25-hydroxy cholecalciferol, or 25(OH)D3, is formed. This, also known as calcidiol, is the inactive form of vitamin D. The kidney performs the critical role of its activation and second hydroxylation to form 1,25-dihydroxycholecalciferol or calcitriol (the active form) (Levey et al., 2007). Therefore, reduced function of kidneys in CKD leads to low levels of 1,25-dihydroxy vitamin D. Reduced levels of 1,25-dihydroxy vitamin D3 cause impaired Ca absorption and bone mineralization (Franca Gois et al., 2018).

19.4   Regulation of 1,25-dihydroxy vitamin D

The active form of vitamin D (1,25-dihydroxy vitamin D3) alone provides essentially no information about the nutritional status of vitamin D. It is important to understand that to identify vitamin D deficiency, the 25-hydroxy vitamin D, the inactive form, is the preferred initial test for assessing vitamin D status. If there is a suspicion of either an excess or a deficiency of 1,25-dihydroxy vitamin D, serum levels should be measured (Table 19.1). In addition to the 25-hydroxy vitamin D testing, 1,25-dihydroxy vitamin is the recommended test for individuals with hypercalcemia or renal failure. To exclude vitamin D toxicity with conditions that can enhance 1,25-dihydroxy vitamin production, such as lymphoma, sarcoidosis, and other granulomatous diseases, both active and inactive forms of vitamin D levels in blood must be assessed in individuals with hypercalcemia.

19.5   Vitamin D deficiency in chronic kidney disease

The levels of circulating 25(OH)D may start to decline from the early stages of CKD, and vitamin D therapy is often prescribed to CKD patients who are deficient. Vitamin D deficiency in CKD patients has been linked to increased all-cause mortality, accelerated kidney disease progression, and albuminuria (Ravani et al., 2009; Wolf et al., 2007).

Table 19.1   Diseases and conditions (in alphabetical order) in which 1,25-dihydroxy D levels are deranged.

Decreased 1,25-dihydroxyvitamin D Levels	Increased 1,25-dihydroxyvitamin D Levels
Autosomal-dominant hypophosphatemic rickets	Hereditary vitamin D-resistant rickets
Advance liver disease	Inflammatory bowel disease
Chronic kidney disease	Lymphoproliferative disorders
HIV protease inhibitors	Primary hyperparathyroidism
Hypoparathyroidism	Sarcoidosis
Magnesium deficiency	Tuberculosis
Nephrotic syndrome	Vitamin D intoxication
Severe 25OHD deficiency	
Tumor-induced osteomalacia	
Vitamin D-dependent rickets type 1	
X-linked hypophosphatemic rickets	

Many factors contribute to the low serum 25(OH)D levels (nutritional indicator of vitamin D) even at initial CKD stages. One such factor is the hyperpigmentation of skin in CKD resulting from uremic toxins, hormonal imbalances in CKD, and iron deposition. Hyperpigmentation in CKD contributes to decreased synthesis of cholecalciferol in the skin. Additionally, factors like dietary limitations in CKD patients, increased catabolism of vitamin D, and significant urinary excretion of vitamin D-binding protein (DBP) and vitamin D metabolites all contribute to vitamin D deficiency (Llach & Yudd, 1998; Rovin et al., 2024).

19.6 Vitamin D and chronic kidney disease—mineral and bone disorder pathogenesis

As for the role of active vitamin D or 1,25-dihydroxy cholecalciferol, it has an important contribution to the pathogenesis of CKD–MBD. Declining glomerular filtration rate as CKD progresses reduces the production of 1,25-dihydroxy cholecalciferol, leading to derangements in Ca and P homeostasis, secondary hyperparathyroidism, and eventually declining BMD (Levin et al., 2007). It contributes to Ca homeostasis by increasing its absorption in the intestine and the kidneys. In the duodenum, 1,25-dihydroxy cholecalciferol binds to the vitamin D receptor and stimulates the production of calcium-binding proteins, increasing the amount of Ca absorbed (Franca Gois et al., 2018). There is lots of evidence that besides bone and kidneys, this active hormone also has paracrine or autocrine functions in the skin, cells of the immune system, parathyroid gland, intestinal epithelium, prostate, and breast.

19.7 Calcium homeostasis and chronic kidney disease—mineral and bone disorder

19.7.1 Total calcium versus ionized calcium

A common biochemical abnormality in individuals with CKD is low calcium concentration or hypocalcemia. Before we discuss the pathogenesis and cause of Ca derangement in CKD, it is important to appreciate the available laboratory test options to assess hypo/hypercalcemia. Calcium testing can be done by assessing total Ca, corrected Ca, or the free form of ionized Ca. Generally, ionised Ca (the free, active form) is often considered a better lab test than total Ca because it more accurately reflects the biologically active form of calcium in the body. Total Ca refers to both ionized Ca and calcium bound to proteins (mainly albumin) and other molecules. On the other hand, ionized Ca is the fraction of Ca that is not bound to proteins, and it is the form that is physiologically active. In CKD patients, particularly when there is protein loss, the levels of total Ca (protein-bound Ca) can be affected. Hypoalbuminemia in patients can lead to a falsely low total Ca value. Therefore, in CKD patients, it is recommended to test for ionized Ca, which is independent of protein levels. For accurate results of ionized Ca preanalytical and analytical factors must be taken care of, as it is the active/free form of Ca (Jafri et al., 2014).

19.8 Calcium and parathyroid gland

Ionized calcium is the form directly sensed by the parathyroid glands to regulate PTH secretion, and PTH, in turn, helps regulate calcium levels by affecting kidney function, bone resorption, and intestinal calcium absorption. The primary calcium-regulating hormone, PTH, is released in its active form before the liver breaks it down into amino-(N-) and carboxy-C-) terminal fragments that are eliminated by the kidneys. Additionally, Ca ions are the main regulators of the secretion of PTH. The Ca ions in blood bind to Ca-sensing G-protein-coupled receptors on parathyroid cells and decrease the release of PTH from the parathyroid gland and vice versa (Brown, 2013). Once released, the main approach that PTH functions is by attaching itself to PTH1 receptors in the kidneys and bones. Parathyroid hormone has the following effects: inhibits calciuria, stimulates phosphaturia, and produces 1,25-dihydroxy vitamin D3. With the help of PTH bone resorption is stimulated by starting the remodeling/modeling process, which also affects osteoblast differentiation, prevents osteoblasts from undergoing apoptosis, inhibits sclerostin expression in osteocytes, and indirectly stimulates osteoclasts by increasing the synthesis of receptor activator of nuclear factor-κB ligands from osteocytes (Al-Jumaili & Al-jumaili, 2024).

Factors contributing to hypocalcemia in CKD include increased P binding to Ca, decreased levels of 1,25-dihydroxyvitamin D3, and skeletal resistance to the effects of PTH (Mosbah, 2019). PTH release increases in response to vitamin D deficiency, counteracting the decrease in Ca absorption. Since Ca ions bind to parathyroid cells' calcium-sensing G-protein-coupled receptors (CaSR) and reduce PTH release, they are the primary regulators of PTH secretion. Signaling through these CaSR has direct effects on the parathyroid gland function (formation and secretion of PTH, and parathyroid gland hyperplasia). Hyperplasia and enlargement of the parathyroid glands have meaningful effects on the disease prognosis (Goodman & Quarles, 2008).

Clinical management strategies of CKD that maintain adequate Ca-dependent signaling through the CaSR may ultimately prove useful in reducing parathyroid gland hyperplasia and in the progression of the disease. Secondary hyperparathyroidism often occurs early in CKD and gets worse over time as the kidneys become less functional. Phosphate retention or hyperphosphatemia also contributes to the pathogenesis of secondary hyperparathyroidism, which starts in the early stages of CKD (Sprague et al., 2021). Secondary hyperparathyroidism contributes to bone demineralization and hence CKD–MBD. To prevent and control demineralization of bones and other detrimental effects of CKD–MBD the management of CKD–MBD should focus on biochemical parameters like hypocalcemia, hyperphosphatemia, and abnormal vitamin D and PTH levels (Ahmad et al., 2025). As we move through this chapter, we will go into more detail on several other hormones besides PTH that interact with vitamin D and are important in the onset and progression of CKD–MBD.

19.9 Role of fibroblast growth factor 23 in phosphate homeostasis

19.9.1 FGF23 release

The kidney is a key player in P homeostasis. A protein belonging to the fibroblast growth factor (FGF) family, FGF23 has a role in the control of serum P levels and its metabolism. Fibroblast growth factor 23 consists of 251 amino acids and is coded by the FGF23 gene on chromosome 12p13 in humans. One of the main target organs of the hormone FGF23 is the kidney (Ferrari et al., 2005). The fibroblast growth factor is formed in response to high P intake, hyperphosphatemia, or an increase in 1,25-dihydroxy vitamin D3 concentration. The primary cells responsible for its synthesis are the osteoblasts and the osteocytes (Mirams et al., 2004).

19.10 Function of FGF23

The main function of FGF23 is to maintain P homeostasis in the body by causing phosphaturia and inhibiting the kidney's ability to synthesize 1,25-dihydroxy vitamin D3 by inhibiting the rate-limiting enzyme 1α-hydroxylase (Yamazaki et al., 2002). Expression of 1α-hydroxylase is mainly localized in proximal renal tubules. Both the N/Pi Type II and the Na/Pi IIc cotransporters are expressed at the apical membrane of proximal tubular cells, which physiologically regulate renal P excretion. Another action of FGF23 on the kidneys is by decreasing the expression of both these cotransporters in the proximal tubule (Sun & Yu, 2023).

In healthy kidneys, FGF23 helps keep P levels within a narrow range by promoting its excretion and reducing vitamin D activation when P levels are high. The effect of FGF23 is through activation of FGF23 receptors. The coreceptor needed for binding of FGF23 to FGF receptors is transmembrane or soluble αKlotho. Because the presence of the coreceptor αKlotho (referred to as Klotho) on target cells is necessary for high-affinity binding of FGF23 to FGF receptors, the endocrine activities of FGF23 in the kidney are αKlotho-dependent at physiological concentrations of the hormone (Wei et al., 2021).

Plasma FGF23 is an early marker of CKD–MBD and is seen to be elevated even before the rise of PTH and P (Isakova et al., 2011). The FGF23 levels rise gradually with declining decreased in glomerular filtration rate. High FGF23 levels further contribute to CKD–MBD by inhibiting proximal tubular cells' production of 1,25-dihydroxyvitamin D3, which reduces intestine absorption of Ca and P. Phosphate excretion per nephron rises because of the parathyroid glands' increased PTH secretion (Komaba & Fukagawa, 2010). Therefore, to maintain a neutral P balance by increasing urinary P excretion, circulating levels of FGF23 and PTH rise in patients with early-stage CKD. In individuals with CKD, the FGF-23-receptor complex, Klotho-fibroblast growth factor receptor 1, is downregulated in the parathyroid gland, which prevents FGF-23 from reducing PTH levels. In other words, FGF23 acts on the kidney to decrease 1,25-dihydroxyvitamin D3 synthesis, which contributes to the secondary hyperparathyroidism of CKD, whereas 1,25-dihydroxyvitamin D3 itself increases FGF-23 transcription (Shigematsu et al., 2004). According to earlier research, cardiovascular problems such as endothelial dysfunction, arterial calcification, stroke, and cardiomyocyte hypertrophy in CKD patients have been associated with over-expression of FGF23 (Ärnlöv et al., 2013).

Increased PTH and FGF23 levels have a major impact on the pathophysiology of CKD–MBD and are associated with several adverse outcomes, including fractures, cardiovascular disease, and death in patients with advanced CKD (Larsson, 2010).

19.11 FGF23 assays

In clinical laboratories, there are primarily two types of assays used to quantify or measure FGF23: the intact FGF23 assay and the C-terminal FGF23 assay. The Intact FGF23 assay measures the biologically active full-length FGF23, which captures both the N-terminal and C-terminal regions and is thought to be more reflective of FGF23 functional activity in the body (Smith et al., 2012). The C-terminal FGF23 assay recognizes both full-length and processed C-terminal fragments of FGF-23, which is the longer form and reflects total FGF23 levels. The majority of studies on CKD–MBD have reported elevated C-terminal FGF23, which comprises both the intact and cleaved versions of the hormone (Sharma et al., 2020). The C-terminal assay is more frequently utilized in clinical and research settings for CKD, even though the intact FGF23 assay is thought to be more specific for assessing biologically active FGF23.

19.12 Utility of biomarkers for diagnosis and management of chronic kidney disease–mineral and bone disorder

19.12.1 Biomarkers for diagnosis and management of chronic kidney disease–mineral and bone disorder

Biomarkers and hormones that can help in the identification of early CKD–MBD having high sensitivity and specificity, are ideal. However, in a real clinical scenario, there is no single biomarker to diagnose CKD–MBD with 100% sensitivity or specificity. Therefore, usually a panel of markers and hormones is used. This may include serum Ca, serum P, vitamin D metabolites, Cr with estimated glomerular filtration rate, PTH, and if available, plasma FGF23. As the function and the glomerular filtration rate of the kidney decline, there is an ongoing worsening in mineral homeostasis (Hou et al., 2018). This results in fluctuations in the levels of hormones and minerals in the bloodstream. The regulation of both early bone modeling at a young age and bone remodeling in adulthood depends greatly on the mineral and endocrine functions that are disturbed in CKD (Felsenfeld et al., 2015). One of the main goals of managing CKD–MBD is to correct biochemical and hormonal abnormalities and maintain them as close to reference limits as feasible to mitigate the consequences of biochemical derangements. A thorough assessment of the abnormalities in mineral metabolism and bone health that result from the chronic decline in glomerular filtration rate is required to diagnose CKD–MBD. The objective must be to detect changes in bone turnover, bone mineralization (Haarhaus et al., 2022).

19.13   Available biomarkers and frequency of testing

The primary goal of managing CKD–MBD is to avoid the complications from secondary hyperparathyroidism. Therefore, validated, quantifiable surrogate measures of metabolic bone disorders associated with CKD are essential for managing the disease. Serum Ca, P, intact PTH, alkaline phosphatase, complemented by FGF23 and 25-hydroxy vitamin D, are the markers generally used for CKD–MBD identification and management (Srisuwarn et al., 2024; Wetmore et al., 2021).

Based on the values and trends of these biochemical markers, as per the current KDIGO guideline treatment, is suggested or modified. The frequency of monitoring serum Ca, P, alkaline phosphatase and PTH in patients with CKD stages G3a (eGFR of 45–59 mL/min, indicating a mild-to-moderate decrease in kidney function) to G5D (eGFR of < 15 mL/min, indicating severe kidney dysfunction) depends on the severity of and the progression of the disease (Levey et al., 2007; Levey et al., 2020). The kidneys' capacity to properly eliminate P load is compromised starting in stage 3 of CKD, which results in hyperphosphatemia, increased PTH, and decreased 1,25-dihydroxyvitamin D, along with corresponding increases in FGF-23 levels. The conversion of 25-hydroxy vitamin D (inactive form) to 1,25-dihydroxyvitamin D (active form) is also compromised, reducing intestinal Ca absorption and increasing PTH (Felsenfeld et al., 2015). Parathyroid hormone, which often helps in P excretion and Ca reabsorption, and FGF-23, the phosphaturic hormone, are not sufficiently absorbed by the kidney. Additionally, there is evidence of tissue-level downregulation of the vitamin D receptor and resistance to the effects of PTH.

The kidney disease: Improving Global Outcomes guidelines recommend different frequencies of laboratory testing for CKD–MBD (as listed below) depending on the magnitude of dysfunction, rate of progression of CKD, and the CKD stage (Ketteler et al., 2017).

• Serum Ca and serum P.
  CKD G3a–G3b: Every 6–12 months.
  CKD G4: Every 3–6 months.
  CKD G5, including G5D: Every 1–3 months.

- Serum/plasma PTH.
  CKD G3a–G3b: Based on baseline level and CKD progression.
  CKD G4: Every 6–12 months.
  CKD G5, including G5D: Every 3–6 months.
- Serum alkaline phosphatase.
  CKD G4–G5D: Every 12 months, or more frequently if PTH is elevated.

As per KDIGO guidelines, to ensure that laboratory results for patients with CKD stages 3–5D are accurately interpreted, clinical laboratories are advised to notify clinicians of the assay method employed and to report any modifications to methodology, sample source, and handling requirements. Complex changes in mineral metabolism are common in CKD patients, and even minor adjustments to laboratory procedures or sample handling might provide inaccurate or unreliable results. The reported values of biomarkers like vitamin D or PTH may be impacted by the differences in sensitivity, specificity, or methodology differences between assay techniques, especially in immunoassays or interassay comparability issues (Lai et al., 2012). Biochemical analyses that are essential for determining the course of CKD–MBD can also differ due to preanalytical factors like modifications in sample handling (specimen storage, temperature, centrifugation) or sample source (plasma vs. serum) (Cheng et al., 2023).

19.14   Utility of bone mineral density and bone turnover markers in chronic kidney disease–mineral and bone disorder

19.14.1   Bone mineral density testing, its advantages and limitations

The risk of fragility fracture is doubled in CKD G3 and up to four times higher in CKD G5D patients than in the general population due to the combination of low bone mass, poor bone microarchitecture, and poor bone quality. Patients with CKD G5D have a four-fold increased chance of death and a seven-fold increased risk of getting another fracture within a year after their last fracture. Routine BMD testing is not advised for individuals with evidence of CKD–MBD since it is not as good at predicting fracture risk as it is in the general population and is unable to distinguish between different forms of renal osteodystrophy. BMD testing is recommended for patients with CKD G3a–G5D with CKD–MBD and/or osteoporosis risk factors to assess fracture risk, potentially impacting treatment decisions (Ginsberg & Ix, 2022). The 2009 KDIGO mineral-bone guideline recommends not routinely performing BMD testing in patients with CKD stages 3–5D with evidence of CKD–MBD, as BMD does not predict fracture risk or renal osteodystrophy type (KDIGO clinical practice guideline for the diagnosis, evaluation, prevention, and treatment of chronic kidney disease-mineral and bone disorder CKD-MBD, 2009). However, multiple prospective studies have consistently demonstrated that low BMD is strongly associated with fracture risk in persons with CKD, and these associations are like those of BMD in persons without CKD. In 2017, the KDIGO updated the CKD–MBD guideline to state that BMD testing should be used to assess fracture risk if results will impact treatment decisions (Ketteler et al., 2017). Nearly all patients with CKD have evidence of CKD–MBD and therefore have a high risk of osteoporosis, making BMD testing a critical element of the management of patients with CKD. When interpreting and using BMD tests in individuals with CKD–MBD, it is important to consider whether osteoporosis is getting worse with time. However, bone turnover and mineralization—which are known to be aberrant in many CKD patients and have obvious therapy implications—cannot be deduced from BMD findings. Other imaging modalities that provide information on bone turnover or architecture, such as positron-emission tomography or high-resolution peripheral quantitative computed tomography, are not widely available.

19.15   Bone turnover markers in chronic kidney disease–mineral and bone disorder

Understanding the importance of biomarkers and their role in the pathophysiology of CKD–MBD is crucial for managing it. Renal osteodystrophy (which is not the focus of this chapter and is not covered in detail here) has various subtypes, including hyperparathyroidism-related bone disease, mixed uremic osteodystrophy, osteomalacia, and adynamic bone disease (Sherrard et al., 1993).

The classification of renal osteodystrophy is established on bone turnover, bone mineralization, and bone volume. Bone histomorphometry (the gold standard test for classifying renal osteodystrophy) is a labor-intensive procedure, limited by equipment availability, specialists, and high costs, and patients may be reluctant to undergo this painful procedure. The significance of bone turnover in the pathogenesis of CKD–MBD was highlighted by this categorization. However, since a bone biopsy is not routinely used for monitoring CKD–MBD patients, there is a need for reliable biomarkers for evaluating, diagnosing, and monitoring patients. To address diagnostic obstacles like these, the KDIGO CKD–MBD clinical practice guideline recommends the use of bone-specific alkaline phosphatase and blood PTH to predict the underlying bone turnover phenotype in renal osteodystrophy. The ease of collecting blood samples for these biomarkers enables clinicians to track the course of the illness and to monitor, trend of markers and tailor the treatment accordingly.

Targeting bone turnover abnormalities is crucial for managing CKD–MBD, as both high and low bone turnover can lead to low bone mass and fracture risk, with different treatment strategies (Iimori et al., 2012). Both PTH and alkaline phosphatase, as markedly high or low, can assist in identifying underlying bone turnover. Bone-derived turnover markers of collagen synthesis (like pro-collagen type I C-terminal pro-peptide) and breakdown (like type I collagen cross-linked telopeptide, cross-laps, pyridinoline, or deoxypyridinoline) may not be routinely measured in these patients and are not thought to be necessary for routine evaluation. Cross-sectional studies have shown inconsistent results regarding the relationship between prevalent fractures in CKD G2–5D and increased PTH, bone ALP, Pro-collagen type 1 N-terminal pro peptide (P1NP), and tartrate-resistant acid phosphatase (TRAP5b). PTH and bone ALP are the most studied markers for predicting fracture incidence (Salam et al., 2018). High serum ALP is more robust in predicting fracture outcomes than high serum PTH. Alkaline phosphatase and bone-specific alkaline phosphatase are biomarkers of bone formation that are not affected by GFR (Sardiwal et al., 2013). Bone-specific alkaline phosphatase has been extensively studied for its utility as a marker of turnover in CKD, including in individuals treated with dialysis. Low concentrations of bone-specific alkaline phosphatase are consistently associated with low bone turnover, helping determine the underlying turnover state (Couttenye et al., 1996). Two turnover bone markers, P1NP and TRAP5b, seem promising markers of bone formation and resorption, but are not widely available in clinical settings (Srisuwarn et al., 2024).

19.16   Conclusion

Together with PTH, FGF23, and 1,25-dihydroxyvitamin D, the kidneys are crucial in controlling the homeostasis and blood levels of P and Ca. This control is compromised in individuals with CKD, which results in CKD–MBD. Biochemical features of CKD–MBD include increased FGF23, reduced 1,25-dihydroxy vitamin D, hyperphosphatemia, secondary hyperparathyroidism, and bone abnormalities. In terms of its etiology, diagnosis, unfavourable clinical consequences, and treatment, CKD–MBD has continued to evolve throughout time. Since there are still information gaps in CKD–MBD despite a great deal of research, more longitudinal studies that compare biomarkers and hormones in clinical usage side by side with novel ones that employ machine learning are required to help manage this condition successfully. In summary, these complex disorders should be identified as early as possible and should be properly managed for better patient outcomes.

References

Ahmad, R., Sarraj, B., & Razzaque, M. S. (2025). Vitamin D and mineral ion homeostasis: Endocrine dysregulation in chronic diseases. *Frontiers in Endocrinology, 16*, 1493986.

Al-Jumaili, R. A., & Al-jumaili, E. F. (2024). Study of the causes of parathyroid hormone imbalance and some biochemical parameter in patients with chronic kidney disease. *Nutrition and Metabolic Diseases, 31*(1), 49–57.

Aljawadi, M. H., Babaeer, A. A., Alghamdi, A. S., Alhammad, A. M., Almuqbil, M. S., & Alonazi, K. F. (2024). Quality of life tools among patients on dialysis: A systematic review. *Pharmaceutical Journal, 32*(3). https://doi.org/10.1016/j.jsps.2024.101958, https://www.sciencedirect.com/science/journal/13190164.

Ärnlöv, J., Carlsson, A. C., Sundstrom, J., Ingelsson, E., Larsson, A., Lind, L., & Larsson, T. E. (2013). Serum FGF23 and risk of cardiovascular events in relation to mineral metabolism and cardiovascular pathology. *Clinical Journal of the American Society of Nephrology, 8*(5), 781–786. https://doi.org/10.2215/CJN.09570912, http://cjasn.asnjournals.org/content/8/5/781.full.pdf+html.

Brown, E. M. (2013). Best practice and research: Clinical endocrinology and metabolism. In *Role of the calcium-sensing receptor in extracellular calcium homeostasis*. United States: Bailliere Tindall Ltd, 27. http://doi.org/10.1016/j.beem.2013.02.006, http://www.elsevier.com/inca/publications/store/6/2/3/0/0/1/index.htt.

Cheng, J., Mu, D., Wang, D., Qiu, L., & Cheng, X. (2023). Preanalytical considerations in parathyroid hormone measurement. *Clinica Chimica Acta, 539*, 259–265. https://doi.org/10.1016/j.cca.2022.12.022.

Couttenye, M. M., D'Haese, P. C., Van Hoof, V. O., Lemoniatou, E., Goodman, W., Verpooten, G. A., & De Broe, M. E. (1996). Low serum levels of alkaline phosphatase of bone origin: A good marker of adynamic bone disease in haemodialysis patients. *Nephrology Dialysis Transplantation, 11*(6), 1065–1072. https://doi.org/10.1093/ndt/11.6.1065.

Felsenfeld, A. J., Levine, B. S., & Rodriguez, M. (2015). Pathophysiology of calcium, phosphorus, and magnesium dysregulation in chronic kidney disease. *Seminars in Dialysis, 28*(6), 564–577. https://doi.org/10.1111/sdi. 12411UnitedStates, http://onlinelibrary.wiley.com/journal/10.1111/(ISSN)1525-139X.

Ferrari, S. L., Bonjour, J. P., & Rizzoli, R. (2005). Fibroblast growth factor-23 relationship to dietary phosphate and renal phosphate handling in healthy young men. *Journal of Clinical Endocrinology and Metabolism, 90*(3), 1519–1524. https://doi.org/10.1210/jc.2004-1039.

Franca Gois, P. H., Wolley, M., Ranganathan, D., & Seguro, A. C. (2018). Vitamin D deficiency in chronic kidney disease: Recent evidence and controversies. *International Journal of Environmental Research and Public Health, 15*(8), 1773. https://doi.org/10.3390/ijerph15081773.

Ginsberg, C., & Ix, J. H. (2022). Diagnosis and management of osteoporosis in advanced kidney disease: A review. *Journal of Kidney Diseases, 79*(3), 427–436. https://doi.org/10.1053/j.ajkd.2021.06.031, http://www.elsevier. com/inca/publications/store/6/2/3/2/7/6/index.htt.

Goodman, W. G., & Quarles, L. D. (2008). Development and progression of secondary hyperparathyroidism in chronic kidney disease: Lessons from molecular genetics. *Kidney International, 74*(3), 276–288. https://doi. org/10.1038/sj.ki.5002287, https://www.journals.elsevier.com/kidney-international.

Haarhaus, M., Cianciolo, G., Barbuto, S., La Manna, G., Gasperoni, L., Tripepi, G., Plebani, M., Fusaro, M., & Magnusson, P. (2022). Alkaline phosphatase: An old friend as treatment target for cardiovascular and mineral bone disorders in chronic kidney disease. *Nutrients, 14*(10), 2124. https://doi.org/10.3390/nu14102124.

Hou, Y. C., Lu, C. L., & Lu, K. C. (2018). Mineral bone disorders in chronic kidney disease. *Nephrology, 23*, 88–94. https://doi.org/10.1111/nep.13457, http://onlinelibrary.wiley.com/journal/10.1111/(ISSN)1440-1797.

Iimori, S., Mori, Y., Akita, W., Kuyama, T., Takada, S., Asai, T., Kuwahara, M., Sasaki, S., & Tsukamoto, Y. (2012). Diagnostic usefulness of bone mineral density and biochemical markers of bone turnover in predicting fracture in CKD stage 5D patients—A single-center cohort study. *Nephrology Dialysis Transplantation, 27*(1), 345–351. https://doi.org/10.1093/ndt/gfr317.

Isakova, T., Wahl, P., Vargas, G. S., Gutiérrez, O. M., Scialla, J., Xie, H., Appleby, D., Nessel, L., Bellovich, K., Chen, J., Hamm, L., Gadegbeku, C., Horwitz, E., Townsend, R. R., Anderson, C. A. M., Lash, J. P., Hsu, C. Y., Leonard, M. B., & Wolf, M. (2011). Fibroblast growth factor 23 is elevated before parathyroid hormone and phosphate in chronic kidney disease. *Kidney International, 79*(12), 1370–1378. https://doi.org/10.1038/ki. 2011.47, https://www.journals.elsevier.com/kidney-international.

Jafri, L., Khan, A. H., & Azeem, S. (2014). Ionized calcium measurement in serum and plasma by ion selective electrodes: Comparison of measured and calculated parameters. *Journal of Clinical Biochemistry, 29*(3), 327–332. https://doi.org/10.1007/s12291-013-0360-x, http://www.springer.com/life+sci/biochemistry+and +biophysics/journal/12291.

KDIGO clinical practice guideline for the diagnosis, evaluation, prevention, and treatment of chronic kidney disease-mineral and bone disorder (CKD-MBD) (2009). Kidney international. *Supplement, 76*(113), 1–130.

Kaur, R., & Singh, R. (2022). Mechanistic insights into CKD-MBD-related vascular calcification and its clinical implications. *Life Sciences, 311*(Pt B), 121148. https://doi.org/10.1016/j.lfs.2022.121148.

Ketteler, M., Block, G. A., Evenepoel, P., Fukagawa, M., Herzog, C. A., McCann, L., Moe, S. M., Shroff, R., Tonelli, M. A., Toussaint, N. D., Vervloet, M. G., & Leonard, M. B. (2017). Executive summary of the 2017 KDIGO Chronic Kidney Disease–Mineral and Bone Disorder (CKD-MBD) Guideline Update: What's changed and why it matters. *Kidney International, 92*(1), 26–36. https://doi.org/10.1016/j.kint.2017.04.006, https://www.journals.elsevier.com/kidney-international.

Komaba, H., & Fukagawa, M. (2010). FGF23–parathyroid interaction: Implications in chronic kidney disease. *Kidney International, 77*(4), 292–298. https://doi.org/10.1038/ki.2009.466.

Lai, J. K. C., Lucas, R. M., Banks, E., & Ponsonby, A.-L. (2012). Variability in vitamin D assays impairs clinical assessment of vitamin D status. *Internal Medicine Journal, 42*(1), 43–50. https://doi.org/10.1111/j.1445-5994.2011.02471.x.

Larsson, T. E. (2010). The role of FGF-23 in CKD-MBD and cardiovascular disease: Friend or foe? *Nephrology Dialysis Transplantation, 25*(5), 1376–1381. https://doi.org/10.1093/ndt/gfp784.

Levey, A. S., Atkins, R., Coresh, J., Cohen, E. P., Collins, A. J., Eckardt, K.-U., Nahas, M. E., Jaber, B. L., Jadoul, M., Levin, A., Powe, N. R., Rossert, J., Wheeler, D. C., Lameire, N., & Eknoyan, G. (2007). Chronic kidney disease as a global public health problem: Approaches and initiatives – A position statement from Kidney Disease Improving Global Outcomes. *Kidney International, 72*(3), 247–259. https://doi.org/10.1038/sj.ki.5002343.

Levey, A. S., Eckardt, K. U., Dorman, N. M., Christiansen, S. L., Hoorn, E. J., Ingelfinger, J. R., Inker, L. A., Levin, A., Mehrotra, R., Palevsky, P. M., Perazella, M. A., Tong, A., Allison, S. J., Bockenhauer, D., Briggs, J. P., Bromberg, J. S., Davenport, A., Feldman, H. I., Fouque, D., ... Winkelmayer, W. C. (2020). Kidney International. In *Nomenclature for kidney function and disease: Report of a Kidney Disease: Improving Global Outcomes (KDIGO) Consensus Conference*. United States: Elsevier B.V, 97. https://doi.org/10.1016/j.kint.2020.02.010, https://www.journals.elsevier.com/kidney-international.

Levin, A., Bakris, G. L., Molitch, M., Smulders, M., Tian, J., Williams, L. A., & Andress, D. L. (2007). Prevalence of abnormal serum vitamin D, PTH, calcium, and phosphorus in patients with chronic kidney disease: Results of the study to evaluate early kidney disease. *Kidney International, 71*(1), 31–38. https://doi.org/10.1038/sj.ki.5002009.

Llach, F., & Yudd, M. (1998). Pathogenic, clinical, and therapeutic aspects of secondary hyperparathyroidism in chronic renal failure. *Journal of Kidney Diseases, 32*(4), S3. https://doi.org/10.1053/ajkd.1998.v32.pm9808139, http://www.elsevier.com/inca/publications/store/6/2/3/2/7/6/index.htt.

Lucca, L. J., Moysés, R. M. A., Hernandes, F. R., & Gueiros, J. E. B. (2021). CKD-MBD diagnosis: Biochemical abnormalities. *Brazilian Journal of Nephrology, 43*, 615–620. https://doi.org/10.1590/2175-8239-JBN-2021-S102, http://www.scielo.br/scielo.php?script=sci_arttext&pid=S0101-28002021000500615&tlng=en.

Mirams, M., Robinson, B. G., Mason, R. S., & Nelson, A. E. (2004). Bone as a source of FGF23: Regulation by phosphate? *Bone, 35*(5), 1192–1199. https://doi.org/10.1016/j.bone.2004.06.014.

Moe, S., Drüeke, T., Cunningham, J., Goodman, W., Martin, K., Olgaard, K., Ott, S., Sprague, S., Lameire, N., & Eknoyan, G. (2006). Definition, evaluation, and classification of renal osteodystrophy: A position statement from Kidney Disease: Improving Global Outcomes (KDIGO). *Kidney International, 69*(11), 1945–1953. https://doi.org/10.1038/sj.ki.5000414.

Mosbah, O. (2019). Chronic kidney disease-mineral and bone disorders (CKD-MBD). *Archives of Nephrology and Urology, 02*(02). https://doi.org/10.26502/anu.2644-2833008.

Mußmächer, N. P. H. (2024). Dose response of PTH and FGF23 to Paricalcitol in patients with end stage renal failure on chronic intermittent haemodialysis (Doctoral dissertation).

Pimentel, A., Ureña-Torres, P., Bover, J., Luis Fernandez-Martín, J., & Cohen-Solal, M. (2021). Bone fragility fractures in CKD patients. *Calcified Tissue International, 108*(4), 539–550. https://doi.org/10.1007/s00223-020-00779-z.

Ravani, P., Malberti, F., Tripepi, G., Pecchini, P., Cutrupi, S., Pizzini, P., Mallamaci, F., & Zoccali, C. (2009). Vitamin D levels and patient outcome in chronic kidney disease. *Kidney International, 75*(1), 88–95. https://doi.org/10.1038/ki.2008.501.

Rovin, B. H., Ayoub, I. M., Chan, T. M., Liu, Z.-H., Mejía-Vilet, J. M., & Floege, J. (2024). KDIGO 2024 Clinical Practice Guideline for the management of LUPUS NEPHRITIS. *Kidney International, 105*(1), S1. https://doi.org/10.1016/j.kint.2023.09.002.

Salam, S., Gallagher, O., Gossiel, F., Paggiosi, M., Khwaja, A., & Eastell, R. (2018). Diagnostic accuracy of biomarkers and imaging for bone turnover in renal osteodystrophy. *Journal of the American Society of Nephrology, 29*(5), 1557–1565. https://doi.org/10.1681/asn.2017050584.

Sardiwal, S., Magnusson, P., Goldsmith, D. J. A., & Lamb, E. J. (2013). Bone alkaline phosphatase in CKD-mineral bone disorder. *American Journal of Kidney Diseases, 62*(4), 810–822. https://doi.org/10.1053/j.ajkd.2013.02.366, http://www.elsevier.com/inca/publications/store/6/2/3/2/7/6/index.htt.

Sharma, S., Katz, R., Bullen, A. L., Chaves, P. H. M., De Leeuw, P. W., Kroon, A. A., Houben, A. J. H. M., Shlipak, M. G., & Ix, J. H. (2020). Intact and c-terminal FGF23 assays-do kidney function, inflammation, and low iron influence relationships with outcomes? *Journal of Clinical Endocrinology and Metabolism, 105*(12). https://doi.org/10.1210/clinem/dgaa665, https://academic.oup.com/jcem.

Sherrard, D. J., Hercz, G., Pei, Y., Maloney, N. A., Greenwood, C., Manuel, A., Saiphoo, C., Fenton, S. S., & Segre, G. V. (1993). The spectrum of bone disease in end-stage renal failure - An evolving disorder. *Kidney International, 43*(2), 436–442. https://doi.org/10.1038/ki.1993.64, https://www.journals.elsevier.com/kidney-international.

Shigematsu, T., Kazama, J. J., Yamashita, T., Fukumoto, S., Hosoya, T., Gejyo, F., & Fukagawa, M. (2004). Possible involvement of circulating fibroblast growth factor 23 in the development of secondary hyperparathyroidism associated with renal insufficiency. *American Journal of Kidney Diseases, 44*(2), 250–256. https://doi.org/10.1053/j.ajkd.2004.04.029.

Simic, P. (2024). Bone and bone derived factors in kidney disease. *Frontiers in Physiology, 15*. https://doi.org/10.3389/fphys.2024.1356069.

Smith, E. R., Cai, M. M., McMahon, L. P., & Holt, S. G. (2012). Biological variability of plasma intact and C-terminal FGF23 measurements. *Journal of Clinical Endocrinology and Metabolism, 97*(9), 3357–3365. https://doi.org/10.1210/jc.2012-1811Australia, http://jcem.endojournals.org/content/97/9/3357.full.pdf+html.

Sprague, S. M., Martin, K. J., & Coyne, D. W. (2021). Phosphate balance and CKD-mineral bone disease. *Kidney International Reports, 6*(8), 2049–2058. https://doi.org/10.1016/j.ekir.2021.05.012.

Srisuwarn, P., Eastell, R., & Salam, S. (2024). Clinical utility of bone turnover markers in chronic kidney disease. *Journal of Bone Metabolism, 31*(4), 264–278. https://doi.org/10.11005/jbm.24.789.

Sun, T., & Yu, X. (2023). FGF23 Actions in CKD-MBD and other Organs During CKD. *Current Medicinal Chemistry, 30*(7), 841–856. https://doi.org/10.2174/0929867329666220627122733.

Waziri, B., Duarte, R., & Naicker, S. (2019). Chronic kidney disease–mineral and bone disorder (CKD-MBD): Current perspectives. *International Journal of Nephrology and Renovascular Disease, 12*, 263–276. https://doi.org/10.2147/IJNRD.S191156, https://www.dovepress.com/getfile.php?fileID=54933.

Wei, X., Huang, X., Liu, N., Qi, B., Fang, S., Zhang, Y., & Michele, C. (2021). Understanding the stony bridge between osteoporosis and vascular calcification: Impact of the FGF23/Klotho axis. *Oxidative Medicine and Cellular Longevity, 2021*(1). https://doi.org/10.1155/2021/7536614.

Wetmore, J. B., Ji, Y., Ashfaq, A., Gilbertson, D. T., & Roetker, N. S. (2021). Testing patterns for CKD-MBD abnormalities in a sample US population. *Kidney International Reports, 6*(4), 1141–1150. https://doi.org/10.1016/j.ekir.2020.12.036, http://www.journals.elsevier.com/kidney-international-reports.

Wolf, M., Shah, A., Gutierrez, O., Ankers, E., Monroy, M., Tamez, H., Steele, D., Chang, Y., Camargo, C. A., Tonelli, M., & Thadhani, R. (2007). Vitamin D levels and early mortality among incident hemodialysis patients. *Kidney International, 72*(8), 1004–1013. https://doi.org/10.1038/sj.ki.5002451.

Yamazaki, Y., Okazaki, R., Shibata, M., Hasegawa, Y., Satoh, K., Tajima, T., Takeuchi, Y., Fujita, T., Nakahara, K., Yamashita, T., & Fukumoto, S. (2002). Increased circulatory level of biologically active full-length FGF-23 in patients with hypophosphatemic rickets/osteomalacia. *The Journal of Clinical Endocrinology & Metabolism, 87*(11), 4957–4960. https://doi.org/10.1210/jc.2002-021105.

CHAPTER 20

Vitamin D and fragility fractures

Saira Perwaiz Iqbal

Infectious Diseases, Department of Medicine, Maimonides Medical Center, Brooklyn, NY, United States

20.1 Introduction

One major health problem that affects the geriatric population and causes a significant economic burden is osteoporosis. Osteoporosis is a skeletal disorder that results in severe microarchitectural deformity due to loss of bone mass over time. As a result, the affected bone becomes porous and excessively weak, so much that even the slightest stress or pressure can cause fractures. Dietary supplementation with micronutrients like calcium and vitamin D has been implicated in improving bone mineral density, thereby reducing the risk of fracture.

20.2 Pathogenesis of osteoporosis

The human skeleton is responsible for supporting body structure, protecting vital organs, and allowing mobility. All these factors rely on bone mass and strength. Therefore, bone cells constantly undergo replacement and remodeling, also known as "bone turnover," where old bone cells are replaced by newer cells to maintain skeletal integrity.

There are three kinds of bone cells that cause remodeling: (1) osteoblasts, which help build new bone, (2) osteoclasts, which destroy old or damaged bone, (3) osteocytes, which form the main bone mass and maintain balance between osteoblastic and osteoclastic activity. In the early years of life, bone formation is greater than bone resorption, hence bone mass increases and peaks at age 20–25 years. After the bone matrix or osteoid is formed, it undergoes mineralization; deposition of calcium and phosphate salts, which further solidifies bone structure to enhance bone density. Vitamin D plays a vital role in maintaining a balance between calcium and phosphate to promote mineralization. After the age of 50 years, bone resorption exceeds bone formation and results in a gradual decline in bone mass over the years. By the age of 80 years, the total bone mass and mineral density reduce to 50% of peak, leading to osteopenia and ultimately osteoporosis, thereby increasing the risk of fragility fractures (Fig. 20.1).

The Impact of Vitamin D on Health and Disease. **DOI:** https://doi.org/10.1016/B978-0-443-34037-6.00035-2

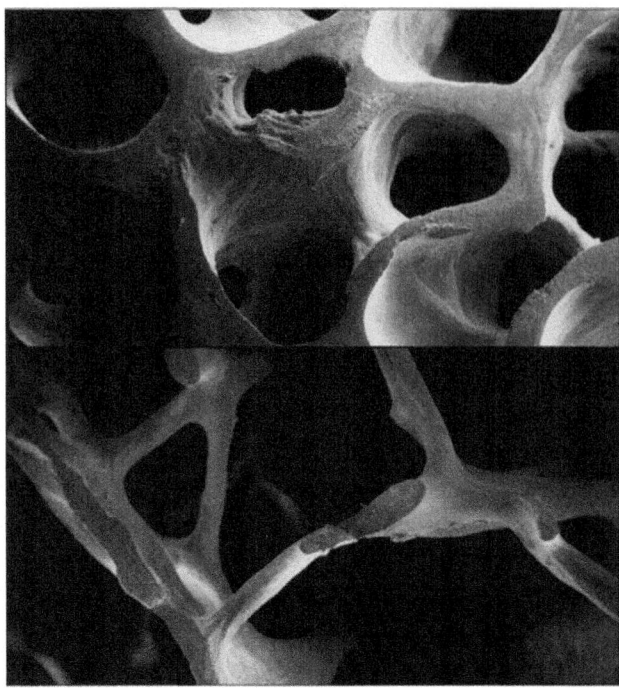

Figure 20.1
Osteoporotic and normal trabecular bone. Comparison of osteoporotic bone (below) with normal bone (above).
Source: *From Dempster, D. W., et al. (1986). A simple method for correlative light and scanning electron microscopy of human iliac crest bone biopsies: Qualitative observations in normal and osteoporotic subjects.* Journal of Bone and Mineral Research, 1, 15–21.

20.3 Fragility fractures

Osteoporotic bone, with its low mineral density, becomes porous and "fragile" over time. Hence, it is highly susceptible to partial or complete breaks in bone called "fragility fractures." Fragility fractures are pathological fractures that occur from minimal trauma, minor events, or stresses that would normally not result in fractures, such as a fall from standing height or even less, and sometimes, no trauma can even be identified. Osteoporosis usually occurs silently without overt symptoms. Often, fragility fractures are the first clinical sign or manifestation of osteoporosis. Fragility fractures can also occur in postmenopausal women without osteoporosis. This signifies a strong relationship between the hormone estrogen and bone health. A rapid decline in estrogen levels in postmenopausal women can predispose them to fragility fractures.

20.4 Epidemiology

Osteoporosis is highly prevalent in the aging population worldwide. A global meta-analysis on worldwide prevalence of osteoporosis, published in the Journal of Orthopedic Surgery and Research in 2021, showed that prevalence was highest in Africa and Europe, then Asia, and comparatively less prevalent in the USA and Australia (Salari et al., 2021). In the year 2019, in Europe alone, 32 million people aged over 50 years were estimated to have osteoporosis and deemed high-risk for fragility fractures (Kanis et al., 2021).

According to a report issued by the International Osteoporosis Foundation, every year around 37 million fragility fractures occur worldwide in individuals over the age of 55 years (Wu et al., 2021). Another way to represent its global impact is that one in every five males and one in every three females, over the age of 50 years, will have an osteoporotic fracture. These numbers forecast a tremendous economic burden in the upcoming years and warrant early intervention.

20.5 Risk factors

Fragility fractures are undesirable consequences of osteoporosis. It is imperative to identify the risk factors that predispose to fragility fractures if they are to be prevented. These factors can be classified into modifiable and nonmodifiable.

The nonmodifiable risk factors are those that cannot be changed or prevented. These are listed below:
- Increasing age.
- Female gender.
- Ethnicity (Caucasians are more susceptible).
- Menopause.
- Prior history of fractures.
- Family history of bone disease.

Modifiable risk factors for fragility fractures are listed below:
1. *Smoking:* Bone health is determined by turnover, the replacement of old cells with new cells to maintain bone strength and integrity. Certain harmful substances in cigarettes can have a detrimental effect on the bone turnover rate. Nicotine is a peripheral vasoconstrictor that slows down blood circulation, and carbon monoxide reduces the oxygen binding capacity of hemoglobin. This impairs healing and regeneration in all tissues, including bone (Xu et al., 2021).
2. *Alcohol use:* Acute alcohol intake affects wound and tissue healing by inhibiting inflammation, the formation of new vessels, and collagen production. Alcohol use has also been implicated in delaying fracture healing by inhibiting osteoblast proliferation (Xu et al., 2021).

3. *Reduced physical activity/sedentary lifestyle:* Physical inactivity is a major risk factor that has significantly increased the incidence of osteoporosis over the last few years. Standing and weight-bearing create mechanical stress on bones that sends signals for bone remodeling and increases bone mineral density. Less weight-bearing bones receive fewer signals and eventually become weaker and fracture-prone. A study carried out on healthy subjects showed that 12 weeks of bed rest reduced bone mineral density at the spine by 2.9% and hip by 3.8% (Zerwekh et al., 1998). Furthermore, studies have shown that bed rest increases bone resorption and decreases bone formation (Park et al., 2020).

4. *Micronutrient deficiency (vitamin D and calcium):* Vitamin D and calcium are known to play an important role in improving bone health. Maintaining adequate calcium intake and correcting the underlying vitamin D deficiency improves bone mineralization, but there is some evidence to suggest that it may also have a role in delaying osteoporosis and reducing the risk of fractures.

5. *Malnutrition and low body weight:* Malnourishment occurs when dietary intake is insufficient or if certain nutritional factors are deficient in the diet, resulting in a lower body mass index (BMI). Protein malnutrition can cause amino acid deficiency. Amino acids are precursors for many biological processes that speed up healing by promoting cellular growth and proliferation. Malnutrition mostly affects older adults over 65 years of age. It increases their risk of falls and obtunds fracture healing to cause nonunion (Meesters et al., 2018).

6. *Malabsorption/Gastrointestinal abnormalities:* Many gastrointestinal diseases, such as malabsorption and maldigestion, lead to osteoporosis. This could be attributable to concurrent nutritional deficiencies or absorption defects (Katz & Weinerman, 2010). A complete list of these GI abnormalities can be seen in Table 20.1.

7. *Eating disorders:* Disorders of eating, such as anorexia and bulimia, cause low bone mineral density and osteoporosis. However, studies have also shown that regardless of age and gender, there is an increased risk of falls and a high incidence of hip fractures in patients with eating orders (Axelsson et al., 2022).

8. *Falls/Gait disturbances:* Older adults and individuals with gait abnormalities are prone to falls and, hence, fragility fractures. Physical therapy and gait exercises may help in reducing falls.

Table 20.1 Gastrointestinal abnormalities that cause secondary osteoporosis.

Celiac disease
Postgastrectomy, short gut syndrome
Pancreatic insufficiency
Gastric bypass
Inflammatory bowel disease
Chronic liver disease (cholestatic and hepatic)
Liver and small bowel transplant
Total parenteral nutrition

9. *Medications:* There are many medications that can reduce bone mineral density (Table 20.2). The most notorious amongst them are corticosteroids that are usually given for asthma or autoimmune disorders. Proton pump inhibitors (PPIs) and antacids can interfere with calcium absorption from the gut. Antiepileptic drugs (AEDs) such as phenytoin, phenobarbital, and carbamazepine induce liver enzymes that inactivate vitamin D and affect calcium homeostasis. Even anticonvulsants that are enzyme noninducers, such as valproate, can also accelerate bone loss. Hence, most studies have shown that prolonged use of AEDs increases the risk of fractures. Medroxyprogesterone acetate (hormonal contraceptive), aromatase inhibitors (anti-androgenic), and gonadotropin-releasing hormone agonists cause a decline in estrogen levels and accelerate bone resorption similar to menopause. Thiazolidinediones (TZDs) are agonists of peroxisome proliferator-activated receptor γ (PPARγ) and treat type 2 diabetes by sensitizing insulin receptors. Since PPARγ is also expressed in stromal cells, it inhibits the formation of osteoblast precursors, causing osteoporosis. Heparin also reduces osteoblast differentiation and also increases bone resorption. Warfarin reduces bone mineralization and increases fractures, but the mechanism is unclear, and studies are inconclusive. Calcineurin inhibitors in combination with steroids can cause fragility fractures in transplant patients. Other drugs, such as selective-serotonin-reuptake inhibitors (SSRIs), also cause bone loss through unclear mechanisms (Panday et al., 2014). For a complete list of medications, see Table 20.2.

20.6 Common sites for fragility fractures

Fragility fractures commonly occur at the spine, hip, and wrist. Lesser common sites include pelvis, ribs, proximal tibia, arms, and shoulders. However, typical fragility fractures that should raise suspicion of severe osteoporosis are seen in the vertebrae, neck of femur, and Colles' fracture of the wrist. Vertebral and hip fractures are serious fractures that are associated with significant morbidity. See Fig. 20.2.

Table 20.2 Medications that cause secondary osteoporosis.

Anticonvulsants (phenobarbital, phenytoin, valproate, topiramate)
Anticoagulants (heparin, warfarin)
Aromatase inhibitors (letrozole, anastrozole)
Calcineurin inhibitors (tacrolimus)
Chemotherapy (methotrexate)
Gonadotropin-releasing hormone agonists and antagonists
Glucocorticoids
Medroxyprogesterone acetate (Depo-Provera)
PPIs
SERMs, e.g., tamoxifen
SSRIs, e.g., fluoxetine
Thiazolidinediones (rosiglitazone, pioglitazone)

PPIs, Proton pump inhibitors; *SERMs*, selective-estrogen receptor modulators; *SSRIs*, selective serotonin reuptake inhibitors.

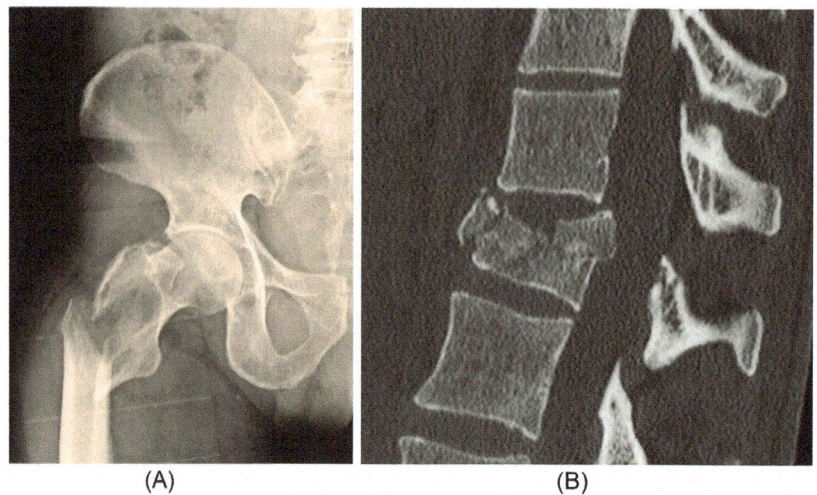

(A)   (B)

Figure 20.2

Fragility fractures. Hip fracture and vertebral compression fracture secondary to osteoporosis.

20.6.1   Vertebral fractures

These are often asymptomatic and diagnosed incidentally on imaging; some may experience back pain and loss of height. Incidence of spinal fractures increases with age in both sexes; however, it is higher in males up to 60 years of age, which could be related to occupational trauma. After the age of 60 years, the incidence is higher in females. The commonly affected vertebrae are mid-thoracic and thoracolumbar. They are diagnosed with dual-energy X-ray absorptiometry scan (DXA), which is discussed in detail below.

20.6.2   Hip fractures

Hip fractures are associated with significant morbidity as they cause immobility and a need for long-term nursing care. Around 75% of hip fractures occur in women, and studies have shown a 10%–20% higher mortality among women. It is diagnosed with radiographs, and early surgical intervention is the treatment of choice unless contraindicated due to comorbidities.

20.6.3   Wrist/forearm fractures

These fractures usually occur when the arms are outstretched to break falls. Most wrist fractures are likely to occur in women, especially over the age of 65 years. On the other hand, around 15% of wrist fractures have been reported in men with no significant effect of increasing age. Hence, a wrist fracture in males is a sensitive marker for skeletal fragility and warrants further investigation.

20.7 Diagnosis and screening for osteoporosis

Screening for osteoporosis is deemed necessary due to its global prevalence and major economic impact. Most developed countries have incorporated screening programs in their healthcare systems for early detection and intervention. The USPSTF (United States Preventive Services Task Force) recommends screening for all women over age 65 years and all postmenopausal women with risk factors for osteoporosis. The National Osteoporosis Foundation (NOF) additionally recommends screening in all men over the age of 70 years because of similar fracture risk. See summarized screening recommendations for osteoporosis in Table 20.3.

The best screening tool for osteoporosis is dual-energy X-ray absorptiometry (DXA) scan, which measures bone strength by low and high-energy photon emissions that calculate bone mineral density (BMD). The higher the density, the stronger the bone. Results are displayed as T-scores defined by the World Health Organization (WHO) as follows:

- T-score greater than or equal to $-1.0 \rightarrow$ Normal.
- T-score between -1.0 and $-2.5 \rightarrow$ Osteopenia.
- T-score less than or equal to $-2.5 \rightarrow$ Osteoporosis.
- T-score less than or equal to -2.5 plus fragility fracture $\rightarrow$ Severe osteoporosis.

Table 20.3 Recommendations for osteoporosis screening.

All women over age 65 years OR men over age 70 years
Women younger than 65 years with:
● Estrogen deficiency
● Hip fracture before age 50 years
● Low BMI < 18.5 kg/m^2
● Premature menopause
Women younger than 65 years OR men younger than 70 years who are/have:
● Current smokers
● Loss of height
● Thoracic kyphosis
Osteopenia or fragility fractures at any age
More than one fracture at any site at any age
Use of glucocorticoid at dose 5 mg or more for > 3 months (receiving or planning to receive)
Men with hypogonadism (> age 18 years)
Chronic medical conditions
● Hyperparathyroidism
● Hyperthyroidism
● Cushing's syndrome
Assessing response to osteoporosis treatment
Follow-up for abnormal BMD in chronic conditions

BMD, Bone mineral density.

In 2008, the World Health Organization (WHO) implemented the Fracture Risk Assessment Tool (FRAX) to calculate the risk of developing a fracture in a 10-year time period (Fujiwara et al., 2008). The National Osteoporosis Foundation (NOF) recommends calculating the FRAX Score of all patients who have T-scores between −1.0 and −2.5 in the hip, spinal, or femoral neck region to quantify their 10-year risk of developing a fracture (Watts, 2011). Clinical factors that are used to determine the FRAX score are listed in Table 20.4.

Once osteoporosis is confirmed, it is recommended to screen for secondary causes of osteoporosis by testing for the following:
• 25-Hydroxy vitamin D level.
• Serum calcium and phosphate.
• Serum creatinine.
• Thyroid-stimulating hormone (TSH).

20.8   Treatment

Once osteoporosis is diagnosed, it is necessary to treat it to prevent its disastrous consequences, like fragility fractures. Treatment can be classified as pharmacological and nonpharmacological.

20.9   Pharmacological treatment

Antiresorptive agents such as bisphosphonates are first-line treatment for osteoporosis. Multiple RCTs have proven that oral and intravenous bisphosphonates significantly reduce

Table 20.4   Determinants of FRAX Score (absolute fracture risk calculation)

Age (between 40 and 90 years)
Sex
Weight
Height
Previous fracture
Fractured hip in parent
Smoking
Use of steroids
Rheumatoid arthritis
Secondary osteoporosis
Alcohol use (3 or more units/day)
Femoral Neck BMD in g/cm^2 (determined by DXA scan)

Source: Kanis, J. A., Johnell, O., Oden, A., Johansson, H., McCloskey, E. V., Melton, L. J. *FRAX™: A tool for assessing fracture risk*. University of Sheffield, UK. Available at: FRAX.

spinal and hip fractures, even in patients with postmenopausal and steroid-induced osteoporosis. They need to be taken with caution because of their untoward GI effects.

Calcitonin and selective-estrogen receptor modulators (SERMs) such as Raloxifene treat postmenopausal osteoporosis but are only useful for compression vertebral fractures. SERMs increase the risk of breast cancer and thrombosis. Calcitonin is also associated with an increased risk of cancer. Teriparatide is a recombinant human parathyroid hormone, and it is used when bisphosphonate therapy fails. Denosumab is a human monoclonal antibody that inhibits osteoclastic activity and reduces spinal, hip, and nonvertebral fractures. It is also safe to use in patients with renal disease.

20.10   Nonpharmacological treatment

Nonpharmacological methods include physical activity to prevent falls, smoking cessation, alcohol use in moderation, dietary modifications, and correcting underlying micronutrient deficiencies. These are also methods of primary prevention.

20.11   Fall prevention

Falls have a stronger association with fractures as compared to low BMD. Therefore, preventing falls in the geriatric population is equally important as treating osteoporosis, if not more. Multiple measures can be undertaken to overcome these factors, which are broadly classified as extrinsic and intrinsic.

Extrinsic factors that contribute to falls inside the house include slippery, uneven surfaces, clutter such as extra furniture, stranded objects, loose cords from electronics, inadequate lighting, and lack of supportive surfaces like handrails.

Intrinsic factors that predispose to falls are related to an individual's health status, such as gait imbalance due to motor or sensory defects, muscle weakness, impaired vision, cognitive decline, chronic diseases, and use of medications that cause dizziness. The USPSTF recommends physical therapy to overcome some of these factors by balance-training and weight-bearing resistance exercises.

20.12   Effect of vitamin D and calcium

Vitamin D and calcium are strongly recommended for improving bone health. Therefore, supplementation with these micronutrients is universally adopted for most bone disorders. However, multiple studies and controlled trials on calcium and vitamin D have been conducted, and they show different results based upon dosage, indications, and duration of treatment. An earlier study performed by Chapuy et al. (1992) in institutionalized elderly females showed that vitamin D supplementation of 800 IU/day reduced the rate of hip fractures by 43% and increased bone densitometry by 2.7% compared to the placebo group. Furthermore, this study later concluded the intervention to be extremely cost-effective (Meier & Kraenzlin, 2011). Based on this study, vitamin D and calcium supplementation became a common practice. A meta-analysis was published in New Zealand in 2020 by Reid and Bolland (2020) that showed that vitamin D supplementation was dependent upon baseline levels of vitamin D. For instance, patients with 25-hydroxy vitamin D level < 30 mol/L, showed a reduction in bone loss with supplements. However, in patients with 25-hydroxy vitamin D level > 30 nmol/L, there was no effect of supplementation. Doses of 400–1000 IU/day are considered safe doses of vitamin D. Trials show that higher doses of vitamin D up to 4000 IU/day accelerate bone loss, increase risk of falls and fractures (Sanders et al., 2010). Calcium supplements, 500–1000 mg, can transiently increase calcium levels in the blood, and this will suppress parathyroid hormone and halt bone resorption for a few months to a year. However, continued supplementation does not show further improvement in bone density or reduction in fractures. Furthermore, calcium supplements are not without side effects. Prolonged use is associated with gastrointestinal disturbances like constipation, increased incidence of urinary calculi, and increased risk of myocardial infarction and stroke (Reid & Bolland, 2020).

Bisphosphonates are the drug of choice for osteoporosis, and they significantly reduce the risk of vertebral and hip fractures even when administered alone. Coadministration of calcium or vitamin D with bisphosphonates also did not increase efficacy any further. However, it is necessary to ensure that serum levels of calcium and vitamin D are adequate prior to using antiresorptive agents such as bisphosphonates or denosumab, as their use can cause severe hypocalcemia (Reid & Bolland, 2020). Another meta-analysis was published in Medicine in 2020, which compared many randomized controlled trials, including the study by Reid and Bolland (2020). This study concluded that vitamin D3 (cholecalciferol) specifically did reduce the incidence of falls, and combination therapy of vitamin D with calcium also reduced the overall risk of fractures. These results were associated with higher daily doses of vitamin D up to 800 IU/day (Thanapluetiwong et al., 2020). These contrasting results from prior meta-analysis by Reid and Bolland are likely due to different cutoff levels of vitamin D and calcium, the number of participants analyzed, and duration of treatment intervention.

20.13 Primary prevention

These are strategies or interventions that are employed to prevent the initial disease event, that is, fragility fracture. First, the population at risk is identified, and then measures are taken to eliminate the risk factors. A few pertinent interventions include physical rehabilitation, exercises, dietary modifications, micronutrient supplementation, fall prevention, and review of medications that cause secondary osteoporosis as listed in Table 20.2. Patients who are on medications that cause secondary osteoporosis, such as antiepileptic drugs, should have a baseline 25-hydroxy vitamin D level ideally before initiation of therapy and then follow-up level every 6–12 monthly to ensure that vitamin D levels are adequate (Meier & Kraenzlin, 2011). It is prudent to replace vitamin D and calcium with daily supplements and encourage weight-bearing exercises while continuing treatment with these medicines.

20.14   Secondary prevention

Individuals who have already sustained a fragility fracture should have all measures done to prevent another fall and fracture. This is secondary prevention. Such patients should receive osteoporosis treatment and interventions to prevent future falls. A history of prior fractures significantly increases the risk of further falls and increases morbidity and mortality among older women. Hence, rehabilitation along with secondary prevention is necessary to improve outcomes.

20.15   Conclusion

Fragility fractures carry significant morbidity that has a negative impact on the healthcare system. Early screening and intervention may provide some relief; however, there are certain gaps in care that must be addressed. Calcium supplementation by itself has not proven to be beneficial; however, there are enough data to support a preventive and protective effect of vitamin D supplementation on reducing rates of fragility fractures. Furthermore, this intervention appears to be highly cost-effective when compared to the immense healthcare costs imposed after fractures' occurrence.

References

Axelsson, K. F., Woessner, M. N., Litsne, H., Wheeler, M., Flehr, A., King, A. J., Kalén, M., Vandenput, L., & Lorentzon, M. (2022). Eating disorders are associated with increased risk of fall injury and fracture in Swedish men and women. *Osteoporosis International, 33*(6), 1347–1355. https://doi.org/10.1007/s00198-022-06312-2.

Chapuy, M. C., Arlot, M. E., Duboeuf, F., Brun, J., Crouzet, B., Arnaud, S., Delmas, P. D., & Meunier, P. J. (1992). Vitamin D3 and calcium to prevent hip fractures in elderly women. *New England Journal of Medicine, 327*(23), 1637–1642. https://doi.org/10.1056/NEJM199212033272305.

Fujiwara, S., Nakamura, T., Orimo, H., Hosoi, T., Gorai, I., Odén, A., & Kanis, J. A. (2008). Development and application of a Japanese model of the WHO fracture risk assessment tool (FRAX™). *Osteoporosis International, 19*, 429–435.

Kanis, J. A., Norton, N., Harvey, N. C., Jacobson, T., Johansson, H., Lorentzon, M., McCloskey, E. V., Willers, C., & Borgström, F. (2021). SCOPE 2021: A new scorecard for osteoporosis in Europe. *Archives of Osteoporosis, 16*(1). https://doi.org/10.1007/s11657-020-00871-9, http://www.springer.com/west/home?SGWID=4-102-70-173658284-0&changeHeader=true.

Katz, S., & Weinerman, S. (2010). Osteoporosis and gastrointestinal disease. *Gastroenterology and Hepatology, 6*(8), 506–517.

Meesters, D. M., Wijnands, K. A. P., Brink, P. R. G., & Poeze, M. (2018). Malnutrition and fracture healing: Are specific deficiencies in amino acids important in nonunion development? *Nutrients, 10*(11), 1597 2018.

Meier, C., & Kraenzlin, M. E. (2011). Antiepileptics and bone health. *Therapeutic Advances in Musculoskeletal Disease, 3*(5), 235–243. https://doi.org/10.1177/1759720X11410769.

Panday, K., Gona, A., & Humphrey, M. B. (2014). Medication-induced osteoporosis: Screening and treatment strategies. *Therapeutic Advances in Musculoskeletal Disease, 6*(5), 185–202. https://doi.org/10.1177/1759720X14546350.

Park, J. H., Moon, J. H., Kim, H. J., Kong, M. H., & Oh, Y. H. (2020). Sedentary lifestyle: Overview of updated evidence of potential health risks. *Korean Journal of Family Medicine, 41*(6), 365.

Reid, I. R., & Bolland, M. J. (2020). Calcium and/or vitamin D supplementation for the prevention of fragility fractures: Who needs it? *Nutrients, 12*(4). https://doi.org/10.3390/nu12041011, https://www.mdpi.com/2072-6643/12/4/1011/pdf.

Salari, N., Ghasemi, H., Mohammadi, L., Behzadi, M. H., Rabieenia, E., & Shohaimi, S. (2021). The global prevalence of osteoporosis in the world: A comprehensive systematic review and meta-analysis. *Journal of Orthopaedic Surgery and Research, 16*, 1–20.

Sanders, K. M., Stuart, A. L., Williamson, E. J., Simpson, J. A., Kotowicz, M. A., Young, D., & Nicholson, G. C. (2010). Annual high-dose oral vitamin D and falls and fractures in older women: A randomized controlled trial. *JAMA: the Journal of the American Medical Association, 303*(18), 1815–1822. https://doi.org/10.1001/jama.2010.594, http://jama.ama-assn.org/cgi/reprint/303/18/1815.

Thanapluetiwong, S., Chewcharat, A., Takkavatakarn, K., Praditpornsilpa, K., & Eiam-Ong, S. (2020). Vitamin D supplement on prevention of fall and fracture: A meta- analysis of randomized controlled trials. *Medicine, 99*(34), e21506.

Watts, N. B. (2011). The fracture risk assessment tool (FRAX®): Applications in clinical practice. *Journal of Women's Health, 20*(4), 525–531. https://doi.org/10.1089/jwh.2010.2294.

Wu, A. M., Bisignano, C., James, S. L., Abady, G. G., Abedi, A., & Abu-Gharbieh, E. (2021). Global, regional, and national burden of bone fractures in 204 countries and territories, 1990–2019: A systematic analysis from the Global Burden of Disease Study 2019. *The Lancet Healthy Longevity, 9*(2), e580–e592.

Xu, B., Anderson, D. B., Eun-Sun, P. A. R. K., Chen, L., & Lee (2021). The influence of smoking and alcohol on bone healing: Systematic review and meta-analysis of non-pathological fractures. *EClinicalMedicine, 42*.

Zerwekh, J. E., Ruml, L. A., Gottschalk, F., & Pak, C. Y. C. (1998). The effects of twelve weeks of bed rest on bone histology, biochemical markers of bone turnover, and calcium homeostasis in eleven normal subjects. *Journal of Bone and Mineral Research, 13*(10), 1594–1601. https://doi.org/10.1359/jbmr.1998.13.10.1594.

CHAPTER 21

Rare disorders of vitamin D metabolism

Aysha Habib Khan[1], and Manju Chandran[2,3]

[1]Department of Pathology & Laboratory Medicine, The Aga Khan University, Karachi, Pakistan
[2]Osteoporosis and Bone Metabolism Unit, Department of Endocrinology, Singapore General Hospital, Singapore [3]DUKE NUS Medical School, Singapore

21.1   Introduction

Historically, vitamin D deficiency was linked to rickets, particularly in socioeconomically disadvantaged populations with limited sunlight exposure and inadequate dietary intake. Over time, clinicians observed that some individuals required unusually high doses of vitamin D, while others remained unresponsive to conventional therapy. These puzzling cases led to the identification of rare genetic disorders affecting vitamin D metabolism and receptor function (Bikle, 2014; Fraser et al., 1973; Christakos et al., 2015).

The first documented evidence of such genetic defects emerged in 1961 when Prader and colleagues described pseudo-deficiency rickets, a condition marked by hypocalcemia, defective bone mineralization, and resistance to standard vitamin D therapy. Today, we recognize that rare vitamin D disorders stem from mutations impacting its activation, receptor function, or degradation, disrupting calcium and phosphate regulation (Prader, Illig & Heierli, 1961; Feldman & Pike, 2005; Bikle, 2014; Jones, 2010).

The study of rare disorders of vitamin D metabolism not only helps in managing affected patients, but also provides insight into the essential role of vitamin D in health and its diverse biological effects. Identifying these disorders early is crucial for preventing severe complications such as rickets, osteomalacia, and growth retardation in children. Treatment often involves high doses of vitamin D or its active metabolites and, in some cases, calcium supplements to manage hypocalcemia. It is very important to know that a disorder of genetic origin may be the cause of the failure of classic treatment in patients with rachitic symptoms. Proper management is essential to maintain bone density and prevent fractures and includes regular monitoring of serum calcium, phosphate, and vitamin D levels to adjust treatment and prevent complications. Diagnosis can be challenging due to genetic variability and environmental influences, underscoring the need for greater awareness among healthcare providers to facilitate early screening and intervention (Fu et al., 1997;

Monkawa et al., 1997; Li et al., 1998; Dardenne et al., 2001; Glorieux & St-Arnaud, 2005; Kim et al., 2007; Rebelos, Tentolouris & Jude, 2023).

With advancements in molecular diagnostics, the understanding of vitamin D metabolism disorders has expanded dramatically. This chapter presents an updated classification system, integrating recent scientific discoveries to enhance comprehension of these rare disorders in both the research and clinical settings. To illustrate the clinical presentation, diagnostic challenges, and management of these rare conditions, we provide a series of case examples. While these cases are not real, they are based on common clinical patterns observed in patients with these disorders, helping to contextualize the impact of these metabolic defects in real-world scenarios.

21.2   Classification of rare disorders of vitamin D metabolism

There are multiple ways to classify these disorders, but the most effective approach is based on genetic mutations that alter biochemical pathways and clinical phenotypes. A precise understanding of these mechanisms is essential for accurate diagnosis and targeted treatment. Table 21.1 outlines the genetic classification, while Table 21.2 summarizes the biochemical and clinical features of these disorders.

21.3   Disorders of vitamin D synthesis

21.3.1   Overview of vitamin D synthesis

Fig. 21.1A shows the synthesis of active vitamin D, which begins with its synthesis in the skin upon exposure of 7 dehydrocholesterol (7-DHC) to ultraviolet B (UVB) in sunlight to form previtamin D. Previtamin D undergoes temperature-dependent isomerization to vitamin D (cholecalciferol). Dietary intake in plant (ergocalciferol) and animal (cholecalciferol) sources of vitamin D complements this endogenous synthesis. Activation of cholecalciferol requires two hydroxylation steps; the first of which occurs in liver microsomes, catalyzed by P450 25-hydroxylase (CYP2R1) enzyme, resulting in the formation of 25-hydroxyvitamin D [25(OH) D(Calcidiol)], which is the primary circulating metabolite and provides the best index of nutritional vitamin D status. The second hydroxylation occurs in the proximal tubule cells in kidneys by mitochondrial cytochrome P450 1-alpha-hydroxylase (CYP27B1), producing 1,25-dihydroxyvitamin D [$1,25(OH)_2D$], the biologically active form that binds to the vitamin D receptor (VDR) to mediate its effects. Renal CYP27B1 is tightly regulated, and its expression and activity are induced by PTH and suppressed by FGF23 (Christakos et al., 2015).

Genetic or acquired defects in any of these steps in the synthesis of vitamin D can lead to a heterogeneous group of the following rare conditions.

Table 21.1 Classification of rare disorders of vitamin D (VD) metabolism based on genetic defects.

Type	OMIM ID	Defect/s	Gene	Location	Effect
I. Disorders of vitamin D synthesis					
Vitamin D-dependent rickets type 1 A	264700	1-Alpha hydroxylase deficiency	CYP27B1	Kidney PCT cells	Impaired renal conversion of 25(OH)D to 1, 25 (OH)$_2$D
Vitamin D-dependent rickets type 1B/ selective pseudo vitamin D deficiency rickets (PDDR)	600081	25-Hydroxylase deficiency	CYP2R1	Liver microsomes	Inadequate conversion of Colecalciferol to 25(OH)D
II. Disorders of signaling/vitamin D receptor function					
Vitamin D-dependent rickets type 2 A/ Hereditary vitamin D-resistant rickets (HVDRR) /hereditary resistance to 1,25(OH)$_2$D/pseudo vitamin D deficiency type IIa (PDRRIIa)	277440	• Complete absence of 1,25(OH)$_2$D binding, • Reduced Vitamin D Receptor (VDR) binding affinity for 1,25(OH)$_2$D, • Disrupted RXR alpha heterodimerization • Interference with cofactor inactivation	VDR	Most tissues of the body	Impaired cellular response to 1,25(OH)$_2$D i.e end organ resistance to 1,25(OH)$_2$D
Vitamin D-dependent rickets type 2B with normal VDR, vitamin D-dependent rickets type 2 with alopecia	600785	Abnormal expression of a hormone response element-binding protein	Unknown nuclear ribonucleoprotein interfering with signal transduction		Interference with the normal function of VDR
III. Increased inactivation of vitamin D metabolites					
Vitamin D-dependent rickets type 3 (VDDR3)	619073	Caused by mutation in the cytochrome P450, subfamily IIIA, polypeptide-4 gene	CYP3A4	Liver	Rapid inactivation of 25 D and 1,25 (OH)$_2$D. 4-beta,25-dihydroxyvitamin D, (the principal product of CYP3A4 metabolism of 25(OH)D) to 1,25 (OH)$_2$D markedly elevated
IV. Disorders of vitamin D hypersensitivity/inactivation					
Infantile hypercalcemia type 1 (IH type 1)	143880	Mutations in the 24-hydroxylase enzyme	CYP24A1	Kidney, intestine, and bone	Impaired inactivation of 1,25(OH)$_2$D and 25(OH)D, results in their accumulation, In adults may manifest as renal stone disease
Infantile hypercalcemia type 2 (IH type 2)	616963	Mutations in renal sodium phosphate cotransporter (NaP1–11a)	SLC34A1	Kidney	Kidney's ability to reabsorb phosphate is impaired leading to increased compensatory increase in 1,25 (OH)$_2$D

Table 21.2 Biochemical and clinical features in rare diseases of vitamin D metabolism.

Disorders	Mode of inheritance	Age at presentation	Biochemical features	Clinical features
VDDR1A	AR	2–4 months of life	Hypocalcemia, hypophosphatemia, increased alkaline phosphatase, secondary hyperparathyroidism, decreased or undetectable 1,25(OH)$_2$D, normal or increased 25(OH)D	Affected individuals present with rickets and osteomalacia despite normal or elevated 25(OH)D levels. Hypotonia, irritability, tetany or seizures & failure to thrive
VDDR1B	AR	6 months -2 years	Low-to-normal serum calcium, hypophosphatemia, increased alkaline phosphatase, normal 1,25(OH)$_2$D decreased 25(OH)D	Features of rickets with poor growth, skeletal deformities, and muscle weakness
VDDR2A	AR	2–8 months of life	Hypocalcemia, increased 1,25(OH)$_2$D	Clinically characterized by alopecia and severe rickets
VDDR2B	AR	infancy	Hypocalcemia, increased 1,25(OH)$_2$D	Idiopathic infantile hypercalcemia, hypercalciuria, nephrocalcinosis, and recurrent kidney stones
VDDR3	AD	2 years	Very low 25 (OH)D and 1,25 (OH)$_2$D despite supplementation. Ratio of 4-beta, 25 (OH)$_2$D to 1,25 (OH)$_2$ D markedly elevated.	Short stature and clinical features of rickets
IH1	AR	Infancy, later childhood, and adulthood	Hypercalcemia, hypercalciuria, elevated or inappropriately normal 1,25 (OH)$_2$D, Suppressed PTH	Nephrocalcinosis, and growth impairment, affected adults may develop extrarenal manifestations, including Ca deposits in joints, cornea.
IH2	AR	Infancy, kidney disease in adults	Hypophosphatemia, phosphaturia, hypercalcemia, suppressed PTH	Features of hypercalcemia, vomiting, failure to thrive, nephrocalcinosis, and nephrolithiasis

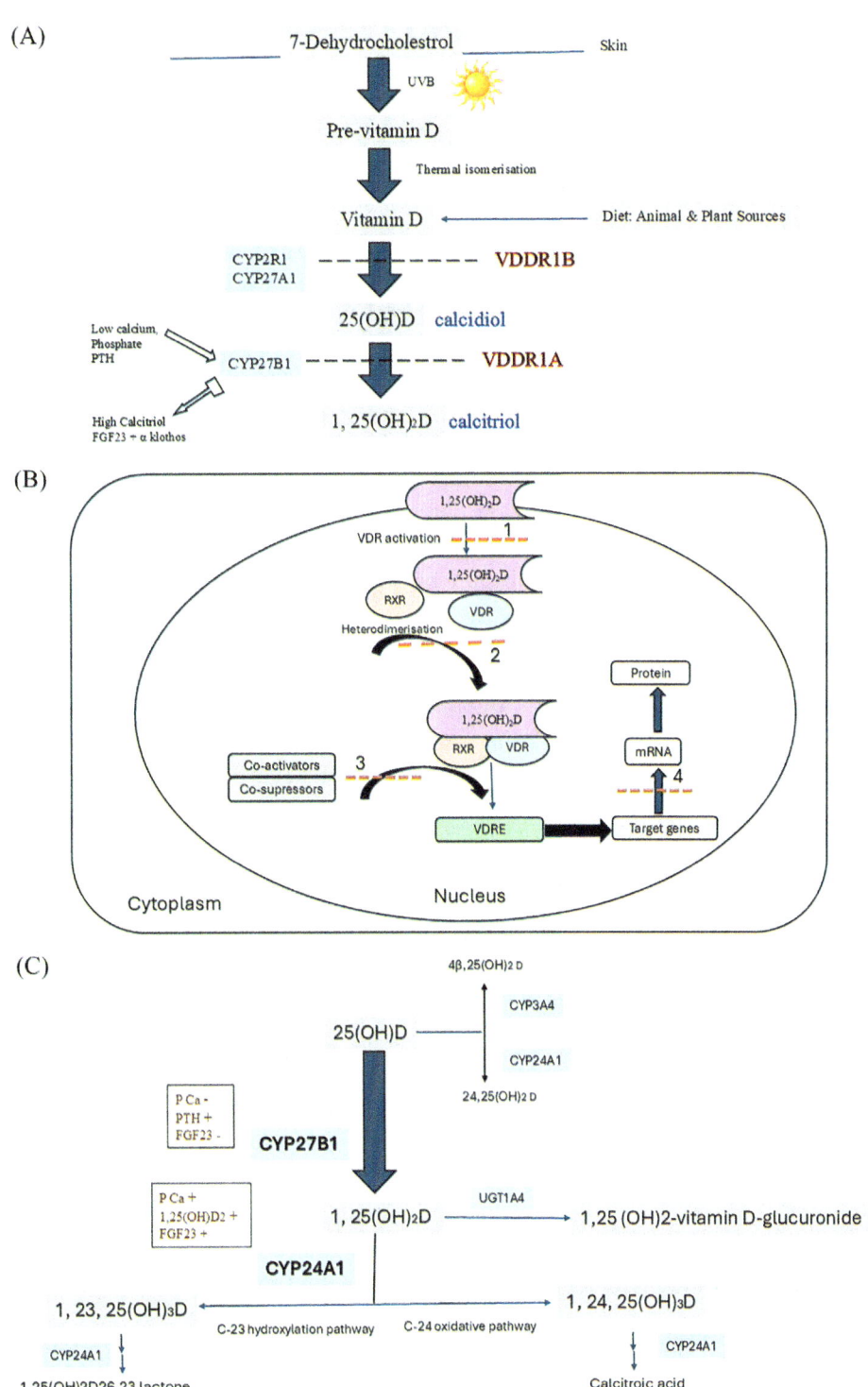

Figure 21.1

Vitamin D metabolism and the overall metabolic control of vitamin D homeostasis.

21.3.2 Vitamin D-dependent rickets type 1 A

Case study: A puzzling case of rickets

Mariam, an 18-month-old girl, was brought to the pediatric endocrinology clinic with persistent muscle weakness, frequent falls, and delayed developmental milestones in walking. Despite early recognition of rickets at 10 months, conventional vitamin D supplementation failed to resolve her symptoms. Physical examination revealed frontal bossing, widening of the wrists, and bowed legs. Laboratory tests showed hypocalcemia, elevated alkaline phosphatase, and undetectable $1,25(OH)_2D$ levels despite normal $25(OH)D$. A skeletal survey confirmed rickets, and genetic testing identified a CYP27B1 mutation. She was started on calcitriol and calcium supplementation, leading to improved muscle strength and radiological healing over the next six months.

Vitamin D-dependent rickets type 1 A (VDDR1A, OMIM 264700) is the most common form of rickets, inherited in an autosomal recessive manner. This condition is caused by mutations in the CYP27B1 gene, which is located on chromosome 12q13. The disorder leads to the inactivation of the enzyme 1-alpha hydroxylase, resulting in decreased serum levels of $1,25(OH)_2D$ and creating a selective deficiency of this active form of vitamin D. Individuals with vitamin D dependency require unusually high doses of vitamin D to maintain remission from the disease (Cui et al., 2012; Meyer et al., 2024).

Affected subjects appear normal at birth. Impaired $1,25(OH)_2D$ activity becomes obvious at 2–24 months. Hypotonia, irritability, tetany or seizures, and failure to thrive are typical in the first few months of life. Typical skeletal features of rickets (e.g., frontal bossing, long-bone deformities, and rib cage abnormalities), as well as impaired growth, become evident within the first two years of life. Delayed tooth eruption, enamel hypoplasia, low trauma fractures, and seizures due to hypocalcemia can occur (Sunkar & Neeharika, 2020; Levine, 2020).

Biochemically, patients exhibit hypocalcemia, hypophosphatemia, and elevated alkaline phosphatase and parathyroid hormone levels. Plasma concentrations of $1,25(OH)_2D$ are low or undetectable. By contrast, plasma concentrations of $25(OH)D$ are normal or increased, likely reflecting the effects of vitamin D supplementation given to combat deficiency and decreased clearance of $25(OH)D$ due to lack of induction of CYP24A1 by the absence of $1,25(OH)_2D$. If untreated, there is progressive skeletal deformity and short stature. With appropriate early diagnosis and appropriate intervention, individuals can achieve normal growth and development. However, in some individuals, despite vitamin D supplementation, fractures, rachitic rosary, growth failure, genu valgum deformity, and hypotonia can occur (Giannakopoulos, Efthymiadou & Chrysis, 2017; Sunkar & Neeharika, 2020).

Patients with VDDR1A respond to supplementation with calcium and activated forms of vitamin D, such as calcitriol and 1 α hydroxyvitamin D3 (alfacalcidiol). Parent vitamin D (ergocalciferol or cholecalciferol) or 25(OH)-vitamin D (calcifediol) can be used at pharmacologic doses but carries a greater risk of inducing hypercalcemia. Calcitriol, effective in physiological doses, is usually administered twice per day due to its relatively short half-life. Treatment with 1 α hydroxyvitamin D3 is similarly effective as this metabolite also overcomes the enzymatic block, and due to its longer half-life than calcitriol, it can be administered once daily. During the first 3–6 months, as the under-mineralized skeleton requires unusually large amounts of calcium, patients should be given calciferol in doses 2–5 times those expected for long-term maintenance. Calcium supplements should also be given during initial treatment to prevent the worsening of hypocalcemia due to the "hungry bones" phenomenon that occurs with remineralization of the skeleton (Haffner et al., 2022; Biasucci, Donini & Cannalire, 2024).

With successful therapy, the fractional absorption of calcium in the intestine remains constant. However, blood and urinary calcium can fluctuate greatly with variations in the dietary intake of calcium; therefore it is recommended to give calcium supplements to ensure a consistent intake of calcium. Treatment must be continued indefinitely. Despite their effectiveness, calcitriol and alfacalcidiol are also often associated with complications such as nephrocalcinosis, hypercalcemia and hypercalciuria (Haffner et al., 2022; Levine, 2020; Biasucci, Donini & Cannalire, 2024).

21.3.3 Vitamin D-dependent rickets type 1B

Case study: Mysteriously persistent hypocalcemia in Nigeria

Ade, a 3-year- old boy presented with short stature, frequent fractures, and delayed dentition. Despite receiving standard vitamin D therapy, his 25(OH)D levels remained abnormally low, and his symptoms persisted. His family history was unremarkable for metabolic bone disorders. Genetic testing identified a CYP2R1 mutation, diagnosing him with VDDR1B. High-dose cholecalciferol was prescribed, and after months of careful monitoring, Ade showed significant improvements in bone strength and growth velocity.

Vitamin D-dependent rickets type 1B (VDDR1B, OMIM 600081) is due to impaired production of 25(OH)D (calcifediol or calcidiol). It is due to mutations in the CYP2R1 gene, located on chromosome 11p15.2 (Fig. 21.1C), that decrease the expression or function of the encoded microsomal cytochrome P450 CYP2R1 enzyme in the liver (principal 25-hydroxylase). The 25-hydroxylase activity is also possessed by CYP27A1, a cytochrome P450 oxidase in mitochondria, commonly known as sterol 27-hydroxylase and involved in the biosynthesis of bile acids (Balsan et al., 1986; Hirst, Hochman & Feldman, 1985; Thacher et al., 2015).

CYP2R1 mutations were first reported in 1994 in two Nigerian siblings with severe rickets despite normal 1,25(OH)$_2$D and subsequently in 2004 and 2012 in Nigerian and Saudi siblings with similar biochemical anomalies. They responded to high-dose vitamin D therapy, emphasizing CYP2R1's residual enzymatic activity or alternative hydroxylation pathways in maintaining partial function. Later, Thacher et al. in 2015 and Molin et al. in 2017 provided critical insights into CYP2R1 mutations, demonstrating semidominant inheritance patterns (Casella et al., 1994; Cheng et al., 2004; Al Mutair, Nasrat & Russell, 2012).

VDDR1B is associated with hypocalcemia, low 25(OH)D, and secondary hyperparathyroidism, with reduced clinical and biochemical response to conventional doses of vitamin D. The clinical phenotype of VDDR1B closely resembles VDDR1A, but in contrast, the magnitude of vitamin D deficiency and clinical severity in subjects with *CYP2R1* mutations exhibits a gene dosage effect with a milder phenotype in patients who carry only one defective allele. The phenotype appears to improve with age, likely due to the acquisition of vitamin D-independent mechanisms for intestinal absorption of calcium mediated perhaps by postpubertal sex hormones. It is also possible that other CYP enzymes that possess 25-hydroxylase activity may assume greater importance as the child matures (Cali & Russell, 1991; Molin et al., 2017; Thacher et al., 2015; Menon et al., 2024).

Management of VDDR1B requires the administration of pharmacologic doses of ergocalciferol or cholecalciferol or physiological doses of calcitriol, plus supplemental calcium. The availability of calcifediol (25 $(OH)D_3$ now permits a superior pharmacological approach that bypasses the defect in 25-hydroxylation and has the advantage of restoring physiological control of mineral metabolism. Serum levels of calcium and PTH should be maintained in the mid-normal range, and treatment will be required for life (Mansour et al., 2023; Levine, 2020).

21.4 Disorders of signaling/vitamin D receptor function

Disorders of vitamin D receptor (VDDR2, OMIM 601769) function are rare genetic conditions that disrupt the body's ability to respond to $1,25(OH)_2D$ for its biological activity. The vitamin D receptor (VDR) is a member of a superfamily of nuclear steroid hormone receptors that regulate gene transcription by interacting with response elements in gene promoters. The two core functional domains of the VDR are the highly conserved NH2-terminal DNA binding domain (DBD) and the more variable COOH-terminal ligand binding domain (LBD), connected through a hinge region. $1,25(OH)_2D$ binding induces a conformational change that facilitates interaction with RXR, and coregulatory complexes required for the transcription of target genes (Fig. 21.1b). VDDR2, that is characterized by resistance to $1,25(OH)_2D$ owing to mutations in the VDR, is denoted as vitamin D-dependent rickets type 2 A (VDDR2A), änd that due to the presence of a nuclear ribonuclear protein that interferes with the vitamin D receptor -DNA interaction, is termed VDDR2B (Fig. 21.1B) (St-Arnaud et al., 1997; Rochel et al., 2000; Malloy, Feldman & Pike, 2005).

21.4.1   Vitamin D-dependent rickets type 2 A

Case study: When high vitamin D doses fail

Anna, a 2-year-old girl, was initially treated with high-dose vitamin D for rickets but failed to show improvement. Her parents noticed that she had sparse scalp hair since infancy. Further testing revealed severe hypocalcemia, secondary hyperparathyroidism, and markedly elevated $1,25(OH)_2D$ levels. Genetic analysis confirmed a VDR mutation, leading to a diagnosis of VDDR2A. Due to her resistance to vitamin D, Anna required long-term intravenous calcium infusions and high-dose oral calcium supplementation to maintain adequate mineralization.

Vitamin D-dependent rickets type 2 A(VDDR2A, OMIM 277440) is due to biallelic loss-of-function mutations in the gene encoding the VDR on chromosome 12q13.11 and, therefore, represents a form of tissue resistance to vitamin D. As many patients with this disorder are unable to respond to any form of vitamin D; it is more appropriately described by the terms hereditary 1,25 $(OH)_2D$-resistant rickets (HVDRR), hereditary resistance to 1,25 $(OH)_2D$, or even pseudo vitamin D-deficiency, type IIA (PDDR IIA) (Hochberg et al., 1984; Chen et al., 1984; Balsan et al., 1986).

VDDR2A manifests as an active metabolic bone disease in early childhood. Patients normal at birth develop features of vitamin D deficiency over the first 2–8 months of life with low calcium, phosphorus, elevated 1,25(OH)2D, and normal or elevated 25(OH)D. More than 50% of the patients have total alopecia or sparse hair, believed to be due to more severe diseases in the vitamin D receptor effector system. The cause is increased expression of the hairless (*Hr*) protein, a transcription factor that regulates hair follicle cycling via interaction with unliganded VDR. Alopecia is associated with VDR mutations that impair DNA binding, RXR heterodimerization, or production of the VDR, while mutations that alter VDR affinity for $1,25(OH)_2D$ or disrupt coactivator interactions do not cause alopecia. Several sporadic cases with mild late-onset disease in adolescence and adulthood have been described that undergo remission when treated (Fraher et al., 1986; Malloy et al., 1990; Malloy et al., 1997; Cockerill et al., 1997; Ahmad et al., 1998).

Management during the first few months of life may require high doses of oral calcium. In some cases, intravenous calcium may be necessary to raise the serum calcium and replenish calcium deficits. Most patients require additional therapy with age as the requirement for calcium increases and vitamin D-independent intestinal absorption of calcium decreases. Children with milder forms of VDDR2A, such as those without alopecia, may have clinical and radiologic improvement with the administration of high-dose vitamin D therapy. Many patients will achieve complete remission after receiving very high doses of calciferol. Among patients with alopecia, about half will be resistant to even the highest doses of colecalciferol; the other half have demonstrated satisfactory calcemic responses at doses that are typically 10 times greater than in those with normal hair. Some patients will be unable to produce sufficient $1,25(OH)_2D$ to overcome the VDR defect but nevertheless will respond to extraordinarily high doses of calcitriol (1,25 $(OH)_2D$) or alpha calcidiol ($1\alpha(OH)D$). These patients should receive consistent daily supplementation with calcium (Blizotes et al., 1988; Panda et al., 2004; Ma et al., 2009).

Those patients who fail to respond to maximal doses of colecalciferol will require intravenous infusions of calcium, over many months to achieve clinically meaningful results. Although fractional calcium absorption is low from early childhood through the end of puberty, during and after puberty, subjects with VDDR2A develop an unusual adaptation that is characterized by an increase in calcium absorption to levels that are even greater than those of normal subjects. Accordingly, many affected patients will be able to maintain normal plasma levels of calcium with more modest oral calcium supplementation or, at least in some cases, even without calcium supplements altogether. Many patients maintain near-normal PTH concentrations and normal bone mineral density, although they continue to have elevated serum concentrations of $1,25(OH)_2D$, suggesting persistent target organ resistance (Sakati et al., 1986; Balsan et al., 1986; Weisman et al., 1987).

21.4.2   Vitamin D-dependent rickets type 2B

Case study: An unusual resistance to vitamin D

A 4-year-old boy named Liam exhibited classic signs of rickets but had an unexpected lack of response to both vitamin D and calcium therapy. Despite an initial suspicion of VDDR2A, genetic testing ruled out VDR mutations. Further investigation involved electrophoretic mobility shift assays (EMSA) and chromatin immunoprecipitation (ChIP) testing, which revealed an interfering ribonucleoprotein binding to the vitamin D response element, thereby preventing normal VDR function. His treatment was modified to include intensified calcium supplementation, leading to gradual radiographic and symptomatic improvements.

Vitamin D-dependent rickets type 2B (VDDR2B, OMIM 600785) resembles VDDR2A, but the molecular defect appears to be overexpression of a nuclear protein that specifically interacts with a DNA response element that binds retinoid X-receptor-VDR heterodimers. This dominant-negative protein appears to be a member of the family of heterogeneous nuclear ribonucleoproteins (hnRNPs), which attenuate gene transcription via their role as hormone response element-binding proteins. VDDR2B appears to be an uncommon condition. The management of rickets is like that described above for VDDR2A (Mechica et al., 1997; Malloy et al., 2001; Li et al., 2001; Chen et al., 2003; Hsieh et al., 2003; Katavetin et al., 2006).

21.5   Increased inactivation of vitamin D metabolites

21.5.1   Overview of inactivation of vitamin D metabolites

$1,25(OH)_2D$ enhances the transcription of the CYP3A4 gene located on chromosome 7q22.1 by a VDR-mediated pathway in the liver and small intestine through the binding of ligand–VDR–RXR heterodimer to response elements. CYP3A4 is a drug-metabolizing cytochrome P450 enzyme, contributing to the clearance of therapeutic agents that undergo metabolic biotransformation in the liver and small intestine. Through induction of hepatic CYP3A4 expression, $1,25(OH)_2D$ can enhance the metabolism and clearance of orally administered drugs that are CYP3A4 substrates. Consequently, vitamin D supplementation, by increasing circulating $1,25 (OH)_2D$ may alter the pharmacokinetics of such drugs. Induction of CYP3A4 älso accelerates vitamin D catabolism, giving rise to vitamin D deficiency. Importantly, induction of CYP3A4 in the small intestine could cause local tissue vitamin D deficiency and possibly directly affect intestinal calcium absorption. On the other hand, induction of hepatic CYP3A4 may alter systemic circulating levels of 25(OH) D through activation of the 4β-hydroxylation pathway. Thus intra- and interindividual differences in circulating vitamin D levels and associated intestinal CYP3A4 activity may contribute to variability in oral drug bioavailability. Osteomalacia can be a serious, debilitating side effect of certain drug therapies.

Mutation in CYP3A4 has been implicated in vitamin D deficiency through accelerated vitamin D inactivation. The resultant phenotype is labeled as vitamin D-dependent rickets type 3 (VDDR3).

21.5.2 Vitamin D-dependent rickets type 3

Case study: Rapid vitamin D breakdown

Sofia, a 6-year-old girl, suffered from persistent rickets despite adequate vitamin D intake. Her biochemical profile revealed normal 25(OH)D but inappropriately low $1,25(OH)_2D$ levels. Genetic sequencing identified a CYP3A4 gain-of-function mutation, confirming VDDR3. She required supraphysiologic doses of vitamin D and close biochemical monitoring to maintain normal calcium and phosphorus levels.

Vitamin D-dependent rickets type 3 (VDDR3, OMIM 619073) phenotype, due to increased inactivation of vitamin D metabolites, was described in 2018, based on a report of two unrelated girls by Roizen et al. The cause was a recurrent gain-of-function mutation (p.I301T) in CYP3A4 in an autosomal dominant mode of inheritance. The first girl presented before 2 years of age with a history of genu varum deformity and unsteady gait. Biochemically reduced calcium and phosphorus with increased alkaline phosphatase and PTH were identified. The second girl did not walk until 4.5 years of age and had been treated unsuccessfully for vitamin D deficiency using conventional dosages. Both girls were of short stature and demonstrated classical features of rickets with detectable vitamin D, low 25(OH)D, and $1,25(OH)_2D$ that increased after administration of very large doses of vitamin D or calcitriol and decreased rapidly thereafter. Both patients required high doses of calcitriol or vitamin D to maintain normal vitamin D metabolites, PTH, calcium, and phosphorus. The third case of VDDR3 was described by Mantoanelli, L et al., in a 2-year-old boy with no family history of rickets. The same CYP3A4 mutation was identified with bone deformities associated with poor growth (Roizen et al., 2018; Al-Ashwal et al., 2023; Mantoanelli et al., 2023).

In vitro studies of the CYP3A4 p.I301T mutation show rapid and extensive inactivation of vitamin D metabolites; hence, the poor response of affected children to normal doses of vitamin D or its analogues requires lifelong treatment with high doses of vitamin D to maintain biochemical and clinical remission as compared to doses in simple vitamin D deficiency.

21.6   Disorders of vitamin D hypersensitivity/inactivation

Abnormalities in vitamin D inactivation pathways have been identified, with hypersensitivity to vitamin D (HVD) implicated in causing disturbed calcium homeostasis during supplementation. 24-Hydroxylase (CYP24A1), is responsible for degradation of 25(OH)D and 1,25(OH)$_2$D to inactive metabolites. CYP24A1 is a mitochondrial inner membrane P450 enzyme expressed in the kidney, bone, skin, and intestine. It catalyzes the conversion of 1,25(OH)$_2$D through multiple hydroxylation steps at C-23 or C-24, resulting in the 1,25(OH)$_2$D-26,23-lactone and in the biliary catabolite calcitroic acid, respectively. Likewise, 25(OH)D is transformed by CYP24A1 to 24, 25 (OH)$_2$D and this is then further converted to the water soluble calcitroic acid. The enzymatic activity of CYP24A1 is inhibited by hypocalcemia, and PTH down-regulates its expression. In addition, the fibroblast growth factor 23 (FGF23), together with its coreceptor α-Klotho, positively modulates CYP24A1 activity in response to hypercalcemia and hyperphosphatemia. In 2011, loss-of-function mutations in the CYP24A1 gene were described. These mutations result in an increase of both 25(OH)D and 1,25(OH)2D levels, which enhance intestinal Ca absorption and bone reabsorption. The consequent hypercalcemic phenotype is the major cause of manifestations of idiopathic infantile hypercalcemia type 1(IH1) (Jones, Prosser & Kaufmann, 2012; Tieu, Tang & Tuckey, 2014; Seth-Vollenweider et al., 2014; Bikle, 2014, 2021; Milan & Ramkumar, 2024).

In addition to CYP24A1, complex cross-talk between the regulatory mechanisms of calcium and phosphate metabolic pathways exists. A protein-coding gene SLC34A1 (solute carrier family 34), involved in active transport of phosphate into cells via sodium-dependent phosphate transporter 2 A (NaPi-IIa), is implicated in the HVD phenotype. NaPi-IIa is located in the renal brush border membrane, reabsorbing phosphate, and is regulated by vitamin D and PTH, together with FGF23 and α-klotho. 1,25(OH)2D3 modulates both intestinal and renal Pi handling, upregulating the NaPi-II cotransporter's expression. In 2016 loss-of-functional mutations in SLC34A1 encoding NaPi-IIa were identified, leading to phosphate wasting. The resultant hypophosphatemia causes suppression of FGF23, and, via inhibition of CYP24A1 catabolic activity and stimulation of CYP27B1, leads to inappropriate 1,25(OH)D2 synthesis. This, in turn, increases calcium absorption into the bloodstream, causing hypercalcemia and hypercalciuria. (Wagner et al., 2014; Levi et al., 2019; Meyer & Pike, 2020; Kowalska et al., 2021; Meyer et al., 2024).

With the exception of CYP24A and SCLA1, specific phenotypes for other candidate genes are also evolving, which makes diagnosis further challenging. For example, mutations in the gene

SLC34A3, encoding the renal phosphate transporter NPT2c, associated with autosomal recessive hypophosphatemic rickets (ARHR) with hypercalciuria (OMIM 241530), were also suggested to have a potential role in HVD phenotype. However, more work is to be done to understand the pathophysiological basis.

21.6.1 Infantile hypercalcemia type 1

Case study: A baby with severe hypercalcemia

James, a 3-month-old infant, was brought to the emergency department with persistent vomiting, irritability, and failure to thrive. His parents reported that he had been unusually fussy, with poor feeding and excessive urination. Laboratory findings revealed severe hypercalcemia, hypercalciuria, and suppressed PTH levels, with markedly elevated $1,25(OH)_2D$. Given his young age and lack of any external vitamin D supplementation, genetic testing was pursued and confirmed biallelic CYP24A1 mutations, diagnosing him with IH1. Treatment involved immediate hydration, administration of bisphosphonates to lower calcium levels, and long-term dietary restrictions on vitamin D and calcium. Over the next several months, James' condition stabilized, and his growth improved with careful monitoring.

Infantile Hypercalcemia Type 1 / Hypercalcemia, Infantile, type 1 (IH 1/HCINF1, OMIM 143880) is a rare condition mainly characterized by severe hypercalcemia, hypercalciuria and suppressed PTH, with a predispositionto nephrolithiaisis and nephrocalcinosis. Typical manifestations include polyuria with dehydration, vomiting, and constipation. Anorexia and weight loss are reported. Affected babies could also exhibit muscular hypotonia and lethargy, with delays in the development of mental and movement abilities. Clinical manifestations may appear later in adult life, with nephrocalcinosis and nephrolithiasis due to long-term subclinical hypercalcemia/ hypercalciuria. Extrarenal manifestations, including Ca deposits in the joints and in the cornea, low bone mineral density, and osteoporosis, principally related to the increase of osteoclast activity, may be seen (Nizar, Cantley & Tang, 2021).

Clinical and biochemical phenotypes are featured by a gene-dose effect. A more severe phenotype is seen in subjects with biallelic genetic variants as compared to mono-allelic carriers, with the latter being asymptomatic or borderline. Moreover, in the heterozygote individuals, the chronic and latent abnormalities of vitamin D metabolism are more likely to predispose to long-term clinical events such as renal stones. In addition to the genetic background, the IH1 manifestations and the phenotypic differences between infants and adult carriers rely on many environmental factors like diet, lifestyle, vitamin D intake, and activity of the other vitamin D enzymes in metabolic pathways. Sunlight exposure and vitamin D supplementation therapy were identified as the two main environmental triggering factors. For instance, higher calcium and vitamin D intake is often recommended in infant diets as well as during pregnancy and lactation to support maternal, fetal, and child health. During gestation, adaptive physiological mechanisms naturally arise to meet fetal demands. However, in women carrying CYP24A1 defects, these physiological changes, together with the recommended additional supplementation, may unmask an underlying IH phenotype and precipitate gestational hypercalcemia maternal hypercalcemia, with possible hypertension and fetal demise. A significant seasonal variation has been observed in IH1 patients with a trend to higher calcium levels and excretion, with lower PTH levels, from April to September (when there is greater exposure to sunlight) as compared to the winter months. A high 25-OH-D3:24,25 $(OH)_2D$ ratio (substrate over product ratio, R ratio), which directly reflects the enzymatic defect, has been specifically associated in patients with biallelic CYP24A1 variants. Comprehensive profiling of 23- and 24-hydroxylated vitamin D metabolites such as 23,25, 26 $(OH)_3D$, 25 (OH)D-26,23- lactone and 1, 24, 25 $(OH)_3D$ underscores the distinct pathophysiology of IH1 and IH2, with markedly reduced levels of these CYP24A1-derived metabolites in IH1 but preserved production in IH2. Taken together, these findings support the conclusion that the dose and as well as the type of vitamin D administration may drastically modulate adverse effects (Jones, 2010).

Patients with CYP24A1 deficiency are advised to strictly monitor, and in some cases restrict, their vitamin D intake. Genetic confirmation of CYP24A1 mutations is therefore important to guide safe vitamin D management strategies. In addition, limiting excessive sun exposure while allowing mild, controlled exposure may help prevent worsening of clinical and biochemical manifestations (Gorvin, 2022).

21.6.2   Infantile hypercalcemia 2

Case study: Persistent hypercalcemia and kidney complications

Emma, a 2-year-old girl, was referred to nephrology due to recurrent kidney stones and persistent hypercalcemia. Her parents noted that she had suffered from frequent urinary tract infections and episodes of severe constipation. Laboratory workup showed suppressed PTH, hypercalciuria, and hypophosphatemia, with renal phosphate wasting. Additional genetic testing revealed mutations in the SLC34A1 gene, confirming a diagnosis of IH2. Treatment included phosphate supplementation, increased fluid intake to reduce nephrocalcinosis risk, and close monitoring of renal function. Over time, Emma's symptoms improved with dietary modifications and careful medical management, although long-term follow-up was necessary to prevent further complications.

Infantile hypercalcemia type 2 (IH2, OMIM 616963) is characterized by the classic symptoms of hypercalcemia and suppressed PTH but also exhibits hypophosphatemia due to the inactivation of NaPi-IIa protein leading to renal phosphate wasting. The consequent status of hypercalcemia, hypercalciuria, and hyperphosphaturia promotes the formation of Ca-Pi crystals and renal calcifications. Subsequently, low serum phosphate and FGF23 increase CYP27B1 expression and 1, 25$(OH)_2D$ activity, while inhibiting CYP24A1 expression and 24-hydroxylase activity, which have the combined effect of increasing 1,25$(OH)_2D$ and hypercalcemia. Extensive studies proved the pathological role of both complete deletion and loss-of-function genetic variants in the *SLC34A1* gene (Schlingmann et al., 2016; Fearn et al., 2018).

To date, pathogenic alleles of *SLC34A1* seem to contribute to both autosomal dominant and autosomal recessive renal stone disease, suggesting the importance of other factors that can influence the clinical features of the disease (Brazier et al., 2023).

21.7 Conclusion

The study of rare disorders of vitamin D metabolism has provided profound insights into the complexities of calcium and phosphate regulation, shaping both diagnostic and therapeutic strategies. These conditions, though individually rare, have substantial clinical consequences if unrecognized or mismanaged. Advances in molecular diagnostics have enabled earlier detection, allowing for personalized treatment approaches that improve long-term outcomes.

Despite advancements, several knowledge gaps remain. More research is needed to better understand the long-term effects of treatment, particularly in cases requiring lifelong management. The potential for gene-targeted therapies and novel pharmacologic interventions also holds promise for improving patient outcomes in the future.

As our understanding of these disorders continues to evolve, interdisciplinary collaboration between basic scientists, pathologists, endocrinologists, nephrologists, geneticists, and pediatricians will be crucial. Increased awareness among clinicians and better screening strategies can ensure that affected individuals receive timely interventions, ultimately enhancing their quality of life.

References

Ahmad, W., Faiyaz ul Haque, M., Brancolini, V., Tsou, H. C., ul Haque, S., Lam, H. M., Aita, V. M., Owen, J., deBlaquiere, M., Frank, J., Cserhalmi-Friedman, P. B., Leask, A., McGrath, J. A., Peacocke, M., Ahmad, M., Ott, J., & Christiano, A. M. (1998). Alopecia universalis associated with a mutation in the human hairless gene. *Science (New York, N.Y.), 279*(5351), 720–724. https://doi.org/10.1126/science.279.5351.720.

Al Mutair, A. N., Nasrat, G. H., & Russell, D. W. (2012). Mutation of the CYP2R1 vitamin D 25-hydroxylase in a Saudi Arabian family with severe vitamin D deficiency. *Journal of Clinical Endocrinology and Metabolism, 97*(10). http://doi.org/10.1210/jc.2012-1340Saudi, http://jcem.endojournals.org/content/97/10/E2022.full.pdf +html, Arabia.

Al-Ashwal, A., Al Zahrani, A., Dammas, N., Aletani, L., & Alhuthil, R. (2023). CYP3A4 mutation causes vitamin D-dependent rickets type 3: A case report in Saudi Arabia. *Cureus, 15*(12). https://doi.org/10.7759/cureus.49976.

Balsan, S., Garabedian, M., Larchet, M., Gorski, A. M., Cournot, G., Tau, C., Bourdeau, A., Silve, C., & Ricour, C. (1986). Long-term nocturnal calcium infusions can cure rickets and promote normal mineralization in hereditary resistance to 1,25-dihydroxyvitamin D. *Journal of Clinical Investigation, 77*(5), 1661–1667. https://doi.org/10.1172/JCI112483.

Biasucci, G., Donini, V., & Cannalire, G. (2024). Rickets types and treatment with vitamin D and analogues. *Nutrients, 16*(3), 416. https://doi.org/10.3390/nu16030416.

Bikle, D. D. (2014). Vitamin D metabolism, mechanism of action, and clinical applications. *Cell Press, United States Chemistry and Biology, 21*(3), 319–329. https://doi.org/10.1016/j.chembiol.2013.12.016, www.elsevier.com/inca/publications/store/6/0/1/2/8/1/index.htt.

Bikle, D. D. (2021). *Vitamin D: Production, metabolism and mechanisms of action, endotext.* MDText.com, Inc.

Bliziotes, M., Yergey, A. L., Nanes, M. S., Muenzer, J., Begley, M. G., Vieira, N. E., Kher, K. K., Brandi, M. L., & Marx, S. J. (1988). Absent intestinal response to calciferols in hereditary resistance to 1, 25-dihydroxyvitamin d: Documentation and effective therapy with high dose intravenous calcium infusions. *Journal of Clinical Endocrinology and Metabolism, 66*(2), 294–300. https://doi.org/10.1210/jcem-66-2-294.

Brazier, F., Courbebaisse, M., David, A., Bergerat, D., Leroy, C., Lindner, M., Maruani, G., Saint Jacques, C., Letavernier, E., Hureaux, M., Vargas-Poussou, R., & Prié, D. (2023). Relationship between clinical phenotype and in vitro analysis of 13 NPT2c/SCL34A3 mutants. *Scientific Reports, 13*(1). https://doi.org/10.1038/s41598-022-25995-5.

Cali, J. J., & Russell, D. W. (1991). Characterization of human sterol 27-hydroxylase. A mitochondrial cytochrome P-450 that catalyzes multiple oxidation reaction in bile acid biosynthesis. *Journal of Biological Chemistry, 266*(12), 7774–7778. https://doi.org/10.1016/s0021-9258(20)89517-9.

Casella, S. J., Reiner, B. J., Chen, T. C., Holick, M. F., & Harrison, H. E. (1994). A possible genetic defect in 25-hydroxylation as a cause of rickets. *The Journal of Pediatrics, 124*(6), 929–932. https://doi.org/10.1016/S0022-3476(05)83184-1.

Chen, H., Hewison, M., Hu, B., & Adams, J. S. (2003). Heterogeneous nuclear ribonucleoprotein (hnRNP) binding to hormone response elements: A cause of vitamin D resistance. *Proceedings of the National Academy of Sciences, 100*(10), 6109–6114. https://doi.org/10.1073/pnas.1031395100.

Chen, T. L., Hirst, M. A., Cone, C. M., Hochberg, Z., Tietze, H. U., & Feldman, D. (1984). 1,25-Dihydroxyvitamin D resistance, rickets, and alopecia: Analysis of receptors and bioresponse in cultured fibroblasts from patients and parents. *Journal of Clinical Endocrinology and Metabolism, 59*(3), 383–388. https://doi.org/10.1210/jcem-59-3-383.

Cheng, J. B., Levine, M. A., Bell, N. H., Mangelsdorf, D. J., & Russell, D. W. (2004). Genetic evidence that the human CYP2R1 enzyme is a key vitamin D 25-hydroxylase. *Proceedings of the National Academy of Sciences of the United States of America, 101*(20), 7711–7715. https://doi.org/10.1073/pnas.0402490101.

Christakos, S., Dhawan, P., Verstuyf, A., Verlinden, L., & Carmeliet, G. (2015). Vitamin D: Metabolism, molecular mechanism of action, and pleiotropic effects. *Physiological Reviews, 96*(1), 365–408. https://doi.org/10.1152/physrev.00014.2015, http://physrev.physiology.org/content/96/1/365.full.pdf.

Cockerill, F. J., Hawa, N. S., Yousaf, N., Hewison, M., O'Riordan, J. L. H., & Farrow, S. M. (1997). Mutations in the vitamin D receptor gene in three kindreds associated with hereditary vitamin D resistant rickets. *Journal of Clinical Endocrinology and Metabolism, 82*(9), 3156–3160. https://doi.org/10.1210/jcem.82.9.4243, http://jcem.endojournals.org.

Cui, N., Xia, W., Su, H., Pang, L., Jiang, Y., Sun, Y., Nie, M., Xing, X., Li, M., Wang, O., Yuan, T., Chi, Y., Hu, Y., Liu, H., Meng, X., & Zhou, X. (2012). Novel mutations of CYP27B1 gene lead to reduced activity of 1α-hydroxylase in Chinese patients. *Bone, 51*(3), 563–569. https://doi.org/10.1016/j.bone.2012.05.006.

Dardenne, O., Prud'homme, J., Arabian, A., Glorieux, F. H., & St-Arnaud, R. (2001). Targeted inactivation of the 25-hydroxyvitamin D3-1α-hydroxylase gene (CYP27B1) creates an animal model of pseudovitamin D-deficiency rickets*. *Endocrinology, 142*(7), 3135–3141. https://doi.org/10.1210/endo.142.7.8281.

Fearn, A., Allison, B., Rice, S. J., Edwards, N., Halbritter, J., Bourgeois, S., Pastor-Arroyo, E. M., Hildebrandt, F., Tasic, V., Wagner, C. A., Hernando, N., Sayer, J. A., & Werner, A. (2018). Clinical, biochemical, and pathophysiological analysis of SLC34A1 mutations. *Physiological Reports, 6*(12). https://doi.org/10.14814/phy2.13715, http://physoc.onlinelibrary.wiley.com/hub/journal/10.1002/(ISSN)2051-817X/.

Feldman, J. W., & Pike (2005). In F. H. Glorieux (Ed.). *Vitamin D. 2*. Elsevier Academic Press.

Fraher, L. J., Karmali, R., Hinde, F. R. J., Hendy, G. N., Jani, H., Nicholson, L., Grant, D., & O'Riordan, J. L. H. (1986). Vitamin D-dependent rickets type II: Extreme end organ resistance to 1,25-dihydroxy vitamin D3 in a patient without alopecia. *European Journal of Pediatrics, 145*(5), 389–395. https://doi.org/10.1007/BF00439245.

Fraser, D., Kooh, S. W., Kind, H. P., Holick, M. F., Tanaka, Y., & Deluca, H. F. (1973). Pathogenesis of hereditary vitamin-D-dependent rickets: An inborn error of vitamin D metabolism involving defective conversion of 25-hydroxyvitamin D to 1α,25-dihydroxyvitamin D. *New England Journal of Medicine, 289*(16), 817–822. https://doi.org/10.1056/NEJM197310182891601.

Fu, G. K., Lin, D., Zhang, M. Y. H., Bikle, D. D., Shackleton, C. H. L., Miller, W. L., & Portale, A. A. (1997). Cloning of human 25-hydroxyvitamin D-1α-hydroxylase and mutations causing vitamin D-dependent rickets type 1. *Molecular Endocrinology, 11*(13), 1961–1970. https://doi.org/10.1210/mend.11.13.0035, http://mend.endojournals.org/.

Giannakopoulos, A., Efthymiadou, A., & Chrysis, D. (2017). A case of vitamin-D-dependent rickets type 1A with normal 1,25-dihydroxyvitamin D caused by two novel mutations of the CYP27B1 gene. *Hormone Research in Paediatrics, 87*(1), 58–63. https://doi.org/10.1159/000446774.

Glorieux, F. H., & St-Arnaud, R. (2005). Vitamin, pseudodeficiency. In *Vitamin D. 2*. Elsevier Academic Press.

Gorvin, C. M. (2022). Genetic causes of neonatal and infantile hypercalcaemia. *Pediatric Nephrology, 37*(2), 289–301. https://doi.org/10.1007/s00467-021-05082-z, https://www.springer.com/journal/467.

Haffner, D., Leifheit-Nestler, M., Grund, A., & Schnabel, D. (2022). Rickets guidance: Part II—Management. *Pediatric Nephrology, 37*(10), 2289–2302. https://doi.org/10.1007/s00467-022-05505-5, link.springer.de/link/service/journals/00467/index.htm.

Hirst, M. A., Hochman, H. I., & Feldman, D. (1985). Vitamin d resistance and alopecia: A kindred with normal 1, 25-dihydroxyvitamin d binding, but decreased receptor affinity for deoxyribonucleic acid. *Journal of Clinical Endocrinology and Metabolism, 60*(3), 490–495. https://doi.org/10.1210/jcem-60-3-490.

Hochberg, Z., Benderli, A., Levy, J., Vardi, P., Weisman, Y., Chen, T., & Feldman, D. (1984). 1,25-dihydroxyvitamin D resistance, rickets, and alopecia. *The American Journal of Medicine, 77*(5), 805–811. https://doi.org/10.1016/0002-9343(84)90516-3.

Hsieh, J. C., Sisk, J. M., Jurutka, P. W., Haussler, C. A., Slater, S. A., Haussler, M. R., & Thompson, C. C. (2003). Physical and functional interaction between the vitamin D receptor and hairless corepressor, two proteins required for hair cycling. *Journal of Biological Chemistry, 278*(40), 38665–38674. https://doi.org/10.1074/jbc.M304886200, http://www.jbc.org/content/by/year.

Jones, G. (2010). *Metabolism and catabolism of vitamin D, its metabolites and clinically relevant analogs*. Springer Science and Business Media LLC, 99–134. http://doi.org/10.1007/978-1-60327-303-9_4 3885.

Jones, G., Prosser, D. E., & Kaufmann, M. (2012). 25-Hydroxyvitamin D-24-hydroxylase (CYP24A1): Its important role in the degradation of vitamin D. *Archives of Biochemistry and Biophysics, 523*(1), 9–18. https://doi.org/10.1016/j.abb.2011.11.003.

Katavetin, P., Katavetin, P., Wacharasindhu, S., & Shotelersuk, V. (2006). A girl with a novel splice site mutation in VDR supports the role of a ligand-independent VDR function on hair cycling. *Hormone Research in Paediatrics, 66*(6), 273–276. https://doi.org/10.1159/000095546.

Kim, C. J., Kaplan, L. E., Perwad, F., Huang, N., Sharma, A., Choi, Y., Miller, W. L., & Portale, A. A. (2007). Vitamin D 1α-hydroxylase gene mutations in patients with 1α-hydroxylase deficiency. *The Journal of Clinical Endocrinology & Metabolism, 92*(8), 3177–3182. https://doi.org/10.1210/jc.2006-2664.

Kowalska, E., Rola, R., Wójcik, M., Łaszcz, N., Płudowski, P., Wierzbicka, A., Janiec, A., Książyk, J., Halat, P., Ciara, E., Obrycki, Ł., Pronicka, E., & Litwin, M. (2021). Analysis of vitamin D3 metabolites in survivors of infantile idiopathic hypercalcemia caused by CYP24A1 mutation or SLC34A1 mutation. *Journal of Steroid Biochemistry and Molecular Biology, 208*. https://doi.org/10.1016/j.jsbmb.2021.105824, www.elsevier.com/locate/jsbmb.

Levi, M., Gratton, E., Forster, I. C., Hernando, N., Wagner, C. A., Biber, J., Sorribas, V., & Murer, H. (2019). Mechanisms of phosphate transport. *Nature Reviews Nephrology, 15*(8), 482–500. https://doi.org/10.1038/s41581-019-0159-y, http://www.nature.com/nrneph/archive/index.html.

Levine, M. A. (2020). Diagnosis and management of vitamin D dependent rickets. *Frontiers in Pediatrics, 8*. Available from: https://doi.org/10.3389/fped.2020.00315, https://www.frontiersin.org/journals/pediatrics.

Li, M., Chiba, H., Warot, X., Messaddeq, N., Gérard, C., Chambon, P., & Metzger, D. (2001). RXRα ablation in skin keratinocytes results in alopecia and epidermal alterations. *Development (Cambridge, England), 128*(5), 675–688. https://doi.org/10.1242/dev.128.5.675, https://journals.biologists.com/dev/.

Li, Y. C., Amling, M., Pirro, A. E., Priemel, M., Meuse, J., Baron, R., Delling, G., & Demay, M. B. (1998). Normalization of mineral ion homeostasis by dietary means prevents hyperparathyroidism, rickets, and osteomalacia, but not alopecia in vitamin D receptor-ablated mice. *Endocrinology, 139*(10), 4391–4396. https://doi.org/10.1210/endo.139.10.6262, https://academic.oup.com/endo/issue.

Ma, N. S., Malloy, P. J., Pitukcheewanont, P., Dreimane, D., Geffner, M. E., & Feldman, D. (2009). Hereditary vitamin D resistant rickets: Identification of a novel splice site mutation in the vitamin D receptor gene and successful treatment with oral calcium therapy. *Bone, 45*(4), 743–746. https://doi.org/10.1016/j.bone.2009.06.003.

Malloy, P. J., Eccleshall, T. R., Gross, C., Van Maldergem, L., Bouillon, R., & Feldman, D. (1997). Hereditary vitamin D resistant rickets caused by a novel mutation in the vitamin D receptor that results in decreased affinity for hormone and cellular hyporesponsiveness. *Journal of Clinical Investigation, 99*(2), 297–304. https://doi.org/10.1172/JCI119158.

Malloy, P. J., Hochberg, Z., Tiosano, D., Pike, J. W., Hughes, M. R., & Feldman, D. (1990). The molecular basis of hereditary 1,25-dihydroxyvitamin D3 resistant rickets in seven related families. *Journal of Clinical Investigation, 86*(6), 2071–2079. https://doi.org/10.1172/JCI114944.

Malloy, P. J., Zhu, W., Zhao, X. Y., Pehling, G. B., & Feldman, D. (2001). A novel inborn error in the ligand-binding domain of the vitamin D receptor causes hereditary vitamin D-resistant rickets. *Molecular Genetics and Metabolism, 73*(2), 138–148. https://doi.org/10.1006/mgme.2001.3181, http://www.elsevier.com/inca/publications/store/6/2/2/9/2/0/index.htt.

Malloy, P. J., Feldman, D., & Pike, J. W. (2005). In F. Glorieux (Ed.). *Vitamin D. 2.* Elsevier Hereditary 1,25-dihydroxyvitamin D resistant rickets.

Mansour, Z. A., Lames, N. S. A., Shahad, A., Tahani, D. A., Zainab, H. A., & Rabia (2023). Overview of studies on: Diagnosis and treatment of vitamin D-dependent rickets. *International Journal of Life Sciences Research, 11*, 30–39.

Mantoanelli, L., de Almeida, C. M., Coelho, M. C. A., Coutinho, M., Levine, M. A., Collett-Solberg, P. F., & Bordallo, A. P. (2023). Vitamin D-dependent rickets type 3: A case report and systematic review. *Calcified Tissue International, 112*(4), 512–517. https://doi.org/10.1007/s00223-022-01051-2, https://www.springer.com/journal/223.

Mechica, J. B., Leite, M. O. R., Mendonca, B. B., Frazzatto, E. S. T., Borelli, A., & Latronico, A. C. (1997). A novel nonsense mutation in the first zinc finger of the vitamin D receptor causing hereditary 1,25-dihydroxyvitamin D3-resistant rickets. *Journal of Clinical Endocrinology and Metabolism, 82*(11), 3892–3894. https://doi.org/10.1210/jcem.82.11.4384, http://jcem.endojournals.org.

Menon, J. C., Kumari, A., Sajjan, S. M., & Dabadghao, P. (2024). Novel mutation in CYP2R1 causing vitamin D-dependent rickets type 1b. *JCEM Case Reports, 2*(3). https://doi.org/10.1210/jcemcr/luae024.

Meyer, M. B., Lee, S. M., Towne, J. M., Cichanski, S. R., Kaufmann, M., Jones, G., & Pike, J. W. (2024). In vivo contribution of Cyp24a1 promoter vitamin D response elements. *Endocrinology, 165*(11). https://doi.org/10.1210/endocr/bqae134.

Meyer, M. B., & Pike, J. W. (2020). Mechanistic homeostasis of vitamin D metabolism in the kidney through reciprocal modulation of Cyp27b1 and Cyp24a1 expression. *The Journal of Steroid Biochemistry and Molecular Biology, 196*, 105500. https://doi.org/10.1016/j.jsbmb.2019.105500.

Milan, K. L., & Ramkumar, K. M. (2024). Regulatory mechanisms and pathological implications of CYP24A1 in Vitamin D metabolism. *Pathology - Research and Practice, 264*, 155684. https://doi.org/10.1016/j.prp.2024.155684.

Molin, A., Wiedemann, A., Demers, N., Kaufmann, M., Do Cao, J., Mainard, L., Dousset, B., Journeau, P., Abeguile, G., Coudray, N., Mittre, H., Richard, N., Weryha, G., Sorlin, A., Jones, G., Kottler, M. L., & Feillet, F. (2017). Vitamin D–Dependent rickets type 1B (25-hydroxylase deficiency): A rare condition or a misdiagnosed condition? *Journal of Bone and Mineral Research, 32*(9), 1893–1899. https://doi.org/10.1002/jbmr.3181, http://onlinelibrary.wiley.com/journal/10.1002/(ISSN)1523-4681.

Monkawa, T., Yoshida, T., Wakino, S., Shinki, T., Anazawa, H., Deluca, H. F., Suda, T., Hayashi, M., & Saruta, T. (1997). Molecular cloning of cDNA and genomic DNA for human 25-hydroxyvitamin D31α-hydroxylase. *Biochemical and Biophysical Research Communications, 239*(2), 527–533. https://doi.org/10.1006/bbrc.1997.7508.

Nizar, R., Cantley, N. W. P., & Tang, J. C. Y. (2021). Infantile hypercalcaemia type 1: A vitamin D-mediated, under-recognised cause of hypercalcaemia. *Endocrinology, Diabetes and Metabolism Case Reports, 2021*(1). https://doi.org/10.1530/EDM-21-0058, https://edm.bioscientifica.com/view/journals/edm/2021/1/EDM21-0058.xml.

Panda, D. K., Miao, D., Bolivar, I., Li, J., Huo, R., Hendy, G. N., & Goltzman, D. (2004). Inactivation of the 25-hydroxyvitamin D 1α-hydroxylase and vitamin D receptor demonstrates independent and interdependent effects of calcium and vitamin D on skeletal and mineral homeostasis. *Journal of Biological Chemistry, 279*(16), 16754–16766. https://doi.org/10.1074/jbc.M310271200.

Prader, A., Illig, R., & Heierli, E. (1961). An unusual form of primary vitamin D-resistant rickets with hypocalcemia and autosomal-dominant hereditary transmission: hereditary pseudo-deficiency rickets. *Helvetica Paediatrica Acta, 16*, 452–468.

Rebelos, E., Tentolouris, N., & Jude, E. (2023). The role of vitamin D in health and disease: A narrative review on the mechanisms linking vitamin D with disease and the effects of supplementation. *Adis, Finland Drugs, 83*(8), 665–685. https://doi.org/10.1007/s40265-023-01875-8, https://www.springer.com/journal/40265.

Rochel, N., Wurtz, J. M., Mitschler, A., Klaholz, B., & Moras, D. (2000). The crystal structure of the nuclear receptor for vitamin D bound to its natural ligand. *Molecular Cell, 5*(1), 173–179. https://doi.org/10.1016/s1097-2765(00)80413-x.

Roizen, J. D., Li, D., O'Lear, L., Javaid, M. K., Shaw, N. J., Ebeling, P. R., Nguyen, H. H., Rodda, C. P., Thummel, K. E., Thacher, T. D., Hakonarson, H., & Levine, M. A. (2018). CYP3A4 mutation causes Vitamin D-dependent rickets type 3. *Journal of Clinical Investigation, 128*(5), 1913–1918. https://doi.org/10.1172/JCI98680, https://www.jci.org/articles/view/98680/pdf.

Sakati, N., Woodhouse, N. J. Y., Niles, N., Harfi, H., De Grange, D. A., & Marx, S. (1986). Hereditary resistance to 1,25-dihydroxyvitamin d: Clinical and radiological improvement during high-dose oral calcium therapy. *Hormone Research in Paediatrics, 24*(4), 280–287. https://doi.org/10.1159/000180568.

Schlingmann, K. P., Ruminska, J., Kaufmann, M., Dursun, I., Patti, M., Kranz, B., Pronicka, E., Ciara, E., Akcay, T., Bulus, D., Cornelissen, E. A. M., Gawlik, A., Sikora, P., Patzer, L., Galiano, M., Boyadzhiev, V., Dumic, M., Vivante, A., Kleta, R., ... Konrad, M. (2016). Autosomal-recessive mutations in SLC34A1 encoDing sodium-phosphate cotransporter 2a cause idiopathic infantile hypercalcemia. *Journal of the American Society of Nephrology, 27*(2), 604–614. https://doi.org/10.1681/ASN.2014101025, http://jasn.asnjournals.org/content/27/2/604.full.pdf+html.

Seth-Vollenweider, T., Joshi, S., Dhawan, P., Sif, S., & Christakos, S. (2014). Novel mechanism of negative regulation of 1,25-dihydroxyvitamin D3-induced 25-hydroxyvitamin D3 24-hydroxylase (Cyp24a1) transcription: Epigenetic modification involving cross-talk between protein-arginine methyltransferase 5 and the SWI/SNF complex. *Journal of Biological Chemistry, 289*(49), 33958–33970. https://doi.org/10.1074/jbc.M114.583302, http://www.jbc.org/content/289/49/33958.full.pdf+html.

St-Arnaud, R., Messerlian, S., Moir, J. M., Omdahl, J. L., & Glorieux, F. H. (1997). The 25-hydroxyvitamin D 1-alpha-hydroxylase gene maps to the pseudovitamin D-deficiency rickets (PDDR) disease locus. *Journal of Bone and Mineral Research, 12*(10), 1552–1559. https://doi.org/10.1359/jbmr.1997.12.10.1552.

Sunkar, S., & Neeharika, D. (2020). CYP2R1 and CYP27A1 genes: An in silico approach to identify the deleterious mutations, impact on structure and their differential expression in disease conditions. *Genomics, 112*(5), 3677–3686. https://doi.org/10.1016/j.ygeno.2020.04.017.

Thacher, T. D., Fischer, P. R., Singh, R. J., Roizen, J., & Levine, M. A. (2015). CYP2R1 mutations impair generation of 25-hydroxyvitamin D and cause an atypical form of vitamin D deficiency. *Journal of Clinical Endocrinology and Metabolism, 100*(7), E1005. https://doi.org/10.1210/jc.2015-1746, http://press.endocrine.org/doi/pdf/10.1210/jc.2015-1746.

Tieu, E. W., Tang, E. K. Y., & Tuckey, R. C. (2014). Kinetic analysis of human CYP24A1 metabolism of vitamin D via the C24-oxidation pathway. *FEBS Journal, 281*(14), 3280–3296. https://doi.org/10.1111/febs.12862, http://www.febsjournal.org/default.asp.

Wagner, C. A., Hernando, N., Forster, I. C., & Biber, J. (2014). The SLC34 family of sodium-dependent phosphate transporters. *Pflugers Archiv European Journal of Physiology, 466*(1), 139–153. https://doi.org/10.1007/s00424-013-1418-6.

Weisman, Y., Bab, I., Gazit, D., Spirer, Z., Jaffe, M., & Hochberg, Z. (1987). Long-term intracaval calcium infusion therapy in end-organ resistance to 1,25-dihydroxyvitamin D. *The American Journal of Medicine, 83*(5), 984–990. https://doi.org/10.1016/0002-9343(87)90666-8.

Vitamin D, pregnancy, and child health

Rehana Rehman[1], and Shaheen Basheer[2]

[1]Department of Biological & Biomedical Sciences, Aga Khan University, Karachi, Pakistan [2]Western Health and Social Care Trust, Obstetrics & Gynaecology, South West Acute Hospital, Enniskillen United Kingdom

22.1 Vitamin D in pregnancy

Vitamin D (VD), a fat-soluble seco-steroid, plays a fundamental role in calcium homeostasis alongside its significant impact on neurological, cardiovascular, immunological, and reproductive health. Satisfactory preconception, conception, pregnancy, and peripartum levels are crucial in controlling fetal embryogenesis, skeletal development, and maintaining calcium levels in the developing fetus.

It is recommended by the UK National Institute for Health and Clinical Excellence (NICE 2014) that all women be commenced on 10 µg (400 IU)–15 µg (600 IU) of VD throughout pregnancy as part of the Healthy Start programme, ideally starting from the preconception period (Larqué et al., 2018).

22.2 Sources of vitamin D

The primary natural source of vitamin D is its synthesis in the skin from solar radiation. Dietary intake contributes minimally (10%–20%) to vitamin D levels due to its limited presence in dietary source Fig. 22.1

Vitamin D is found to some extent in the following dietary sources:
- Oily fish—salmon and sardines.
- Liver—(not a recommended source during pregnancy).
- Red meat.
- Egg yolk.
- Fortified food—margarine, breakfast cereals.

22.3 Metabolism of vitamin D and its effects

Vitamin D exists in two forms (Arshad et al., 2022) Fig. 22.1:

The Impact of Vitamin D on Health and Disease. DOI: https://doi.org/10.1016/B978-0-443-34037-6.00034-0

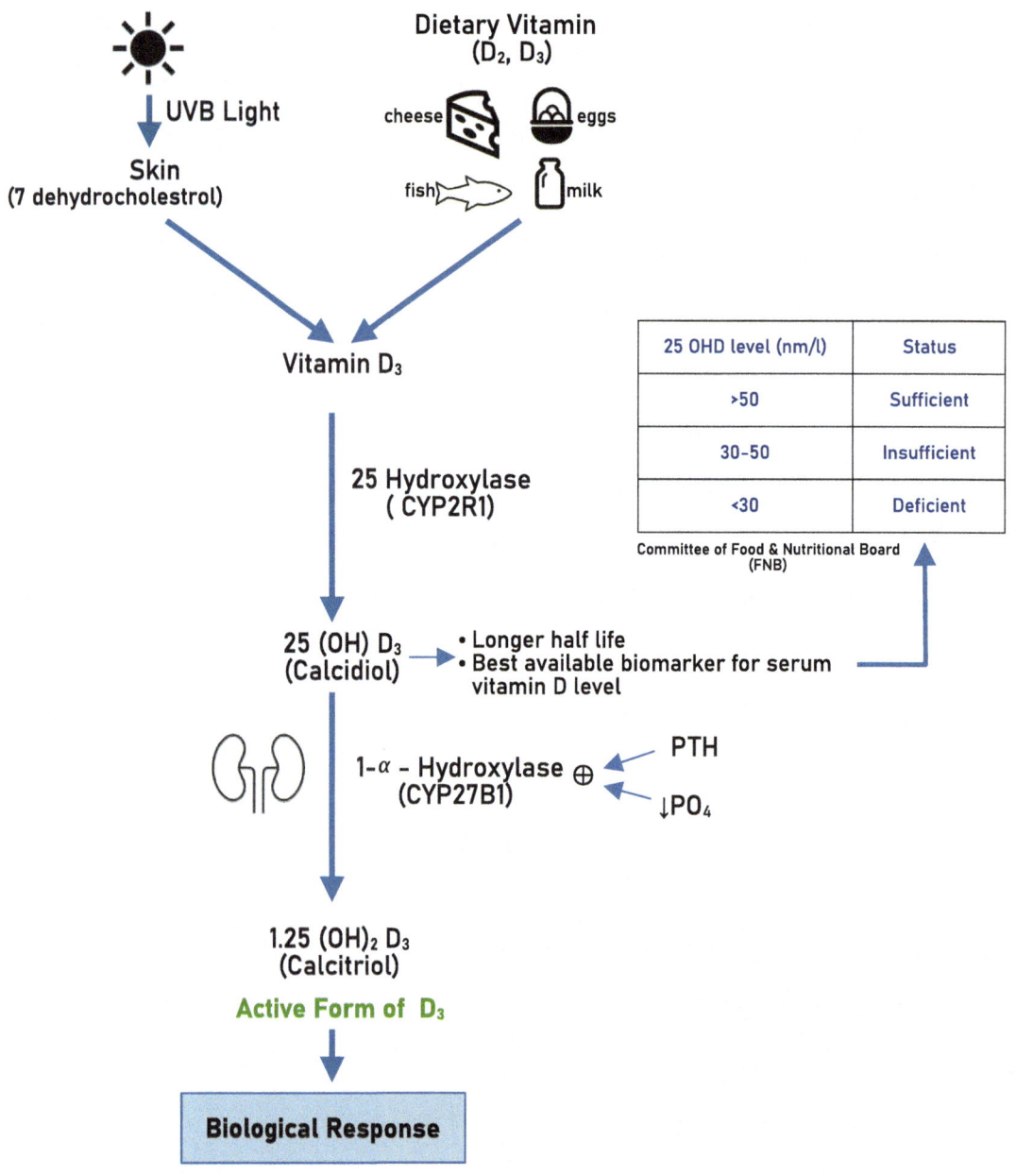

Figure 22.1
Synthesis of the active form of vitamin D.

1. **Vitamin D2 (Ergocalciferol)**—25-hydroxy vitamin D (25 OHD)—inactive form of vitamin D.
2. **Vitamin D3 (Cholecalciferol)**—1, 25 Hydroxy vitamin D (1,25 OH2 D)—active form of vitamin D.

22.4 Metabolism of vitamin D in the placenta

The placenta not only plays a fundamental role in fetal development by mediating nutritional transport, but it is also essential for immunotolerance adaptations to maintain a healthy pregnancy, as well as contributing to vitamin D homeostasis.

The developing fetus is reliant on the maternal vitamin D supply, which is transported through the placenta. The inactive form of vitamin D, 25(OH)D3, from maternal circulation reaches the placenta by endocytosis, where it is 1st metabolized to 24,25-dihydroxy vitamin D3 by 24-hydroxylase (CYP24A1) and then converted to active 1,25-dihydroxy vitamin D [1,25(OH)2 D3] by the action of placental 1α-hydroxylase (CYP27B1). Both forms of vitamin D (24,25-dihydroxy vitamin D3 and 1,25-dihydroxy vitamin D [1,25(OH)2 D3) are discharged into the maternal and fetal circulations (Ashley et al., 2022). Hence, vitamin D metabolism during pregnancy primarily occurs in the placenta Fig. 22.2.

As the fetus grows, there are increasing requirements for vitamin D. Its level rises with advancing gestation, as evidenced by a two to three-fold increase in levels seen during the second and third trimesters in comparison with the nonpregnant state.

22.5 Maternal and fetal effects of vitamin D

VD affects maternal as well as fetal well-being in various ways, as shown in Fig. 22.3. Maintaining an optimum level of VD is essential for safe feto-maternal outcomes, whereas insufficiency or deficiency results in adverse effects. Vitamin D deficiency (VDD) is an emerging global issue that influences maternal health and fetal outcomes (Menon et al., 2020). Pregnant women are at increased risk of VDD, with reported prevalence is 7%–98% which is associated with pregnancy complications (Urrutia & Thorp, 2012) (Fig. 22.3).

22.5.1 Maternal effects

• Preeclampsia and vitamin D.

Preeclampsia is defined as a pathological condition of raised blood pressure (> 140/90 mmHg) diagnosed after 20 weeks of pregnancy, along with proteinuria (PCR > 30 mg/mmol) and/or multiorgan involvement such as liver dysfunction, hematological disturbances, renal, and neurological problems (AlSubai et al., 2023). A correlation of hypovitaminosis D and an increased risk of preeclampsia through various mechanisms, including the following (Giourga et al., 2023):

1. **Angiogenic factors**: VD controls the release of angiogenic factors in plasma, thus stabilising blood pressure.
2. **Calcium regulation**: VD regulates serum calcium levels. Reduced plasma calcium concentration in VDD results in parathyroid hormone stimulation and renin secretion, which lead to vasoconstriction and, consequently, high blood pressure.

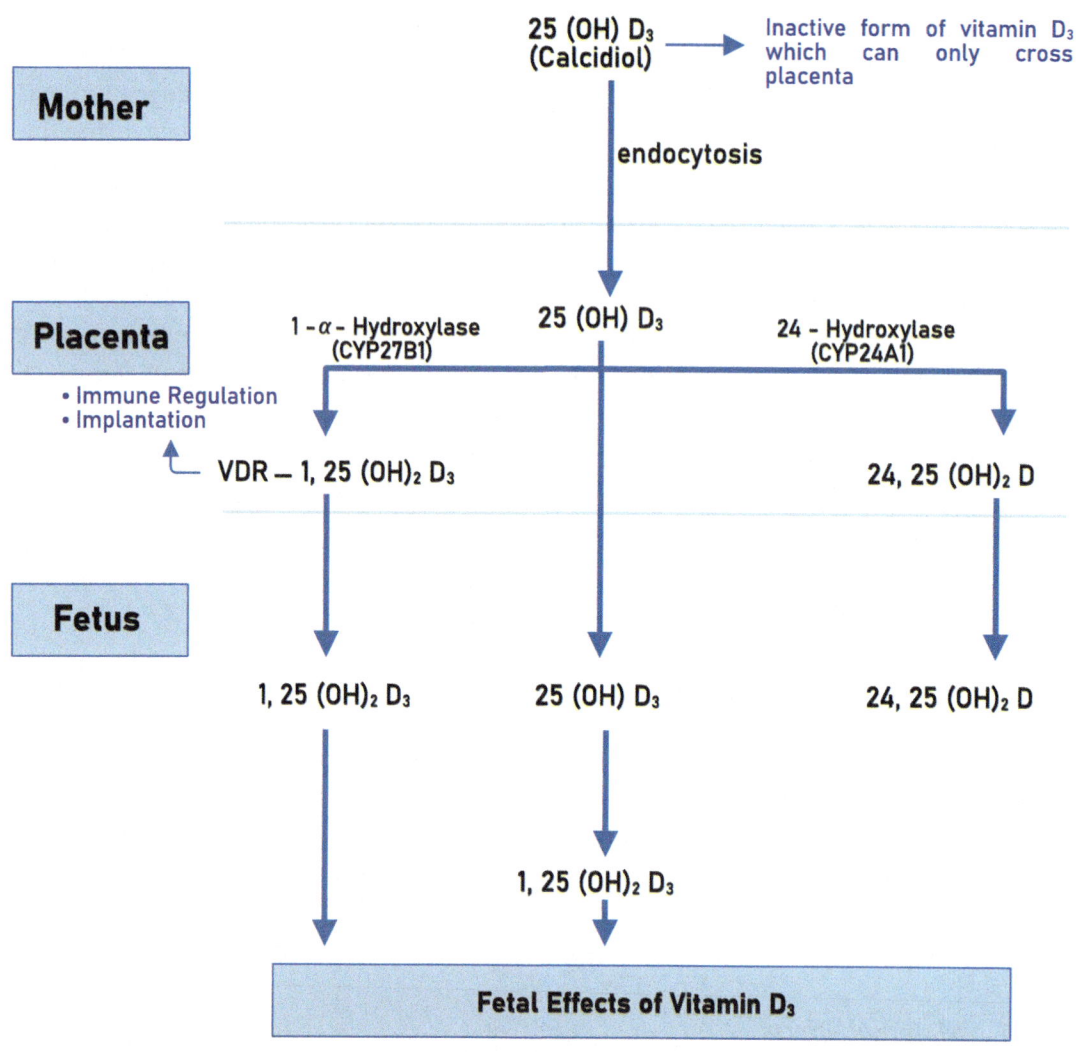

Figure 22.2
Metabolism of vitamin D in placenta.

There is a direct implication of hypovitaminosis D and a substantial probability of preeclampsia, as extrapolated from a study by Gernand et al. (2017). Nevertheless, there is conflicting evidence from other studies demonstrating no profound relation between increased consumption of VD and reduction in the possibility of hypertensive complications.

- Impaired glucose tolerance in pregnancy.

Gestational diabetes is a condition that arises during pregnancy, marked by significant insulin resistance due to hormones released by the placenta. A positive correlation intervening low VD levels is associated with reduced glucose tolerance and diabetes in

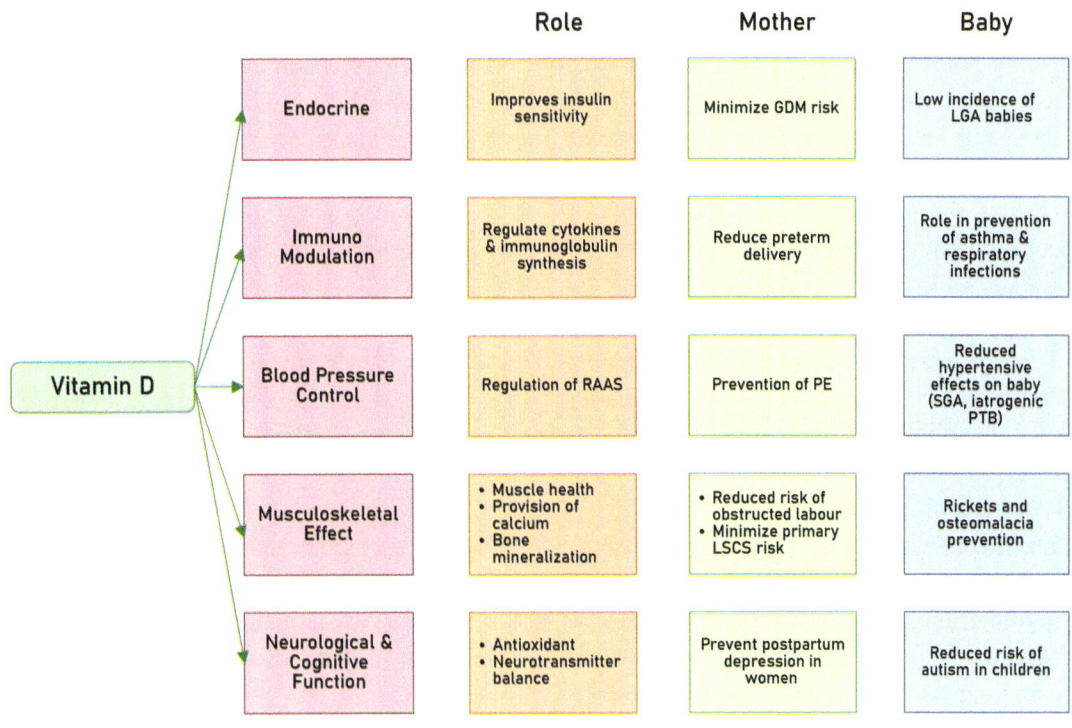

Role	Mother	Baby
Endocrine — Improves insulin sensitivity	Minimize GDM risk	Low incidence of LGA babies
Immuno Modulation — Regulate cytokines & immunoglobulin synthesis	Reduce preterm delivery	Role in prevention of asthma & respiratory infections
Blood Pressure Control — Regulation of RAAS	Prevention of PE	Reduced hypertensive effects on baby (SGA, iatrogenic PTB)
Musculoskeletal Effect — • Muscle health • Provision of calcium • Bone mineralization	• Reduced risk of obstructed labour • Minimize primary LSCS risk	Rickets and osteomalacia prevention
Neurological & Cognitive Function — • Antioxidant • Neurotransmitter balance	Prevent postpartum depression in women	Reduced risk of autism in children

Figure 22.3

Role of vitamin D and its effect on the fetus and mother.

nonpregnant as well as pregnant women. The primary action of VD in glucose metabolism is by enhancing insulin sensitivity and controlling insulin secretion through its action on pancreatic β cells (Arshad et al., 2022). Suboptimum levels or any alteration in its receptors on pancreatic β cells would result in diabetes. Whether the same mechanism is attributed to GDM (gestational diabetes mellitus) risk in VDD pregnant women is still unclear.

Recent research has explained a low vitamin D level, increased maternal insulin resistance, and small-for-gestational-age babies. Different results are observed due to multiple confounders, such as ethnicity, study design, and the threshold value for describing vitamin D deficiency. It is advisable to sufficiently maintain VD levels during pregnancy (especially during the 2nd and 3rd trimesters) to curtail GDM risk and related impediments.

• Preterm birth (PTB).

Preterm birth is the birth of a baby at less than 37 weeks of gestation (Barbosa et al., 2024). It is the predominant cause of neonatal admission to the "Special Care Baby Unit (SCBU) and Neonatal Intensive Care Unit (NICU)." Preterm birth results from composite factors such as immunologic, genetic, nutritional, and environmental influences. Inflammation and immune dysregulation are also linked to preterm birth (Tahsin et al., 2023). VD is of paramount importance in immune regulation as it is an integral part of the innate immunity, aiding in the production of host defence peptides. Additionally, multiple studies investigating polymorphisms in the VDreceptor gene (VDR) in the placenta have found a positive association between these polymorphisms and the risk of PTB. A substantial decrease in PTB risk was observed in other studies involving pregnant women with serum VD concentrations more than 40 ng/ml (Arshad et al., 2022).

Despite the above evidence, the impact of VD on preterm delivery, accounting for other confounding factors, needs to be researched. This is necessary because some retrospective studies have produced contrary results.

• Caesarean section.

There is a higher plausibility of caesarean delivery in pregnant women with VDD due to its direct effect on the method of delivery and aforementioned concomitant maternal complications of preeclampsia and preterm births. The risk of caesarean section increased from 18.6% at normal VD levels to 47.22% in VDD women, as observed in some studies (Amiri et al., 2023).

The mechanisms linking 25(OH)D levels to a high risk of caesarean section are multifaceted and not entirely understood. Synchronous contractions of uterine smooth muscles and myometrium, crucial for the initiation of labor, are partially dependent on VD status. Moderate and severe VD deficiencies are linked with increased odds of requiring a caesarean section compared to individuals with normal VD levels.

This association can potentially be explained by the presence of VD receptors in skeletal muscle besides their action on muscle contractions. VDD is complicated by proximal muscle weakness and unsatisfactory muscle function and strength. Furthermore, 25(OH)D regulates calcium levels, which are crucial for smooth muscle contraction for the onset of labour. Sufficient serum calcium levels are vital for labor to begin, and inadequate VD adversely affects musculoskeletal performance, contributing to specific causes of caesarean delivery, such as cephalopelvic disproportion (CPD) or failed labor advancement. Therefore, VD's role in uterine muscle contraction is linked to its involvement with intracellular VD receptors and alterations in calcium homeostasis.

• Postpartum depression (PPD).

Postpartum depression (postnatal depression), affecting 20%–40% of women, is a major depressive disorder occurring with the onset of pregnancy and within 4 weeks postnatally (Amini et al., 2019). It has a meaningful influence on the mother-baby association. Pregnant women with inadequate VD levels are prone to have PPD, as deduced from various studies. VD plays a substantial role as a neurosteroid in maintaining cognitive functions by affecting the neurotransmitters production, activating neuroreceptors, serving as an antioxidant, and being implicated in the neuronal signaling system between cells (Szpunar, 2020). The Endocrine Society advocates a higher dose of VD (2000 IU) during the antenatal period plus breastfeeding to address the increased requirements and to combat PPD symptoms.

22.6 VDD in pregnancy and its effects on baby

22.6.1 Small for gestational age

Small for gestational age (SGA) babies remain described by way of babies with an estimated weight less than the 10th percentile (Morris et al., 2024). Pooled analyses of various interventional studies have produced contradictory results, with some advocating VD supplementation during the antenatal period to reduce the risk of SGA and low birth weight (LBW) babies (Perichart-Perera et al., 2022), while other studies show no significant correspondence between vitamin D levels and mean birth weights.

However, corroborated evidence confirms that VD supplementation positively affects fetal weight and anthropometric measurements, showing a considerable increase in birth weight, body length, and head circumference. Despite this evidence, more randomized controlled trials (RCTs) are required to precisely define the risks and benefits of this intervention.

22.6.2 Asthma and respiratory infections

Researches have investigated the influence of VD levels during pregestational and gestational periods on susceptibility to asthma and other respiratory infections. Proposed mechanisms whereby VD plays a role in this context include (Tibrewal et al., 2023):

1. Regulation of mesenchymal and epithelial cells of alveoli.
2. Pronounced alteration in a proinflammatory and antiinflammatory environment in response to infective stimuli after vitamin D supplementation.
3. Presence of VDR (vitamin D receptors) in Type 2 Alveolar cells (responsible for surfactant production).
4. Immunomodulatory effect of VD.

Therefore, conserving acceptable levels of VD is of paramount importance to prevent respiratory infections in newborns.

22.6.3 Bone health

Fetal skeletal development begins between 8 and 12 weeks of gestation, involving necessary processes in chondrification, bone ossification, and diarthroses formation. There is an alteration in maternal calcitropic hormones, parathyroid-related peptides, and 1,25-dihydroxy vitamin D [1,25(OH)2D], to facilitate the availability of calcium (Ca^{2+}) to meet fetal demands. Abnormal neonatal calcium homeostasis is observed in expecting mothers with suboptimal VD levels and secondary hyperparathyroidism. Sufficient serum VD level in gravid women in vital in regulation calcium levels and fetal osteogenesis. Low bone mineral content (BMC) is prevalent in VDD parturients, which in severe cases results in neonatal rickets, which is deficient bone mineralization with subsequent bone softening and skeletal deformities. Untreated VDD could lead to intellectual disabilities, hungry bone syndrome, tetanus, abnormal dentition, and heart diseases.

The MAVIDOS study observed possible constructive effects of maternal VD supplementation throughout pregnancy on the bone mass of offspring (Moon et al., 2021). The current recommendation from the UK NICE guidelines advocates the use of 400 IU/day of cholecalciferol during pregnancy and breastfeeding. In contrast, supplementation with 600 IU/day during this period has been suggested by the "Institute of Medicine and the Global Consensus on Prevention and Management of Nutritional Rickets."

22.6.4 Autism and neurodevelopment

Autism spectrum disorder (ASD) is a composite of neurobehavioral conditions that involves limited interests, frequent and stereotyped behaviors, and difficulties in social communication and interaction, which results in remarkable debilitation in performing core functions (Siddiqui et al., 2024). As per the World Health Organization, approximately 1 in 160 children are affected by ASD.

There is subtle evidence indicating that children with ASD have severe VDD compared to typically developing children. Additionally, VDD has a significant correlation with the severity of ASD. Calcitriol, a neuroactive hormone, plays a critical part in neurological development and early cognitive development. The following mechanisms are hypothesized to explain how VD impacts on fetal neurocognitive development:
- Antiinflammatory properties.
- Promoting the synthesis of neurotrophic factors that are critical for neurodevelopment, such as Nerve Growth Factor (NGF) and Glial cell-derived neurotrophic factor (GDNF).
- Reducing the likelihood of seizures.
- Maintaining adequate levels of important neurotransmitters, for example, glutathione and serotonin.
- Enhancing neural cell proliferation and neurotransmission, thereby potentially influencing neurodevelopmental processes.

The influence of VD status and ASD has been extensively studied, but it is not yet fully understood. More randomised controlled trials (RCTs) are awaited to further reconnoitre and clarify this relationship.

22.7 Risk factors for vitamin D deficiency and screening

Pregnant women should be comprehensively counselled regarding the risks of VDD to their own health and to the developing fetus. During antenatal visits, women should be screened for risk factors leading to insufficient VD levels. Although routine serum screening is not endorsed by current NICE guidelines, considering the remarkable impact of VDD on maternal and child health, it is advisable to offer screening to females at high risk of this necessary vitamin deficiency or those with hypocalcaemia and symptoms attributable to severe deficiency (e.g., generalized musculoskeletal pain, proximal muscle weakness, gait abnormality, and hyperalgesia). Women who are deemed vitamin D deficient should be commenced on more than normal dose of vitamin D supplementation.

Some of the depicted predisposing factors for suboptimal vitamin D levels are (Joshi & Uday, 2023):
• Living in high latitudes.
• Overly use of sunscreen.
• Pigmented skin.
• Covered clothing.
• Old age à reduce synthesis.
• High BMI (> 30) à sequestration of VD in Adipose tissues.
• Chronic dermatological, hepatic, or renal diseases à reduced UVB absorption, reduced vitamin D synthesis.
• Pregnancy and childhood à increasing demand.
• Drug intake (Glucocorticoids, Anticonvulsants, and few antibiotics)—increases degradation of vitamin D.

22.8   Treatment

The "National Institute for Health and Care Excellence (NICE)" and the Institute of Medicine (IOM) recommend all pregnant women to start vitamin D supplements at a dose of 400 IU (NICE) and 600 IU (IOM) from the preconception period, continuing throughout pregnancy and until postpartum to avert the adverse effects of vitamin D deficiency (VDD) (Mithal & Kalra, 2014). This is because reliance on dietary VD can only provide 5 µg/day (200 IU/day) (Guideline: Vitamin D supplementation in pregnant women, 2012). Women with VDD should be commenced on vitamin D3 1000–2000 IU/day, as noted in the MAVIDOS study in the United Kingdom. This approach has shown a remarkable decrease in pregnancy complications (Larqué et al., 2018).

The "Royal College of Obstetricians and Gynaecologists (RCOG) Scientific Impact Paper" recommends treating vitamin D-deficient pregnant women with a higher dose of VD (either cholecalciferol 20,000 IU/week or ergocalciferol 10,000 IU twice weekly) for a period of 4–6 weeks. While no adverse effects were noticed with this higher dose, some studies on the use of weekly VD macrodoses during pregnancy in countries with endemic vitamin D deficiency suggested a nonphysiological rise (very high and close to safe serum upper limits) in VD levels within a day or two after the macrodose, followed by a gradual decline. Consequently, daily VD supplements are proposed to achieve the desired level in a controlled manner during pregnancy.

Advanced doses of VD should be meticulously checked and supervised by an obstetrician to intercept the risk of hypercalcaemia, which may result from excessive VD supplementation or as a manifestation of Williams syndrome, where circulating 25(OH)D has an amplified response to orally administered VD. Hypercalcemia can result in gastrointestinal problems (nausea and vomiting, constipation), myasthenia, neurological disturbances, pain, anorexia, dehydration, micturition frequency, polydipsia, and nephrolithiasis.

Thereby, all pregnant women consuming macro doses of VD should have serial serum calcium levels monitored. Treatment with calcifediol 25(OH)D is not approved for use in pregnancy (Larqué et al., 2018). There are no current studies to support its use or to clarify its safety and tolerance (Ashley et al., 2022).

VD supplements should only be used after a consultant obstetrician's advice in women with sarcoidosis, renal disease, inflammatory bowel disease, or any other malabsorption conditions (Fig. 22.4).

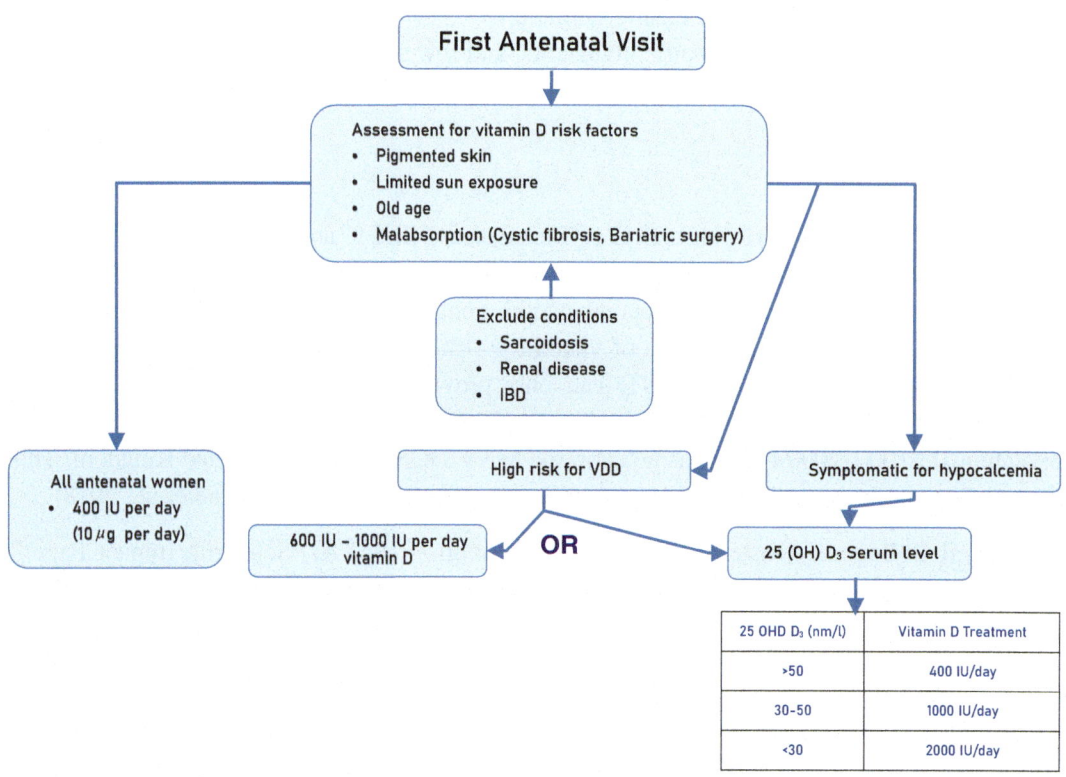

Figure 22.4
Antenatal assessment and management of vitamin D deficiency during pregnancy.

AI disclosure

During the preparation of this work, the authors used ChatGPT for grammatical corrections. After using this tool/ service, the authors reviewed and edited the content as needed and took full responsibility for the content of the publication.

References

AlSubai, A., Baqai, M. H., Agha, H., Shankarlal, N., Javaid, S. S., Jesrani, E. K., Golani, S., Akram, A., Qureshi, F., Ahmed, S., & Saran, S. (2023). Vitamin D and preeclampsia: A systematic review and meta-analysis. *SAGE Open Medicine, 11.* https://doi.org/10.1177/20503121231212093, https://journals.sagepub.com/home/ SMO.

Amini, S., Jafarirad, S., & Amani, R. (2019). Postpartum depression and vitamin D: A systematic review. *Critical Reviews in Food Science and Nutrition, 59*(9), 1514–1520. https://doi.org/10.1080/10408398.2017.1423276, https://www.tandfonline.com/loi/bfsn20.

Amiri, M., Rostami, M., Sheidaei, A., Fallahzadeh, A., & Ramezani Tehrani, F. (2023). Mode of delivery and maternal vitamin D deficiency: An optimized intelligent Bayesian network algorithm analysis of a stratified randomized controlled field trial. *Scientific Reports, 13*(1). https://doi.org/10.1038/s41598-023-35838-6.

Arshad, R., Sameen, A., Murtaza, M. A., Sharif, H. R., Iahtisham-Ul-Haq, Dawood, S., Ahmed, Z., Nemat, A., & Manzoor, M. F. (2022). Impact of vitamin D on maternal and fetal health: A review. *Food Science and Nutrition, 10*(10), 3230–3240. https://doi.org/10.1002/fsn3.2948, onlinelibrary.wiley.com/journal/10.1002/% 28ISSN%292048-7177.

Ashley, B., Simner, C., Manousopoulou, A., Jenkinson, C., Hey, F., Frost, J. M., Rezwan, F. I., White, C. H., Lofthouse, E. M., Hyde, E., Cooke, L. D. F., Barton, S., Mahon, P., Curtis, E. M., Moon, R. J., Crozier, S. R., Inskip, H. M., Godfrey, K. M., Holloway, J. W., ... Cleal, J. K. (2022). Placental uptake and metabolism of 25(OH)vitamin D determine its activity within the fetoplacental unit. *eLife, 11.* https://doi.org/10.7554/eLife. 71094, https://elifesciences.org/articles/71094.

Barbosa, O., Sim-Sim, M., Silvestre, M. P., Pedro, C., & Cruz, D. (2024). Effects of vitamin D levels during pregnancy on prematurity: A systematic review protocol. *BMJ Publishing Group, Portugal BMJ Open, 14*(2). https://doi.org/10.1136/bmjopen-2023-076702, http://bmjopen.bmj.com/content/early/by/section.

Gernand, A. D., Simhan, H. N., Baca, K. M., Caritis, S., & Bodnar, L. M. (2017). Vitamin D, pre-eclampsia, and preterm birth among pregnancies at high risk for pre-eclampsia: An analysis of data from a low-dose aspirin trial. *BJOG: An International Journal of Obstetrics and Gynaecology, 124*(12), 1874–1882. https://doi.org/ 10.1111/1471-0528.14372.

Giourga, C., Papadopoulou, S. K., Voulgaridou, G., Karastogiannidou, C., Giaginis, C., & Pritsa, A. (2023). Vitamin D deficiency as a risk factor of preeclampsia during pregnancy. *Multidisciplinary Digital Publishing Institute (MDPI), Greece Diseases, 11*(4). https://doi.org/10.3390/diseases11040158, https://www.mdpi.com/ journal/diseases.

Guideline: Vitamin D supplementation in pregnant women. World Health Organization, (2012).

Joshi, M., & Uday, S. (2023). Vitamin D deficiency in chronic childhood disorders: Importance of screening and prevention. *Multidisciplinary Digital Publishing Institute (MDPI), United Kingdom Nutrients, 15*(12). https:// doi.org/10.3390/nu15122805, http://www.mdpi.com/journal/nutrients/.

Larqué, E., Morales, E., Leis, R., & Blanco-Carnero, J. E. (2018). Maternal and foetal health implications of vitamin D status during pregnancy. *Annals of Nutrition and Metabolism, 72*(3), 179–192. https://doi.org/10. 1159/000487370, https://www.karger.ch/journals/anm/anm_jh.htm.

Menon, M., Sridevi, T. A., Mohan, T., & Patil, A. B. (2020). Vitamin D deficiency and its correlation with pregnancy outcome. *International Journal of Reproduction, Contraception, Obstetrics and Gynecology, 9*(4), 1493. https://doi.org/10.18203/2320-1770.ijrcog20201211.

Mithal, A., & Kalra, S. (2014). Vitamin D supplementation in pregnancy. *Indian Journal of Endocrinology and Metabolism, 18*(5), 593. https://doi.org/10.4103/2230-8210.139204.

Moon, R. J., Curtis, E. M., Woolford, S. J., Ashai, S., Cooper, C., & Harvey, N. C. (2021). The importance of maternal pregnancy vitamin D for offspring bone health: Learnings from the MAVIDOS trial. *Therapeutic Advances in Musculoskeletal Disease, 13*. https://doi.org/10.1177/1759720X211006979, http://tab.sagepub.com/content/by/year.

Morris, R. K., Johnstone, E., Lees, C., Morton, V., & Smith, G. (2024). Investigation and care of a small-for-gestational-age fetus and a growth restricted fetus (green-top guideline no. 31). *Inc, Undefined BJOG: An International Journal of Obstetrics and Gynaecology, 131*(9), e31. https://doi.org/10.1111/1471-0528.17814, http://obgyn.onlinelibrary.wiley.com/hub/journal/10.1111/(ISSN)1471-0528/.

Perichart-Perera, O., Avila-Sosa, V., Solis-Paredes, J. M., Montoya-Estrada, A., Reyes-Muñoz, E., Rodríguez-Cano, A. M., González-Leyva, C. P., Sánchez-Martínez, M., Estrada-Gutierrez, G., & Irles, C. (2022). Vitamin D deficiency, excessive gestational weight gain, and oxidative stress predict small for gestational age newborns using an artificial neural network model. *MDPI, Mexico Antioxidants, 11*(3). https://doi.org/10.3390/antiox11030574, https://www.mdpi.com/2076-3921/11/3/574/pdf.

Siddiqui, R. W., Siddiqui, T. W., & Siddiqui, S. W. (2024). Vitamin D and autism spectrum disorder: An intriguing association. *Emirates Annals of Child Neurology, 32*(2), 83–91. https://doi.org/10.26815/acn.2023.00353, https://www.annchildneurol.org/upload/pdf/acn-2023-00353.pdf.

Szpunar, M. J. (2020). Association of antepartum Vitamin D deficiency with postpartum depression: A clinical perspective. *Public Health Nutrition, 23*(7), 1173–1178. https://doi.org/10.1017/S136898001800366X, http://journals.cambridge.org/PHN.

Tahsin, T., Khanam, R., Chowdhury, N. H., Hasan, A. S. M. T., Hosen, M. B., Rahman, S., Roy, A. K., Ahmed, S., Raqib, R., & Baqui, A. H. (2023). Vitamin D deficiency in pregnancy and the risk of preterm birth: A nested case–control study. *BMC Pregnancy and Childbirth, 23*(1). https://doi.org/10.1186/s12884-023-05636-z, https://bmcpregnancychildbirth.biomedcentral.com/.

Tibrewal, C., Modi, N. S., Bajoria, P. S., Dave, P. A., Rohit, R. K., Patel, P., Gandhi, S. K., Gutlapalli, S. D., Gottlieb, P., & Nfonoyim, J. (2023). Therapeutic potential of vitamin D in management of asthma: A literature review. *Cureus, 15*(7). https://doi.org/10.7759/cureus.41956.

Urrutia, R. P., & Thorp, J. M. (2012). Vitamin D in pregnancy: Current concepts. *Current Opinion in Obstetrics and Gynecology, 24*(2), 57–64. https://doi.org/10.1097/GCO.0b013e3283505ab3.

CHAPTER 23

Vitamin D and Mental Health: From Neurobiology to Clinical Outcomes

Aisha Noorullah, Nargis Asad, and Shahina Pirani

Department of Psychiatry, Aga Khan University, Karachi, Pakistan

23.1 Introduction

Psychiatric disorders are widespread, affecting populations globally (Rehm & Shield, 2019), with over 1 billion individuals impacted by mental or addictive disorders (Rehm & Shield, 2019). These disorders are major contributors to disability and significant risk factors for premature death (Charlson et al., 2015). The COVID-19 pandemic has intensified the psychological challenges faced by patients, healthcare workers, and the general population (Vindegaard & Benros, 2020). Psychological distress is closely linked to unemployment, and for those who are employed, it significantly contributes to a reduction in productivity (Canavan et al., 2013). In 2019, psychiatric disorders were responsible for approximately 418 million disability-adjusted life years (DALYs), accounting for 16% of the global total (Arias et al., 2022).

Vitamin D, a fat-soluble vitamin (Reddy & Jialal, 2018) crucial for bone health, also influences blood pressure, glycemic control, and immune function (Hewison, 2012). Deficiencies in vitamin D are linked to a range of health conditions, including cancer, infectious diseases, and autoimmune disorders (Holick & Chen, 2008). Emerging scientific evidence suggests a growing impact of vitamin D on mental health.

Globally, vitamin D deficiency remains a widespread issue, affecting around 1 billion people (Cui et al., 2023), with approximately 50% of the world's population experiencing vitamin D insufficiency (Nair & Maseeh, 2012). This persistent high prevalence is likely to significantly impact the global disease burden (Cui et al., 2023).

Calcitriol (1,25(OH)2-vitamin D), the biologically active form of vitamin D, is a seco-steroid (Pérez-López, 2007) with a partially open ring structure. It exerts profound endocrine, paracrine, and autocrine effects by binding to its specific receptor, the vitamin D receptor (VDR). Calcitriol affects neurotransmitter synthesis and degradation, regulates various neurotrophic factors (Groves & Burne, 2017), and enhances the brain's antioxidant defenses (Wrzosek et al., 2013). The primary biomarker for assessing vitamin D status is the serum concentration of 25-hydroxyvitamin D [25(OH)D], which reflects both dietary intake and

The Impact of Vitamin D on Health and Disease. DOI: https://doi.org/10.1016/B978-0-443-34037-6.00007-8

cutaneous synthesis of the vitamin. Adequate levels of 25(OH)D are crucial for maintaining physiological functions and mitigating the risk of deficiency-related disorders (Giustina et al., 2024). Vitamin D, obtained from both dietary sources and sun exposure, is initially stored in fat cells and then transported into the bloodstream by vitamin D-binding protein. Vitamin D3 (cholecalciferol) is inactive until it undergoes conversion in the liver to 25-hydroxyvitamin D3 (25-(OH) D3), and subsequently in the kidneys to its active form, 1,25-dihydroxyvitamin D3 (1,25-di (OH)D3) (DeLuca, 2004).

23.2   Mechanisms linking vitamin D to psychiatric disorders

Several mechanisms have been proposed to explain the link between vitamin D and various psychiatric disorders. The widespread distribution of vitamin D receptors throughout the brain (Stumpf et al., 1982) suggests a potential role for vitamin D in these conditions. These receptors are present in nearly every tissue and cell (Eyles et al., 2005), including critical regions associated with depression (Eyles et al., 2013), such as the hippocampus, prefrontal cortex, hypothalamus, cingulate gyrus, substantia nigra, thalamus, and amygdala, a key limbic system component crucial for emotion and behavior. Vitamin D deficiency has been associated with reduced brain tissue and hippocampal volumes, as shown by MRI scans in a cross-sectional study (Croll et al., 2021).

Vitamin D plays a significant role in neurotransmitter regulation, critical to understanding its link to psychiatric disorders. Abnormalities in neurotransmitters such as serotonin (5-HT), norepinephrine (NE), dopamine (DA), glutamate, and brain-derived neurotrophic factor (BDNF) are recognized as biological contributors to depression. Vitamin D helps maintain extracellular serotonin concentrations in the brain, influencing the development and progression of neuropsychiatric disorders (Sabir et al., 2018). Additionally, calcitriol, the active form of vitamin D, regulates the expression of tyrosine hydroxylase (Puchacz et al., 1996), an enzyme crucial for synthesizing epinephrine, NE, and DA, thereby potentially impacting the pathophysiology of psychiatric disorders. Calcitriol also enhances cholinergic function by increasing the activity of choline acetyltransferase (Sonnenberg et al., 1986), the key enzyme in acetylcholine synthesis, while inhibiting acetylcholinesterase (Stio et al., 1995), which prolongs acetylcholine's synaptic transmission.

Beyond neurotransmitter regulation, vitamin D is also involved in neuroprotective functions and structural brain integrity. It plays a critical role in regulating neurotrophic factors such as BDNF, neurotrophins (NT-3), glial-derived neurotrophic factor (GDNF), and nerve growth factor (NGF) (Brown et al., 2003). Dysregulation of these factors has been associated with various psychiatric disorders, including depression (Angelucci et al., 2003) and schizophrenia (Shoval & Weizman, 2005). For example, NGF is crucial for brain development and may help prevent degeneration of the cholinergic system in Alzheimer's disease (Cattaneo et al., 2008). Calcitriol also exerts neuroprotective effects by modulating calcium levels within and outside neurons, reducing calcium-induced toxicity (Kalueff et al., 2004). Furthermore, vitamin D protects the brain against oxidative damage by upregulating the expression of γ-glutamyl transpeptidase, an enzyme that supports glutathione production, thereby increasing the brain's most important antioxidant levels (Garcion et al., 1999).

Numerous studies have shown that vitamin D is essential for brain development, with its deficiency leading to altered brain morphology, including enlarged ventricles and reduced cortical thickness, as seen in schizophrenia (Almeras et al., 2007). The observed interaction between vitamin D and glucocorticoid receptors in hippocampal cells suggests a potential connection between vitamin D and the hypothalamic–pituitary–adrenal (HPA) axis (Obradovic et al., 2006). Considering the well-established role of the HPA axis in the development of depression, this interaction implies that vitamin D might influence depressive symptoms by modulating HPA axis regulation (Pariante & Lightman, 2008).

Inflammation is recognized as a contributing factor in depression (Dregan et al., 2019), and several randomized controlled trials have shown that vitamin D can reduce levels of inflammatory cytokines (Cannell et al., 2014).

Vitamin D may improve psychological symptoms through various mechanisms, including activating brain receptors involved in behavior regulation, stimulating the release of neurotrophins, and offering protection against oxidative damage and inflammation (Paul Cherniack et al., 2009). Additionally, vitamin D's effects on glutamate may influence neural calcium levels, impacting calcium signaling pathways by regulating calcium pumps and buffers (Berridge, 2017). Its structural resemblance to cholesterol and ergosterol contributes to its membrane antioxidant properties (Wiseman, 1993).

In summary, the involvement of vitamin D in these brain processes strongly indicates its potential role in psychiatric disorders.

23.2.1 Vitamin D and depression

Research has increasingly highlighted the association between vitamin D deficiency and depression, indicating that individuals experiencing depressive disorder often exhibit lower serum vitamin D levels. Vitamin D concentrations were 8.4% lower in participants experiencing a current episode of depression as compared to those without depression among the young adult US population (Ganji et al., 2010). Similarly, a large population-based study conducted in the Netherlands found that both major and minor depression in older adults was linked to lower serum 25-hydroxyvitamin D (25(OH)D) levels. This study underscores the correlation between depression severity and vitamin D deficiency, suggesting that addressing vitamin D deficiency could be a potentially treatable factor in managing depression among older individuals (Hoogendijk et al., 2009). Further supporting this link, a recent prospective study demonstrated that both vitamin D deficiency and insufficiency may serve as risk factors for the onset of new depression in middle-aged adults (40–69 years). Vitamin D deficiency, and to a lesser extent insufficiency, could also predict persistent depressive symptoms in individuals who are already experiencing depression (Ronaldson et al., 2022). This prospective association is drawn from large-scale data from the UK Biobank. Another large, prospective cohort study from the Netherlands Study of Depression and Anxiety (NESDA), spanning participants aged 18–65 years, found that low 25(OH)D levels were linked to the presence and severity of depressive disorders, suggesting that hypovitaminosis D may be an underlying biological vulnerability for depression (Milaneschi et al., 2014). Moreover, a systematic review and meta-analysis of observational studies and randomized controlled trials revealed a significant association between low vitamin D levels and depression (Anglin et al., 2013).

Although the baseline status of participants varied between studies, some involving healthy individuals and others focusing on those with depression (current or in remission), and across various age groups, the overall evidence points to a significant relationship between vitamin D levels and depression. Both conditions are prevalent globally (vitamin D deficiency and depression), and an association between them has public health implications, indicating a potential strategy for reducing depression through vitamin D supplementation (Anglin et al., 2013). More extensive clinical studies are necessary to confirm these observations and further elucidate the relationship between vitamin D and depression (Li et al., 2019).

Conversely, not all studies support this association. For example, Pan et al. (2009) found no significant link between 25(OH)D concentrations and depression in Chinese adults aged 50–70 years. Similarly, a cross-sectional study involving university students from 39 different countries did not find a significant association between vitamin D deficiency and depression (Kouider et al., 2019).

In terms of symptomatology, decreased libido, a common symptom of depression, doesn't align with the serotonin deficit theory as increased serotonin typically reduces sexual activity, which is a known side effect of serotonin-based antidepressants (Higgins et al., 2010). In contrast, vitamin D treatment does not cause this side effect and may enhance reproductive functions (Wehr et al., 2010), making a deficiency in vitamin D a more plausible explanation for this aspect of depressive symptoms. Additionally, major depressive episodes (MDE) have been associated with cognitive impairments, particularly in the cognitive inhibition process, as measured by the Stroop test. Studies have shown that patients experiencing MDE with hypovitaminosis D may be more susceptible to cognitive impairment, further linking vitamin D deficiency with the cognitive symptoms of depression (Belzeaux et al., 2018). These connections suggest that vitamin D could play a significant role in the broader symptomatology of depression.

The key findings on the relationship between vitamin D and depression are summarized in Box 23.1.

> **BOX 23.1 Key findings on vitamin D and depression.**
> - People with vitamin D deficiency are significantly more likely to have depression than those with adequate vitamin D levels.
> - It remains unclear whether vitamin D deficiency causes depression or if depression leads to vitamin D deficiency.
> - Randomized controlled trials are needed to determine if the link between vitamin D and depression is causal.
> - The association has been observed across various age groups.
> - Given the widespread occurrence of both vitamin D deficiency and depression, this connection could have important public health implications.

23.2.2   Vitamin D and seasonal affective disorder

Sun exposure patterns have shifted worldwide due to lifestyle changes, such as increased time spent indoors, sedentary activities, and sunscreen use. In parallel, the prevalence of major depression (Witters, 2023) in the United States has risen, and autism spectrum disorder (ASD) (Autism prevalence higher, according to data from 11 ADDM communities, 2023) has become more prevalent. These trends may be relevant to vitamin D, light exposure, and mental health.

Vitamin D has been effective in treating seasonal affective disorder (SAD). A small-scale randomized controlled trial found 100,000 I.U. of vitamin D to be more effective at alleviating depressive symptoms than three weeks of light therapy. This suggests that vitamin D may be important in treating SAD. Further research is needed to confirm these findings (Gloth et al., 1999). The efficacy of vitamin D is closely related to its dosage and the resulting blood levels. Studies that have failed to demonstrate its efficacy in improving mood symptoms likely used insufficient doses, leading to inadequate blood levels; 800 IU of vitamin D was used among elderly women (Dumville et al., 2006).

23.2.3   Vitamin D in early life and schizophrenia

Disturbances in early brain development increase the risk of psychiatric disorders, such as schizophrenia. The normal progression of brain development can be disrupted by insufficient levels of various biological substances and micronutrients, including vitamin D. Vitamin D deficiency during fetal development and early childhood increases the risk of developing schizophrenia later in life (Brown & Susser, 2008). Factors like being born in winter or spring (Davies et al., 2000), higher latitudes (Saha et al., 2006) having darker skin, and low fish consumption (Kinney et al., 2009) are all associated with a higher risk of vitamin D deficiency, which may contribute to the development of schizophrenia. Schizophrenia is more commonly observed in individuals who grew up in urban areas, where sun exposure is typically lower compared to rural environments (Pedersen & Mortensen, 2001). Research also indicates that vitamin D supplementation in early life may reduce this risk, particularly among men (McGrath et al., 2003).

A population-based case–control study, utilizing Danish national health registers and a neonatal biobank, found that both low and high concentrations of neonatal vitamin D are associated with an increased risk of developing schizophrenia (McGrath et al., 2010). This raises the possibility that optimal vitamin D levels may play a protective role during early life.

Vitamin D supplementation in pregnant women and/or their offspring who are at high risk of vitamin D deficiency has the potential to lower the incidence of schizophrenia in their children. However, based on the available evidence, it cannot be recommended as a preventive strategy (Albiñana et al., 2022). This is an area of ongoing focus for research.

23.2.4   Vitamin D and adult schizophrenia

In Sweden, low serum levels of 25-hydroxyvitamin D (25-OHD) have been reported in psychiatric outpatients diagnosed with schizophrenia (Humble et al., 2010). A systematic review and meta-analysis of observational studies found a strong association between vitamin D deficiency and schizophrenia (Valipour et al., 2014). Low blood levels of vitamin D might contribute to the development of schizophrenia, or both conditions could co-occur due to shared genetic factors (Yüksel et al., 2014).

Cognitive dysfunctions are core features of psychotic spectrum disorders and have a substantial impact on the daily functioning of the patients. Vitamin D deficiency has been linked to decreased processing speed and verbal fluency in patients with schizophrenia (Nerhus et al., 2017). A systematic review found that low vitamin D levels were inversely associated with more severe clinical symptoms, particularly in negative psychotic symptoms and cognitive functioning, in individuals with psychosis. However, due to the variability between studies and the observational design of most included articles, causality could not be determined (Tsiglopoulos et al., 2021). Vitamin D deficiency has also been observed in individuals with first-episode psychosis (FEP) compared to matched controls, with one-third of people being vitamin D deficient at the time of their first episode of illness (Crews et al., 2013).

Given vitamin D's neuroprotective properties and the possible connection between developmental vitamin D deficiency and an elevated risk of psychosis, along with the impact of early psychosis on lifestyle and dietary habits, more research is essential to investigate this relationship thoroughly.

Many factors may contribute to low vitamin D levels in individuals with schizophrenia:
• During the prodromal phase (George et al., 2017) of schizophrenia, individuals withdraw from their daily activities and interests. It often leads to reduced sunlight exposure, subsequently leading to vitamin D deficiency, which is further compounded by unhealthy dietary habits.

- Vitamin D acts as a negative acute-phase reactant (Waldron et al., 2013), with levels potentially dropping during systemic inflammatory responses, which are common in acute schizophrenia but do not fully explain the deficiency seen in stable cases of psychosis.

The key findings on the relationship between vitamin D and schizophrenia are summarized in Box 23.2.

23.2.5 Vitamin D and bipolar affective disorder

Elevated levels of vitamin D binding protein (DBP) have been found in individuals with bipolar affective disorder compared to those in the nonmood symptoms (control group) and major depressive disorder. DBP was used as a marker because it is a homolog of glia maturation factor beta (GMFβ) and was identified in human plasma (Petrov et al., 2018). The elevated levels of DBP in the blood of adolescents with bipolar affective disorder could suggest two possibilities: either DBP contributes to the development of bipolar affective disorder in adolescents, or it is a factor associated with the condition. DBP shows potential as a candidate marker for bipolar disorder, and its validation in larger cohorts of patients with mood disorders is recommended (Petrov et al., 2018).

Individuals with bipolar affective disorder consistently display increased levels of circulating proinflammatory cytokines throughout various phases of the condition (Bai et al., 2014). This connection suggests that inflammation could contribute to the pathophysiology of bipolar affective disorder. Vitamin D is known for its anti-inflammatory properties (AlGhamdi et al., 2022), suggesting that it may play a protective role in bipolar affective disorder by helping to mitigate inflammation.

A recent study found no significant differences in the serum concentrations of 25-hydroxyvitamin D [25(OH)D], 24,25-dihydroxyvitamin D [24,25(OH)2D], or the vitamin D metabolic ratio (VMR) between bipolar affective disorder patients and healthy controls. However, the researchers observed an inverse correlation between Young Mania Rating Scale (YMRS) scores and both 24,25(OH)2D levels and the VMR. (Späth et al., 2023), Interestingly, this study was conducted with bipolar affective disorder patients who were primarily in a euthymic state, exhibiting only subthreshold symptoms.

BOX 23.2 Key findings on vitamin D and schizophrenia.

- Low levels of vitamin D, particularly during early development, are associated with an increased risk of schizophrenia.
- Vitamin D deficiency in individuals with schizophrenia is linked to poorer cognitive performance, especially in processing speed and verbal fluency.
- While observational studies suggest a connection between vitamin D levels and schizophrenia, causality remains unclear, and further research is essential.

In conclusion, while vitamin D has been explored in the context of bipolar disorder, the current evidence highlights the need for long-term assessments and evaluations across different phases of the disorder to gain a more comprehensive understanding of the relationship between vitamin D and the clinical progression of bipolar disorder.

23.2.6   Vitamin D and autism spectrum disorders

Vitamin D and ASD are associated in children and adolescents (Şengenç et al., 2020). Vitamin D deficiency or insufficiency was found in approximately 95% of all patients (Şengenç et al., 2020). This conclusion was drawn from children and adolescents who had an ASD without any additional chronic illness, and the study included a wide range of age groups from 3 to 18 years. Cannell & Grant (2013) have discussed several plausible explanations linking vitamin D deficiency with autism. Low prenatal vitamin D levels may impair fetal brain development, and genetic variations in vitamin D metabolism, such as in the CYP27B1 gene, could increase the risk of autism. Environmental factors like reduced sun exposure, especially in darker-skinned individuals, might exacerbate this deficiency. All these factors guide that maintaining optimal vitamin D levels during pregnancy and early childhood may mitigate some autism risk factors.

Autism in genetically predisposed children may be triggered by environmental factors, with a positive association with increased precipitation (Waldman et al., 2008). Vitamin D deficiency, among many others, is one such potential trigger (Cannell & Grant, 2013). Increased precipitation often results in increased indoor activity, leading to reduced sunlight exposure, the primary source of vitamin, which could lead to higher rates of vitamin D deficiency. As a result of Vitamin D deficiency, levels of calcitriol may be reduced, an essential neurosteroid in brain development, which could influence the risk of autism. Over the last many years, as public health messages have encouraged reduced sun exposure, autism prevalence has risen. Vitamin D deficiency is widespread among infants and toddlers in the United States and other countries (Gordon et al., 2008).

Vitamin D is essential for repairing DNA damage and shielding against oxidative stress. Therefore, vitamin D deficiency can lead to higher mutation rates and inhibit DNA repair processes. A higher concordance rate for autism exists in monozygotic compared to dizygotic twins. De novo mutations could help explain the significance. This suggests potential strategies for preventing autism, such as tackling widespread vitamin D deficiency and reducing exposure to known mutagens (Kinney et al., 2010).

23.2.7   Vitamin D and attention deficit hyperactivity disorder

Children with attention deficit hyperactivity disorder (ADHD) may be more likely to have lower levels of vitamin D along with other minerals, it cannot be concluded that these lower levels are the cause of ADHD (Villagomez & Ramtekkar, 2014). A lower prevalence of

ADHD is reported in regions with high sunlight exposure, based on both US and non-US data (Arns et al., 2013). This may be attributed to the improved circadian rhythm, which is associated with ADHD.

Evidence linking vitamin D deficiency to ADHD is established through systematic reviews and meta-analyses. The included studies in these systematic reviews and meta-analyses, though showing small overall effect sizes, consistently demonstrate an association between lower vitamin D levels and ADHD (Khoshbakht et al., 2018; Kotsi et al., 2019). Future studies with improved designs are recommended, such as prospective cohorts and randomized controlled trials, to explore the causal relationship between Vitamin D and ADHD. Adequate prenatal exposure to vitamin D may reduce the risk of ADHD and autism traits in adult life (García-Serna & Morales, 2020).

Vitamin D supplementation as adjunctive therapy to methylphenidate has been shown to improve evening symptoms of ADHD (Mohammadpour et al., 2018). Additionally, it reduced impulsivity post-intervention (vitamin D supplementation; 1000 IU) (Naini et al., 2018), while no differences in attention and response inhibition were detected. Future research is needed to clarify the effects of vitamin D as a monotherapy in ADHD and to better understand its underlying mechanisms.

23.2.8   Vitamin D and cognitive function

Vitamin D deficiency has been linked to impaired performance on several cognitive measures in the elderly age group (Wilkins et al., 2006). The significant positive correlation between 25(OH)D levels and mini-mental state examination (MMSE) scores suggests that vitamin D may have a specific role in supporting cognitive function in older adults (Przybelski & Binkley, 2007). Furthermore, vitamin D deficiency may also act as a risk factor for Alzheimer's disease (AD) (Chai et al., 2019; Jayedi et al., 2019). The severity of deficiency is associated with an increased risk of dementia, with greater deficiency leading to a higher risk. Additionally, dietary patterns and specific components have been linked to dementia. A systematic review and meta-analysis of cohort studies found that low vitamin D levels are particularly associated with cognitive decline (Cao et al., 2016). Emerging evidence also indicates that low levels of vitamin D could potentially increase the risk of developing vascular dementia in patients with type II diabetes (Geng et al., 2022).

The potential cognitive benefits of vitamin D could be attributed to several mechanisms. These include its role in increasing acetylcholine concentration in the brain by enhancing acetylcholine transferase activity (Sonnenberg et al., 1986), boosting neurotrophin synthesis (Garcion et al., 2002), and reducing free radicals, which protect brain tissue from oxidative damage. Additionally, vitamin D's role in calcium homeostasis (Kalueff et al., 2004) may offer protection against neurodegeneration and related cognitive impairments.

Collectively, evidence implies that vitamin D deficiency could worsen the progression of Alzheimer's disease and vascular dementia. It is essential to highlight that while these findings are compelling, further research is needed to clarify the precise mechanisms involved.

23.2.9   COVID-19 and vitamin D

Vitamin D deficiency played a role in stress-related depression during the COVID-19 pandemic (Ceolin et al., 2021). One of the possible mechanisms can be reduced exposure to sunlight (essential for vitamin D synthesis), due to lockdowns and social distancing measures.

Long COVID was found among patients with lower baseline and follow-up levels of 25-hydroxyvitamin D compared to those without long COVID, potentially reinforcing the role of vitamin D in infectious health emergencies (Di Filippo et al., 2023).

23.2.10   Vitamin D and age group

Vitamin D deficiency has been reported in all age groups, ranging from infants and children to adults and the elderly (Milaneschi et al., 2010), and is not limited to any nation, race, or ethnicity (González-Gross et al., 2012).

23.2.11   Women and vitamin D

Multiple studies have demonstrated a significant association between vitamin D deficiency and increased risk of depression during and after pregnancy.

Lower vitamin D levels in early pregnancy have been associated with an increased risk of depression during pregnancy (Brandenbarg et al., 2012; Cassidy-Bushrow et al., 2012). Further research in China also underscored the relationship between low vitamin D levels and increased rates of postpartum depression (Fu et al., 2015). Among women at risk for depression, low vitamin D levels in early pregnancy are linked to increased depressive symptoms during both the early and late stages of pregnancy (Williams et al., 2016).

The available evidence collectively highlights the importance of maintaining adequate vitamin D levels in reducing the risk of depression during pregnancy and the postpartum period.

23.2.12   Effects of vitamin D supplementation on psychiatric disorders

Vitamin supplementation plays an essential role in mental health disorders (Mörkl et al., 2020; Sangle et al., 2020), particularly depression, and has gained significant scientific attention.

Vitamin D supplementation has been effective in reducing depressive symptoms in adolescents (Bahrami et al., 2018; Högberg et al., 2012) with low baseline serum 25(OH)D levels, as well as in adults with major depressive disorder (MDD) and chronic liver disease, two commonly comorbid conditions (Stokes et al., 2016). The antidepressant effects of vitamin D have been observed in both adolescents and adults. While these findings highlight the positive association between vitamin D and the amelioration of depressive symptoms, the underlying mechanisms and differential effects, particularly across age groups and genders, remain areas for further investigation.

Vitamin D also has a beneficial role in improving maternal mental health during and after pregnancy. The study by Vaziri et al. (2016) demonstrated that vitamin D supplementation significantly reduced perinatal depression symptoms (at 38–40 weeks of gestation) and postpartum depression (at 4 and 8 weeks after birth). Screening for and addressing vitamin D deficiency during pregnancy can improve the psychological well-being of mothers.

Greater levels of vitamin D may be required in individuals with severe vitamin D deficiency for its antidepressant effects (Sharifi et al., 2019). However, in otherwise healthy individuals, including those who are obese or overweight (Mousa et al., 2018) without clinically significant depressive symptoms, vitamin D deficiency does not appear to increase the risk of depression. Therefore, vitamin D supplementation may not be necessary for reducing depressive symptoms in this population.

Research findings on the broader impact of vitamin D on mental health are mixed (Gowda et al., 2015; Li et al., 2014; Okereke et al., 2020). A meta-analysis (Wang et al., 2024) examining vitamin D supplementation in adults with primary depression and 25(OH)D levels above 50 nmol/L identified improvements in depressive symptoms, while other systematic reviews (Guzek et al., 2021) have not consistently supported a strong positive effect of vitamin D on mental health. Some of these inconsistencies may be attributed to flaws in the study designs (Spedding, 2014). Meta-analysis found that vitamin D supplementation was effective in alleviating depressive symptoms in studies with sound methodology, whereas studies with biological flaws yielded inconclusive results. This suggests that the quality of the study design is critical in determining the efficacy of vitamin D as a treatment for depression.

Vitamin D supplementation also shows beneficial effects in ameliorating anxiety symptoms, aligning with the broader evidence suggesting its influence on mental health outcomes (Eid et al., 2019).

The efficacy of vitamin D supplementation in the elderly has shown inconclusive results. Some studies demonstrate its benefits while others do not (Alavi et al., 2019; De Koning et al., 2019). It is important to consider several factors contributing to low vitamin D levels in elderly individuals, including reduced skin capacity for synthesizing vitamin D precursors, decreased sunlight exposure, changes in body fat, impaired kidney function, and insufficient dietary intake.

Most existing research on vitamin D supplementation primarily focuses on its effects on depression, with less comprehensive evidence supporting its benefits for other psychiatric disorders. For example, less encouraging results have been found for improving symptoms of bipolar depression (Marsh et al., 2017) and schizophrenia (Sheikhmoonesi et al., 2016).

The available evidence on vitamin D supplementation must be interpreted with caution. It is not recommended as a first-line treatment for managing or preventing psychiatric disorders (Menon et al., 2020). Several factors need to be considered to achieve the therapeutic effects of vitamin D supplementation. There is no consensus on the optimal serum 25(OH)D concentration for alleviating depressive symptoms. Higher levels of 25(OH)D may be required for neuropsychiatric disorders, as the typical threshold of 50 nmol/L might not be sufficient for neuroprotective effects, as seen in conditions like multiple sclerosis (Häusler & Weber, 2019). Another consideration is the therapeutic window of vitamin D; lower levels may be less effective, but higher levels can lead to hypercalcemia, which may alter immune responses (Häusler & Weber, 2019). There is also no consensus on the optimal doses and duration of vitamin D supplementation, though studies frequently discuss on the 8-week duration (Cheng et al., 2020). Higher doses over a shorter duration may be effective. Interestingly, like antidepressants, which have a delayed onset of action (Cipriani et al., 2018), vitamin D effects may also take several weeks to manifest.

Available research strongly supports vitamin D's therapeutic potential (AlGhamdi et al., 2024). However, its impact may vary across different age groups and conditions. Correctly identifying and treating vitamin D deficiency could lead to better health outcomes (Humble et al., 2012). Exploring vitamin D augmentation with other medications is an area of research that may offer insights into its synergistic and antagonistic effects (Mikola et al., 2023). More robust studies with better designs are required to confirm these findings.

23.2.13   Effect of vitamin D supplementation on biomarkers of oxidative stress

Psychiatric disorders are often associated with elevated oxidative stress and inflammatory conditions (Maes et al., 2011). In addition to the beneficial effects of vitamin D supplementation on mental health, it also impacts inflammation and oxidative stress biomarkers. It significantly increases glutathione (GSH) and total antioxidant capacity (TAC), both are biomarkers of oxidative stress, and reduces C-reactive protein (CRP), an inflammatory biomarker (Jamilian et al., 2019). An increase in GSH enhances antioxidant capacity, helping to protect against oxidative damage. At the same time, a reduction in CRP lowers inflammation, which may reduce the risk of metabolic syndrome, a common issue in psychiatric patients due to heightened inflammatory responses (Penninx & Lange, 2018).

The key findings on vitamin D supplementation in psychiatric disorders are summarized in Box 23.3.

23.2.14   Prevalence of vitamin D deficiency in psychiatric settings

Low vitamin D levels are frequently associated with psychiatric disorders, and supplementation has been shown to provide benefits, as discussed in earlier sections of the chapter. Shifting the focus, we now examine the prevalence of vitamin D deficiency among patients in various psychiatric settings.

> **BOX 23.3 Key findings on vitamin D supplementation in psychiatric disorders.**
> - Vitamin D supplementation has been effective in reducing depressive symptoms across various age groups, including adolescents, adults, and the elderly.
> - The exact mechanism by which vitamin D supplementation exerts its effect in ameliorating psychiatric symptoms is not fully understood.
> - Pregnant women, deficient in Vitamin D, will experience improvements in perinatal and postpartum depression through vitamin D supplementation.
> - Studies on vitamin D's impact on mental health have yielded mixed results due to flaws in study design, varying population characteristics, and differing environmental factors across studies.
> - Vitamin D supplementation raises glutathione (GSH) and lowers C-reactive protein (CRP), enhancing antioxidant protection and reducing inflammation.
> - Vitamin D supplementation is generally well-tolerated but more robust randomized controlled trials are required to determine its therapeutic potential across different conditions and populations.

Numerous studies indicate that there is a significant proportion of psychiatric inpatients (Faivre et al., 2019; Seiler et al., 2022) and outpatients (Thapa et al., 2020) who exhibit insufficient or deficient levels of vitamin D, with varying degrees across different psychiatric conditions.

The relationship between vitamin D deficiency in inpatient psychiatric patients is complex. Low vitamin D levels in psychiatric patients may result from social withdrawal (Mulcahy et al., 2016), reduced sun exposure, dietary restrictions, and obesity (which can dimimish circulatory levels) (Buscemi et al., 2021), affecting the vitamin's distribution in the body. Additionally, weight gain from atypical antipsychotic medications can further reduce vitamin D levels.

It is difficult to ascertain whether vitamin D deficiency contributes to the onset of psychiatric orders or is a consequence of the illness itself. Understanding this relationship is essential as it will guide the management approaches to psychiatric disorders. This highlights the need for routine screening and management of vitamin D deficiency as a potential adjunctive treatment in psychiatric settings.

23.2.15   Risk factors for vitamin D deficiency

Risk factors for vitamin D deficiency include a variety of demographic, socioeconomic, and lifestyle factors.

Among the US population (Ganji et al., 2010) certain groups exhibit a higher prevalence of deficiency, including women, non-Hispanic Black individuals, those living below the poverty line, individuals who do not consume supplements, residents of the South or West regions, and urban areas, and those with a higher BMI. Interestingly, many of these risk factors, such as being female (Andrade et al., 2003), living in poverty (Ridley et al., 2020), and obesity (Blasco et al., 2020), are also associated with an increased risk of depression. This overlap suggests a potential link between vitamin D deficiency and depression, highlighting the importance of addressing these shared risk factors.

South Asian women suffer disproportionately from vitamin D deficiency compared to men (Siddiqee et al., 2021). One possible explanation is the wearing of concealing and excessive clothing, which limits sun exposure (Masood & Iqbal, 2008a). Given the higher prevalence of common mental disorders (Naveed et al., 2020) and vitamin D deficiency in South Asia (Siddiqee et al., 2021), a potential underlying mechanism connecting the two warrants further exploration.

Betel chewing may also exacerbate the effects of vitamin D deficiency, an addictive habit common throughout South Asian communities (Ogunkolade et al., 2006). Poor diet, cultural practices of the region, and poverty are some of the important reasons for vitamin D deficiency in South Asia (Masood & Iqbal, 2008b).

The level of vitamin D in any population is ultimately influenced by the amount and intensity of sunlight exposure, which is affected by various factors, with geographical location being a significant determinant (Yeum et al., 2016). People in tropical regions receive more sunlight throughout the year compared to those in subtropical regions. South Asian countries with both tropical and subtropical regions on their maps, such as Bangladesh and India, experience varying levels of vitamin D deficiency. This contrasts with countries like Pakistan, which is primarily subtropical with lower sunlight availability.

In conclusion, understanding the wide array of risk factors contributing to vitamin D deficiency is critical for addressing its potential health implications, particularly in vulnerable populations.

23.3 Gaps and future research directions for vitamin D and mental health

Box 23.4 summarizes the complexity and gaps in the current research on vitamin D and mental health.

Box 23.5 summarizes the future research directions required to address the complexity and gaps in the existing evidence on the role of vitamin D in mental health.

BOX 23.4 Key issues in the evidence regarding vitamin D and mental health.

- **Inconsistent baseline measurements:** Psychiatric disorders are assessed using different tools across studies.
- **Challenges in causality:** Observational studies struggle to establish causality due to uncontrolled confounding factors.
- **Small sample sizes:** Many studies lack sufficient sample sizes, limiting the strength of findings.
- **Physiological differences:** Study populations vary in age, baseline nutritional status, and gender, complicating comparisons.
- **Blood collection and analysis:** Differences in the timing of blood collection and the assays used for serum vitamin D analysis create variability in results.
- **Outcome assessments:** Diverse methods for evaluating outcomes make generalization difficult.
- **Illness severity and outcomes:** Variations in the severity of psychiatric disorders (e.g., mild, moderate, severe depression) and vitamin D deficiency levels lead to differing outcomes.
- **Insufficient evidence for public health recommendations:** Currently, there is inadequate evidence to support vitamin D supplementation for treating psychiatric disorders.
- **Variability in supplementation protocols:** Studies have used varying dosages, durations, and routes of administration, often with brief follow-up periods.

BOX 23.5 Future research directions to address gaps in vitamin D and mental health.

- Research is needed to understand further the underlying mechanisms linking vitamin D to psychiatric disorders and to determine whether vitamin D deficiency in the psychiatric population is a consequence of psychiatric disorders or contributes to their pathogenesis.
- The therapeutic potential of vitamin D supplementation in individuals with psychiatric disorders requires further exploration, with randomized controlled trials needed to investigate its impact on the management of these conditions and deepen our understanding of this complex area.
- A larger, nationally representative sample across diverse geographies is needed.
- Some factors are common to both depression and vitamin D deficiency, with biopsychosocial elements contributing to both conditions and their associated health outcomes, warranting further exploration.
- The global health impact of climate change, particularly sun exposure, presents an interesting area for exploration in the context of vitamin D and mental health.
- Research should include consistency in study groups, outcomes, and behavioral assessments.
- Standardized protocols for vitamin D supplementation are needed for more reliable comparisons, including strategies for preventing deficiency and protocols for addressing it when detected or suspected.
- Research should explore the role of vitamin D in infectious health emergencies to determine its potential as a preventive strategy for mitigating long-term neuropsychiatric sequelae.
- Studies are needed across all age groups to capture differences in physiological and pathological mechanisms related to vitamin D deficiency.

23.4   Conclusion

Vitamin D plays a crucial role in brain function, and its deficiency may contribute to psychological issues through various mechanisms, potentially influencing the onset of psychiatric disorders. The coexistence of vitamin D deficiency and psychiatric disorders can negatively impact overall health. Identifying and addressing vitamin D deficiency, particularly in low- and middle-income countries, is a cost-effective strategy that may enhance treatment outcomes and improve patient quality of life. Routine evaluation of vitamin D levels should be considered, with future research guiding best practices for its integration into psychiatric care.

References

AlGhamdi, S. A. (2024). Effectiveness of vitamin D on neurological and mental disorders. *Diseases, 12*(6), 2024. https://doi.org/10.3390/diseases12060131, https://www.mdpi.com/journal/diseases.

AlGhamdi, S. A., Enaibsi, N. N., Alsufiani, H. M., Alshaibi, H. F., Khoja, S. O., & Carlberg, C. (2022). A single oral vitamin D3 bolus reduces inflammatory markers in healthy Saudi males. *International Journal of Molecular Sciences, 23*(19). https://doi.org/10.3390/ijms231911992, http://www.mdpi.com/journal/ijms.

Alavi, N. M., Khademalhoseini, S., Vakili, Z., & Assarian, F. (2019). Effect of vitamin D supplementation on depression in elderly patients: A randomized clinical trial. *Clinical Nutrition, 38*(5), 2065–2070. https://doi.org/10.1016/j.clnu.2018.09.011, http://www.elsevier-international.com/journals/clnu/.

Albiñana, C., Boelt, S. G., Cohen, A. S., Zhu, Z., Musliner, K. L., Vilhjálmsson, B. J., & McGrath, J. J. (2022). Developmental exposure to vitamin D deficiency and subsequent risk of schizophrenia. *Schizophrenia Research, 247*, 26–32. https://doi.org/10.1016/j.schres.2021.06.004, http://www.elsevier.com/locate/schres.

Almeras, L., Eyles, D., Benech, P., Laffite, D., Villard, C., Patatian, A., Boucraut, J., Mackay-Sim, A., McGrath, J., & Féron, F. (2007). Developmental vitamin D deficiency alters brain protein expression in the adult rat: Implications for neuropsychiatric disorders. *Proteomics, 7*(5), 769–780. https://doi.org/10.1002/pmic.200600392.

Andrade, L., Caraveo-Anduaga, J. J., Berglund, P., Bijl, R. V., Graaf, R. D., Vollebergh, W., Dragomirecka, E., Kohn, R., Keller, M., Kessler, R. C., Kawakami, N., Kiliç, C., Offord, D., Ustun, T. B., & Wittchen, H. U. (2003). The epidemiology of major depressive episodes: Results from the International Consortium of Psychiatric Epidemiology (ICPE) Surveys. *International Journal of Methods in Psychiatric Research, 12*(1), 3–21. https://doi.org/10.1002/mpr.138.

Angelucci, F., Aloe, L., Jiménez-Vasquez, P., & Mathé, A. A. (2003). Lithium treatment alters brain concentrations of nerve growth factor, brain-derived neurotrophic factor and glial cell line-derived neurotrophic factor in a rat model of depression. *International Journal of Neuropsychopharmacology, 6*(3), 225–231. https://doi.org/10.1017/S1461145703003468.

Anglin, R. E. S., Samaan, Z., Walter, S. D., & McDonald, S. D. (2013). Vitamin D deficiency and depression in adults: Systematic review and meta-analysis. *British Journal of Psychiatry, 202*(2), 100–107. https://doi.org/10.1192/bjp.bp.111.106666.

Arias, D., Saxena, S., & Verguet, S. (2022). Quantifying the global burden of mental disorders and their economic value. *eClinicalMedicine, 54*, 101675. https://doi.org/10.1016/j.eclinm.2022.101675.

Arns, M., Van Der Heijden, K. B., Arnold, L. E., & Kenemans, J. L. (2013). Geographic variation in the prevalence of attention-deficit/hyperactivity disorder: The sunny perspective. *Biological Psychiatry, 74*(8), 585–590. https://doi.org/10.1016/j.biopsych.2013.02.010.

Autism prevalence higher, according to data from 11 ADDM communities. (2023). Centers for Disease Control and Prevention. https://www.cdc.gov/media/releases/2023/p0323-autism.html.

Bahrami, A., Mazloum, S. R., Maghsoudi, S., Soleimani, D., Khayyatzadeh, S. S., Arekhi, S., Arya, A., Mirmoosavi, S. J., Ferns, G. A., Bahrami-Taghanaki, H., & Ghayour-Mobarhan, M. (2018). High Dose Vitamin D Supplementation Is Associated With a Reduction in Depression Score Among Adolescent Girls: A Nine-Week Follow-Up Study. *Journal of Dietary Supplements, 15*(2), 173–182. https://doi.org/10.1080/ 19390211.2017.1334736.

Bai, Y. M., Su, T. P., Tsai, S. J., Wen-Fei, C., Li, C. T., Pei-Chi, T., & Mu-Hong, C. (2014). Comparison of inflammatory cytokine levels among type I/type II and manic/hypomanic/euthymic/depressive states of bipolar disorder. *Journal of Affective Disorders, 166*, 187–192. https://doi.org/10.1016/j.jad.2014.05.009, http://www.elsevier.com/locate/jad.

Belzeaux, R., Annweiler, C., Bertrand, J. A., Beauchet, O., Pichet, S., Jollant, F., Turecki, G., & Richard-Devantoy, S. (2018). Association between hypovitaminosis D and cognitive inhibition impairment during major depression episode. *Journal of Affective Disorders, 225*, 302–305. https://doi.org/10.1016/j.jad.2017.08.047.

Berridge, M. J. (2017). Vitamin D and depression: Cellular and regulatory mechanisms. *Pharmacological Reviews, 69*(2), 80–92.

Blasco, B. V., García-Jiménez, J., Bodoano, I., & Gutiérrez-Rojas, L. (2020). Obesity and depression: Its prevalence and influence as a prognostic factor: A systematic review. *Psychiatry Investigation, 17*(8), 715–724. https://doi.org/10.30773/pi.2020.0099, http://www.psychiatryinvestigation.org/upload/pdf/pi-2020-0099.pdf.

Brandenbarg, J., Vrijkotte, T. G. M., Goedhart, G., & van Eijsden, M. (2012). Maternal early-pregnancy vitamin D status is associated with maternal depressive symptoms in the amsterdam born children and their development cohort. *Psychosomatic Medicine, 74*(7), 751–757. https://doi.org/10.1097/psy.0b013e3182639fdb.

Brown, A. S., & Susser, E. S. (2008). Prenatal nutritional deficiency and risk of adult schizophrenia. *Schizophrenia Bulletin, 34*(6), 1054–1063. https://doi.org/10.1093/schbul/sbn096.

Brown, J., Bianco, J. I., McGrath, J. J., & Eyles, D. W. (2003). 1,25-Dihydroxyvitamin D3 induces nerve growth factor, promotes neurite outgrowth and inhibits mitosis in embryonic rat hippocampal neurons. *Neuroscience Letters, 343*(2), 139–143. https://doi.org/10.1016/S0304-3940(03)00303-3, http://www.elsevier.com/locate/neulet.

Buscemi, S., Buscemi, C., Corleo, D., De Pergola, G., Caldarella, R., Meli, F., Randazzo, C., Milazzo, S., Barile, A. M., Rosafio, G., Settipani, V., Gurrera, S., Borzì, A. M., & Ciaccio, M. (2021). Obesity and circulating levels of vitamin D before and after weight loss induced by a very low-calorie ketogenic diet. *Nutrients, 13*(6), 1829. https://doi.org/10.3390/nu13061829.

Canavan, M. E., Sipsma, H. L., Adhvaryu, A., Ofori-Atta, A., Jack, H., Udry, C., Osei-Akoto, I., & Bradley, E. H. (2013). Psychological distress in Ghana: Associations with employment and lost productivity. *International Journal of Mental Health Systems, 7*(1). https://doi.org/10.1186/1752-4458-7-9, http://www.ijmhs.com/content/7/1/9.

Cannell, J. J., & Grant, W. B. (2013). What is the role of vitamin D in autism? *Dermato-Endocrinology, 5*(1), 199–204. https://doi.org/10.4161/derm.24356, http://www.landesbioscience.com/journals/dermatoendocrinology/2012DE0206R.pdf.

Cannell, J. J., Grant, W. B., & Holick, M. F. (2014). Vitamin D and inflammation. *Dermato-Endocrinology, 6*(1). https://doi.org/10.4161/19381980.2014.983401, http://www.tandfonline.com/toc/kder20/current.

Cao, L., Tan, L., Wang, H. F., Jiang, T., Zhu, X. C., Lu, H., Tan, M. S., & Yu, J. T. (2016). Dietary patterns and risk of dementia: A systematic review and meta-analysis of cohort studies. *Molecular Neurobiology, 53*(9), 6144–6154. https://doi.org/10.1007/s12035-015-9516-4, http://www.springer.com/biomed/neuroscience/journal/12035.

Cassidy-Bushrow, A. E., Peters, R. M., Johnson, D. A., Li, J., & Rao, D. S. (2012). Vitamin d nutritional status and antenatal depressive symptoms in African American women. *Journal of Women's Health, 21*(11), 1189–1195. https://doi.org/10.1089/jwh.2012.3528.

Cattaneo, A., Capsoni, S., Paoletti, F., & Chohan, M. O. (2008). Towards non invasive nerve growth factor therapies for Alzheimer's disease. *Journal of Alzheimer's Disease, 15*(2), 255–283. https://doi.org/10.3233/jad-2008-15210.

Ceolin, G., Mano, G. P. R., Hames, N. S., Antunes, Ld. C., Brietzke, E., Rieger, D. K., Moreira, J. D., & Vitamin, D. (2021). Depressive symptoms, and Covid-19 pandemic. *Frontiers in Neuroscience, 15*. https://doi.org/10. 3389/fnins.2021.670879, https://www.frontiersin.org/journals/neuroscience#.

Chai, B., Gao, F., Wu, R., Dong, T., Gu, C., Lin, Q., & Zhang, Y. (2019). Vitamin D deficiency as a risk factor for dementia and Alzheimer's disease: An updated meta-analysis. *BMC Neurology, 19*(1). https://doi.org/10. 1186/s12883-019-1500-6.

Charlson, F. J., Baxter, A. J., Dua, T., Degenhardt, L., Whiteford, H. A., & Vos, T. (2015). Excess mortality from mental, neurological and substance use disorders in the Global Burden of Disease Study 2010. *Epidemiology and Psychiatric Sciences, 24*(2), 121–140. https://doi.org/10.1017/s2045796014000687.

Cheng, Y. C., Huang, Y. C., & Huang, W. L. (2020). The effect of vitamin D supplement on negative emotions: A systematic review and meta-analysis. *Depression and Anxiety, 37*(6), 549–564. https://doi.org/10.1002/da. 23025, http://onlinelibrary.wiley.com/journal/10.1002/(ISSN)1520-6394.

Cipriani, A., Furukawa, T. A., Salanti, G., Chaimani, A., Atkinson, L. Z., Ogawa, Y., Leucht, S., Ruhe, H. G., Turner, E. H., Higgins, J. P. T., Egger, M., Takeshima, N., Hayasaka, Y., Imai, H., Shinohara, K., Tajika, A., Ioannidis, J. P. A., & Geddes, J. R. (2018). Comparative efficacy and acceptability of 21 antidepressant drugs for the acute treatment of adults with major depressive disorder: A systematic review and network meta-analysis. *The Lancet, 391*(10128), 1357–1366. https://doi.org/10.1016/S0140-6736(17)32802-7, http://www. journals.elsevier.com/the-lancet/.

Crews, M., Lally, J., Gardner-Sood, P., Howes, O., Bonaccorso, S., Smith, S., Murray, R. M., Di Forti, M., & Gaughran, F. (2013). Vitamin D deficiency in first episode psychosis: A case–control study. *Schizophrenia Research, 150*(2-3), 533–537. https://doi.org/10.1016/j.schres.2013.08.036.

Croll, P. H., Boelens, M., Vernooij, M. W., van de Rest, O., Zillikens, M. C., Ikram, M. A., & Voortman, T. (2021). Associations of vitamin D deficiency with MRI markers of brain health in a community sample. *Clinical Nutrition, 40*(1), 72–78. https://doi.org/10.1016/j.clnu.2020.04.027, http://www.elsevier-international.com/journals/clnu/.

Cui, A., Zhang, T., Xiao, P., Fan, Z., Wang, H., & Zhuang, Y. (2023). Global and regional prevalence of vitamin D deficiency in population-based studies from 2000 to 2022: A pooled analysis of 7.9 million participants. *Frontiers in Nutrition, 10*. https://doi.org/10.3389/fnut.2023.1070808.

Davies, G. J., Welham, J., Torrey, E. F., & McGrath, J. (2000). Season of birth effect and latitude: A systematic review and meta-analysis of Northern hemisphere schizophrenia studies. *Schizophrenia Research, 41*(1), 62. https://doi.org/10.1016/s0920-9964(00)90437-7.

De Koning, E. J., Lips, P., Penninx, B. W. J. H., Elders, P. J. M., Heijboer, A. C., Den Heijer, M., Bet, P. M., Van Marwijk, H. W. J., & Van Schoor, N. M. (2019). Vitamin D supplementation for the prevention of depression and poor physical function in older persons: The D-Vitaal study, a randomized clinical trial. *American Journal of Clinical Nutrition, 110*(5), 1119–1130. https://doi.org/10.1093/ajcn/nqz141, http://www.ajcn.org/contents-by-date.2005.shtml.

DeLuca, H. F. (2004). Overview of general physiologic features and functions of vitamin D. *The American Journal of Clinical Nutrition, 80*(6), 1689S. https://doi.org/10.1093/ajcn/80.6.1689s.

Di Filippo, L., Frara, S., Nannipieri, F., Cotellessa, A., Locatelli, M., Rovere Querini, P., & Giustina, A. (2023). Low vitamin D levels are associated with long COVID syndrome in COVID-19 survivors. *The Journal of Clinical Endocrinology & Metabolism, 108*(10), e1106–e1116.

Dregan, A., Matcham, F., Harber-Aschan, L., Rayner, L., Brailean, A., Davis, K., Hatch, S., Pariante, C., Armstrong, D., Stewart, R., & Hotopf, M. (2019). Common mental disorders within chronic inflammatory disorders: a primary care database prospective investigation. *Annals of the Rheumatic Diseases, 78*(5), 688–695. https://doi.org/10.1136/annrheumdis-2018-214676.

Dumville, J. C., Miles, J. N. V., Porthouse, J., Cockayne, S., Saxon, L., & King, C. (2006). Can vitamin D supplementation prevent winter-time blues? A randomised trial among older women. *Journal of Nutrition, Health and Aging, 10*(2), 151–153. http://www.springerlink.com/content/121281/.

Eid, A., Khoja, S., AlGhamdi, S., Alsufiani, H., Alzeben, F., Alhejaili, N., Tayeb, H. O., & Tarazi, F. I. (2019). Vitamin D supplementation ameliorates severity of generalized anxiety disorder (GAD). *Metabolic Brain Disease, 34*(6), 1781–1786. https://doi.org/10.1007/s11011-019-00486-1, http://www.wkap.nl/journalhome.htm/0885-7490.

Eyles, D. W., Smith, S., Kinobe, R., Hewison, M., & McGrath, J. J. (2005). Distribution of the Vitamin D receptor and 1α-hydroxylase in human brain. *Journal of Chemical Neuroanatomy, 29*(1), 21–30. https://doi.org/10.1016/j.jchemneu.2004.08.006.

Eyles, D. W., Burne, T. H. J., & McGrath, J. J. (2013). Vitamin D, effects on brain development, adult brain function and the links between low levels of vitamin D and neuropsychiatric disease. *Frontiers in Neuroendocrinology, 34*(1), 47–64. https://doi.org/10.1016/j.yfrne.2012.07.001.

Faivre, S., Roche, N., Lacerre, F., & Dealberto, M. J. (2019). Vitamin D deficiency in a psychiatric population and correlation between vitamin D and CRP. *L'Encephale, 45*(5), 376–383. https://doi.org/10.1016/j.encep.2019.02.005, http://www.elsevier.com/wps/find/journaldescription.cws_home/709657/description#description.

Fu, C. W., Liu, J. T., Tu, W. J., Yang, J. Q., & Cao, Y. (2015). Association between serum 25-hydroxyvitamin D levels measured 24 hours after delivery and postpartum depression. *BJOG: An International Journal of Obstetrics and Gynaecology, 122*(12), 1688–1694. https://doi.org/10.1111/1471-0528.13111China, http://obgyn.onlinelibrary.wiley.com/hub/journal/10.1111/(ISSN)1471-0528/.

Ganji, V., Milone, C., Cody, M. M., McCarty, F., & Wang, Y. T. (2010). Serum vitamin D concentrations are related to depression in young adult US population: The third National Health and Nutrition Examination Survey. *International Archives of Medicine, 3*(1). https://doi.org/10.1186/1755-7682-3-29.

Garcion, E., Sindji, L., Leblondel, G., Brachet, P., & Darcy, F. (1999). 1,25-Dihydroxyvitamin D3 Regulates the Synthesis of γ-Glutamyl Transpeptidase and Glutathione Levels in Rat Primary Astrocytes. *Journal of Neurochemistry, 73*(2), 859–866. https://doi.org/10.1046/j.1471-4159.1999.0730859.x.

Garcion, E., Wion-Barbot, N., Montero-Menei, C. N., Berger, F., & Wion, D. (2002). New clues about vitamin D functions in the nervous system. *Trends in Endocrinology and Metabolism, 13*(3), 100–105. https://doi.org/10.1016/S1043-2760(01)00547-1.

García-Serna, A. M., & Morales, E. (2020). Neurodevelopmental effects of prenatal vitamin D in humans: Systematic review and meta-analysis. *Molecular Psychiatry, 25*(10), 2468–2481. https://doi.org/10.1038/s41380-019-0357-9.

Geng, T., Lu, Q., Wan, Z., Guo, J., Liu, L., Pan, A., & Liu, G. (2022). Association of serum 25-hydroxyvitamin D concentrations with risk of dementia among individuals with type 2 diabetes: A cohort study in the UK Biobank. *PLoS Medicine, 19*(1), e1003906.

George, M., Maheshwari, S., Chandran, S., Manohar, J. S., & Sathyanarayana Rao, T. S. (2017). Understanding the schizophrenia prodrome. *Indian Journal of Psychiatry, 59*(4), 505–509. https://doi.org/10.4103/psychiatry.IndianJPsychiatry_464_17, http://www.indianjpsychiatry.org.

Giustina, A., Bilezikian, J. P., Adler, R. A., Banfi, G., Bikle, D. D., Binkley, N. C., Bollerslev, J., Bouillon, R., Brandi, M. L., Casanueva, F. F., Di Filippo, L., Donini, L. M., Ebeling, P. R., Fuleihan, G. E. H., Fassio, A., Frara, S., Jones, G., Marcocci, C., Martineau, A. R., ... Virtanen, J. K. (2024). Consensus statement on vitamin D status assessment and supplementation: Whys, whens, and hows. *Endocrine Reviews, 45*(5), 625–654. https://doi.org/10.1210/endrev/bnae009, https://academic.oup.com/edrv/issue.

Gloth, F. M., Alam, W., & Hollis, B. (1999). Vitamin D vs broad spectrum phototherapy in the treatment of Seasonal Affective Disorder. *Journal of Nutrition, Health and Aging, 3*(1), 5–7. http://www.springerlink.com/content/121281/.

González-Gross, M., Valtueña, J., Breidenassel, C., Moreno, L. A., Ferrari, M., Kersting, M., De Henauw, S., Gottrand, F., Azzini, E., Widhalm, K., Kafatos, A., Manios, Y., & Stehle, P. (2012). Vitamin D status among adolescents in Europe: The Healthy Lifestyle in Europe by Nutrition in Adolescence study. *British Journal of Nutrition, 107*(5), 755–764. https://doi.org/10.1017/S0007114511003527.

Gordon, C. M., Feldman, H. A., Sinclair, L., Williams, A. L., Kleinman, P. K., Perez-Rossello, J., & Cox, J. E. (2008). Prevalence of vitamin D deficiency among healthy infants and toddlers. *Archives of Pediatrics and Adolescent Medicine, 162*(6), 505–512. https://doi.org/10.1001/archpedi.162.6.505, http://archpedi.ama-assn.org/cgi/reprint/162/6/505.

Gowda, U., Mutowo, M. P., Smith, B. J., Wluka, A. E., & Renzaho, A. M. N. (2015). Vitamin D supplementation to reduce depression in adults: Meta-analysis of randomized controlled trials. *Nutrition (Burbank, Los Angeles County, Calif.), 31*(3), 421–429. https://doi.org/10.1016/j.nut.2014.06.017, http://www.elsevier.com/locate/nut.

Groves, N. J., & Burne, T. H. J. (2017). The impact of vitamin D deficiency on neurogenesis in the adult brain. *Neural Regeneration Research, 12*(3), 393–394. https://doi.org/10.4103/1673-5374.202936, http://www.nrronline.org/.

Guzek, D., Kołota, A., Lachowicz, K., Skolmowska, D., Stachoń, M., & Głąbska, D. (2021). Association between vitamin D supplementation and mental health in healthy adults: A systematic review. *Journal of Clinical Medicine, 10*(21), 5156. https://doi.org/10.3390/jcm10215156.

Hewison, M. (2012). Vitamin D and immune function: An overview. *Proceedings of the Nutrition Society, 71*(1), 50–61. https://doi.org/10.1017/s0029665111001650.

Higgins, A., Nash, M., & Lynch, A. M. (2010). Antidepressant-associated sexual dysfunction: Impact, effects, and treatment. *Drug, Healthcare and Patient Safety, 2*(1), 141–150. https://doi.org/10.2147/DHPS.S7634Ireland, http://www.dovepress.com/getfile.php?fileID=7635.

Holick, M. F., & Chen, T. C. (2008). Vitamin D deficiency: A worldwide problem with health consequences. *The American Journal of Clinical Nutrition, 87*(4), 1080S. https://doi.org/10.1093/ajcn/87.4.1080s.

Hoogendijk, W., Beekman, A., Deeg, D., Lips, P., & Penninx, B. (2009). Depression is associated with decreased 25-hydroxyvitamin-D and increased parathyroid hormone levels in old age. *European Psychiatry, 24*(S1). https://doi.org/10.1016/s0924-9338(09)70550-4.

Humble, M. B., Gustafsson, S., & Bejerot, S. (2010). Low serum levels of 25-hydroxyvitamin D (25-OHD) among psychiatric out-patients in Sweden: Relations with season, age, ethnic origin and psychiatric diagnosis. *Journal of Steroid Biochemistry and Molecular Biology, 121*(1-2), 467–470. https://doi.org/10.1016/j.jsbmb.2010.03.013.

Häusler, D., & Weber, M. S. (2019). Vitamin D supplementation in central nervous system demyelinating disease—Enough is enough. *International Journal of Molecular Sciences, 20*(1). https://doi.org/10.3390/ijms20010218, https://www.mdpi.com/1422-0067/20/1/218/pdf.

Högberg, G., Gustafsson, S. A., Hällström, T., Gustafsson, T., Klawitter, B., & Petersson, M. (2012). Depressed adolescents in a case-series were low in vitamin D and depression was ameliorated by vitamin D supplementation. *Acta Paediatrica, 101*(7), 779–783. https://doi.org/10.1111/j.1651-2227.2012.02655.x.

Jamilian, H., Amirani, E., Milajerdi, A., Kolahdooz, F., Mirzaei, H., Zaroudi, M., & Asemi (2019). The effects of vitamin D supplementation on mental health, and biomarkers of inflammation and oxidative stress in patients with psychiatric disorders: A systematic review and meta-analysis of randomized controlled trials. *Progress in Neuro-Psychopharmacology and Biological Psychiatry, 94*.

Jayedi, A., Rashidy-Pour, A., & Shab-Bidar, S. (2019). Vitamin D status and risk of dementia and Alzheimer's disease: A meta-analysis of dose-response. *Nutritional Neuroscience, 22*(11), 750–759.

Kalueff, A. V., Eremin, K. O., & Tuohimaa, P. (2004). Mechanisms of neuroprotective action of vitamin D 3. *Biochemistry (Moscow), 69*(7), 738–741. https://doi.org/10.1023/B:BIRY.0000040196.65686.2f.

Khoshbakht, Y., Bidaki, R., & Salehi-Abargouei, A. (2018). Vitamin D status and attention deficit hyperactivity disorder: A systematic review and meta-analysis of observational studies. *Advances in Nutrition, 9*(1), 9–20.

Kinney, D. K., Teixeira, P., Hsu, D., Napoleon, S. C., Crowley, D. J., Miller, A., Hyman, W., & Huang, E. (2009). Relation of Schizophrenia prevalence to latitude, climate, fish consumption, infant mortality, and skin color: A role for prenatal vitamin D deficiency and infections? *Schizophrenia Bulletin, 35*(3), 582–595. https://doi.org/10.1093/schbul/sbp023.

Kinney, D. K., Barch, D. H., Chayka, B., Napoleon, S., & Munir, K. M. (2010). Environmental risk factors for autism: Do they help cause de novo genetic mutations that contribute to the disorder? *Medical Hypotheses, 74*(1), 102–106. https://doi.org/10.1016/j.mehy.2009.07.052.

Kotsi, E., Kotsi, E., & Perrea, D. N. (2019). Vitamin D levels in children and adolescents with attention-deficit hyperactivity disorder (ADHD): A meta-analysis. *ADHD Attention Deficit and Hyperactivity Disorders, 11*(3), 221–232. https://doi.org/10.1007/s12402-018-0276-7, http://www.springer.com/springerwiennewyork/medicine/journal/12402.

Kouider, D. A. R., Hassan, N. A. G., & Al-Worafi, Y. M. (2019). A study investigating the association between vitamin D and depression among university students in 39 countries. *Biomedical Research, 30*(4), 655–659.

Li, G., Mbuagbaw, L., Samaan, Z., Falavigna, M., Zhang, S., Adachi, J. D., Cheng, J., Papaioannou, A., & Thabane, L. (2014). Efficacy of vitamin D supplementation in depression in adults: A systematic review. *Journal of Clinical Endocrinology and Metabolism, 99*(3), 757–767. https://doi.org/10.1210/jc.2013-3450, http://press.endocrine.org/doi/pdf/10.1210/jc.2013-3450.

Li, H., Sun, D., Wang, A., Pan, H., Feng, W., Ng, C. H., Ungvari, G. S., Tao, L., Li, X., Wang, W., Xiang, Y. T., & Guo, X. (2019). Serum 25-hydroxyvitamin D levels and depression in older adults: A dose–response meta-analysis of prospective cohort studies. *American Journal of Geriatric Psychiatry, 27*(11), 1192–1202. https://doi.org/10.1016/j.jagp.2019.05.022, http://www.sciencedirect.com/science/journal/10647481.

Maes, M., Galecki, P., Chang, Y. S., & Berk, M. (2011). A review on the oxidative and nitrosative stress (O&NS) pathways in major depression and their possible contribution to the (neuro)degenerative processes in that illness. *Progress in Neuro-Psychopharmacology and Biological Psychiatry, 35*(3), 676–692. https://doi.org/10.1016/j.pnpbp.2010.05.004.

Marsh, W. K., Penny, J. L., & Rothschild, A. J. (2017). Vitamin D supplementation in bipolar depression: A double blind placebo controlled trial. *Journal of Psychiatric Research, 95*, 48–53. https://doi.org/10.1016/j.jpsychires.2017.07.021, www.elsevier.com/locate/jpsychires.

Masood, S. H., & Iqbal, M. P. (2008a). Prevalence of vitamin D deficiency in South Asia. *Angiogenesis, 1*(11), 12.

Masood, S. H., & Iqbal, M. P. (2008b). Prevalence of vitamin D deficiency in South Asia. *Pakistan Journal of Medical Sciences, 24*(6), 891–897. http://www.pjms.com.pk/issues/octdec208/pdf/review01.pdf.

McGrath, J. J., Kaisa, S., Hakko, H., Jokelainen, J., Jones, P. B., Jarvelin, M. R., & Isohanni, M. (2003). Vitamin D supplementation during the first year of life and risk of schizophrenia: A Finnish birth-cohort study. *Schizophrenia Research, 60*(1), 44–45.

McGrath, J. J., Eyles, D. W., Pedersen, C. B., Anderson, C., Ko, P., Burne, T. H., Norgaard-Pedersen, B., Hougaard, D. M., & Mortensen, P. B. (2010). Neonatal vitamin D status and risk of schizophrenia: A population-based case-control study. *Archives of General Psychiatry, 67*(9), 889–894. https://doi.org/10.1001/archgenpsychiatry.2010.110Australia, http://archpsyc.ama-assn.org/cgi/reprint/67/9/889.

Menon, V., Kar, S., Suthar, N., & Nebhinani, N. (2020). Vitamin D and depression: A critical appraisal of the evidence and future directions. *Indian Journal of Psychological Medicine, 42*(1), 11–21. https://doi.org/10.4103/IJPSYM.IJPSYM_160_19, http://www.ijpm.info/.

Mikola, T., Marx, W., Lane, M. M., Hockey, M., Loughman, A., Rajapolvi, S., Rocks, T., O'Neil, A., Mischoulon, D., Valkonen-Korhonen, M., Lehto, S. M., & Ruusunen, A. (2023). The effect of vitamin D supplementation on depressive symptoms in adults: A systematic review and meta-analysis of randomized controlled trials. *Critical Reviews in Food Science and Nutrition, 63*(33), 11784–11801. https://doi.org/10.1080/10408398.2022.2096560, https://www.tandfonline.com/loi/bfsn20.

Milaneschi, Y., Shardell, M., Corsi, A. M., Vazzana, R., Bandinelli, S., Guralnik, J. M., & Ferrucci, L. (2010). Serum 25-hydroxyvitamin D and depressive symptoms in older women and men. *The Journal of Clinical Endocrinology & Metabolism, 95*(7), 3225–3233.

Milaneschi, Y., Hoogendijk, W., Lips, P., Heijboer, A. C., Schoevers, R., van Hemert, A. M., ... Penninx, B. W. J. H. (2014). The association between low vitamin D and depressive disorders. *Molecular Psychiatry, 19*(4), 444–451.

Mohammadpour, N., Jazayeri, S., Tehrani-Doost, M., Djalali, M., Hosseini, M., Effatpanah, M., Davari-Ashtiani, R., & Karami, E. (2018). Effect of vitamin D supplementation as adjunctive therapy to methylphenidate on ADHD symptoms: A randomized, double blind, placebo-controlled trial. *Nutritional Neuroscience, 21*(3), 202–209. https://doi.org/10.1080/1028415X.2016.1262097, http://www.tandfonline.com/loi/ynns20#.VvukQLdf1Hh.

Mousa, A., Naderpoor, N., de Courten, M. P. J., & de Courten, B. (2018). Vitamin D and symptoms of depression in overweight or obese adults: A cross-sectional study and randomized placebo-controlled trial. *The Journal of Steroid Biochemistry and Molecular Biology, 177*, 200–208. https://doi.org/10.1016/j.jsbmb.2017.08.002.

Mulcahy, K. B., Trigoboff, E., Opler, L., & Demler, T. L. (2016). Physician prescribing practices of vitamin D in a psychiatric hospital. *Innovations in Clinical Neuroscience, 13*.

Mörkl, S., Wagner-Skacel, J., Lahousen, T., Lackner, S., Holasek, S. J., Bengesser, S. A., Painold, A., Holl, A. K., & Reininghaus, E. (2020). The role of nutrition and the gut-brain axis in psychiatry: A review of the literature. *Neuropsychobiology, 79*(1), 80–88. https://doi.org/10.1159/000492834, http://www.karger.com/journals/nps/nps_jh.htm.

Naini, A. A., Fasihi, F., Najafi, M., Ghazvini, M. R., & Hasanzadeh, A. (2018). The effects of vitamin D supplementation on ADHD (Attention Deficit Hyperactivity Disorder) 1996-2021 in 6–13 year-old students: A randomized, double-blind, placebo-controlled study. *European Journal of Integrative Medicine, 25*, 28–33.

Nair, R., & Maseeh, A. (2012). Vitamin D: The sunshine vitamin. *Journal of Pharmacology and Pharmacotherapeutics, 3*(2), 118–126. https://doi.org/10.4103/0976-500X.95506.

Naveed, S., Waqas, A., Chaudhary, A. M. D., Kumar, S., Abbas, N., Amin, R., Jamil, N., & Saleem, S. (2020). Prevalence of common mental disorders in South Asia: A systematic review and meta-regression analysis. *Frontiers in Psychiatry, 11*, 573150. https://doi.org/10.3389/fpsyt.2020.573150, http://www.frontiersin.org/Psychiatry.

Nerhus, M., Berg, A. O., Simonsen, C., Haram, M., Haatveit, B., Dahl, S. R., Gurholt, T. P., Bjella, T. D., Ueland, T., Andreassen, O. A., & Melle, I. (2017). Vitamin D deficiency associated with cognitive functioning in psychotic disorders. *Journal of Clinical Psychiatry, 78*(7), e750. https://doi.org/10.4088/JCP.16m10880, http://www.psychiatrist.com/JCP/article/_layouts/ppp.psych.controls/BinaryViewer.ashx?Article=/JCP/article/Pages/2017/v78n07/16m10880.aspx&Type=Article.

Obradovic, D., Gronemeyer, H., Lutz, B., & Rein, T. (2006). Cross-talk of vitamin D and glucocorticoids in hippocampal cells. *Journal of Neurochemistry, 96*(2), 500–509. https://doi.org/10.1111/j.1471-4159.2005.03579.x.

Ogunkolade, W. B., Boucher, B. J., Bustin, S. A., Burrin, J. M., Noonan, K., Mannan, N., & Hitman, G. A. (2006). Vitamin D metabolism in peripheral blood mononuclear cells is influenced by chewing "betel nut" (Areca catechu) and vitamin D status. *Journal of Clinical Endocrinology and Metabolism, 91*(7), 2612–2617. https://doi.org/10.1210/jc.2005-2750, http://jcem.endojournals.org/cgi/reprint/91/7/2612.

Okereke, O. I., Reynolds, C. F., Mischoulon, D., Chang, G., Vyas, C. M., Cook, N. R., Weinberg, A., Bubes, V., Copeland, T., Friedenberg, G., Lee, I. M., Buring, J. E., & Manson, J. E. (2020). Effect of long-term vitamin d3supplementation vs placebo on risk of depression or clinically relevant depressive symptoms and on change in mood scores: A randomized clinical trial. *American Medical Association, United States JAMA - Journal of the American Medical Association, 324*(5), 471–480. https://doi.org/10.1001/jama.2020.10224, http://jama.jamanetwork.com/journal.aspx.

Pan, A., Lu, L., Franco, O. H., Yu, Z., Li, H., & Lin, X. (2009). Association between depressive symptoms and 25-hydroxyvitamin D in middle-aged and elderly Chinese. *Journal of Affective Disorders, 118*(1-3), 240–243. https://doi.org/10.1016/j.jad.2009.02.002.

Pariante, C. M., & Lightman, S. L. (2008). The HPA axis in major depression: Classical theories and new developments. *Trends in Neurosciences, 31*(9), 464–468. https://doi.org/10.1016/j.tins.2008.06.006.

Paul Cherniack, E., Troen, B. R., Florez, H. J., Roos, B. A., & Levis, S. (2009). Some new food for thought: the role of vitamin D in the mental health of older adults. *Current Psychiatry Reports, 11*(1), 12–19.

Pedersen, C. B., & Mortensen, P. B. (2001). Evidence of a dose-response relationship between urbanicity during upbringing and schizophrenia risk. *Archives of General Psychiatry, 58*(11), 1039–1046. https://doi.org/10.1001/archpsyc.58.11.1039, http://archpsyc.jamanetwork.com/journal.aspx.

Penninx, B. W. J. H., & Lange, S. M. M. (2018). Metabolic syndrome in psychiatric patients: Overview, mechanisms, and implications. *Dialogues in Clinical Neuroscience, 20*(1), 63–73. https://doi.org/10.31887/dcns.2018.20.1/bpenninx.

Petrov, B., Aldoori, A., James, C., Yang, K., Algorta, G. P., Lee, A., Zhang, L., Lin, T., Awadhi, R. A., Parquette, J. R., Samogyi, A., Arnold, L. E., Fristad, M. A., Gracious, B., & Ziouzenkova, O. (2018). Bipolar disorder in youth is associated with increased levels of Vitamin D-binding protein. *Translational Psychiatry, 8*(1), 61. https://doi.org/10.1038/s41398-018-0109-7, http://www.nature.com/tp/index.html.

Przybelski, R. J., & Binkley, N. C. (2007). Is vitamin D important for preserving cognition? A positive correlation of serum 25-hydroxyvitamin D concentration with cognitive function. *Archives of Biochemistry and Biophysics, 460*(2), 202–205. https://doi.org/10.1016/j.abb.2006.12.018.

Puchacz, E., Stumpf, W. E., Stachowiak, E. K., & Stachowiak, M. K. (1996). Vitamin D increases expression of the tyrosine hydroxylase gene in adrenal medullary cells. *Molecular Brain Research, 36*(1), 193–196. https://doi.org/10.1016/0169-328X(95)00314-I, http://www.elsevier.com/locate/molbrainres.

Pérez-López, F. R. (2007). Vitamin D: The secosteroid hormone and human reproduction. *Gynecological Endocrinology, 23*(1), 13–24.

Reddy, P., & Jialal, I. (2018). Biochemistry, fat soluble vitamins. https://europepmc.org/article/NBK/nbk534869.

Rehm, J., & Shield, K. D. (2019). Global burden of disease and the impact of mental and addictive disorders. *Current Psychiatry Reports, 21*(2). https://doi.org/10.1007/s11920-019-0997-0, http://www.springerlink.com/content/1523-3812/.

Ridley, M., Rao, G., Schilbach, F., & Patel, V. (2020). Poverty, depression, and anxiety: Causal evidence and mechanisms. *Science (New York, N.Y.), 370*(6522). https://doi.org/10.1126/science.aay0214.

Ronaldson, A., Arias De La Torre, J., Gaughran, F., Bakolis, I., Hatch, S. L., Hotopf, M., & Dregan, A. (2022). Prospective associations between vitamin D and depression in middle-aged adults: Findings from the UK Biobank cohort. *Kingdom Psychological Medicine, 52*(10), 1866–1874. https://doi.org/10.1017/S0033291720003657, http://journals.cambridge.org/action/displayJournal?jid=PSM.

Sabir, M. S., Haussler, M. R., Mallick, S., Kaneko, I., Lucas, D. A., Haussler, C. A., Whitfield, G. K., & Jurutka, P. W. (2018). Optimal vitamin D spurs serotonin: 1,25-dihydroxyvitamin D represses serotonin reuptake transport (SERT) and degradation (MAO-A) gene expression in cultured rat serotonergic neuronal cell lines. *Genes and Nutrition, 13*(1). https://doi.org/10.1186/s12263-018-0605-7, http://www.springerlink.com/content/1555-8932.

Saha, S., Chant, D. C., Welham, J. L., & McGrath, J. J. (2006). The incidence and prevalence of schizophrenia varies with latitude. *Acta Psychiatrica Scandinavica, 114*(1), 36–39. https://doi.org/10.1111/j.1600-0447.2005.00742.x.

Sangle, P., Sandhu, O., Aftab, Z., Anthony, A. T., & Khan, S. (2020). Vitamin B12 supplementation: Preventing onset and improving prognosis of depression. *Cureus.* https://doi.org/10.7759/cureus.11169.

Şengenç, E., Kıykım, E., & Saltik, S. (2020). Vitamin D levels in children and adolescents with autism. *Journal of International Medical Research, 48*(7) 0300060520934638.

Seiler, N., Tsiglopoulos, J., Keem, M., Das, S., & Waterdrinker, A. (2022). Prevalence of vitamin D deficiency among psychiatric inpatients: A systematic review. *International Journal of Psychiatry in Clinical Practice, 26*(4), 330–336. https://doi.org/10.1080/13651501.2021.2022701.

Sharifi, A., Vahedi, H., Nedjat, S., Mohamadkhani, A., & Hosseinzadeh Attar, M. J. (2019). Vitamin D decreases beck depression inventory score in patients with mild to moderate ulcerative colitis: A double-blind randomized placebo-controlled trial. *Journal of Dietary Supplements, 16*(5), 541–549. https://doi.org/10.1080/19390211.2018.1472168, http://www.tandfonline.com/loi/ijds20.

Sheikhmoonesi, F., Zarghami, M., Mamashli, S., Charati, J. Y., Hamzehpour, R., Fattahi, S., Azadbakht, R., Kashi, Z., Ala, S., Moshayedi, M., Alinia, H., & Hendouei, N. (2016). Effectiveness of vitamin d supplement therapy in chronic stable schizophrenic male patients: A randomized controlled trial. *Iranian Journal of Pharmaceutical Research, 15*(4), 941–950. http://ijpr.sbmu.ac.ir/article_1942_cba34aeb9ea94e6f644cca1b82086437.pdf.

Shoval, G., & Weizman, A. (2005). The possible role of neurotrophins in the pathogenesis and therapy of schizophrenia. *European Neuropsychopharmacology, 15*(3), 319–329. https://doi.org/10.1016/j.euroneuro.2004.12.005.

Siddiqee, M. H., Bhattacharjee, B., Siddiqi, U. R., & MeshbahurRahman, M. (2021). High prevalence of vitamin D deficiency among the South Asian adults: a systematic review and meta-analysis. *BMC Public Health, 21*(1), 1–18. https://doi.org/10.1186/s12889-021-11888-1, http://www.biomedcentral.com/bmcpublichealth.

Sonnenberg, J., Luine, V. N., Krey, L. C., & Christakos, S. (1986). 1,25-Dihydr oxyvitamin D3 treatment results in increased choline acetyltransferase activity in specific brain nuclei. *Endocrinology, 118*(4), 1433–1439. https://doi.org/10.1210/endo-118-4-1433.

Spedding, S. (2014). Vitamin D and depression: A systematic review and meta-analysis comparing studies with and without biological flaws. *Nutrients, 6*(4), 1501–1518. https://doi.org/10.3390/nu6041501.

Späth, Z., Tmava-Berisha, A., Fellendorf, F. T., Stross, T., Maget, A., Platzer, M., Bengesser, S. A., Häussl, A., Zwigl, I., Birner, A., Queissner, R., Stix, K., Wels, L., Lenger, M., Dalkner, N., Zelzer, S., Herrmann, M., & Reininghaus, E. Z. (2023). Vitamin D status in bipolar disorder. *Nutrients, 15*(22). https://doi.org/10.3390/nu15224752, http://www.mdpi.com/journal/nutrients/.

Stio, M., Lunghi, B., Celli, A., & Treves, C. (1995). Vitamin D - related modification of enzyme activities in synaptosomes and mitochondria isolated from rat cerebral cortex. *Biochemistry and Molecular Biology International, 37*(5), 813–820.

Stokes, C. S., Grünhage, F., Baus, C., Volmer, D. A., Wagenpfeil, S., Riemenschneider, M., & Lammert, F. (2016). Vitamin D supplementation reduces depressive symptoms in patients with chronic liver disease. *Clinical Nutrition, 35*(4), 950–957. https://doi.org/10.1016/j.clnu.2015.07.004, http://www.elsevier-international.com/journals/clnu/.

Stumpf, W. E., Sar, M., Clark, S. A., & Deluca, H. F. (1982). Brain target sites for 1,25-dihydroxyvitamin D3. *Science (New York, N.Y.), 215*(4538), 1403–1405. https://doi.org/10.1126/science.6977846.

Thapa, A., Karki, M., & Thapa, A. (2020). Vitamin-D deficiency among psychiatric outpatients attending tertiary care hospital. *Journal of College of Medical Sciences-Nepal, 16*(4), 195–200. https://doi.org/10.3126/jcmsn.v16i4.34460.

Tsiglopoulos, J., Pearson, N., Mifsud, N., Allott, K., & O'Donoghue, B. (2021). The association between vitamin D and symptom domains in psychotic disorders: A systematic review. *Schizophrenia Research, 237*, 79–92. https://doi.org/10.1016/j.schres.2021.08.001.

Valipour, G., Saneei, P., & Esmaillzadeh, A. (2014). Serum vitamin D levels in relation to schizophrenia: A systematic review and meta-analysis of observational studies. *The Journal of Clinical Endocrinology & Metabolism, 99*(10), 3863–3872. https://doi.org/10.1210/jc.2014-1887.

Vaziri, F., Nasiri, S., Tavana, Z., Dabbaghmanesh, M. H., Sharif, F., & Jafari, P. (2016). A randomized controlled trial of vitamin D supplementation on perinatal depression: In Iranian pregnant mothers. *BMC Pregnancy and Childbirth, 16*(1). https://doi.org/10.1186/s12884-016-1024-7, http://www.biomedcentral.com/bmcpregnancychildbirth/.

Villagomez, A., & Ramtekkar, U. (2014). Iron, Magnesium, vitamin D, and zinc deficiencies in children presenting with symptoms of attention-deficit/hyperactivity disorder. *Children, 1*(3), 261–279. https://doi.org/10.3390/children1030261.

Vindegaard, N., & Benros, M. E. (2020). COVID-19 pandemic and mental health consequences: Systematic review of the current evidence. *Brain, Behavior, and Immunity, 89*, 531–542. https://doi.org/10.1016/j.bbi.2020.05.048, http://www.elsevier.com/inca/publications/store/6/2/2/8/0/0/index.htt.

Waldman, M., Nicholson, S., Adilov, N., & Williams, J. (2008). Autism prevalence and precipitation rates in California, Oregon, and Washington counties. *Archives of Pediatrics and Adolescent Medicine, 162*(11), 1026–1034. https://doi.org/10.1001/archpedi.162.11.1026, http://archpedi.ama-assn.org/cgi/reprint/162/11/1026.

Waldron, J. L., Ashby, H. L., Cornes, M. P., Bechervaise, J., Razavi, C., Thomas, O. L., Chugh, S., Deshpande, S., Ford, C., & Gama, R. (2013). Vitamin D: A negative acute phase reactant. *Journal of Clinical Pathology, 66*(7), 620–622. https://doi.org/10.1136/jclinpath-2012-201301, http://jcp.bmj.com/content/66/7/620.full.pdf.

Wang, R., Xu, F., Xia, X., Xiong, A., Dai, D., Ling, Y., Sun, R., Qiu, L., Ding, Y., & Xie, Z. (2024). The effect of vitamin D supplementation on primary depression: A meta-analysis. *Journal of Affective Disorders, 344*, 653–661. https://doi.org/10.1016/j.jad.2023.10.021.

Wehr, E., Pilz, S., Boehm, B. O., März, W., & Obermayer-Pietsch, B. (2010). Association of vitamin D status with serum androgen levels in men. *Clinical Endocrinology, 73*(2), 243–248. https://doi.org/10.1111/j.1365-2265.2009.03777.x.

Wilkins, C. H., Sheline, Y. I., Roe, C. M., Birge, S. J., & Morris, J. C. (2006). Vitamin D deficiency is associated with low mood and worse cognitive performance in older adults. *American Journal of Geriatric Psychiatry, 14*(12), 1032–1040. https://doi.org/10.1097/01.JGP.0000240986.74642.7c, http://www.sciencedirect.com/science/journal/10647481.

Williams, J. A., Romero, V. C., Clinton, C. M., Vazquez, D. M., Marcus, S. M., Chilimigras, J. L., & Mozurkewich, E. L. (2016). Vitamin D levels and perinatal depressive symptoms in women at risk: A secondary analysis of the mothers, omega-3, and mental health study. *BMC Pregnancy and Childbirth, 16*, 1–9.

Wiseman, H. (1993). Vitamin D is a membrane antioxidant Ability to inhibit iron-dependent lipid peroxidation in liposomes compared to cholesterol, ergosterol and tamoxifen and relevance to anticancer action. *FEBS Letters, 326*(1-3), 285–288. https://doi.org/10.1016/0014-5793(93)81809-e.

Witters, D. (2023). US depression rates reach new highs. Gallup. https://news.gallup.com/poll/505745/depression-rates-reach-new-highs.aspx.

Wrzosek, M., Łukaszkiewicz, J., Wrzosek, M., Jakubczyk, A., Matsumoto, H., Piątkiewicz, P., ... Nowicka, G. (2013). Vitamin D and the central nervous system. *Pharmacological Reports: PR, 65*(2), 271–278.

Yeum, K. J., Song, B. C., & Joo, N. S. (2016). Impact of geographic location on vitamin D status and bone mineral density. *International Journal of Environmental Research and Public Health, 13*(2). https://doi.org/10.3390/ijerph13020184, http://www.mdpi.com/1660-4601/13/2/184/pdf.

Yüksel, R. N., Altunsoy, N., Tikir, B., Cingi Külük, M., Unal, K., Goka, S., Aydemir, C., & Goka, E. (2014). Correlation between total vitamin D levels and psychotic psychopathology in patients with schizophrenia: Therapeutic implications for add-on vitamin D augmentation. *Therapeutic Advances in Psychopharmacology, 4*(6), 268–275. https://doi.org/10.1177/2045125314553612 appraisal of the evidence and future directions.

CHAPTER 24

Vitamin D and aging

Rabia Mahmood Khan[1,2,3]**, and Mahwish Nida**[4]

[1]*Community Rehabilitation GP, Community Hospital, Oxford University Health and Care Trust, Oxford, United Kingdom* [2]*Bartlemas Surgery, Oxford, United Kingdom* [3]*Witney Community Hospital, Oxford University Health and Care Trust; Bartlemas Surgery, Manzil Way, Cowley, Oxfordshire, United Kingdom* [4]*Geratology, Oxford University Hospital, Oxford, United Kingdom*

24.1   Introduction

Aging is known to lead to reduced absorption, conversion, and utilization of vitamin D (VD) in the body. A causal association between aging and VD deficiency is difficult to establish. VD deficiency could be due to various processes related to aging, like reduced skin function and hydroxylation of VD, or it could be a result of chronic health conditions in older people. Studies done on older people have shown that overall, the requirement for VD changes as we age (Suter & Vetter, 1994).

As would have already been highlighted in previous chapters, vitamin D is available as ergocalciferol (vitamin D_2) and cholecalciferol (vitamin D_3). The sources that can provide VD include VD-rich food, oral or injectable supplements, and daylight. Foods which supply adequate amounts of vitamin D are oily fish such as cod liver oil, swordfish, and salmon (vitamin D_3) and ultraviolet-exposed mushrooms (vitamin D_2). Other products include fortified milk, orange juices, and cereals (Hossein-Nezhad & Holick, 2013).

After absorption from the gut, VD is carried through the circulation in an inactive form to the kidneys, where its morphology and functioning are changed through hydroxylation so that it can exert its effect in various organ systems.

However, older people are at risk of not getting enough VD, especially when they are confined indoors. Skin production of VD makes a much more contribution, and it can be reduced by high altitudes, winter months, darker skin color, sunscreen use, and age associated reduction of dermal production of VD (Tanaka et al., 2024). A recent study showed that there was a 13% decline in dermal production per decade, which meant that VD production in people of 70 years of age was approximately half of that in those at 20 years of age (Lips et al., 2020). Hence, elderly people need to be encouraged to add vitamin D supplementation through the above sources improve their overall health status. NICE recommends daily

The Impact of Vitamin D on Health and Disease. DOI: https://doi.org/10.1016/B978-0-443-34037-6.00010-8

supplements of vitamin D for older people more than 65 years of age, especially in care home settings, who are less exposed to sunlight (NICE).

On review of the literature, most of the data on the role of VD has been focused to demonstrate its effects on bone metabolism and its regulation to maintain healthy bones and skeletal systems. This research on VD was accelerated when its supplementation was found to prevent experimentally created rickets (Mellanby et al., 1919). Slowly and gradually, more research on this vitamin highlighted its immune regulatory function, which is perhaps older than its role in calcium homeostasis (Bouillon & Suda, 2014). For example, cod liver oil, a substance with high levels of vitamin D3, as well as UVB exposure, were both discovered to be a treatment as well as preventative for tuberculosis, a bacterial infection (Grad, 2004; Holick, 1981), and the risk of autoimmune diseases, such as multiple sclerosis, was negatively correlated with sufficient VD levels (Schwartz, 1992).

24.2   Vitamin D insufficiency and deficiency in older people

The most common screening test for the assessment of the VD status among all age groups, including older people living at home or in sheltered or nursing homes, is plasma 25 OH D measurements. The definition of VD deficiency, insufficiency, and sufficiency, according to the Endocrine Society's Clinical Practice Guideline is serum concentrations of 25(OH) D < 20 ng/mL (< 50 nmol/L), 21–29 ng/mL (51–74 nmol/L), and 30–100 ng/mL (75–250 nmol/L), respectively (Holick et al., 2011). A survey was done by Lips (2001) to assess the VD status in several countries, including the USA, Europe, and Australia, to name a few. The survey showed that VD insufficiency is not only a common phenomenon in geriatric populations residing in communities, irrespective of the country of location. It seemed to be a universal occurrence in older people living in nursing homes. When compared with the mean values of the old aged healthy patients, European people were found to have lower VD levels on average as compared to the USA. Similarly, the VD levels among the older people with hip fractures were low in Europe compared to the USA and Australia, respectively. There are other studies that have also highlighted the higher prevalence of low plasma VD concentrations in hip fracture patients compared to their age-matched controls (Knorring et al., 1982; Lips et al., 1982).

24.3   Aging and frailty

Aging is a natural process whereby molecular and cellular damage accumulation leads to the weakening of the whole human body. But what confuses the mind is, if aging is universal, then how would one 80 years old be sprightly while another appear fatigued and exhausted? Is age really just a number, or other powers are at play? Is fitness the only determinant of good health or nutritional supplementation play a role as well?

Aging can be broadly considered as healthy aging and pathological aging. Pathological aging is associated with a high occurrence of comorbidities and frailty, both of which can impact functional status and contribute to the development of geriatric syndromes like falls and fractures. VD is seen as having a critical role in healthy aging, where people with low levels have been shown to be more functionally dependent with a higher chance of admission to hospital and long-term care facilities (Kupisz-Urbańska et al., 2021).

Frailty is an age-related clinical condition of reduced reserves and resistance to stressors. It is mainly a result of age associated declines across a multitude of physiological systems that might be recognized by five key clinical manifestations: unintentional weight loss, asthenia, fatigue, sluggish pace, and reduced activity levels (Fried et al., 2001). In frailty, a small, insignificant event or illness, for example, urinary tract infection, can have longterm implications on health. Frailty has been shown to have a higher frequency in the elderly and corresponds to the underlying longterm nutritional status (Cruz-Jentoft & Woo, 2019). In addition, as we age, the risk of developing chronic diseases such as coronary artery disease or CVD, COPD, osteoporosis (OP), and osteoarthritis (OA) significantly increases. Many older adults experience multiple comorbidities along with frailty, particularly after reaching 60 years of age, necessitating a diverse approach to treatment for an effective longterm management.

Several studies highlight VD and frailty association. For example, in the Women's Health and Aging Study II, Buta et al. (2017) found that menopausal womens' risk of developing frailty tripled over a mean period of 8.5 years if serum VD levels were < 10 ng/mL. A meta analysis and systematic review was conducted by Zhou et al. (2016) to describe the positive correlation between low vitamin D (25(OH)D) level and frailty. Studies were reviewed, and the results suggested that low levels of vitamin D were significantly associated with the risk of frailty. In addition, results of subgroup analysis indicated that females with low levels of VD were significantly associated with a higher risk of frailty.

Sarcopenia, or reduced muscle mass and function in older age, is considered one of the etiological factors of frailty due to its close connection with the development of geriatric syndromes and impaired quality of life. In sarcopenia, vitamin D deficiency, exacerbated by malnutrition and reduced exposure to sunlight in older patients, is associated with altered muscular processes like reduced mitochondrial function, increased fat deposition, increased protein breakdown, and termination of cell cycle or senility (Bollen et al., 2022). Interventional and observational research has shown that VD supplementation may improve muscle vigor and ability to move with some form of independence, with marked results seen in those with VD deficiency or adults aged ≥65 years. There are other interventional studies that show how older adults on VD3 treatment, especially taking 800–1000 IU daily, had improved power in the lower limbs (Beaudart et al., 2014; Muir & Montero-Odasso, 2011; Rejnmark, 2011). A meta analysis to analyze the role of VD supplementation in affecting sarcopenia showed that parameters like muscular mass and strength measured by hand grip strength (HGS) and timed get up and go test (TUGT) did not improve with low doses of VD. However, they concluded that more research is needed with higher doses of VD supplements, as it has been shown to improve HGS and TUGT. It has been hypothesized that this effect could be due to lower VD receptors in older people, which could be mitigated by higher doses of VD supplements. In addition, as sarcopenia is a result of various environmental and genetic factors, only VD supplements would not be sufficient to treat sarcopenia in its entirety. The international clinical practice guidelines for sarcopenia also suggest utilizing VD supplements along with high protein intake and exercise training for its treatment (Widajanti et al., 2024).

High burden of chronic health conditions and resultant polypharmacy in older adults also constitute a major clinical consideration in pathological aging. Both these problems show correlation to low VD levels and hence negative consequences associated with advancing age. This effect of VD is usually carried out via its complex action on chronic inflammation, high oxidative stress, and reduced immune function in older adults. Its causal association is not well established though (Sohl et al., 2012; Wimalawansa, 2023). According to recent endocrine society guidelines, VD should be offered empirically to all older adults more than 75 years of age due to its inverse relationship with mortality in this age group. As mentioned before, this guideline is also in accordance with NICE recommendation of VD supplementation in all patients residing in long-term care facilities (Demay et al., 2024; NICE, 2017).

In addition to muscle weakness, patients with low VD levels complain of generalized tiredness as well (Gowda et al., 2015; Shaffer et al., 2014). Although there is limited data to support VD supplementation on combating lethargy in the community (Havdahl et al., 2019), a randomized controlled trial (RCT) found that supplementation with VD, significantly lowered the likelihood of lethargy in VD-deficient adults (Nowak et al., 2016).

24.4   Cognitive dysfunction

One important aspect of healthy aging is preservation of cognition, which is vital for older people to maintain their independence for day to day activities. Neurodegenerative conditions, including Alzheimer's disease and Parkinson's disease, affect millions of people worldwide. Multiple observational, longitudinal studies, as well as meta analyses, have been carried out to show the link between vitamin D and cognitive dysfunction. Dementia associated with neurodegenerative conditions has been associated with low VD levels, as well as the milder aspect of this spectrum, called mild cognitive impairment, has also been shown to bear a positive relationship with vitamin D deficiency. Various modifiable and nonmodifiable risk factors and etiological theories have been put forward in this regard, including the relationship of vitamin D levels with age, gender, ethnicity, seasonal variations, other nutritional supplements, etc. Even with the availability of the above data, it is difficult to establish if Vit D presents as a cause or effect of cognitive dysfunction (Landel et al., 2016).

The neuro protective and neuro modulating role of Vit D in cognitive dysfunction is put forward by the presence of the following:

- Widespread expression of VD receptors (VDR) in the brain, especially areas associated with learning and memory, that is, hippocampus, hypothalamus, cortex, and sub cortex (Annweiler et al., 2015).
- Association of VDR gene polymorphism with cognitive impairment in Alzheimer's disease (AD), Parkinson's disease (PD), and multiple sclerosis (MS) (Schlögl & Holick, 2014).
- The ability of the brain to utilize vitamin D in various cellular processes, which plays an important part in neurosynaptic plasticity and dopaminergic transmission. It has also been considered that VD may act in the nervous system as neuro steroid and may act in an autocrine or paracrine fashion on adjacent tissues (Bivona et al., 2021).
- Reduction of oxidative stress, inflammation, and immune responses in the nervous and cardiovascular system, which is achieved through the complex role of vitamin D in these areas. All of these processes are closely linked to atherosclerosis and stroke, which then contribute toward vascular dementia and mild cognitive impairment (Pál et al., 2023).
- Various mechanisms through which vitamin D affects the modulation of Serotonin. Serotonin is well known to contribute to the development of executive functions of the brain (Patrick & Ames, 2015).
- Indirect action of vitamin D on amyloid beta protein synthesis and degradation, as shown by in vitro studies, that is, reduction of amyloid-β precursor transcription and enhancement of phagocytosis of amyloid β peptide in the brain (Cheng et al., 2016).
- Amyloid beta and its interaction with the ApoE4 allele are a well-known risk factor for AD. Observation of VD deficiency has been linked with late-onset Alzheimer's dementia in people with cognitive dysfunction who are noncarriers of ApoE 4 (Dursun et al., 2016; Wisniewski & Drummond, 2020).
- Neuroimaging of patients with VD deficiency has shown brain and hippocampal atrophy (Croll et al., 2021).

Despite the availability of the above evidence, the exact pathogenesis of vitamin D deficiency in relation to cognitive dysfunction still needs to be evaluated further.

The critical level of vitamin D that affects cognitive function remains still unclear. Various studies on cognitive dysfunction have presented data on vitamin D sufficiency, VD insufficiency, and severe VD deficiency. Unfortunately, different studies have used different serum cutoffs to define the vitamin D status in the body, which makes it hard to establish a clear association of a particular level of deficiency to cognitive dysfunction (Gáll & Székely, 2021).

The methods by which vitamin D is measured are also not standard. Serum level of 25 hydroxy VD is the most commonly used screening test to measure VD levels, while liquid chromatography spectrometric analysis is considered a gold standard to measure vitamin D levels.

To make matters more complicated, the above uncertainties regarding the level and methods of measurement of VD are not helped by the fact that there is no agreed test to ascertain the cognitive dysfunction, which also encompasses mild, moderate, and severe cognitive diseases. The DSM-5 proposes six cognitive domains of cognitive dysfunction which include complex attention, executive function, learning and memory, language, perceptual motor control, and social cognition (Ganguli et al., 2011), which of these cognitive domains are associated with vitamin D deficiency is difficult to predict as studies have shown mixed results. Moreover, these studies have used different cognitive tests with different cutoffs for the diagnosis of cognitive impairment and dementia in patients having VD deficiency.

Cheng et al. discovered a weak positive association between levels of VD and overall scores on MoCA, as well as between language and abstract domains of MoCA (Cheng et al., 2022). In another study in the Asian population, 4AT assessment showed a correlation of low VD levels with global cognitive impairment, especially semantic memory and orientation (Annweiler et al., 2016).

The Benton Visual Retention Test, used to assess visual memory, has been linked with moderate to severe VD deficiency (Kuma et al., 2016). Significant effects of severe vitamin D deficiency have been demonstrated on the AFT used for verbal fluency and the DSST used for the speed at processing information and switching attention (Guo et al., 2024).

Addenbrooke's cognitive examination III assessment in patients with low VD levels has also shown lower scores in attention and verbal fluency domains of cognitive function (Ghosh et al., 2024).

In contrast to the above, there is plenty of data that shows no changes in cognitive domains with low vitamin D levels. For instance, in one study, the memory tests like 6CIT, MMSE, CFT, and AMTS showed no link between cognition and VD deficiency (Barmaki et al., 2023). Another study showed that adequate Vit D level was associated with better cognitive test results, including MMSEKC, Trail Making test, and digit span test. However, after adjustment for other variables linked to cognitive impairment, results were not statistically significant (Lee et al., 2020)

After reviewing all of the above, it is not surprising that many studies looking at the effect of vitamin D supplementation on cognitive functions have yielded both positive and negative results. There are significant variations in the materials and methodologies, including dose, duration, and timing of vitamin D supplementation in these studies that have made it more challenging to demonstrate a conclusive benefit of such supplements on cognitive dysfunction (Sultan et al., 2020).

As dementia is a progressive condition with limited treatment options, it is important to explore any modifiable risk factors that could treat or slow the cognitive dysfunction in such patients. A study on supplementation of nutrients and phytonutrients, including vitamin D, has shown some benefit not only on dementia but also on mild cognitive impairment (Lewis et al., 2021). Omega3 fatty acids, along with vitamin D supplements, have been thought to affect behavioral problems by modulating serotonin pathways in the brain (Macpherson et al., 2019).

Another study has suggested using a multidomain model to improve cognitive impairment which included aerobic exercises and vitamin D. However, the same study showed that the VD supplement alone had no impact on cognition (Montero-Odasso et al., 2023).

Another systematic literature review on the data published in the last 20 years has shown a positive correlation of VD on cognitive impairment in patients > 65 years (Fu et al., 2024). It is also suggested that ethnic differences should be considered while deciding for VD supplementation in people with cognitive dysfunction and behavioral issues (Dhana et al., 2023).

24.5 Osteoporosis

Osteoporosis is a worldwide phenomenon and the most common cause of pathological fractures in the elderly. According to WHO, osteoporosis can be diagnosed in nearly 6.3% of men and 21.2% of women more than 50 years of age globally, with the risk of osteoporotic damage, estimated to be tripled in this age group. Applying the available data shows that worldwide, approximately 500 million men and women could be affected (Kanis et al., 2008). The probability of osteoporosis increases with certain characteristics like insufficient use of foods containing calcium and VD, sedentary lifestyle, smoking, age above 50 years, female, especially when menopausal, hereditary, and low BMI (Pasco et al., 2006).

Although available evidence is enough to support the beneficial effects of VD supplementation on bone mineral density and prevention of osteoporotic fractures yet several studies have found that the above correlation is possible only when VD deficiency is corrected with high doses of VD. There are cohort studies to suggest association of incident fracture risk with other vitamin deficiencies as well (Kuroda et al., 2019). Hence, the nutritional status of the elderly is important in preventing fractures.

A Cochrane systematic review examined many randomized control trials of VD and its related products and their role in preventing fractures in people more than 65 years of age or postmenopausal women (Avenell et al., 2009). No effective correlation was found between VD intake and fracture prevention of the hip or vertebra; however, supplementing calcium with VD was seen to show a decrease in the risk of fragility fractures in institutionalized elderly. Seven randomized control trials from both the United States and Europe (DIPART,

2010) also show similar results in the analysis of over 68,000 adults. Participants who received VD and calcium supplementation together had a reduced risk of all fractures, whereas participants who only received VD supplementation showed no significant change in fracture risk.

Another review examined the past 15 years of literature on VD and falls and found that VD supplementation of at least 800 IUs effectively decreased the risk of falls in the geriatric population (Annweiler et al., 2010). In addition, VD was also linked with steadiness when walking and improvement in functional status, and hence reduced number of falls.

According to the American Geriatric Society Work group (American Geriatrics Society Workgroup on Vitamin D Supplementation for Older Adult. Recommendations abstracted from the American Geriatrics Consensus Statement on Vitamin D for prevention of falls and their consequences, 2014) serum VD level of 30 ng/mL is recommended as a minimum goal to achieve in older people, particularly those living with frailty. The report highlighted that unless there was a risk for hypercalcemia as a result of progressive chronic renal disease or sarcoidosis, the daily intake of 1000 IUs per day was not harmful.

24.6 Cardiovascular disorders

It is not unreasonable to briefly highlight the effects of vitamin D on cardiovascular health in old age as a reminder in this chapter.

Various mechanisms by which VD plays its role have been postulated, though most studies have failed to establish a clear causal association. VD deficiency has been connected to poor cardiovascular health. An abundance of VD receptors and 1 alpha hydroxylase in extra skeletal organs, especially the heart and blood vessels, suggests that many cardiovascular diseases can be theoretically explained by vitamin D deficiency. These mechanisms include a complex relationship between oxidative stress, endothelial dysfunction, inflammation, and the renin angiotensin aldosterone system, which ultimately leads to atherosclerosis and contributes to the development of cardiovascular dysfunction in older people (Latic & Erben, 2020).

Dhealth trial suggests that vitamin D supplementation along with standard treatment might be helpful in reducing the risk of cardiovascular events, especially acute coronary syndromes and angina in older people. However, there is no absolute risk reduction with vitamin D supplementation only. Other large studies, including VITAL (vitamin D and Omega-2 Trial) and ViDA (vitamin D assessment study), have shown no benefit of VD supplements on cardiovascular disorders, which include coronary diseases and stroke (Thompson et al., 2023). Another meta analysis showed a positive effect of vitamin D on high blood pressure and cardiac failure but no effect on stroke and myocardial ischemia (Ford et al., 2014). This effect can be explained by an antiinflammatory role of VD in the pathogenesis of heart failure (Virtanen et al., 2023).

In another study, high dose VD treatment showed promising effects against atrial fibrillation in older people (Virtanen et al., 2023).

24.7   Prevention of vitamin D deficiency

Several ways can help improve VD in the elderly: food fortification and supplementation with tablets. Sun exposure is difficult to rely on, especially in the winter season and at high latitudes. Also, it can increase the risk of skin cancers in the elderly.

24.8   Food fortification

Fortification of food items ensures that the population receives an appropriate dispersion, independent of eating habits. It is recommended that food for the elderly should be fortified with about 20 µg Vit D, equivalent to eight hundred International Units per day, for prevention of deficiencies. Studies in various Danish populations highlighted this point. They showed that if the edible fats or breads and cereal were enriched with 35 µg vit D/100 g or 10 µg vit D/100 g, respectively, it would ensure that half of the geriatric population would receive 20 µg/day of Vit D from diet and fortification combined, keeping the average baseline dietary vit D intake well above average (Mosekilde et al., 2005).

So far, there are no clinical trials that show any correlation between fortification and prevention of falls risks, low impact fractures, or CVD disease risk. However, it does have an impact on hip fracture prevention and muscle strength improvement (Lips et al., 1987).

24.9   Supplementation

There is evidence to support that supplementation of the geriatric population with 20 µg (800 IU) of vit D in combination with 1000–12,000 mg of calcium for 18 months reduces the chances of hip and non vertebral fractures as well as falls, by improving bone mass in postmenopausal women (Chapuy et al., 1992).

24.10   Learning points

Evaluation and replacement of vitamin D should be an essential part of the assessment of any chronic health condition in older people. Special consideration should be given to older patients presenting with frailty and geriatric syndromes like cognitive issues, falls, and fractures. It is worth remembering that vitamin D only constitutes one piece of a big puzzle in the optimization of the health status of an older person, so a holistic approach by physicians is always crucial in such scenarios.

24.11 Conclusion

VD is a readily available and inexpensive nutritional supplement that could represent the key to understand and treat various serious health conditions associated with negative consequences in old age.

References

American Geriatrics Society Workgroup on Vitamin D Supplementation for Older Adult. Recommendations abstracted from the American Geriatrics Consensus Statement on Vitamin D for prevention of falls and their consequences. (2014). *Journal of the American Geriatrics Society, 62*, 147. https://doi.org/10.1111/jgs.12631. 10.1111/jgs.12631.

Annweiler, C., Dursun, E., Féron, F., Gezen-Ak, D., Kalueff, A. V., Littlejohns, T., Llewellyn, D. J., Millet, P., Scott, T., Tucker, K. L., Yilmazer, S., & Beauchet, O. (2015). Vitamin D and cognition in older adults': Updated international recommendations. *Journal of Internal Medicine, 277*(1), 45–57. https://doi.org/10.1111/joim.12279.

Annweiler, C., Milea, D., Whitson, H. E., Cheng, C. Y., Wong, T. Y., Ikram, M. K., Lamoureux, E. L., & Sabanayagam, C. (2016). Vitamin D insufficiency and cognitive impairment in Asians: A multi-ethnic population-based study and meta-analysis. *Journal of Internal Medicine, 280*(3), 300–311. https://doi.org/10.1111/joim.12491, http://www.blackwellpublishing.com/journals/JIM.

Annweiler, C., Montero-Odasso, M., Schott, A. M., Berrut, G., Fantino, B., & Beauchet, O. (2010). Fall prevention and vitamin D in the elderly: An overview of the key role of the non-bone effects. *Journal of Neuroengineering and Rehabilitation, 7*(1). https://doi.org/10.1186/1743-0003-7-50.

Avenell, A., Gillespie, W. J., Gillespie, L. D., & O'Connell, D. (2009). Vitamin D and vitamin D analogues for preventing fractures associated with involutional and post-menopausal osteoporosis. *Cochrane Database of Systematic Reviews, 2*. https://doi.org/10.1002/14651858.CD000227.pub3, http://www.mrw.interscience.wiley.com/cochrane/clsysrev/articles/CD000227/pdf_fs.html.

Barmaki, O., Mansour, A., Moodi, M., Mirahmad, M., Fakhrzadeh, H., Arzaghi, M., Khorashadi, M., Khodabakhshi, H., Esmaeili, A. A., Sharifzadeh, G., Zarban, A., Sharifi, F., & Sajjadi-Jazi, S. M. (2023). Serum vitamin D status and cognitive function in Iranian older adults: Evidence from the Birjand Longitudinal Aging Study. *Journal of Nutrition, 153*(8), 2312–2319. https://doi.org/10.1016/j.tjnut.2023.06.033, https://www.sciencedirect.com/journal/the-journal-of-nutrition/about/aims-and-scope.

Beaudart, C., Buckinx, F., Rabenda, V., Gillain, S., Cavalier, E., Slomian, J., Petermans, J., Reginster, J.-Y., & Bruyère, O. (2014). The effects of vitamin D on skeletal muscle strength, muscle mass, and muscle power: A systematic review and meta-analysis of randomized controlled trials. *The Journal of Clinical Endocrinology & Metabolism, 99*(11), 4336–4345. https://doi.org/10.1210/jc.2014-1742.

Bivona, G., Sasso, B. L., Gambino, C. M., Giglio, R. V., Scazzone, C., Agnello, L., & Ciaccio, M. (2021). The role of vitamin D as a biomarker in alzheimer's disease. *Brain Sciences, 11*(3), 1–7. https://doi.org/10.3390/brainsci11030334, https://www.mdpi.com/2076-3425/11/3/334.

Bollen, S. E., Bass, J. J., Fujita, S., Wilkinson, D., Hewison, M., & Atherton, P. J. (2022). The Vitamin D/Vitamin D receptor (VDR) axis in muscle atrophy and sarcopenia. *Cellular Signalling, 96*, 110355. https://doi.org/10.1016/j.cellsig.2022.110355.

Bouillon, R., & Suda, T. (2014). Vitamin D: Calcium and bone homeostasis during evolution. *BoneKEy Reports, 3*. https://doi.org/10.1038/bonekey.2013.214.

Buta, B., Choudhury, P. P., Xue, Q. L., Chaves, P., Bandeen-Roche, K., Shardell, M., Semba, R. D., Walston, J., Michos, E. D., Appel, L. J., McAdams-DeMarco, M., Gross, A., Yasar, S., Ferrucci, L., Fried, L. P., & Kalyani, R. R. (2017). The association of vitamin D deficiency and incident frailty in older women: The role of cardiometabolic diseases. *Journal of the American Geriatrics Society, 65*(3), 619–624. https://doi.org/10.1111/jgs.14677, http://www.blackwellpublishing.com/journal.asp?ref=0002-8614&site=1.

Chapuy, M. C., Arlot, M. E., Duboeuf, F., Brun, J., Crouzet, B., Arnaud, S., Delmas, P. D., & Meunier, P. J. (1992). Vitamin D3 and calcium to prevent hip fractures in elderly women. *New England Journal of Medicine, 327*(23), 1637–1642. https://doi.org/10.1056/NEJM199212033272305.

Cheng, Z., Lin, J., & Qian, Q. (2016). Role of vitamin D in cognitive function in chronic kidney disease. *Nutrients, 8*(5), 291. https://doi.org/10.3390/nu8050291.

Cheng, L., Dong, R., Song, C., Li, X., Zhang, L., Shi, M., Lv, C., Wang, L., Kou, J., Xie, H., Feng, W., & Zhao, H. (2022). Mediation effects of IL-1β and IL-18 on the association between vitamin D levels and mild cognitive impairment among Chinese older adults: A case–control study in Taiyuan, China. *Frontiers in Aging Neuroscience, 14*. https://doi.org/10.3389/fnagi.2022.836311.

Croll, P. H., Boelens, M., Vernooij, M. W., van de Rest, O., Zillikens, M. C., Ikram, M. A., & Voortman, T. (2021). Associations of vitamin D deficiency with MRI markers of brain health in a community sample. *Clinical Nutrition, 40*(1), 72–78. https://doi.org/10.1016/j.clnu.2020.04.027, http://www.elsevier-international.com/journals/clnu/.

Cruz-Jentoft, A. J., & Woo, J. (2019). Nutritional interventions to prevent and treat frailty. *Current Opinion in Clinical Nutrition & Metabolic Care, 22*(3), 191–195. https://doi.org/10.1097/mco.0000000000000556.

Demay, M. B., Pittas, A. G., Bikle, D. D., Diab, D. L., Kiely, M. E., Lazaretti-Castro, M., Lips, P., Mitchell, D. M., Murad, M. H., Powers, S., Rao, S. D., Scragg, R., Tayek, J. A., Valent, A. M., Walsh, J. M. E., & McCartney, C. R. (2024). Vitamin D for the prevention of disease: An endocrine society clinical practice guideline. *Journal of Clinical Endocrinology and Metabolism, 109*(8), 1907–1947. https://doi.org/10.1210/clinem/dgae290, https://academic.oup.com/jcem.

Dhana, K., Barnes, L. L., Agarwal, P., Liu, X., Dhana, A., Desai, P., Aggarwal, N., Evans, D. A., & Rajan, K. B. (2023). Vitamin D intake and cognitive decline in Blacks and Whites: The role of diet and supplements. *Alzheimer's & Dementia, 19*(4), 1135–1142. https://doi.org/10.1002/alz.12729.

DIPART. (2010). Vitamin D Individual Patient Analysis of Randomized Trials) Group. Patient level pooled analysis of 68 500 patients from seven major vitamin D fracture trials in US and Europe. *BMJ (Clinical Research ed.), 340*. https://doi.org/10.1136/bmj.b5463.10.1136/bmj.b5463.

Dursun, E., Alaylıoğlu, M., Bilgiç, B., Hanağası, H., Lohmann, E., Atasoy, I. L., Candaş, E., Araz, Ö. S., Önal, B., Gürvit, H., Yılmazer, S., & Gezen-Ak, D. (2016). Vitamin D deficiency might pose a greater risk for ApoEε4 non-carrier Alzheimer's disease patients. *Neurological Sciences, 37*(10), 1633–1643. https://doi.org/10.1007/s10072-016-2647-1, http://link.springer.de/link/service/journals/10072/index.htm.

Ford, J. A., MacLennan, G. S., Avenell, A., Bolland, M., Grey, A., & Witham, M. (2014). Cardiovascular disease and vitamin D supplementation: Trial analysis, systematic review, and meta-analysis. *The American Journal of Clinical Nutrition, 100*(3), 746–755. https://doi.org/10.3945/ajcn.113.082602.

Fried, L. P., Tangen, C. M., Walston, J., Newman, A. B., Hirsch, C., Gottdiener, J., Seeman, T., Tracy, R., Kop, W. J., Burke, G., & McBurnie, M. A. (2001). Frailty in older adults: Evidence for a phenotype. *Journals of Gerontology - Series A Biological Sciences and Medical Sciences, 56*(3), M146. https://doi.org/10.1093/gerona/56.3.m146, http://biomedgerontology.oxfordjournals.org/.

Fu, Q., DeJager, J., & Gardner, E. M. (2024). Supplementation and mitigating cognitive decline in older adults with or without mild cognitive impairment or dementia: A systematic review. *Nutrients, 16*(20). https://doi.org/10.3390/nu16203567, http://www.mdpi.com/journal/nutrients/.

Gáll, Z., & Székely, O. (2021). Role of vitamin D in cognitive dysfunction: New molecular concepts and discrepancies between animal and human findings. *Nutrients, 13*(11), 3672. https://doi.org/10.3390/nu13113672.

Ganguli, M., Blacker, D., Blazer, D. G., Grant, I., Jeste, D. V., Paulsen, J. S., Petersen, R. C., & Sachdev, P. S. (2011). Classification of neurocognitive disorders in DSM-5: A work in progress. *American Journal of*

Geriatric Psychiatry, 19(3), 205–210. https://doi.org/10.1097/JGP.0b013e3182051ab4, http://www.sciencedirect.com/science/journal/10647481.

Ghosh, A., Monisha, S., Sunny, A. S., Diwakar, L., & Issac, T. G. (2024). Prevalence and patterns of vitamin D deficiency and its role in cognitive functioning in a cohort from South India. *Scientific Reports, 14*(1). https://doi.org/10.1038/s41598-024-62010-5, https://www.nature.com/srep/.

Gowda, U., Mutowo, M. P., Smith, B. J., Wluka, A. E., & Renzaho, A. M. N. (2015). Vitamin D supplementation to reduce depression in adults: Meta-analysis of randomized controlled trials. *Nutrition (Burbank, Los Angeles County, Calif.), 31*(3), 421–429. https://doi.org/10.1016/j.nut.2014.06.017, http://www.elsevier.com/locate/nut.

Grad, R. (2004). Cod and the consumptive: A brief history of cod-liver oil in the treatment of pulmonary tuberculosis. *Pharmacy in History, 46*(3), 106–120.

Guo, J., Mo, H., Zuo, L., & Zhang, X. (2024). Association of physical activity and vitamin D deficiency with cognitive impairment in older adults: A population based cross-sectional analysis. *Frontiers in Nutrition, 11*. https://doi.org/10.3389/fnut.2024.1390903.

Havdahl, A., Mitchell, R., Paternoster, L., & Davey Smith, G. (2019). Investigating causality in the association between vitamin D status and self-reported tiredness. *Scientific Reports, 9*(1). https://doi.org/10.1038/s41598-019-39359-z.

Holick, M. F. (1981). The cutaneous photosynthesis of previtamin D3: A unique photoendocrine system. *Journal of Investigative Dermatology, 77*(1), 51–58. https://doi.org/10.1111/1523-1747.ep12479237.

Holick, M. F., Binkley, N. C., Bischoff-Ferrari, H. A., Gordon, C. M., Hanley, D. A., Heaney, R. P., Murad, M. H., & Weaver, C. M. (2011). Evaluation, treatment, and prevention of vitamin D deficiency: An endocrine society clinical practice guideline. *Journal of Clinical Endocrinology and Metabolism, 96*(7), 1911–1930. https://doi.org/10.1210/jc.2011-0385, http://jcem.endojournals.org/content/96/7/1911.full.pdf+html.

Hossein-Nezhad, A., & Holick, M. F. (2013). Vitamin D for health: A global perspective. *Mayo Clinic Proceedings, 88*(7), 720–755. https://doi.org/10.1016/j.mayocp.2013.05.011, http://www.journals.elsevier.com/mayo-clinic-proceedings.

Kanis, J. A., McCloskey, E. V., Johansson, H., Oden, A., Melton, L. J., & Khaltaev, N. (2008). A reference standard for the description of osteoporosis. *Bone, 42*(3), 467–475. https://doi.org/10.1016/j.bone.2007.11.001.

Knorring, J. V., Slätis, P., Weber, T. H., & Helenius, T. (1982). Serum levels of 25-hydroxyvitamin D, 24,25-dihydroxyvitamin D and parathyroid hormone in patients with femoral neck fracture in Southern Finland. *Clinical Endocrinology, 17*(2), 189–194. https://doi.org/10.1111/j.1365-2265.1982.tb01578.x.

Kuma, E., Soni, M., Littlejohns, T. J., Ranson, J. M., Van Schoor, N. M., Deeg, D. J. H., Comijs, H., Chaves, P. H. M., Kestenbaum, B. R., Kuller, L. H., Lopez, O. L., Becker, J. T., Langa, K. M., Henley, W. E., Lang, I. A., Ukoumunne, O. C., & Llewellyn, D. J. (2016). Vitamin D and memory decline: Two population-based prospective studies. *Journal of Alzheimer's Disease, 50*(4), 1099–1108. https://doi.org/10.3233/JAD-150811, https://www.iospress.nl/journal/journal-of-alzheimers-disease/.

Kupisz-Urbańska, M., Płudowski, P., & Marcinowska-Suchowierska, E. (2021). Vitamin D deficiency in older patients—Problems of sarcopenia, drug interactions, management in deficiency. *Nutrients, 13*(4), 1247. https://doi.org/10.3390/nu13041247.

Kuroda, T., Uenishi, K., Ohta, H., & Shiraki, M. (2019). Multiple vitamin deficiencies additively increase the risk of incident fractures in Japanese postmenopausal women. *Osteoporosis International, 30*(3), 593–599. https://doi.org/10.1007/s00198-018-4784-2.

Landel, V., Annweiler, C., Millet, P., Morello, M., Féron, F., & Wion, D. (2016). Vitamin D, cognition and Alzheimer's disease: The therapeutic benefit is in the D-Tails. *Journal of Alzheimer's Disease, 53*(2), 419–444. https://doi.org/10.3233/JAD-150943, https://www.iospress.nl/journal/journal-of-alzheimers-disease/.

Latic, N., & Erben, R. G. (2020). Vitamin D and cardiovascular disease, with emphasis on hypertension, atherosclerosis, and heart failure. *International Journal of Molecular Sciences, 21*(18), 1–15. https://doi.org/10.3390/ijms21186483, https://www.mdpi.com/1422-0067/21/18/6483/pdf.

Lee, D. H., Chon, J., Kim, Y., Seo, Y. K., Park, E. J., Won, C. W., & Soh, Y. (2020). E. Bush, Association between Vitamin D deficiency and cognitive function in the elderly Korean population: A Korean frailty and aging cohort study. *Medicine (United States), 99*(8). https://doi.org/10.1097/MD.0000000000019293, https://journals.lww.com/md-journal/pages/default.aspx.

Lewis, Poles, Shaw, Karhu, Khan, Lyons, Sacco, & McDaniel (2021). The effects of twenty-one nutrients and phytonutrients on cognitive function: A narrative review. *Journal of clinical and translational research, 7*(4), 575–620.

Lips, P. (2001). Vitamin D deficiency and secondary hyperparathyroidism in the elderly: Consequences for bone loss and fractures and therapeutic implications. *Endocrine Reviews, 22*(4), 477–501. https://doi.org/10.1210/edrv.22.4.0437.

Lips, P., Bilezikian, J. P., & Bouillon, R. (2020). Vitamin D: Giveth to those who needeth. *JBMR Plus, 4*(1). https://doi.org/10.1002/jbm4.10232, https://asbmr.onlinelibrary.wiley.com/journal/24734039.

Lips, P., Van Ginkel, F. C., Jongen, M. J. M., Rubertus, F., Van der Vijgh, W. J. F., & Netelenbos, J. C. (1987). Determinants of vitamin D status in patients with hip fracture and in elderly control subjects. *American Journal of Clinical Nutrition, 46*(6), 1005–1010. https://doi.org/10.1093/ajcn/46.6.1005.

Lips, P., Netelenbos, J. C., Jongen, M. J. M., van Ginkel, F. C., Althuis, A. L., van Schaik, C. L., van der Vijgh, W. J. F., Vermeiden, J. P. W., & van der Meer, C. (1982). Histomorphometric profile and vitamin d status in patients with femoral neck fracture. *Metabolic Bone Disease and Related Research, 4*(2), 85–93. https://doi.org/10.1016/0221-8747(82)90021-2.

Macpherson, H., Brownell, S., Duckham, R. L., Meyer, B., Mirzaee, S., & Daly, R. M. (2019). Multifaceted intervention to enhance cognition in older people at risk of cognitive decline: study protocol for the Protein Omega-3 and Vitamin D Exercise Research (PONDER) study. *BMJ Open, 9*(5), e024145. https://doi.org/10.1136/bmjopen-2018-024145.

Mellanby, E., Cantab, M. A., McMollum, E. V., Simmonds, N., Becker, J. E., & Shipley, P. G. (1919). Studies on experimental rickets: An experimental demonstration of the existence of a vitamin which promotes calcium deposition. *The Journal of Biological Chemistry, 2*, 293–298.

Montero-Odasso, M., Zou, G., Speechley, M., Almeida, Q. J., Liu-Ambrose, T., Middleton, L. E., Camicioli, R., Bray, N. W., Li, K. Z. H., Fraser, S., Pieruccini-Faria, F., Berryman, N., Lussier, M., Shoemaker, J. K., Son, S., & Bherer, L. (2023). Effects of exercise alone or combined with cognitive training and vitamin D supplementation to improve cognition in adults with mild cognitive impairment: A randomized clinical trial. *JAMA Network Open, 6*(7), E2324465. https://doi.org/10.1001/jamanetworkopen.2023.24465, https://jamanetwork.com/journals/jamanetworkopen.

Mosekilde, L., Brot, C., Hyldstrup, L., Mortensen, L. S., Mølgård, C., Rasmussen, S. E., Mejborn, L. B., & Rasmussen (2005). Arbejdsgruppe nedsat af Danmarks Fødevareforskning. D-vitaminstatus i den danske befolkning bør forbedres [The vitamin D status of the Danish population needs to be improved]. *Ugeskrift for Laeger, 167*.

Muir, S. W., & Montero-Odasso, M. (2011). Effect of vitamin D supplementation on muscle strength, gait and balance in older adults: A systematic review and meta-analysis. *Journal of the American Geriatrics Society, 59*(12), 2291–2300. https://doi.org/10.1111/j.1532-5415.2011.03733.x.

NICE 2017 https://www.nice.org.uk/guidance/ph56.

Nowak, A., Boesch, L., Andres, E., Battegay, E., Hornemann, T., Schmid, C., Bischoff-Ferrari, H. A., Suter, P. M., & Krayenbuehl, P. A. (2016). Effect of vitamin D3 on self-perceived fatigue A double-blind randomized placebo-controlled trial. *Medicine (United States), 95*(52). https://doi.org/10.1097/MD.0000000000005353, http://journals.lww.com/md-journal.

Pasco, J. A., Seeman, E., Henry, M. J., Merriman, E. N., Nicholson, G. C., & Kotowicz, M. A. (2006). The population burden of fractures originates in women with osteopenia, not osteoporosis. *Osteoporosis International, 17*(9), 1404–1409. https://doi.org/10.1007/s00198-006-0135-9.

Patrick, R. P., & Ames, B. N. (2015). Vitamin D and the omega-3 fatty acids control serotonin synthesis and action, part 2: Relevance for ADHD, bipolar disorder, schizophrenia, and impulsive behavior. *FASEB Journal, 29*(6), 2207–2222. https://doi.org/10.1096/fj.14-268342, http://www.fasebj.org/content/29/6/2207.full.pdf+html.

Pál, É., Ungvári, Z., Benyó, Z., & Várbíró, S. (2023). Role of vitamin D deficiency in the pathogenesis of cardiovascular and cerebrovascular diseases. *Nutrients, 15*(2). https://doi.org/10.3390/nu15020334, http://www.mdpi.com/journal/nutrients/.

Rejnmark, L. (2011). Effects of vitamin D on muscle function and performance: A review of evidence from randomized controlled trials. *Therapeutic Advances in Chronic Disease, 2*(1), 25–37. https://doi.org/10.1177/2040622310381934.

Schlögl, M., & Holick, M. F. (2014). Vitamin D and neurocognitive function. *Clinical Interventions in Aging, 9*, 559–568. https://doi.org/10.2147/CIA.S51785, http://www.dovepress.com/getfile.php?fileID=19519.

Schwartz, G. G. (1992). Multiple sclerosis and prostate cancer: What do their similar geographies suggest? *Neuroepidemiology, 11*(4-6), 244–254. https://doi.org/10.1159/000110937.

Shaffer, J. A., Edmondson, D., Wasson, L. T., Falzon, L., Homma, K., Ezeokoli, N., Li, P., & Davidson, K. W. (2014). Vitamin d supplementation for depressive symptoms: A systematic review and meta-analysis of randomized controlled trials. *Psychosomatic Medicine, 76*(3), 190–196. https://doi.org/10.1097/PSY.0000000000000044, http://www.psychosomaticmedicine.org/.

Sohl, E., Van Schoor, N. M., De Jongh, R. T., De Vries, O. J., & Lips, P. (2012). The impact of medication on vitamin D status in older individuals. *European Journal of Endocrinology, 166*(3), 477–485. https://doi.org/10.1530/EJE-11-0917Netherlands, http://www.eje-online.org/content/166/3/477.full.pdf+html.

Sultan, S., Taimuri, U., Basnan, S. A., Ai-Orabi, W. K., Awadallah, A., Almowald, F., & Hazazi, A. (2020). Low vitamin D and its association with cognitive impairment and dementia. *Journal of Aging Research, 2020*, 1–10. https://doi.org/10.1155/2020/6097820.

Suter, P. M., & Vetter, W. (1994). BEDEUTUNG VON UND BEDARF AN VITAMINEN IM ALTER. *Praxis, 83*(10), 262–266.

Tanaka, K., Ao, M., Tamaru, J., & Kuwabara, A. (2024). Vitamin D insufficiency and disease risk in the elderly. *Journal of Clinical Biochemistry and Nutrition, 74*(1), 9–16. https://doi.org/10.3164/jcbn.23-59.

Thompson, B., Waterhouse, M., English, D. R., McLeod, D. S., Armstrong, B. K., Baxter, C., Duarte Romero, B., Ebeling, P. R., Hartel, G., Kimlin, M. G., Rahman, S. T., Van Der Pols, J. C., Venn, A. J., Webb, P. M., Whiteman, D. C., & Neale, R. E. (2023). Vitamin D supplementation and major cardiovascular events: D-Health randomised controlled trial. *BMJ (Clinical Research ed.)*. https://doi.org/10.1136/bmj-2023-075230, http://www.bmj.com/.

Virtanen, J. K., Hantunen, S., Lamberg-Allardt, C., Manson, J. A. E., Nurmi, T., Uusitupa, M., Voutilainen, A., & Tuomainen, T.-P. (2023). The effect of vitamin D3 supplementation on atrial fibrillation in generally healthy men and women: The Finnish Vitamin D Trial. *American Heart Journal, 264*, 177–182. https://doi.org/10.1016/j.ahj.2023.05.024.

Widajanti, N., Hadi, U., Soelistijo, S. A., Syakdiyah, N. H., Rosaudyn, R., & Putra, H. B. P. (2024). The effect of vitamin D supplementation to parameter of sarcopenia in elderly people: A systematic review and meta-analysis. *Canadian Geriatrics Journal, 24*(1), 63–75. https://doi.org/10.5770/cgj.27.694, https://cgjonline.ca/index.php/cgj/article/view/694.

Wimalawansa, S. J. (2023). Controlling chronic diseases and acute infections with vitamin D sufficiency. *Nutrients, 15*(16). https://doi.org/10.3390/nu15163623, http://www.mdpi.com/journal/nutrients/.

Wisniewski, T., & Drummond, E. (2020). APOE-amyloid interaction: Therapeutic targets. *Neurobiology of Disease, 138*, 104784. https://doi.org/10.1016/j.nbd.2020.104784.

Zhou, J., Huang, P., Liu, P., Hao, Q., Chen, S., Dong, B., & Wang, J. (2016). Association of vitamin D deficiency and frailty: A systematic review and meta-analysis. *Maturitas, 94*, 70–76. https://doi.org/10.1016/j.maturitas.2016.09.003.

CHAPTER 25

Vitamin D and infectious diseases

Nosheen Nasir, Kiren Habib, and Iffat Khanum

Section of Adult Infectious Diseases, Department of Medicine, Aga Khan University, Karachi, Sindh, Pakistan

25.1 Vitamin D and bacterial infections

25.1.1 Introduction

Vitamin D (VD) is involved in several important activities, such as cardiovascular hemostasis, antitumor activity, immunomodulation of innate and adaptive responses, and microbial clearance (Cutuli et al., 2022). VD plays a vital role in the clearance of microbial agents by supporting the innate immune system for early recognition of pathogens. It helps in the production of antimicrobial peptides like cathelicidin and defensin, which directly target pathogens. The biological effect of VD is exerted mainly through VD receptors. The nuclear VD receptors (VDR) are present in many tissues and cells, like the liver, skin, and brain. They are also present in almost all immune cells, like macrophages, monocytes, and lymphocytes. These receptors enable VD to regulate the differentiation and proliferation of immune cells (Zmijewski & Carlberg, 2020). To help maintain immunological homeostasis, VD promotes the production of antiinflammatory cytokines like IL-10 and decreases the production of proinflammatory cytokines like IL-12 and TNF-α (Cutuli et al., 2024). VD also affects B-cell proliferations, leading to decreased production of antibodies and autoantibodies and contribute to the decrease in the development of autoimmune diseases (Sîrbe et al., 2022). Hence, the deficiency of VD can predispose to bacterial infections.

A recent meta-analysis found the global prevalence of VD deficiency (VDD) (serum 25(OH) D < 30 nmol/L) around 15.7%, with the highest prevalence found in the Eastern Mediterranean region, LMICs, people living in high latitudes, and female gender (Cui et al., 2023). The highest prevalence of VDD was found in Pakistan (73%; 95% CI: 63%–83%) followed by Bangladesh (67%; 95% CI: 50%–83%), India (67%; 95% CI: 61%–73%), Nepal (57%; 95% CI: 53%–60%), and Sri Lanka (48%; 95% CI: 41%–55%), respectively (Siddiqee et al., 2021).

Sepsis is considered a medical emergency as it is associated with high mortality and morbidity. It is caused by the dysregulated immune response to infections and causes multiorgan dysfunction (Wayland et al., 2024). According to a recent meta-analysis, there

The Impact of Vitamin D on Health and Disease. **DOI:** https://doi.org/10.1016/B978-0-443-34037-6.00015-7

were 11 million sepsis-related mortalities with a global incidence of 48.9 million cases per year (Rudd et al., 2020). There is a growing body of evidence that supports the fact that VDD is associated with increased susceptibility to sepsis. A large population-based study shows a correlation between a higher long-term risk of community-acquired sepsis and low baseline plasma 25(OH)D concentrations (Kempker et al., 2019). According to another meta-analysis, the pooled odds ratio of sepsis in participants with VDD compared with controls was 1.78 (95% confidence interval [CI] = 1.55 to 2.03, $P < .01$) (Upala et al., 2015). In addition to increased susceptibility, severe Vit D deficiency also increases in-hospital mortality, 14-day and 28-day mortality in patients with sepsis (Seok et al., 2023). In a study conducted by Stefano et al., severe VDD was found to be associated with increased mortality (OR = 2.69 (95% CI 1.03–7.00), $P = .043$), lower chances of hospital discharge (sub-HR = 0.66 (95% CI 0.44–0.98)), increased 28-day adjusted mortality (HR = 3.06 (95% CI 1.05–8.94), $P = .04$) and lower chances of discharge [sub-HR = 0.51 (95% CI 0.32–0.81)] (Malinverni et al., 2022). Yang et al. found that in patients with sepsis, although VD supplement during an intensive care unit (ICU) stay did not affect the length of hospital or ICU stay, it was associated with better prognosis, as demonstrated by decreased in-hospital, 28-day, and 90-day mortality rates as well as lower disease severity-related scores (Yang et al., 2023). A recent meta-analysis including 16 randomized controlled trials with 2449 critically ill patients also found an association of VD supplementation with lower mortality (Menger et al., 2022). In contrast, another meta-analysis did not show any additional benefit of administration of VD in critically ill patients with respect to morbidity and mortality (Lan et al., 2020). A large randomised controlled trial is needed to specifically evaluate the impact of VD supplementation on the outcomes of patients with sepsis and septic shock.

25.2 Vitamin D and respiratory tract infections

A large cross-sectional study with 6789 participants, who had measurements of 25(OH)D, available from the age of 45 years found that after adjustment for socioeconomic factors, lifestyle and adiposity, there was a 7% reduction in the risk of infections by each 10 nmol/L increase in 25(OH)D (test for trend $P = .001$) (Berry et al., 2011). A meta-analysis also found that people with VDD experienced a significantly increased risk of CAP (OR = 1.64, 95% CI: 1.00, 2.67) (Zhou et al., 2019). VDD does not only predisposes to infection, but it is also found to be associated with increased severity of pneumonia, increased risk of complications like sepsis, acute respiratory distress syndrome (ARDS), and a higher rate of mortality (Sarhan & Elrifai, 2021).

In a meta-analysis of RCTs, VD supplementation significantly increased levels of serum 25(OH)D and reduced the incidence rate of repeat episodes of pneumonia (RR = 0.68; 95% CI, 0.50–0.93; $I^2 = 83\%$) (Yang et al., 2021). The VIDCAPS randomised controlled trial concluded that adjunctive VD supplementation along with standard of care did not improve overall outcomes in adult hospitalized patients with community-acquired pneumonia (CAP) (Slow et al., 2018). There is a need of additional well-designed population-based studies to assess the effect of VD supplementation as an effective adjuvant therapy for pneumonia and its related complications.

25.3 Vitamin D and genitourinary infections

VDD also predisposes to urinary tract infections and recurrent urinary tract infections (UTIs) (Mercy et al., 2024; "Vitamin D deficiency linked to recurrent UTI, 2013). According to a systematic review by Deng et al., VDD can increase the risk of urinary tract infection (pooled OR = 3.01, 95% CI = 2.31–3.91) (Deng et al., 2019). VD induces the production of antimicrobial peptides like cathelicidin and claudin-4, which maintain the integrity of uroepithelial cells and also regulate the inflammatory response, thus preventing damage to the urinary bladder mucosa and invasion by pathogens (Mohanty et al., 2020). In a study by Nseir et al., mean serum levels of VD was notably decreased in women with recurrent UTI ($P < .001$) and on multivariate analysis, a serum VD level of < 15 ng/ml was predictive of recurrent UTI (OR 4.00, 95% CI 3.40–4.62; $P < .001$) (Nseir et al., 2013).

VDD is also prevalent in patients with end-stage renal disease (ESRD) and renal transplants. Incidence of UTI is more prevalent in patients with VDD in the posttransplant period up to many years, and VDD is considered an independent risk factor for UTI after renal transplant (Kalluri et al., 2017; Kwon et al., 2015).

In a randomized controlled trial with 511 participants, supplementation of VD3 (20,000 IU per week) over 5 years decreased the incidence of UTI as compared to the control group ($P < .02$), irrespective of baseline serum 25(OH)D level (Jorde et al., 2016).

Another randomized, triple-blind placebo placebo-controlled trial did not find any significant impact of VD supplementation on the prevention of recurrent episodes of UTI among children and adolescents (Merrikhi et al., 2018). Large-scale longitudinal studies are needed to establish the role of VD supplementation and optimal dosing strategies in the prevention of UTIs among different age groups.

VDD can also predispose to the risk of *Chlamydia trachomatis* infection and treatment failure (Liu et al., 2024). Bacterial vaginosis (BV) results from the overgrowth of anaerobic bacteria and increases the risk of sexually transmitted infections. Along with other risk factors, deficiency of VD is also associated with increased risk of development of BV (Ma et al., 2022; Mojtahedi et al., 2023).

25.4   Vitamin D and bone infections

In addition to its role in maintaining bone integrity, VD's immunomodulatory properties contribute to infection prevention in bone and joint tissues. A recent literature review identified an association of low levels of VD and bone infections, but the role of VD supplementation in the prevention of infections is unclear.

A systematic review did not find any significant benefit of optimizing VD levels to improve outcomes, including the risk of infection, after hip and knee arthroplasty (Zargaran et al., 2021). In a large prospective multicenter study of patients with total knee and hip arthroplasty, preoperative supplementation of VD levels in patients with VDD was found to be useful in decreasing postoperative complications such as surgical site infection and postoperative cellulitis (Birinci et al., 2024). There is a need for randomized controlled trials to validate results. The necessity of preoperative correction of VD levels to achieve better functional results and minimize the risk of infection following hip and knee arthroplasty remains inconclusive. The extent of exposure to low VD levels and comparison between outliers needs further evaluation (Kenanidis et al., 2020).

25.5   Vitamin D and tuberculosis

Most of the people who develop tuberculosis (TB) disease each year are in 30 high TB-burden countries, which accounted for 87% of the global total in 2023. Five countries accounted for 56% of the worldwide total: India (26%), Indonesia (10%), China (6.8%), the Philippines (6.8%), and Pakistan (6.3%) (Organization, 2024).

The role of VD in the management of TB was first identified by researchers approximately 200 years ago. Subsequent studies have further confirmed its importance, leading to the recognition that VDD should be corrected as part of TB treatment (Junaid & Rehman, 2019). Several studies also found that low serum vitamin D level is significantly associated with acquiring active TB infection (Huang et al., 2017; Zeng et al., 2015).

VD appears to play an important role against mycobacterial infection through different mechanisms. It has both proinflammatory and antiinflammatory roles. It enhances antimicrobial actions by promoting bacterial destruction, autophagy, and macrophage activation while stimulating Th1 and Th2 responses. On the other hand, it regulates inflammation by expanding T-reg lymphocytes, stabilizing endothelial barriers, and balancing cytokine production without compromising antimicrobial activity (Papagni et al., 2022).

A study from Egypt showed a very high prevalence of VDD in patients with extrapulmonary TB (EPTB) (in comparison to healthy controls). Furthermore, supplementation of VD3 was linked to improved treatment outcomes, such as clinical improvement, weight gain, and improvement in inflammatory markers (Eletreby et al., 2024). Low VD levels are also prevalent in patients with PTB, also linked to more serious illness, high degree of smear positivity, and extensive lung parenchymal involvement (Jaimni et al., 2021; Kafle et al., 2021).

According to the World Health Organization (WHO), latent TB infection (LTBI) is defined as *"a persistent immune response to the Mycobacterium TB antigens without any signs of active tuberculosis"* (Organization, 2015). The association of VDD and latent TB infection (LTBI) remains uncertain. A meta-analysis suggested a potential relationship between serum VD level and the risk of LTBI that relatively higher serum VD levels are associated with a reduced risk of LTBI over time. However, another meta-analysis did not find any significant association between VD levels and the incidence of LTBI, nor does a high vitamin level serve as a protective factor against LTBI (Cao et al., 2022).

A double-blinded randomized control trial revealed that VD supplementation in patients with pulmonary TB (PTB) did not seem to have any favorable impact in terms of the prevention of relapse and time to sputum smear and culture conversion (Sinha et al., 2023). Whether VD supplementation can prevent TB infection or the progression of LTBI to active disease is still debatable and needs to be confirmed by further studies like RCTs (Cao et al., 2022; Meng et al., 2024).

VD plays a significant role in immunomodulation, and its deficiency has been associated with an increased susceptibility to bacterial infections such as respiratory tract infections (RTIs) and sepsis. Although a few studies showed a potential benefit of VD supplementation, these findings cannot be generalized due to variability in study design, serum VD level, and different dosage regimens. Future large-scale, longitudinal, and randomized controlled trials are needed to clarify the clinical implications of VD supplementation, define optimal dosing strategies, and identify populations that may derive the greatest benefit in decreasing the risk of bacterial infections.

25.6 Vitamin D and viral infections

25.6.1 Introduction

Viral infections are a cause for global health concern, with pathogens like influenza causing widespread illness each year, leading to morbidity and mortality. The body's immune response is important in protecting against these infections and recovering from illness.

VD is a fat-soluble vitamin mainly obtained from sunlight and certain food items. It has been associated with skeletal health but is now known to play multiple roles in the human body, including enhancing the immune response. VD receptors (VDRs) can be found in almost all cells in the body, including the mononuclear cells, and on various sites in the genome

(Bhalla et al., 1983; Bikle, 2014). It has been shown to modulate the activity at Toll-like receptors (TLRs) and by doing so it mediates the immune response (Siddiqui et al., 2020).

25.7   Vitamin D and rhinoviruses

Human rhinovirus is a common cause of upper RTI affecting both children and adults, leading to an increase in medical visits and absence from school and work (Nichol et al., 2005; Roelen et al., 2011). A study looking at the effect of vitamin D on rhinovirus infection showed that although vitamin D supplementation had no effect on the replication of the virus, the supplementation of vitamin D increased the secretion of chemokines. Chemokines help recruit immune cells to the infection site and thus may affect how VD helps to regulate antiviral response to rhinovirus infection (Brockman-Schneider et al., 2014).

25.8   Vitamin D and influenza

Influenza is one of the common viral infections affecting both adults and children globally and is associated with an increased economic burden in terms of medical visits, missed workdays, and school. Elderly, obese adults and those with comorbid conditions can develop severe infections, which may be lethal (Osterholm et al., 2012). A study from Norway, linked influenza-related mortality to low VD levels, and another study has shown a higher incidence of VDD in adults affected by influenza (Moan et al., 2014; Osterholm et al., 2012).

VD supplementation has been shown to lower the incidence of influenza in children in one study compared to those receiving a placebo (Loeb et al., 2019). While studies have shown a benefit of vitamin D supplementation in preventing influenza-like illness (Huang et al., 2022; van Helmond et al., 2023; Zhu et al., 2021), others have shown no correlation between the two (Godan Hauptman et al., 2021), with one study even reporting a negative correlation (Jorde et al., 2012).

25.9   Vitamin D and dengue

Dengue is a vector-borne infection caused by the dengue virus (DENV). It is endemic in several tropical countries but is now becoming widespread. Increased production of cytokines and a high viral load have been linked to severe infection. Pang et al. have shown that in the presence of vitamin D, DENV infection is restricted by influencing DENV binding to cells. In addition to this, the production of proinflammatory cytokines like TNFα, IL-1 β, and IL-10 is significantly lower in DENV-infected macrophages that have been treated with vitamin D as compared to those without VD treatment (Pang et al., 2007).

25.10   Vitamin D and HIV

VDD is common in HIV patients, with up to 64.9% patients (63 out of 97) in one study presenting with deficiency (Coelho et al., 2015). Several studies have reported higher mortality in patients with HIV who have vitamin D deficiency (Haug et al., 1994; Mehta et al., 2010; Sudfeld et al., 2012; Viard et al., 2011). This may be due to the role of VD in immune regulation. VD causes the production of cathelicidin and defensin β 2, which are both antimicrobial peptides. Levels of VD below 20 ng/mL suppress the cathelicidin response, which impairs immunity and may lead to opportunistic infections (Sudfeld et al., 2012).

VD also helps in regulating CD4 functions (Mehta et al., 2010). VD supplementation may be an important adjuvant therapy to help increase CD4 counts in patients on antiretroviral therapy. One study showed less recovery of CD4 levels in those with VDD at 18 months of HAART (Ezeamama et al., 2016). VD supplementation can also help prevent fractures and maintain bone marrow density (BMD) in patients with HIV, especially those on antiretroviral drugs, which reduce BMD, like tenofovir (Hileman et al., 2016).

25.11   Vitamin D and hepatitis C

Hepatitis C is a single-stranded RNA virus. It is one of the foremost causes of liver-related mortality. It is often asymptomatic but can cause chronic liver disease and lead to irreversible liver damage and cirrhosis. VDD has been seen quite commonly in patients with chronic hepatitis C. Several studies have shown that supplementation of VD along with antiviral therapy for hepatitis C is associated with a sustained virological response (SVR) as well (Abu-Mouch et al., 2011; Bitetto et al., 2011; Nimer & Mouch, 2012). Peta et al. in their study observed that interaction of VD at its receptors on fibroblasts can affect proliferation, gene expression, and migration of fibroblasts as well as protection from oxidative damage and reduction of inflammation in stellate cells of the liver (Petta et al., 2010).

VD levels may also be used as a prognostic marker in cirrhosis in hepatitis C, with levels under 7.2 ng/mL associated with high mortality rates (Licata et al., 2019). Sun exposure, VD supplementation, geographical area, and race must be considered when considering VD levels as a prognostic marker (Fuleihan & -H, 2010).

25.12   Vitamin D and Sars-CoV-2

In 2019, SARS-CoV-2, a coronavirus, emerged as a new pathogen that led to the COVID-19 pandemic. Acute respiratory distress syndrome (ARDS) is the leading cause of death in COVID-19, which was also reported with SARS-CoV and MERS-CoV (Xu et al., 2020). Once inhaled, the virus moves down the respiratory tract and triggers an immune response in the lungs. It requires ACE2 as a receptor, which binds to its surface and facilitates entry into the target cell. This leads to downregulation of ACE2 expression and loss of counterregulation of the RAS (Paz Ocaranza et al., 2020). This loss of regulation causes the accumulation of angiotensin II and renin synthesis, leading to the release of chemokines and cytokines, which cause the cytokine storm. VD can inhibit NFκB activation and thus lead to a decrease in the inflammatory response to the virus in the respiratory epithelium. VD thus acts by counteracting the renin expression and RAS activity caused by SARS-CoV2 and the cytokine storm (Channappanavar & Perlman, 2017; Coperchini et al., 2020). VD also reinforces the innate cellular immunity at the macrophage level by activation of TLR 2/1. This results in expression of cathelicidin and defensins (Snijder et al., 2006). Several studies have reported that critically ill patients with COVID-19 admitted in ICU's had lower VD levels as compared to those admitted in non-ICU settings (Allegra et al., 2020; Entrenas Castillo et al., 2020). Hence, it has a potential role in the clinical course and prognosis of the infection, which needs to be better explored through longitudinal studies (Allegra et al., 2020).

25.13   Vitamin D and fungal infections

25.13.1   Introduction

Over the last 30 years, fungal infections have become more common globally. Fungal infections are a leading cause of disease, particularly in immunocompromised and hospitalized patients with severe underlying conditions. Invasive fungal infections (IFI) provide a significant medical issue, with an estimated 6.5 million cases per year, resulting in 3.8 million fatalities. These infections are caused by pathogens like Aspergillus spp., Candida spp., Mucorales spp., Cryptococcus spp., and other fungal species (Sedik et al., 2024). Invasive Candidiasis is most widespread in critical care units (ICUs), where it occurs ten times more frequently than in medical and surgical wards, accounting for 70%–90% of all ICU fungal infections (Noppè et al., 2024).

VD has numerous immunomodulatory properties and contributes to pulmonary defence, immunity, and inflammation. Its receptor is found on peripheral blood mononuclear cells, dendritic cells, and activated T lymphocytes. VD modulates cytokines and suppresses the Th2 response, linking VDD to allergies. VD3 has immune effects such as promoting cathelicidin secretion, which is an antimicrobial peptide, reducing chemokine synthesis, inhibiting dendritic cell activation, and altering T-cell activation (Charoenngam & Holick, 2020).

VDD has emerged as a significant global public health concern, affecting populations across various regions, including tropical and subtropical areas. Beyond its widespread prevalence, VDD may compromise immune function, increasing the risk and severity of numerous infectious diseases, including fungal infections (Gois et al., 2017).

25.14   Vitamin D and Candida infections

Candidiasis is the most common fungal infection in humans and can occur both topically and systemically, affecting several parts of the body. While C. albicans is the primary cause of disseminated candidiasis, other Candida species have also been implicated. 1,25(OH)2D3 modulates the innate host response to C. albicans by altering proinflammatory cytokine responses in vitro and ex vivo. It has a significant antiinflammatory effect on Candida infection due to its influence on key pattern recognition receptors (PRRs) such as Toll-like receptors TLR2, TLR4, Dectin-, and mannose receptors (Khoo et al., 2011). Prolonged antifungal therapy has led to the emergence of resistant clinical isolates in previously susceptible strains. C. albicans and C. tropicalis were previously thought to be susceptible to fluconazole. However, recent findings have indicated resistance to fluconazole in some centres, leading to clinical therapeutic failure. The emergence of azole resistance in Candida species necessitates the development of new antifungal methods for drug-resistant strains. In vitro studies have shown antifungal effects of vitamin D3, particularly against Candida albicans (Bouzid et al., 2017). VD3 steroid nature causes disruption of membrane sterols, which can lead to cell lysis. Sterols can directly affect eukaryotic membrane cells, including fungal cells that contain ergosterol. VD3 high liposolubility may alter cell membrane integrity, contributing to its antifungal impact. This led to a placebo-controlled clinical trial to evaluate if supplementing VD could reduce candidaemia and candiduria infections in PICU patients using broad-spectrum antibiotics. The study found that oral supplementation with VD was able to significantly reduce the incidence of invasive candidiasis in critically ill children (Xie et al., 2019).

25.15   Vitamin D and Aspergillosis

Recent research indicates that VD3 is crucial for respiratory health. Asthma patients with higher VD3 levels had lower hospitalisation rates and used less antiinflammatory drugs. VD3 levels have a negative correlation with upper RTIs, particularly in asthmatic individuals. Numerous studies have focused on the role of VD3 in upper airway allergic rhinitis. According to Wjst and Hypponen, individuals with low VD3 serum levels were more likely to suffer from allergic rhinitis (Wjst & Hyppönen, 2007).

Previous research suggests that patients with VD3 deficiency are more likely to develop allergic fungal rhinosinusitis (AFRS). This suggests that VD3 plays a crucial role in the immunopathology of chronic rhinosinusitis (CRS) with nasal polyps (CRSwNP). VDD is a global health issue, potentially contributing to the rise in AFRS and other sinus issues. VD3 may be a cost-effective choice for lowering inflammation, either alone or in combination with other therapies (Mostafa et al., 2016).

Allergic bronchopulmonary aspergillosis (ABPA) is a pulmonary condition characterized by hypersensitivity reactions to Aspergillus fumigatus, which colonizes the tracheobronchial tree of patients with asthma and cystic fibrosis (CF). The illness is characterized by poorly managed asthma, recurring pulmonary opacities, and bronchiectasis. Research has shown that CD11c+, thymic stromal lymphopoietin-activated dendritic cells from patients with ABPA and CF trigger strong Th2 cytokine responses from CD4+ T-cells and VD therapy in vitro has been shown to reduce these responses. VD levels are lower in people with ABPA, which might worsen CF. VD insufficiency may contribute to the development of ABPA, which complicates CF. Patients with cystic fibrosis have malabsorption, which can lead to VD insufficiency, unlike asthmatic patients. It is unclear if ABPA causes VD insufficiency, which can worsen asthma. A study comparing VD levels (25[OH]D) in asthmatic individuals with and without ABPA found that vitamin D deficiency was equally prevalent in asthmatic patients with or without ABPA and was not associated with asthma control and severity of bronchiectasis in patients with ABPA (Agarwal et al., 2018). Moreover, a clinical trial demonstrated that supplemental VD did not provide any additional benefit in the clinical or immunological response to glucocorticoid therapy for acute-stage ABPA complicating asthma (Dodamani et al., 2019).

25.16 Vitamin D and cryptococcosis

Cryptococcal meningitis (CM) is a significant opportunistic illness associated with HIV and the primary cause of death in AIDS patients living in low-resource settings. A South African study compared 25(OH)-VD levels in 150 patients with CM and 150 HIV-infected matched controls to evaluate the relationship between VD levels and illness severity, immunological response, and microbiological clearance. This study found a 74% prevalence of VDD, defined as plasma 25(OH)-VD ~50 nmol/L though it failed to find a correlation between VDD and microbiological clearance. Furthermore, there was no significant correlation between 25(OH)-VD levels and fungal load or cytokine profile in cerebral fluid (Jarvis & Harrison, 2007).

25.17 Conclusion

Currently, many questions remain unanswered about the role of VDD as a potential risk factor for fungal infections. Future research could investigate the mechanisms by which VD influences the inflammatory response, the relationship between VDD and fungal infections, and whether VD supplementation improves outcomes in patients with fungal infections.

References

Abu-Mouch, S., Fireman, Z., Jarchovsky, J., Zeina, A. R., & Assy, N. (2011). Vitamin D supplementation improves sustained virologic response in chronic hepatitis C (genotype 1)-naïve patients. *World Journal of*

Gastroenterology, 17(47), 5184–5190. https://doi.org/10.3748/wjg.v17.i47.5184, http://www.wjgnet.com/1007-9327/pdf/v17/i47/5184.pdf.

Agarwal, R., Sehgal, I. S., Dhooria, S., Aggarwal, A. N., Sachdeva, N., Bhadada, S. K., Garg, M., Behera, D., & Chakrabarti, A. (2018). Vitamin D levels in asthmatic patients with and without allergic bronchopulmonary aspergillosis. *Mycoses, 61*(6), 344–349. https://doi.org/10.1111/myc.12744, http://onlinelibrary.wiley.com/journal/10.1111/(ISSN)1439-0507.

Allegra, A., Tonacci, A., Pioggia, G., Musolino, C., & Gangemi, S. (2020). Vitamin deficiency as risk factor for SARS-CoV-2 infection: Correlation with susceptibility and prognosis. *European Review for Medical and Pharmacological Sciences, 24*(18), 9721–9738. https://doi.org/10.26355/eurrev_202009_23064, https://www.europeanreview.org/article/23064.

Berry, D. J., Hesketh, K., Power, C., & Hyppönen, E. (2011). Vitamin D status has a linear association with seasonal infections and lung function in British adults. *British Journal of Nutrition, 106*(9), 1433–1440. https://doi.org/10.1017/S0007114511001991.

Bhalla, A. K., Amento, E. P., Clemens, T. L., Holick, M. F., & Krane, S. M. (1983). Specific high-affinity receptors for 1,25-dihydroxyvitamin d3in human peripheral blood mononuclear cells: Presence in monocytes and induction in t lymphocytes following activation. *Journal of Clinical Endocrinology and Metabolism, 57*(6), 1308–1310. https://doi.org/10.1210/jcem-57-6-1308.

Bikle, D. D. (2014). Vitamin D metabolism, mechanism of action, and clinical applications. *Chemistry and Biology, 21*(3), 319–329. https://doi.org/10.1016/j.chembiol.2013.12.016, http://www.elsevier.com/inca/publications/store/6/0/1/2/8/1/index.htt.

Birinci, M., Hakyemez, Ö. S., Geçkalan, M. A., Mutlu, M., Yildiz, F., Bilgen, Ö. F., & Azboy, İ. (2024). Effect of vitamin D deficiency on periprosthetic joint infection and complications after primary total joint arthroplasty. *Journal of Arthroplasty, 39*(9), S151. https://doi.org/10.1016/j.arth.2024.05.012, https://www.sciencedirect.com/science/journal/08835403.

Bitetto, D., Fabris, C., Fornasiere, E., Pipan, C., Fumolo, E., Cussigh, A., Bignulin, S., Cmet, S., Fontanini, E., Falleti, E., Martinella, R., Pirisi, M., & Toniutto, P. (2011). Vitamin D supplementation improves response to antiviral treatment for recurrent hepatitis C. *Transplant International, 24*(1), 43–50. https://doi.org/10.1111/j.1432-2277.2010.01141.x.

Bouzid, D., Merzouki, S., Bachiri, M., Ailane, S. E., & Zerroug, M. M. (2017). Vitamin D 3 a new drug against Candida albicans. *Journal de Mycologie Médicale, 27*(1), 79–82. https://doi.org/10.1016/j.mycmed.2016.10.003.

Brockman-Schneider, R. A., Pickles, R. J., & Gern, J. E. (2014). Effects of vitamin D on airway epithelial cell morphology and rhinovirus replication. *PLoS ONE, 9*(1). https://doi.org/10.1371/journal.pone.0086755, http://www.plosone.org/article/fetchObject.action?uri=info%3Adoi%2F10.1371%2Fjournal.pone.0086755&representation=PDF.

Cao, Y., Wang, X., Liu, P., Su, Y., Yu, H., & Du, J. (2022). Vitamin D and the risk of latent tuberculosis infection: A systematic review and meta-analysis. *BMC Pulmonary Medicine, 22*(1). https://doi.org/10.1186/s12890-022-01830-5.

Channappanavar, R., & Perlman, S. (2017). Pathogenic human coronavirus infections: Causes and consequences of cytokine storm and immunopathology. *Seminars in immunopathology, 39*(5), 529–539. https://doi.org/10.1007/s00281-017-0629-x.

Charoenngam, N., & Holick, M. F. (2020). Immunologic effects of vitamin d on human health and disease. *Nutrients, 12*(7), 1–28. https://doi.org/10.3390/nu12072097, https://www.mdpi.com/2072-6643/12/7/2097/pdf.

Coelho, L., Cardoso, S. W., Luz, P. M., Hoffman, R. M., Mendonça, L., Veloso, V. G., Currier, J. S., Grinsztejn, B., & Lake, J. E. (2015). Vitamin D3 supplementation in HIV infection: Effectiveness and associations with antiretroviral therapy. *Nutrition Journal, 14*(1). https://doi.org/10.1186/s12937-015-0072-6, http://www.nutritionj.com/home/.

Coperchini, F., Chiovato, L., Croce, L., Magri, F., & Rotondi, M. (2020). The cytokine storm in COVID-19: An overview of the involvement of the chemokine/chemokine-receptor system. *Cytokine & Growth Factor Reviews, 53*, 25–32. https://doi.org/10.1016/j.cytogfr.2020.05.003.

Cui, A., Zhang, T., Xiao, P., Fan, Z., Wang, H., & Zhuang, Y. (2023). Global and regional prevalence of vitamin D deficiency in population-based studies from 2000 to 2022: A pooled analysis of 7.9 million participants. *Frontiers in Nutrition, 10*. https://doi.org/10.3389/fnut.2023.1070808.

Cutuli, S. L., Cascarano, L., Tanzarella, E. S., Lombardi, G., Carelli, S., Pintaudi, G., Grieco, D. L., De Pascale, G., & Antonelli, M. (2022). Vitamin D status and potential therapeutic options in critically ill patients: A narrative review of the clinical evidence. *Diagnostics, 12*(11). https://doi.org/10.3390/diagnostics12112719, http://www.mdpi.com/journal/diagnostics/.

Cutuli, S. L., Ferrando, E. S., Cammarota, F., Franchini, E., Caroli, A., Lombardi, G., Tanzarella, E. S., Grieco, D. L., Antonelli, M., & De Pascale, G. (2024). Update on vitamin D role in severe infections and sepsis. *Journal of Anesthesia, Analgesia and Critical Care, 4*(1). https://doi.org/10.1186/s44158-024-00139-5, https://link.springer.com/journal/44158.

Deng, Q. F., Chu, H., Wen, Z., & Cao, Y. S. (2019). Vitamin D and urinary tract infection: A systematic review and meta-analysis. *Annals of Clinical and Laboratory Science, 49*(1), 134–142. http://www.annclinlabsci.org.

Dodamani, M. H., Muthu, V., Thakur, R., Pal, A., Sehgal, I. S., Dhooria, S., Aggarwal, A. N., Garg, M., Chakrabarti, A., & Agarwal, R. (2019). A randomised trial of vitamin D in acute-stage allergic bronchopulmonary aspergillosis complicating asthma. *Mycoses, 62*(4), 320–327. https://doi.org/10.1111/myc.12879, http://onlinelibrary.wiley.com/journal/10.1111/(ISSN)1439-0507.

Eletreby, R., Elsharkawy, A., Mohamed, R., Hamed, M., Kamal Ibrahim, E., & Fouad, R. (2024). Prevalence of vitamin D deficiency and the effect of vitamin D3 supplementation on response to anti-tuberculosis therapy in patients with extrapulmonary tuberculosis. *BMC infectious diseases, 24*(1). https://doi.org/10.1186/s12879-024-09367-0.

Entrenas Castillo, M., Entrenas Costa, L. M., Vaquero Barrios, J. M., Alcalá Díaz, J. F., López Miranda, J., Bouillon, R., & Quesada Gomez, J. M. (2020). Effect of calcifediol treatment and best available therapy versus best available therapy on intensive care unit admission and mortality among patients hospitalized for COVID-19: A pilot randomized clinical study. *Journal of Steroid Biochemistry and Molecular Biology, 203*. https://doi.org/10.1016/j.jsbmb.2020.105751, http://www.elsevier.com/locate/jsbmb.

Ezeamama, A. E., Guwatudde, D., Wang, M., Bagenda, D., Kyeyune, R., Sudfeld, C., Manabe, Y. C., & Fawzi, W. W. (2016). Vitamin-D deficiency impairs CD4+T-cell count recovery rate in HIV-positive adults on highly active antiretroviral therapy: A longitudinal study. *Clinical Nutrition, 35*(5), 1110–1117. https://doi.org/10.1016/j.clnu.2015.08.007, http://www.elsevier-international.com/journals/clnu/.

Fuleihan, G. E.-H. (2010). Vitamin D deficiency in the Middle East and its health consequences.

Godan Hauptman, A., Lukić-Grlić, A., Vraneš, J., Milošević, M., & Gagro, A. (2021). The effect of standard-dose wintertime vitamin D supplementation on influenza infection in immunized nursing home elderly residents. *Croatian Medical Journal, 62*(5), 495–503. https://doi.org/10.3325/cmj.2021.62.495.

Gois, P. H. F., Ferreira, D., Olenski, S., & Seguro, A. C. (2017). Vitamin D and infectious diseases: Simple bystander or contributing factor? *Nutrients, 9*(7). https://doi.org/10.3390/nu9070651, http://www.mdpi.com/2072-6643/9/7/651/pdf.

Haug, C., Müller, F., Aukrust, P., & Frøland, S. S. (1994). Subnormal serum concentration of 1, 25-vitamin d in human immunodeficiency virus infection: Correlation with degree of immune deficiency and survival. *Journal of Infectious Diseases, 169*(4), 889–893. https://doi.org/10.1093/infdis/169.4.889.

van Helmond, N., Brobyn, T. L., LaRiccia, P. J., Cafaro, T., Hunter, K., Roy, S., Bandomer, B., Ng, K. Q., Goldstein, H., Mitrev, L. V., Tsai, A., Thwing, D., Maag, M. A., & Chung, M. K. (2023). Vitamin D3 supplementation at 5000 IU daily for the prevention of influenza-like illness in healthcare workers: A pragmatic randomized clinical trial. *Nutrients, 15*(1), 180. https://doi.org/10.3390/nu15010180.

Hileman, C. O., Overton, E. T., & McComsey, G. A. (2016). Vitamin D and bone loss in HIV. *Current Opinion in HIV and AIDS, 11*(3), 277–284. https://doi.org/10.1097/COH.0000000000000272, http://journals.lww.com/co-hivandaids/pages/default.aspx.

Huang, S. J., Wang, X. H., Liu, Z. D., Cao, W. L., Han, Y., Ma, A. G., & Xu, S. F. (2017). Vitamin D deficiency and the risk of tuberculosis: A meta-analysis. *Drug Design, Development and Therapy, 11*, 91–102. https:// doi.org/10.2147/DDDT.S79870, https://www.dovepress.com/getfile.php?fileID=34242.

Huang, Y. N., Chi, H., Chiu, N. C., Huang, C. Y., Li, S. T., Wang, J. Y., & Huang, D. T. N. (2022). A randomized trial of vitamin D supplementation to prevent seasonal influenza and enterovirus infection in children. *Journal of Microbiology, Immunology, and Infection, 55*(5), 803–811. https://doi.org/10.1016/j.jmii.2022.01.003, http://www.elsevier.com/wps/find/journaldescription.cws_home/722895/description#description.

Jaimni, V., Shasty, B. A., Madhyastha, S. P., Shetty, G. V., Acharya, R. V., Bekur, R., & Doddamani, A. (2021). Association of vitamin D deficiency and newly diagnosed pulmonary tuberculosis. *Pulmonary Medicine, 2021.* https://doi.org/10.1155/2021/5285841, http://www.hindawi.com/journals/pm/.

Jarvis, J. N., & Harrison, T. S. (2007). HIV-associated cryptococcal meningitis. *AIDS (London, England), 21*(16), 2119–2129. https://doi.org/10.1097/QAD.0b013e3282a4a64d.

Jorde, R., Witham, M., Janssens, W., Rolighed, L., Borchhardt, K., De Boer, I. H., Grimnes, G., & Hutchinson, M. S. (2012). Vitamin D supplementation did not prevent influenza-like illness as diagnosed retrospectively as diagnosed retrospectively by questionnaires in subjects participating in randomized clinical trials. *Scandinavian Journal of Infectious Diseases, 44*(2), 126–132. https://doi.org/10.3109/00365548.2011.621446.

Jorde, R., Sollid, S. T., Svartberg, J., Joakimsen, R. M., Grimnes, G., & Hutchinson, M. Y. S. (2016). Prevention of urinary tract infections with vitamin D supplementation 20,000 IU per week for five years. Results from an RCT including 511 subjects. *Infectious Diseases, 48*(11-12), 823–828. https://doi.org/10.1080/23744235. 2016.1201853, http://www.tandfonline.com/loi/infd20#.VrgcOLdf1Fo.

Junaid, K., & Rehman, A. (2019). Impact of vitamin D on infectious disease-tuberculosis-a review. *Clinical Nutrition Experimental, 25*, 1–10. https://doi.org/10.1016/j.yclnex.2019.02.003.

Kafle, S., Basnet, A. K., Karki, K., Thapa Magar, M., Shrestha, S., & Yadav, R. S. (2021). Association of vitamin D deficiency with pulmonary tuberculosis: A systematic review and meta-analysis. *Cureus, 13*(9). https://doi. org/10.7759/cureus.17883.

Kalluri, H. V., Sacha, L. M., Ingemi, A. I., Shullo, M. A., Johnson, H. J., Sood, P., Tevar, A. D., Humar, A., & Venkataramanan, R. (2017). Low vitamin D exposure is associated with higher risk of infection in renal transplant recipients. *Clinical Transplantation, 31*(5). https://doi.org/10.1111/ctr.12955, http://www.wiley. com/bw/journal.asp?ref=0902-0063.

Kempker, J. A., Panwar, B., Judd, S. E., Jenny, N. S., Wang, H. E., & Gutierrez, O. M. (2019). Plasma 25-hydroxyvitamin D and the longitudinal risk of sepsis in the REGARDS Cohort. *Oxford Clinical Infectious Diseases, 68*(11), 1926–1931. https://doi.org/10.1093/cid/ciy794, http://cid.oxfordjournals.org/content/by/ year.

Kenanidis, E., Kakoulidis, P., Karponis, D., & Tsiridis, E. (2020). < p > The effect of perioperative vitamin D levels on the functional, patient-related outcome measures and the risk of infection following hip and knee arthroplasty: A systematic review < /p > *Patient Related Outcome Measures, 11*, 161–171. https://doi.org/10. 2147/prom.s261251.

Khoo, A. L., Chai, L. Y. A., Koenen, H. J. P. M., Kullberg, B. J., Joosten, I., Van Der Ven, A. J. A. M., & Netea, M. G. (2011). 1,25-Dihydroxyvitamin D3 modulates cytokine production induced by *Candida albicans*: Impact of seasonal variation of immune responses. *Journal of Infectious Diseases, 203*(1), 122–130. https:// doi.org/10.1093/infdis/jiq008Netherlands, http://jid.oxfordjournals.org/content/203/1/122.full.pdf+html.

Kwon, Y. E., Kim, H., Oh, H. J., Park, J. T., Han, S. H., Ryu, D. R., Yoo, T. H., & Kang, S. W. Vitamin D deficiency is an independent risk factor for urinary tract infections after renal transplants. https://journals.lww. com/md-journal/pages/default.aspx.

Lan, S. H., Lai, C. C., Chang, S. P., Lu, L. C., Hung, S. H., & Lin, W. T. (2020). Vitamin D supplementation and the outcomes of critically ill adult patients: A systematic review and meta-analysis of randomized controlled trials. *Scientific Reports, 10*(1). https://doi.org/10.1038/s41598-020-71271-9, http://www.nature.com/srep/ index.html.

Licata, A., Minissale, M. G., Montalto, F. A., & Soresi, M. (2019). Is vitamin D deficiency predictor of complications development in patients with HCV-related cirrhosis? *Internal and emergency medicine, 14*(5),

735–737. https://doi.org/10.1007/s11739-019-02072-w, http://www.springer.com/italy/home?SGWID=6-102-70-173668106-0&changeHeader=true.

Liu, S., Zhao, T., & Liu, Q. (2024). Vitamin D effects on Chlamydia trachomatis infection: A case-control and experimental study. *Frontiers in Cellular and Infection Microbiology, 14.* https://doi.org/10.3389/fcimb.2024.1366136.

Loeb, M., Dang, A. D., Thiem, V. D., Thanabalan, V., Wang, B., Nguyen, N. B., Tran, H. T. M., Luong, T. M., Singh, P., Smieja, M., Maguire, J., & Pullenayegum, E. (2019). Effect of Vitamin D supplementation to reduce respiratory infections in children and adolescents in Vietnam: A randomized controlled trial. *Influenza and other respiratory viruses, 13*(2), 176–183. https://doi.org/10.1111/irv.12615, http://onlinelibrary.wiley.com/journal/10.1111/(ISSN)1750-2659.

Ma, L., Zhang, Z., Li, L., Zhang, L., Lin, Z., & Qin, H. (2022). Vitamin D deficiency increases the risk of bacterial vaginosis during pregnancy: Evidence from a meta-analysis based on observational studies. *Frontiers in Nutrition, 9.* https://doi.org/10.3389/fnut.2022.1016592.

Malinverni, S., Ochogavia, Q., Lecrenier, S., Scorpinniti, M., Preiser, J. C., Cotton, F., Mols, P., & Bartiaux, M. (2022). Severe vitamin D deficiency in patients admitted to the emergency department with severe sepsis is associated with an increased 90-day mortality. *Emergency Medicine Journal, 40*(1), 36–41. https://doi.org/10.1136/emermed-2021-211973, http://emj.bmj.com/.

Mehta, S., Giovannucci, E., Mugusi, F. M., Spiegelman, D., Aboud, S., Hertzmark, E., Msamanga, G. I., Hunter, D., & Fawzi, W. W. (2010). Vitamin D status of HIV-infected women and its association with hiv disease progression, anemia, and mortality. *PLoS ONE, 5*(1). https://doi.org/10.1371/journal.pone.0008770, http://www.plosone.org/article/fetchObjectAttachment.action?uri=info%3Adoi%2F10.1371%2Fjournal.pone.0008770&representation=PDF United States.

Meng, J., Li, X., Xiong, Y., Wu, Y., Liu, P., & Gao, S. (2024). The role of vitamin D in the prevention and treatment of tuberculosis: A meta-analysis of randomized controlled trials. *Infection.* https://doi.org/10.1007/s15010-024-02446-z.

Menger, J., Lee, Z. Y., Notz, Q., Wallqvist, J., Hasan, M. S., Elke, G., Dworschak, M., Meybohm, P., Heyland, D. K., & Stoppe, C. (2022). Administration of vitamin D and its metabolites in critically ill adult patients: an updated systematic review with meta-analysis of randomized controlled trials. *Critical Care, 26*(1). https://doi.org/10.1186/s13054-022-04139-1, https://ccforum.biomedcentral.com/.

Mercy, D. J., Girigoswami, A., & Girigoswami, K. (2024). Relationship between urinary tract infections and serum vitamin D level in adults and children—A literature review. *Molecular Biology Reports, 51*(1). https://doi.org/10.1007/s11033-024-09888-6, https://www.springer.com/journal/11033.

Merrikhi, A., Ziaei, E., Shahsanai, A., Kelishadi, R., & Maghami-Mehr, A. (2018). Is Vitamin D supplementation effective in prevention of recurrent urinary tract infections in the pediatrics? A randomized triple-masked controlled trial. *Advanced Biomedical Research, 7*(1), 150. https://doi.org/10.4103/abr.abr_149_18.

Moan, J. E., Dahlback, A., Ma, L. W., & Juzeniene, A. (2014). Influenza, solar radiation and vitamin D. *Dermato-Endocrinology, 1*(6), 308–310. https://doi.org/10.4161/derm.1.6.11357.

Mohanty, S., Kamolvit, W., Hertting, O., & Brauner, A. (2020). Vitamin D strengthens the bladder epithelial barrier by inducing tight junction proteins during *E. coli* urinary tract infection. *Cell and Tissue Research, 380*(3), 669–673. https://doi.org/10.1007/s00441-019-03162-z.

Mojtahedi, S. F., Mohammadzadeh, A., Mohammadzadeh, F., Jalili Shahri, J., & Bahri, N. (2023). Association between bacterial vaginosis and 25-Hydroxy vitamin D: a case-control study. *BMC Infectious Diseases, 23*(1). https://doi.org/10.1186/s12879-023-08120-3, https://bmcinfectdis.biomedcentral.com/.

Mostafa, B. E. D., Taha, M. S., Abdel Hamid, T., Omran, A., & Lotfi, N. (2016). Evaluation of vitamin D levels in allergic fungal sinusitis, chronic rhinosinusitis, and chronic rhinosinusitis with polyposis. *International Forum of Allergy and Rhinology, 6*(2), 185–190. https://doi.org/10.1002/alr.21585, http://onlinelibrary.wiley.com/journal/10.1002/(ISSN)2042-6984.

Nichol, K. L., Heilly, S. D., & Ehlinger, E. (2005). Colds and influenza-like illnesses in university students: Impact on health, academic and work performance, and health care use. *Clinical Infectious Diseases, 40*(9), 1263–1270. https://doi.org/10.1086/429237.

Nimer, A., & Mouch, A. (2012). Vitamin D improves viral response in hepatitis C genotype 2-3 naïve patients. *World Journal of Gastroenterology, 18*(8), 800–805. https://doi.org/10.3748/wjg.v18.i8.800, http://www.wjgnet.com/1007-9327/pdf/v18/i8/800.pdf.

Noppè, E., Eloff, J. R. P., Keane, S., & Martin-Loeches, I. (2024). A narrative review of invasive candidiasis in the intensive care unit. *Therapeutic Advances in Pulmonary and Critical Care Medicine, 19.* https://doi.org/10.1177/29768675241304684.

Nseir, W., Taha, M., Nemarny, H., & Mograbi, J. (2013). The association between serum levels of vitamin D and recurrent urinary tract infections in premenopausal women. *International Journal of Infectious Diseases, 17*(12), e1121. https://doi.org/10.1016/j.ijid.2013.06.007.

Pang, T., Cardosa, M. J., & Guzman, M. G. (2007). Of cascades and perfect storms: The immunopathogenesis of dengue haemorrhagic fever-dengue shock syndrome (DHF/DSS). *Immunology and Cell Biology, 85*(1), 43–45. https://doi.org/10.1038/sj.icb.7100008.

Osterholm, M. T., Kelley, N. S., Sommer, A., & Belongia, E. A. (2012). Efficacy and effectiveness of influenza vaccines: A systematic review and meta-analysis. *The Lancet Infectious Diseases, 12*(1), 36–44. https://doi.org/10.1016/S1473-3099(11)70295-X.

Papagni, R., Pellegrino, C., Di Gennaro, F., Patti, G., Ricciardi, A., Novara, R., Cotugno, S., Musso, M., Guido, G., Ronga, L., Stolfa, S., Bavaro, D. F., Romanelli, F., Totaro, V., Lattanzio, R., De Iaco, G., Palmieri, F., Saracino, A., & Gualano, G. (2022). Impact of vitamin D in prophylaxis and treatment in tuberculosis patients. *International Journal of Molecular Sciences, 23*(7), 3860. https://doi.org/10.3390/ijms23073860.

Paz Ocaranza, M., Riquelme, J. A., García, L., Jalil, J. E., Chiong, M., Santos, R. A. S., & Lavandero, S. (2020). Counter-regulatory renin–angiotensin system in cardiovascular disease. *Nature Research, Chile Nature Reviews Cardiology, 17*(2), 116–129. https://doi.org/10.1038/s41569-019-0244-8, http://www.nature.com/nrcardio/archive/index.html.

Petta, S., Cammà, C., Scazzone, C., Tripodo, C., Di Marco, V., Bono, A., Cabibi, D., Licata, G., Porcasi, R., Marchesini, G., & Craxí, A. (2010). Low vitamin D serum level is related to severe fibrosis and low responsiveness to interferon-based therapy in genotype 1 chronic hepatitis C†. *Hepatology, 51*(4), 1158–1167. https://doi.org/10.1002/hep.23489.

Roelen, C. A. M., Koopmans, P. C., Notenbomer, A., & Groothoff, J. W. (2011). Job satisfaction and short sickness absence due to the common cold. *Work, 39*(3), 305–313. https://doi.org/10.3233/WOR-2011-1178.

Rudd, K. E., Johnson, S. C., Agesa, K. M., Shackelford, K. A., Tsoi, D., Kievlan, D. R., Colombara, D. V., Ikuta, K. S., Kissoon, N., Finfer, S., Fleischmann-Struzek, C., Machado, F. R., Reinhart, K. K., Rowan, K., Seymour, C. W., Watson, R. S., West, T. E., Marinho, F., Hay, S. I., ... Naghavi, M. (2020). Global, regional, and national sepsis incidence and mortality, 1990–2017: analysis for the Global Burden of Disease Study. *The Lancet, 395*(10219), 200–211. https://doi.org/10.1016/S0140-6736(19)32989-7, http://www.journals.elsevier.com/the-lancet/.

Sarhan, T. S., & Elrifai, A. (2021). Serum level of vitamin D as a predictor for severity and outcome of pneumonia. *Clinical Nutrition, 40*(4), 2389–2393. https://doi.org/10.1016/j.clnu.2020.10.035, http://www.elsevier-international.com/journals/clnu/.

Sedik, S., Wolfgruber, S., Hoenigl, M., & Kriegl, L. (2024). Diagnosing fungal infections in clinical practice: A narrative review. *Expert review of anti-infective therapy, 22*(11), 935–949. https://doi.org/10.1080/14787210.2024.2403017.

Seok, H., Kim, J., Choi, W. S., & Park, D. W. (2023). Effects of vitamin D deficiency on sepsis. *Nutrients, 15*(20). https://doi.org/10.3390/nu15204309, http://www.mdpi.com/journal/nutrients/.

Siddiqee, M. H., Bhattacharjee, B., Siddiqi, U. R., & MeshbahurRahman, M. (2021). High prevalence of vitamin D deficiency among the South Asian adults: A systematic review and meta-analysis. *BMC public health, 21*(1). https://doi.org/10.1186/s12889-021-11888-1, http://www.biomedcentral.com/bmcpublichealth.

Siddiqui, M., Manansala, J. S., Abdulrahman, H. A., Nasrallah, G. K., Smatti, M. K., Younes, N., Althani, A. A., & Yassine, H. M. (2020). Immune modulatory effects of vitamin d on viral infections. *Nutrients, 12*(9), 1–16. https://doi.org/10.3390/nu12092879, https://www.mdpi.com/2072-6643/12/9/2879/pdf.

Sinha, S., Thukral, H., Shareef, I., Desai, D., Singh, B. K., Das, B. K., Dhooria, S., Sarin, R., Singla, R., Meena, S. K., Pandey, R. M., Pandey, S., Sethi, S., Kajal, A., Yadav, R., Aggarwal, A. N., Bhadada, S., & Behera, D. (2023). Prevention of relapse in drug sensitive pulmonary tuberculosis patients with and without vitamin D3 supplementation: A double blinded randomized control clinical trial. *PLoS ONE, 18*(3). https://doi.org/10.1371/journal.pone.0272682, https://journals.plos.org/plosone/article/file?id=10.1371/journal.pone.0272682&type=printable.

Slow, S., Epton, M., Storer, M., Thiessen, R., Lim, S., Wong, J., Chin, P., Tovaranonte, P., Pearson, J., Chambers, S. T., Murdoch, D. R., Jardine, D., Pithie, A., Warren, C., Faville, S., Shankar, A., Cameron, E., Evans, T., Mooi, P., ... Liu, M. (2018). Effect of adjunctive single high-dose vitamin D3 on outcome of community-acquired pneumonia in hospitalised adults: The VIDCAPS randomised controlled trial. *Scientific Reports, 8*(1). https://doi.org/10.1038/s41598-018-32162-2, http://www.nature.com/srep/index.html.

Snijder, E. J., Van Der Meer, Y., Zevenhoven-Dobbe, J., Onderwater, J. J. M., Van Der Meulen, J., Koerten, H. K., & Mommaas, A. M. (2006). Ultrastructure and origin of membrane vesicles associated with the severe acute respiratory syndrome coronavirus replication complex. *Journal of Virology, 80*(12), 5927–5940. https://doi.org/10.1128/JVI.02501-05.

Sudfeld, C. R., Wang, M., Aboud, S., Giovannucci, E. L., Mugusi, F. M., & Fawzi, W. W. (2012). Vitamin D and HIV progression among Tanzanian adults initiating antiretroviral therapy. *PLoS ONE, 7*(6). https://doi.org/10.1371/journal.pone.0040036, http://www.plosone.org/article/fetchObjectAttachment.action?uri=info%3Adoi%2F10.1371%2Fjournal.pone.0040036&representation=PDF United States.

Sîrbe, C., Rednic, S., Grama, A., & Pop, T. L. (2022). An update on the effects of vitamin D on the immune system and autoimmune diseases. *International Journal of Molecular Sciences, 23*(17). https://doi.org/10.3390/ijms23179784, http://www.mdpi.com/journal/ijms.

Upala, S., Sanguankeo, A., & Permpalung, N. (2015). Significant association between vitamin D deficiency and sepsis: A systematic review and meta-analysis. *BMC Anesthesiology, 15*(1). https://doi.org/10.1186/s12871-015-0063-3.

Viard, J. P., Souberbielle, J. C., Kirk, O., Reekie, J., Knysz, B., Losso, M., Gatell, J., Pedersen, C., Bogner, J. R., Lundgren, J. D., & Mocroft, A. (2011). Vitamin D and clinical disease progression in HIV infection: Results from the EuroSIDA study. *AIDS (London, England), 25*(10), 1305–1315. https://doi.org/10.1097/QAD.0b013e328347f6f7.

Vitamin D deficiency linked to recurrent UTI. (2013). *Nature Reviews Urology, 10*(10), 556. https://doi.org/10.1038/nrurol.2013.190.

Wayland, J., Teixeira, J. P., & Nielsen, N. D. (2024). Sepsis in 2024: A review. *Anaesthesia and Intensive Care Medicine, 25*(10), 642–651. https://doi.org/10.1016/j.mpaic.2024.06.010, https://www.sciencedirect.com/science/journal/14720299.

W.H. Organization (2015). *Guidelines on the management of latent tuberculosis infection.* (2015).

W.H. Organization (2024). *Global tuberculosis report 2024.*

Wjst, M., & Hyppönen, E. (2007). Vitamin D serum levels and allergic rhinitis. *Allergy, 62*(9), 1085–1086. https://doi.org/10.1111/j.1398-9995.2007.01437.x.

Xie, J., Zhu, L., Zhu, T., Jian, Y., Ding, Y., Zhou, M., & Feng, X. (2019). Vitamin D-supplemented yogurt drink reduces Candida infections in a paediatric intensive care unit: a randomised, placebo-controlled clinical trial. *Journal of Human Nutrition and Dietetics, 32*(4), 512–517. https://doi.org/10.1111/jhn.12634.

Xu, Z., Shi, L., Wang, Y., Zhang, J., Huang, L., Zhang, C., Liu, S., Zhao, P., Liu, H., Zhu, L., Tai, Y., Bai, C., Gao, T., Song, J., Xia, P., Dong, J., Zhao, J., & Wang, F. S. (2020). Pathological findings of COVID-19 associated with acute respiratory distress syndrome. *The Lancet Respiratory Medicine, 8*(4), 420–422. https://doi.org/10.1016/S2213-2600(20)30076-X, http://www.elsevier.com/journals/the-lancet-respiratory-medicine/2213-2600.

Yang, B., Zhu, Y., Zheng, X., Li, T., Niu, K., Wang, Z., Lu, X., Zhang, Y., & Shen, C. (2023). Vitamin D supplementation during intensive care unit stay is associated with improved outcomes in critically ill patients with sepsis: A cohort study. *Nutrients, 15*(13), 2924. https://doi.org/10.3390/nu15132924.

Yang, C., Lu, Y., Wan, M., Xu, D., Yang, X., Yang, L., Wang, S., & Sun, G. (2021). Efficacy of high-dose vitamin D supplementation as an adjuvant treatment on pneumonia: Systematic review and a meta-analysis of randomized controlled studies. *Nutrition in Clinical Practice, 36*(2), 368–384. https://doi.org/10.1002/ncp. 10585.

Zargaran, A., Zargaran, D., & Trompeter, A. J. (2021). The role of vitamin D in orthopaedic infection: A systematic literature review. *Bone and Joint Open, 2*(9), 721–727. https://doi.org/10.1302/2633-1462.29.BJO-2020-0192.R1, https://online.boneandjoint.org.uk/bjo/about.

Zeng, J., Wu, G., Yang, W., Gu, X., Liang, W., Yao, Y., Song, Y., Cardona, P.-J., & Serum, A. (2015). Vitamin D level < 25nmol/L pose high tuberculosis risk: A meta-analysis. *PLoS ONE, 10*(5), e0126014. https://doi.org/10.1371/journal.pone.0126014.

Zhou, Y. F., Luo, B. A., & Qin, L. L. (2019). Y. Shidoji, The association between Vitamin D deficiency and community-acquired pneumonia: A meta-analysis of observational studies. *Medicine (United States), 98*(38). https://doi.org/10.1097/MD.0000000000017252, https://journals.lww.com/md-journal/pages/default.aspx.

Zhu, Zhu, Gu, Zhan, Chen, & Li (2021). Association between vitamin D and influenza: Meta-analysis and systematic review of randomized controlled trials. *Frontiers in Nutrition, 8*. https://doi.org/10.3389/fnut.2021. 799709.

Zmijewski, M. A., & Carlberg, C. (2020). Vitamin D receptor(s): In the nucleus but also at membranes? *Experimental Dermatology, 29*(9), 876–884. https://doi.org/10.1111/exd.14147, http://onlinelibrary.wiley.com/journal/10.1111/(ISSN)1600-0625.

CHAPTER 26

Vitamin D in Physiotherapy: unlocking new frontiers in recovery and rehabilitation

Fatima Syed[1], Bushra Madad Ali Malik[2], and Rehana Rehman[3]

[1]*Department of Pathology, Fazaia Ruth Pfau Medical College, Karachi, Pakistan* [2]*Department of Health, Physical Education and Sport Sciences, University of Karachi, Karachi, Pakistan* [3]*Department of Biological & Biomedical Sciences, Aga Khan University, Karachi, Pakistan*

26.1 Introduction

Physiotherapy is a science-based healthcare profession dedicated to optimizing movement and functional potential, enhancing the quality of life through prevention, treatment, and rehabilitation. According to World Physiotherapy, it employs evidence-based physical approaches to address not just physical but also mental and social well-being, underscoring the importance of clinical expertise and informed decision-making in practice (World Physiotherapy, 2024). The Australian Physiotherapy Council emphasizes a holistic approach in the therapeutic management of pain and movement disorders, striving to improve the health and welfare of individuals and communities (Australian Physiotherapy Council).

Traditionally recognized for its role in bone health—particularly in calcium regulation and osteoporosis prevention—Vitamin D's influence extends to muscle strength, neuromuscular coordination, immune modulation, and inflammation reduction (Christensen et al., 2004; Holick, 2007). These diverse physiological effects position vitamin D as a potentially transformative tool in enhancing physiotherapy outcomes.

26.1.1 Musculoskeletal health and vitamin D

Vitamin D plays a critical role in maintaining musculoskeletal health, influencing bone density, muscle function, and overall physical performance. A deficiency in vitamin D can lead to various musculoskeletal disorders, including osteoporosis, osteomalacia, and increased risk of fractures (Webb, 2006). As physiotherapists strive to enhance recovery and rehabilitation outcomes, understanding the implications of vitamin D on musculoskeletal health is paramount.

The Impact of Vitamin D on Health and Disease. DOI: https://doi.org/10.1016/B978-0-443-34037-6.00001-7

26.1.2 Vitamin D's role in bone health

Vitamin D is essential for calcium absorption and bone mineralization, directly influencing bone density and strength. Numerous studies have shown that adequate vitamin D levels are associated with improved bone health and a reduced risk of fractures. For instance, research conducted by Tella and Gallagher found that Vitamin D supplementation significantly decreases the incidence of falls and fractures in elderly populations, highlighting the importance of monitoring Vitamin D status in this demographic (Tella & Gallagher, 2014). Furthermore, a systematic review by Rejnmark concluded that vitamin D supplementation reduces the risk of falls by 19%, providing substantial evidence for its protective effects on skeletal health (Rejnmark, 2017) (Fig. 26.1).

26.1.3 Muscle function and performance

In addition to its impact on bone health, vitamin D is crucial for optimal muscle function. Deficiency in vitamin D has been linked to muscle weakness and increased fall risk, particularly in older adults. A study by Beaudart et al. (2014) demonstrated that low vitamin D levels correlate with decreased muscle strength and mobility (Beaudart et al., 2014). Furthermore, evidence suggests that vitamin D supplementation can improve muscle performance and reduce

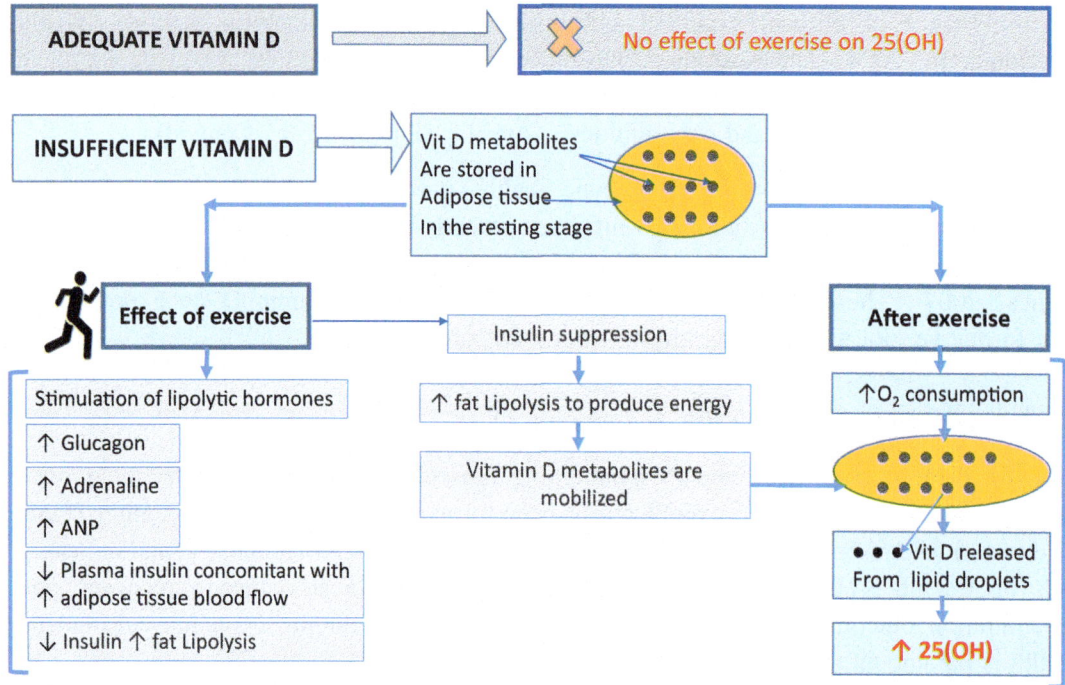

Figure 26.1
Physiology of exercise interventions on vitamin D status and mobilization.

the risk of falls among older adults (Sanders et al., 2010). As physiotherapists incorporate resistance training and balance exercises into rehabilitation protocols, addressing Vitamin D levels becomes integral to enhancing patient outcomes.

26.1.4   Implications for physiotherapy practice

Physiotherapists are well-positioned to assess and manage vitamin D deficiency in patients, particularly those with musculoskeletal conditions. Regular screening for Vitamin D levels can help identify individuals at risk and facilitate timely interventions. For patients presenting with osteoporosis or a history of falls, integrating Vitamin D supplementation into rehabilitation programs may enhance recovery and reduce the likelihood of adverse events.

Recent research highlights the multifaceted role of vitamin D in musculoskeletal health. For example, a study by Aroda (2022) indicated that vitamin D supplementation improved functional outcomes and quality of life in patients with chronic musculoskeletal pain (Aroda, 2022). Additionally, understanding the complex interplay between vitamin D, calcium metabolism, and muscle function is essential for optimizing treatment strategies and promoting recovery in individuals with musculoskeletal disorders.

In summary, vitamin D is a vital nutrient influencing musculoskeletal health, and physiotherapists must prioritize its assessment and management within rehabilitation frameworks. By ensuring optimal vitamin D levels, practitioners can enhance bone density, muscle function, and overall recovery outcomes for their patients. Only chronic endurance exercise training can significantly increase serum 1,25(OH)2D, and the effect may be sex-dependent. Exercise may influence 25(OH)D levels in the circulation by regulating either the vitamin D metabolites stored in tissues or the utilization by target tissues. Evidence from different studies is given in Table 26.1. (Farag et al., 2018; Gao et al., 2022; Lithgow, Florida-James, & Leggate, 2018; Malandish et al., 2020; Mieszkowski et al., 2018; Zhang & Cao, 2022)

26.1.5   Vitamin D and neurological rehabilitation

Vitamin D has garnered increasing attention for its potential role in enhancing neuroplasticity and supporting recovery in patients with neurological conditions. As physiotherapists seek innovative approaches to improve rehabilitation outcomes, understanding how vitamin D influences brain health, cognitive recovery, and neuronal repair opens up exciting avenues for patient care.

26.1.5.1   Vitamin D's role in neuroplasticity

Emerging research indicates that vitamin D may play a pivotal role in neuroplasticity—the brain's ability to adapt and reorganize itself, particularly following injury. Vitamin D receptors are found throughout the brain, and its active form, calcitriol, has been shown to influence various neurotrophic factors and signaling pathways critical for neuronal growth and

Table 26.1 Evidence of positive effect of chronic endurance exercise interventions on 25(OH)D levels.

Study	Participants	Age range	Type of physical activity	Results
Farag et al. (2018)	Endurance PA and Vit D supplementation (2000IU) per day on lipid profile in metabolic syndrome patients	40–45 years	Endurance PA: 30min a day for 12 weeks	25(OH)D: significantly increased
Mieszkowski et al. (2018)	The effect of Nordic walking training with Vit D (800IU) per day supplementation on postural control and muscle strength in the elderly	67–73 years	Nordic walking training: 12 weeks, two hours, three times a week.	$25(OH)D_3$: significantly increased
Mieszkowski et al. (2018)	Nordic walking training in elderly women with 4000 IU/day vitamin D supplementation	68–73 years	Nordic walking training: 12 weeks, three times a week.	$25(OH)D_3$: significantly increased after 12 weeks
Malandish et al. (2020)	The effect of training on electrocardiogram and cardiac biomarkers in postmenopausal women	53–57 years	40 min of walking or jogging on a treadmill	25(OH)D: significantly increased
Gao et al. (2022)	Effect of high-intensity interval training on pulmonary function and exercise capacity in individuals with chronic obstructive pulmonary disease	Not specific	High-Intensity Interval Training	25(OH)D: significantly increased
Lithgow et al. (2018)	Effect of training and Vit D supplementation on the glycemic control of overweight and obese adults	34–44 years	Intervention: 6 weeks, 3 sessions /week, 10 repetitions of 1 min intervals	$25(OH)D_3$: significantly increased

Source: Data from Zhang, J., Cao, Z. B. (2022). Exercise: A possibly effective way to improve vitamin D nutritional status. *Nutrients*, *14*(13), 2652. 10.3390/nu14132652. PMID: 35807833; PMCID: PMC9268447.

repair (Xuan et al., 2016). By enhancing synaptic plasticity and promoting the survival of neurons, vitamin D may support cognitive recovery and overall brain health.

In conditions such as stroke and spinal cord injury, where neuroplastic changes are essential for functional recovery, maintaining optimal vitamin D levels could be a key factor in facilitating rehabilitation. Studies suggest that patients with higher vitamin D levels tend to exhibit better functional outcomes, possibly due to the vitamin's influence on neurogenesis and the restoration of neuronal connections (Kessels, 2018).

26.1.5.2   Stroke rehabilitation

The rehabilitation of stroke patients poses significant challenges, as the brain's ability to rewire itself is often impaired. However, optimizing vitamin D levels during the rehabilitation process may improve motor recovery through enhanced neuromuscular reconditioning (Munch, 2019). Physiotherapists can play an essential role in assessing vitamin D levels in stroke patients and recommending appropriate supplementation when necessary. By integrating vitamin D management into rehabilitation protocols, practitioners may enhance their patients' recovery trajectories, helping them regain independence and improve their quality of life.

26.1.5.3 Impact on chronic pain and neuropathy

Neuropathic pain is a common and often debilitating issue faced by patients undergoing neurological rehabilitation. Recent studies have highlighted the potential of Vitamin D supplementation to reduce neuropathic pain, offering hope for improved management strategies in this challenging area (Koenig et al., 2015; Theiler, 2014). Vitamin D's antiinflammatory properties and its role in regulating pain pathways may contribute to pain relief, providing a dual benefit of alleviating discomfort while supporting the overall rehabilitation process (Mautone, 2014).

For physiotherapists working with patients suffering from chronic pain, understanding the role of vitamin D can facilitate more comprehensive treatment plans. By addressing both the physiological and psychosocial aspects of rehabilitation, physiotherapists can help patients navigate their recovery more effectively.

Recent research has shown that vitamin D supplementation can significantly improve ambulation and lower extremity motor function in stroke patients. A study conducted by Karasu and Karataş (2021) demonstrated that patients receiving vitamin D during rehabilitation exhibited greater improvements in functional ambulation and Brunnstrom recovery stage scores compared to those who did not receive supplementation (Karasu & Karataş, 2021). Notably, these benefits were particularly pronounced in patients undergoing rehabilitation within the first 3 months poststroke, suggesting a critical window for vitamin D's therapeutic effects (Manzoli, 2020). Furthermore, the coexistence of heterotopic ossification of the elbow and vitamin D deficiency following stroke raises important considerations regarding treatment approaches, as calcium and vitamin D treatment may mitigate deficiencies but could also exacerbate ossification (Mullooly, 2018).

Additionally, a systematic review by Sallehuddin (2022) emphasized the effectiveness of nonpharmacological interventions, such as specific physical and vibration therapies, in reducing bone loss among poststroke patients (Sallehuddin, 2022). While these interventions showed promise in improving bone mineral density, they also resulted in a higher incidence of falls, highlighting the need for careful monitoring. The review noted a lack of studies exploring vitamin D or protein supplementation as adjuncts to these interventions, indicating a critical gap in research. Together, this evidence underscores vitamin D's potential role in enhancing rehabilitation outcomes by facilitating neuromuscular recovery, promoting motor function, and addressing complications like heterotopic ossification, while also integrating nonpharmacological strategies to optimize bone health.

26.1.6   Vitamin D in cardiovascular physiotherapy

This section introduces vitamin D's emerging role in cardiovascular health and how it can enhance physiotherapy interventions for patients with cardiovascular conditions such as heart disease, hypertension, and postmyocardial infarction recovery. Research increasingly underscores that vitamin D is vital not only for bone health but also for cardiovascular function and rehabilitation (Pack et al., 2015).

26.1.6.1   Cardiovascular muscle function

Investigating vitamin D's role in supporting cardiac muscle function, this section explores its impact on recovery following heart surgeries. Evidence suggests that adequate vitamin D levels are linked to improved cardiac muscle performance, which is crucial for patients recovering from myocardial infarction or heart surgery (Holick, 2008). By addressing vitamin D deficiency, physiotherapists may enhance cardiac recovery and optimize overall rehabilitation outcomes (Falola, 2013).

26.1.6.2   Vascular health and exercise tolerance

Vitamin D's influence on vascular health cannot be overlooked. This section delves into how Vitamin D supports blood vessel health, improves circulation, and enhances exercise tolerance in patients undergoing cardiac rehabilitation

26.2   Conclusion

In conclusion, vitamin D plays a pivotal role in enhancing musculoskeletal health, neurological rehabilitation, and cardiovascular recovery, offering promising avenues for physiotherapy practice. Its multifaceted benefits extend beyond bone health, significantly impacting muscle function, recovery from neurological disorders, and cardiovascular rehabilitation.

The evidence presented underscores the importance of adequate vitamin D levels for optimal physiological functioning and recovery. In musculoskeletal health, vitamin D supplementation can enhance muscle strength, improve balance, and reduce the risk of falls, thereby playing a crucial role in rehabilitation programs for individuals with musculoskeletal disorders. Similarly, in neurological rehabilitation, vitamin D has emerged as a critical factor influencing recovery outcomes in stroke patients, contributing to functional improvements and quality of life.

Moreover, the implications of vitamin D for cardiovascular health cannot be overlooked. Adequate levels of Vitamin D are associated with better cardiovascular outcomes, suggesting that physiotherapy interventions focusing on vitamin D status may enhance recovery and rehabilitation strategies for patients with heart conditions.

As we continue to unravel the complex interactions between vitamin D and various physiological systems, it is essential for physiotherapists to integrate vitamin D assessment and management into their practice. Future research should aim to elucidate the optimal dosages and strategies for vitamin D supplementation, further exploring its role in diverse populations.

Incorporating vitamin D into physiotherapy protocols not only supports recovery and rehabilitation but also empowers patients to take charge of their health, paving the way for improved outcomes and enhanced well-being. This chapter highlights the necessity for an interdisciplinary approach that combines nutrition, exercise, and physiotherapy, promoting a holistic framework for patient care.

References

Aroda, V. (2022). The role of vitamin D supplementation in chronic musculoskeletal pain: a systematic review. *Journal of Pain Research, 15*, 1941–1954. https://doi.org/10.2147/JPR.S359425.

Australian Physiotherapy Council. Guidelines for the accreditation of physiotherapy practitioner programs leading to specialisation [Internet]. Canberra (AU): Australian Physiotherapy Council; 2024 [cited 2025 Aug 4]. https://australian.physio/sites/default/files/College/Guidelines_for_the_accreditation_of_physiotherapy_practitioners_programs_leading_to_specialisation.pdf.

Beaudart, C., Buckinx, F., Rabenda, V., et al. (2014). The role of vitamin D in the prevention of falls: a systematic review and meta-analysis of randomized controlled trials. *Journal of Aging Research, 2014*, 1–9. https://doi.org/10.1155/2014/306405.

Christensen, J. H., Siggaard, C., Corydon, T. J., Robertson, G. L., Gregersen, N., Bolund, L., & Rittig, S. (2004). Differential cellular handling of defective arginine vasopressin (AVP) prohormones in cells expressing mutations of the AVP gene associated with autosomal dominant and recessive familial neurohypophyseal diabetes insipidus. *The Journal of Clinical Endocrinology & Metabolism, 89*(9), 4521–4531. https://doi.org/10.1210/jc.2003-031813.

Falola, M. (2013). Takotsubo cardiomyopathy: Overrepresentation of cases. *American Journal of Cardiology, 111*(6). https://doi.org/10.1016/j.amjcard.2012.12.030.

Farag, H. A. M., Hosseinzadeh-Attar, M. J., Muhammad, B. A., Esmaillzadeh, A., & Bilbeisi, A. H. E. (2018). Comparative effects of vitamin D and vitamin C supplementations with and without endurance physical activity on metabolic syndrome patients: a randomized controlled trial. *Diabetology & Metabolic Syndrome, 10*(1). https://doi.org/10.1186/s13098-018-0384-8.

Gao, M., Huang, Y., Wang, Q., Liu, K., & Sun, G. (2022). Effects of high-intensity interval training on pulmonary function and exercise capacity in individuals with chronic obstructive pulmonary disease: A meta-analysis and systematic review. *Advances in Therapy, 39*(1), 94–116. https://doi.org/10.1007/s12325-021-01920-6, http://www.springer.com/springer+healthcare/journal/12325.

Holick, M. F. (2007). Medical progress: Vitamin D deficiency. *New England Journal of Medicine, 357*(3), 266–281. https://doi.org/10.1056/NEJMra070553, http://content.nejm.org/cgi/reprint/357/3/266.pdf.

Holick, M. F. (2008). Vitamin D: A D-Lightful health perspective. *Nutrition Reviews, 66*(2), S182–S194. https://doi.org/10.1111/j.1753-4887.2008.00104.x.

Karasu, & Karataş, G. (2021). The effects of vitamin D on functional recovery after stroke: a double-blind randomized clinical trial. *Stroke; a Journal of Cerebral Circulation, 52*(5), 1727–1735. https://doi.org/10.1161/STROKEAHA.120.032551.

Kessels, A. G. (2018). Vitamin D and stroke: A review. *Current Neurology and Neuroscience Reports, 18*(5). https://doi.org/10.1007/s11910-018-0872-3.

Koenig, J., Jarczok, M. N., Ellis, R. J., Warth, M., Hillecke, T. K., & Thayer, J. F. (2015). Lowered parasympathetic activity in apparently healthy subjects with self-reported symptoms of pain: Preliminary results from a pilot study. *Pain Practice, 15*(4), 314–318. https://doi.org/10.1111/papr.12177.

Lithgow, H. M., Florida-James, G., & Leggate, M. (2018). The combined effect of high-intensity intermittent training and vitamin D supplementation on glycemic control in overweight and obese adults. *Physiological Reports, 6*(9). https://doi.org/10.14814/phy2.13684, http://physoc.onlinelibrary.wiley.com/hub/journal/10.1002/(ISSN)2051-817X/.

Malandish, A., Tartibian, B., Sheikhlou, Z., Afsargharehbagh, R., & Rahmati, M. (2020). The effects of short-term moderate intensity aerobic exercise and long-term detraining on electrocardiogram indices and cardiac biomarkers in postmenopausal women. *Journal of Electrocardiology, 60*, 15–22. https://doi.org/10.1016/j.jelectrocard.2020.03.004, http://www.elsevier.com/inca/publications/store/6/2/3/3/0/8/index.htt.

Manzoli, L. (2020). Vitamin D and functional recovery after stroke: A meta-analysis. *Journal of Stroke and Cerebrovascular Diseases: the Official Journal of National Stroke Association, 29*(5). https://doi.org/10.1016/j.jstrokecerebrovasdis.2019.104765.

Mautone, C. (2014). The relationship between vitamin D and pain. *Pain Physician, 17*(4), 469–482.

Mieszkowski, J., Niespodziński, B., Kochanowicz, A., Gmiat, A., Prusik, K., Prusik, K., Kortas, J., Ziemann, E., & Antosiewicz, J. (2018). The effect of nordic walking training combined with vitamin D supplementation on postural control and muscle strength in elderly people—A randomized controlled trial. *International Journal of Environmental Research and Public Health, 15*(9), 1951. https://doi.org/10.3390/ijerph15091951.

Mullooly, M. (2018). Heterotopic ossification in stroke patients: An observational study of vitamin D status and treatment. *Journal of Stroke, 20*(1), 55–62. https://doi.org/10.1177/1747493017719344.

Munch, G. (2019). Vitamin D: A key factor in stroke recovery. *Neural Regeneration Research, 14*(7), 1132–1133. https://doi.org/10.4103/1673-5374.253245.

Pack, Q. R., Dudycha, K. J., Roschen, K. P., Thomas, R. J., & Squires, R. W. (2015). Safety of early enrollment into outpatient cardiac rehabilitation after open heart surgery. *The American Journal of Cardiology, 115*(4), 548–552. https://doi.org/10.1016/j.amjcard.2014.11.040.

Rejnmark, L. (2017). Vitamin D supplementation for prevention of cancer and cardiovascular disease: A systematic review. *Endocrine-Related Cancer, 24*(1), 1–15. https://doi.org/10.1530/ERC-16-0258.

Sallehuddin, N. (2022). Non-pharmacological interventions for improving bone health in post-stroke patients: A systematic review. *BMC Geriatrics, 22*(1). https://doi.org/10.1186/s12877-022-02756-2.

Sanders, K. M., Stuart, A. L., Williamson, E. J., Simpson, J. A., Kotowicz, M. A., Young, D., & Nicholson, G. C. (2010). Annual high-dose oral vitamin D and falls and fractures in older women. *JAMA: the Journal of the American Medical Association, 303*(18), 1815. https://doi.org/10.1001/jama.2010.594.

Tella, S. H., & Gallagher, J. C. (2014). Vitamin D deficiency and its clinical consequences. *Endocrine Practice: Official Journal of the American College of Endocrinology and the American Association of Clinical Endocrinologists, 20*(9), 977–989. https://doi.org/10.4158/EP14195.RA.

Theiler, R. (2014). Vitamin D and chronic pain: Is there a connection? *Clinical and Experimental Rheumatology, 32*(6), 856–863.

Webb, A. R. (2006). Who, what, where and when—Influences on cutaneous vitamin D synthesis. *Progress in Biophysics and Molecular Biology, 92*(1), 17–25. https://doi.org/10.1016/j.pbiomolbio.2006.02.004.

World Physiotherapy (2024). What is physiotherapy? [Internet]. London, UK: World Physiotherapy. https://world.physio/resources/what-is-physiotherapy.

Xuan, D., Han, Q., Tu, Q., Zhang, L., Yu, L., Murry, D., Tu, T., Tang, Y., Lian, J. B., Stein, G. S., Valverde, P., Zhang, J., & Chen, J. (2016). Epigenetic modulation in periodontitis: interaction of adiponectin and JMJD3-IRF4 axis in macrophages. *Journal of Cellular Physiology, 231*(5), 1090–1096. https://doi.org/10.1002/jcp.25201.

Zhang, J., & Cao, Z.-B. (2022). Exercise: A possibly effective way to improve vitamin D nutritional status. *Nutrients, 14*(13), 2652. https://doi.org/10.3390/nu14132652.

Optimising health with vitamin D: Clinical tools, public solutions, and future possibilities

CHAPTER 27

Testing and measurement of Vitamin D

Lena Jafri[1], Ya Chee Lim[2], and Sibtain Ahmed[1]

[1]Section of Chemical Pathology, Department of Pathology and Laboratory Medicine, Aga Khan University, Karachi, Sindh, Pakistan [2]PAPRSB Institute of Health Sciences, Universiti Brunei Darussalam, Bandar Seri Begawan, Brunei-Muara, Brunei

27.1 Introduction

Vitamin D deficiency is considered a global nutritional issue and is evaluated by measuring or quantifying the inactive form of vitamin D that is 25-hydroxy vitamin D (25(OH)D (Cashman, 2020). The only way to evaluate vitamin D deficiency in an individual is to measure their circulating level of 25(OH)D. The major source of vitamin D, being the sun, and hence also known as sunshine vitamins. However, literature shows that it is recognized not only for its importance of bone health in children and adults but also for other health advantages like reducing the risk of chronic diseases, including autoimmune diseases, chronic infections, malignancies (breast, colon, and prostate), and cardiovascular disease (Holick, 1996). Mostly the 25(OH)D test is requested for diagnosis of vitamin D deficiency; in case of differential diagnosis of causes of rickets or osteomalacia; for monitoring vitamin D replacement therapy, and to diagnose vitamin D toxicity of hypervitaminosis D.

Determination of the right cutoff to define vitamin D deficiency has always been a topic of debate and discussion in scientific meetings and published literature. Another area of discussion has been the standardization of vitamin D assays and their comparison. There are a number of assays used to measure the levels of 25(OH)D in blood. Standardization of vitamin D assays has been in discussion to ensure reliable and accurate vitamin D values across different assays and methodologies. Accurate measurement is important for clinical decisions regarding vitamin D deficiency and treatment.

As 25(OH)D is the primary laboratory investigation done to assess nutritional vitamin D deficiency, this chapter will discuss various methodologies and assays available for vitamin D testing, particularly for 25(OH)D only, and their strengths and limitations. Please note that 1,25-dihydroxyvitamin D (1,25(OH)$_2$D), the active form of vitamin D, is a completely different metabolite and laboratory test with its own set of challenges and clinical indications. This active

The Impact of Vitamin D on Health and Disease. **DOI:** https://doi.org/10.1016/B978-0-443-34037-6.00019-4

form of the vitamin is not an indicator of vitamin D deficiency and is typically not used as a nutritional biomarker. 1,25(OH)₂D testing is indicated in diseased states like kidney diseases, and in clinical contexts to evaluate calcium metabolism disorders where its regulation may be deranged.

27.2 Vitamin D metabolites and indication for measurement

The two primary purposes of 25(OH)D analytical testing are to assess an individual's vitamin D nutritional status and monitor therapeutic levels. 25(OH)D exists in two forms: 25(OH)D2 and 25(OH)D3, and it is crucial to understand which form is being tested to ensure accurate monitoring, especially in therapeutic settings. When using protein binding tests or immunoassays, one must confirm whether the antibody reacts equally with both forms of vitamin D, as this could impact the accuracy of the test (Atef, 2018).

For example, if the goal is to monitor therapy with 25(OH)D2, the test should specifically measure 25(OH)D2 levels. However, accurately determining 25(OH)D2 remains challenging despite advances in testing methodologies. This difficulty arises from various factors, including the simultaneous measurement of both 25(OH)D2 and 25(OH)D3, which can complicate the interpretation of results (Rahme et al., 2018). Additionally, the hydrophobic nature of 25(OH)D necessitates its separation from carrier proteins such as vitamin D binding protein (VDBP), albumin, and lipoproteins, further complicating the analysis (Stokes et al., 2018). These complexities contribute to the ongoing challenges in reliably measuring 25(OH)D2 for therapeutic monitoring and hence witnessed a variety of methodological and technical advances over the past 50 years. Additional challenges in vitamin D testing have been described in Table 28.1.

27.3 Global landscape of vitamin D methods of analysis underuse

The vitamin D external quality assessment scheme (DEQAS), which monitors method comparability across 54 countries, reports that in October 2017, approximately 76% of the 871 participating laboratories measured their 25(OH)D using an automated immunoassay, 18% using liquid chromatography–tandem mass spectrometry (LC–MS/MS), 3% using a manual immunoassay, and 2% using high performance liquid chromatography (HPLC) (Dirks et al., 2018). However, with the advent of the chemiluminescence immunoassays, the numbers are evolving widely, aided by the ease of automation, rapid turnaround time (TAT), and cost effectiveness (Chen et al., 2020).

27.4 Competitive protein binding assays

The first-generation assays for vitamin D measurement emerged in the 1970s, primarily using competitive protein binding (CPB) techniques for the Nicholas advantage analyzer (Haddad & Chyu, 1971). These assays relied on the competition between endogenous 25(OH)D and

Table 27.1 Challenges associated with the accuracy and reliability of 25-hydroxy vitamin D levels.

Preanalytical issues	Analytical issues	Postanalytical issues
Matrix effect may affect the concentration of vitamin D. Serum values and plasma values may differ	Lack of standardization of assays	Incorrect use of the reference range of cutoff of vitamin D
Incorrect sample handling and storage can cause falsely low levels	Assay variability	Interpretation in light of the patients health and other associated diseases should be done. Clinicians should also carefully consider the broader clinical context when interpreting vitamin D test results, including biological, seasonal, and lifestyle factors
	Interferences from substances like biotin	Use of incorrect units or misinterpretation of values because of incorrect units. Vitamin D testing may be done in ng/ml or nmol/L
Hemolysis or lipemia can also interfere with assay accuracy	Falsely high levels due to cross reactivity with substances of similar structure as 25(OH)D	Population-based cutoffs or reference ranges correlate poorly with serum 25(OH)D concentrations that are associated with biologically and clinically relevant vitamin D effects and are therefore of limited clinical value
	Some assays may not detect very low or very high levels Occasionally, drugs used to treat seizures, particularly phenytoin (epanutin), can interfere with the liver's production of 25-hydroxyvitamin D	

radiolabeled 25(OH)D for binding to vitamin D-binding protein (DBP). The bound and free fractions were separated, and the bound fraction was measured to infer a total 25(OH)D concentration. This method is simple, cost-effective, and ideal for researchers with limited resources. Its ability to work with small sample sizes makes it suitable for rare or difficult-to-obtain specimens. It is particularly useful in early-stage clinical research, where generating preliminary data is more important than precise quantification. This approach provides valuable insights while conserving resources for future advanced studies (Haddad & Chyu, 1971). The method exhibits cross-reactivity with other vitamin D metabolites, potentially resulting in overestimation of levels. It lacks specificity for distinguishing between the D2 and D3 forms, which differ in their bioavailability and physiological efficacy. Additionally, the reliance on labor-intensive and manual processes increases susceptibility to operator variability and errors (Hollis, 2004).

Belsey et al. created a new CBPA in 1974 when researchers expressed a strong desire to streamline the CPBA for circulating 25(OH)D. Using 3H-25(OH)D3, this second-generation CPBA aimed to do away with both individual sample recovery and chromatographic sample purification. However, matrix issues resulting from the extraction of samples with ethanol prevented researchers from validating and adopting the Belsey assay (Belsey et al., 1974). Nonchromatographic CPBA measurements of circulating 25(OH)D were attempted to be validated for a number of years before being abandoned in 1978. Dorantes et al. released the publication that put a stop to nonchromatographic CPBAs for 25(OH)D (Dorantes et al., 1978).

27.5 High performance liquid chromatography

In 1977, the first HPLC tests for 25OHD based on direct UV detection were published (Matsuyama et al., 1979). Chromatography on Sephadex/silica gel columns was performed after a laborious chloroform methanol extraction, and then HPLC with UV detection was performed. Improved internal standard material, reversed-phase HPLC primarily using C18 columns, improved sample extraction using chloroform–methanol and methanol–hexane, and sample extraction using semiautomated technology using acetonitrile postsample precipitation were the main improvements in HPLC methods (Horst et al., 1981; Liel et al., 1988). These methods reduced HPLC run times to less than 10 minutes, increasing sample throughput (Lensmeyer et al., 2006). In addition, Horst et al. (1981) demonstrated a tremendous correlation between UV detection-based HPLC and competitive protein binding analysis (Horst et al., 1981).

Considered one of the most flexible methods for measuring vitamin D, HPLC is high throughout and cost-effective. HPLC enables differentiation between the various forms of vitamin D due to its sensitivity (Tripathi et al., 2022). The limits of detection for vitamin D2 are 2.4 ng/mL, while for vitamin D3 are 0.94 ng/mL (Palaiogiannis et al., 2017).

27.6 Radioimmunoassay

One of the earliest reports of the utilization of radioimmunoassay for vitamin D measurement is by Haddad & Walgate (1976). This initial development is a radioimmunoassay for the binding protein of vitamin D and its metabolites. Radioactive isotope Iodine-125 is the tracer used for this radioimmunoassay (Haddad & Chyu, 1971). The RIAs revolutionised vitamin D measurement by introducing specificity through the use of antibodies (Hollis & Napoli, 1985). RIAs employ antibodies specific to 25(OH)D, improving the ability to discriminate between the target analyte and other metabolites. A radioactive label provided a measurable signal. This assay further formed the basis for a subsequent chemiluminescent detection–based system. The method offers several advantages, including increased sensitivity and specificity compared to CPBA, making it a more reliable option for clinical applications. Its enhanced performance has contributed to broader adoption in clinical laboratories, where accuracy and consistency are essential for patient care and diagnostic decision-making.

The assay involves a 90-minute room temperature incubation with the first antiserum, a 20-minute incubation with a second antiserum, and centrifugation to separate the bound from free fractions. For 25-hydroxy cholecalciferol, the assay's detection limit was 2.8 µg/L. Results from a liquid-chromatographic method that involved selective UV detection of 25-hydroxy calciferol in plasma showed good agreement with the current test (Hollis et al., 1993). However, the method also has notable limitations. Cross-reactivity with other hydroxylated metabolites, such as $24,25(OH)_2D$, can affect the accuracy of results. Additionally, its reliance on radioactive materials raises concerns regarding safety, disposal, and regulatory compliance. Furthermore, the limited ability to differentiate between the D_2 and D_3 forms of vitamin D poses a challenge, particularly in populations that rely heavily on fortified foods or supplements with varying forms of the vitamin (Hollis et al., 1993).

27.7 Enzyme-linked immunosorbent assay

ELISA further updated the measurement of vitamin D by providing a practical, nonradioactive alternative to earlier methods like RIA and CPBA. Microtiter wells coated with sheep polyclonal anti-25-OHD antibody were used in the test. Endogenous 25-OHD that has been separated from DBP in the patient sample competes with biotin-labeled 25-OHD for antibody binding. Following incubation and washing, the biotin-labeled 25-OHD is bound by avidin labeled with horseradish peroxidase. Following a wash, tetramethylbenzidine is added to the unbound avidin, causing horseradish peroxidase to produce a chromogenic product. As the usual chromogenic substrate or reagent used for visualization is 3,3',5,5'-Tetramethylbenzidine (TMB), the wavelength to read the absorbance will be at 405 nm. The concentration of 25-OHD in the sample has an inverse relationship with the amount of color generated. Cross reactivity for 25-OHD2 has been documented using this test (Zerwekh, 2008; Carter, 2012). Over time, ELISA's role in vitamin D assessment has been complemented by more advanced methods, but it remains a widely used and trusted tool, especially in resource-limited laboratories (Alonso et al., 2023). 25-OHD vitamin D ELISA Kits are commonly available for measurement these days.

27.8 Chemiluminescence immunoassay

Subsequently, using chemiluminescent-labeled antibodies to increase sensitivity and precision, chemiluminescence immunoassay (CLIA) has emerged as a popular technique for determining vitamin D levels (Herrmann, 2023). When combined with automated platforms, CLIA enables quick and effective sample processing, which makes it ideal for population-level research evaluating vitamin D deficiency and extensive clinical testing. When compared to more conventional techniques like ELISA and radioimmunoassay (RIA), CLIA offers the advantages of high sensitivity and specificity in vitamin D testing. Even at low concentrations, these characteristics guarantee more precise measurement of vitamin D levels (Ersfeld et al., 2004).

The completely automated chemiluminescence advantage 25(OH)D assay system was first made available by Nichols Diagnostics in 2001 (Ersfeld et al., 2004). This assay system involves immediately adding unextracted serum or plasma to a mixture that contains 25(OH) D3-coated magnetic particles, human DBP, and anti-DBP labeled with acridinium esters. Keep in mind that human DBP was the main binding agent. This assay was therefore a CPBA, similar to the manual process that (Belsey et al., 1974). The primary distinction between both methods was that Belsey used ethanol to deproteinize the material prior to assaying it. The Belsey assay's calibrators were in ethanol. The developers of this assay believed that the serum or plasma sample delivered straight into the assay equipment would be replicated by the calibrators in a serum-based matrix.

The DiaSorin Corporation introduced the fully automated chemiluminescence Liaison 25(OH)D test System in 2004. This test was a true RIA approach since it used an antibody as the principal binding agent rather than human DBP, which was different from the advantage assay. This assay reports a total 25(OH)D concentration and is cospecific for both 25(OH)D$_2$ and 25(OH) D$_3$. It is frequently utilized in sizeable clinical reference laboratories across the globe and has achieved considerable recognition (Ersfeld et al., 2004). Successively, in the second decade of the 2000s then entered Roche Diagnostics Total 25-OH vitamin D in human serum and plasma can be quantitatively determined using the vitamin D total test, a competitive electrochemiluminescence (ECLIA) protein binding method. A vitamin D binding protein (VDBP), which binds to both 25-OH D3 and 25-OH D2, is used as the capture protein in the procedure (Roche Diagnostics, Germany, Mannheim) (Abdel-Wareth et al., 2013). This assay showed a negative bias for the D$_2$ component when compared to the HPLC, which is more pronounced at higher D$_2$ concentrations. This bias is less apparent when D$_3$ is present and may affect the classification of vitamin D sufficiency or insufficiency, particularly in patients on D$_2$ supplementation. However, the bias has minimal impact on clinical decisions, making it clinically acceptable (Farrell et al., 2012). Notably, both CLIA and ECLIA tests provide faster processing times and greater ease of automation, making them ideal for high-volume clinical laboratories. Their ability to handle large sample volumes efficiently enhances their utility in clinical settings.

Liquid chromatography–tandem mass spectrometry (LC–MS/MS) 1979 saw the first publication of an isotope dilution–mass fragmentography test for 1,25(OH)2D (Bjorkhem et al., 1979). Following the addition of [26-2H3]-1,25(OH)2D3 and purification by liquid chromatography, 20 mL of serum was extracted using chloroform–methanol. After being purified, the substance was transformed into trimethylsilyl ether and subjected to GC–MS analysis. With a CV of 5%, the lower limit of quantification (LLOQ) was 13 pmol/L (5 pg/mL); nevertheless, the assay's broad applicability was constrained by the large sample volume (Bjorkhem et al., 1979). LC–MS/MS tests in clinical laboratories often show higher sensitivity, accuracy, and repeatability when compared to earlier techniques for vitamin D metabolites.

The LC–MS/MS is frequently considered to as the "gold standard" technique for measuring vitamin D metabolites due to these benefits (Hollis, 2008; Carter, 2009; El-Khoury et al., 2011). The National Health and Nutritional Examination Survey (NHANES) has suggested LC–MS/MS as the method for determining 25(OH)D since 2008 (Yetley et al., 2010). NHANES looked into 25(OH)D analysis errors using immunoassays and recommended using LC–MS/MS instead of Diasorin RIA going forward (Yetley et al., 2010). Additionally, scientists were advised by the UK Food Standards Agency (FSA) to employ LC–MS/MS rather than alternative techniques (Hunty et al., 2010). APCI (atmospheric pressure chemical ionization) and ESI (electrospray ionization) are the two ionization methods for vitamin D that are most frequently used. Although the exact ion production mechanism varies, both methods ionize at atmospheric pressures. Whereas APCI produces ions through ion/molecule processes in the gas phase, ESI primarily involves ionization in the liquid phase (Xu et al., 2005; Jessome & Volmer, 2006). Moreover, the methods by Tai, Bedner, and Phinney and Stepman et al. were chosen as reference measurement procedures (RMPs) for 25(OH)D2 and 25(OH)D3 metabolites by the Joint Committee on Traceability in Laboratory Medicine (JCTLM), which is in charge of reference materials and RMPs (Tai et al., 2010; Stepman et al., 2011). Both methods are based on isotope-dilution LC–MS/MS without derivatization. More recently, using artificial vitamin D-free whole blood calibration, Müller et al. developed an LC–MS/MS approach in 2017 for the simultaneous detection of 3α-25(OH)3 and 3β-25(OH)D3 in dried blood spots (DBS). Samples of DBS were taken from infants or from some bigger adult cohort studies. Using the LC–MS/MS approach, they were able to compare the 3α-25(OH)3 and 3β-25(OH)D3 concentrations from DBS to serum samples with acceptable method performance characteristics (Müller et al., 2017).

One of the main drawbacks of MS analysis is the matrix effect. Measurement inaccuracies brought on by matrix effects can be corrected through quantification using internal standard (IS) calibration. Stable isotope-labelled (SIL) ISs have been used in the analytical method for vitamin D analysis (Yin et al., 2019), which has further enhanced the analytical advancements in tandem MS analysis. The clinical definition of vitamin D status may change due to the detection of C3-epi-25(OH)D3, which could result in overestimation and possibly undertreatment. Even when C-3 epimers are present, 25(OH)D can be accurately detected using a well-designed tandem mass spectrometry method (Singh et al., 2006). Keeping this in view, the LC–MS/MS has also been endorsed by the Nutritional Laboratory at the CDC and the National Laboratory in the UK for health and nutrition surveys due to its ability to distinguish between various forms of vitamin D in plasma across all age groups. To perform high-throughput studies, high productivity, and quick turnaround times in clinical laboratories, LC–MS/MS frequently requires a high level of technical skill (Zhang & Rockwood, 2015; Clarke et al., 2013; Seger, 2012;

Elpa et al., 2020), making the technique less suitable to the automation framework. In clinical laboratories, almost all LC–MS/MS-based assays are laboratory-developed tests (LDTs). LDTs usually require more time and resources from creation to deployment, QC monitoring, and maintenance than FDA-approved and self-contained clinical analyzers based on immunoassays. This has an impact on the testing turnaround time as a whole. With the advent of automated LC–MS/MS-based assays, a paradigm shift in vitamin D testing platforms is on the horizon (Greaves, 2024).

27.9   Supercritical fluid chromatography

Supercritical fluid chromatography (SFC) emerged as an alternative to conventional normal-phase liquid chromatography (NPLC) (Petruzziello et al., 2017). Supercritical fluid refers to a fluid that possesses both gaseous and liquid properties at the same time, "due to their proximity at a critical point" in terms of pressure and temperature. A commonly used supercritical fluid is carbon dioxide (Di Maio et al., 2021). It offered improved selectivity and sensitivity for profiling a wide range of analytes, including highly liposoluble vitamin D species, which NPLC struggles to quantify accurately in complex biological samples (Petruzziello et al., 2017). However, it required specialized equipment and expertize, which limited its accessibility in many laboratories. The need for supercritical fluids (typically CO_2) as the mobile phase also posed challenges in terms of cost, handling, and the need for pressurized systems. Utilisation of supercritical fluid chromatography in tandem with mass spectrometry for measurement of vitamin D has been done and reported by several research groups (Jumaah et al., 2016; Jenkinson et al., 2018; Oberson et al., 2020; Liu et al., 2019).

27.10   Capillary electrophoresis

Capillary electrophoresis (CE) was first introduced as "free-zone electrophoresis in glass capillaries" by Jorgenson and Lukacs in 1981 (Jorgenson & Lukacs, 1981). Separation of charged molecules has been obtained in high resolution by zone electrophoresis in open tubular capillaries. The separations are even more effective as the high-voltages pulse within the small diameter capillaries (Jorgenson & Lukacs, 1983). CE has been widely used for vitamin analysis as it reduces pretreatment time and low cost (Schepdael, 2023). Various CE separation techniques, including micellar electrokinetic chromatography (MEKC), capillary electrochromatography (CEC), electrokinetic chromatography (EKC), and microemulsion electrokinetic chromatography (MEEKC), have been utilized to analyze vitamin D species in pharmaceuticals and animal feed (Jiao et al., 2016; Kamankesh et al., 2018; Saber-Tehrani et al., 2014; Shahdousti & Aghamohammadi, 2018). Nevertheless, UV detection was the mainstay of the documented CE techniques for vitamin D assay (CE-UV). Due to the short light path in CE and the modest injection volume, CE-UV's detection sensitivity was inadequate, which restricted its practical use.

27.11 Emerging technologies and point of care tests

27.11.1 Biosensors

Due to their exceptional sensitivity, compact size, and less harmful environmental impact, sensors are increasingly vital in analytical applications. Several sensors have been designed for detecting vitamin D, including four affinity-based biosensors developed by Carlucci et al. for measuring 25(OH)D3 (Carlucci et al., 2013). Among these, an electrochemical biosensor demonstrated high sensitivity, with a detection limit of 10 ng/mL and a linear range from 20 to 200 ng/mL. This advancement holds promise for the creation of portable, automated point-of-care devices for vitamin D testing. However, issues including poor selectivity and reproducibility prevent these sensors from being used more widely. The current sensors can only identify one kind of vitamin D or a class of vitamin D compounds in pharmaceuticals or high-concentration solutions. The development of commercial instruments that can concurrently identify several vitamin D species in actual samples may be the main goal of future research to offer robust POCT, especially for community testing.

27.12 Smart phones

Using an immunoassay technique based on gold nanoparticles, Lee et al. created a smartphone platform in 2014 for the colorimetric detection of 25(OH)D in serum (Lee et al., 2014). The platform included a test strip, application software, and a smartphone attachment. The creation of multianalyte detection systems may enable the simultaneous analysis of numerous vitamins, minerals, and other biomarkers, enhancing the accessibility and personalization of health monitoring. This will be made possible by improvements in smartphone capabilities, sensors, and application software with future research. However, there is still a dearth of experimental and comparative data despite prior research efforts to create portable and mobile microfluidics-based technologies for vitamin D testing. 25 (OH)D Assays—the need for standardization.

Since there are numerous vitamin D assays available, variations in the reported 25(OH) vitamin D values for identical samples were noted between assays, emphasizing on the need for standardization. It has also been recognized that there is substantial within-assay variation in 25(OH)D measurement and even greater between-assay variability. The International Federation for Clinical Chemistry and Laboratory Medicine has worked hard in recent years to encourage laboratory assay standardization, which is crucial to obtaining findings that are comparable across various manufacturers and techniques (Bone Metabolism C-BM, 2019). A method is deemed standardized if the bias is less than 5% and the coefficient of variation is less than 10%, according to the 2010 vitamin D standardization program, which was created to enhance the standardization of 25(OH)D assays (Phinney et al., 2017; Sempos et al., 2017). Together with the NIH, the National Institute of Standards launched a vitamin D quality assurance program in 2010. Participants' data submitted using their preferred approach is compared to the NIST standard (LC–MS/MS) (Bedner et al., 2020). The DEQAS, operating by CDC standardization, has been monitoring laboratories assaying 25(OH)D quarterly. Additionally, the College of American Pathologists (CAP) also offered resources for competency exams to ensure standardized external quality assessment. Moreover, the CDC launched the vitamin D standardization-certification program. Participation in the CDC's standardization-certification program is recommended for all test producers (Sempos et al., 2018). This is particularly crucial for assay measurement systems that are currently in development, as well as the manufacturer's internal reference procedure.

27.13   Conclusion and future perspectives

Measuring vitamin D levels continues to pose significant challenges for researchers, laboratories, and healthcare providers. One key issue is the ongoing debate over the optimal 25(OH)D concentration that defines vitamin D deficiency or serves as a threshold for initiating treatment for insufficiency. Another challenge is the considerable variability across different assays and laboratories. Despite 10 years of standardization efforts, the measurement of vitamin D still faces problems with cross-reactivity and matrix effects. In the near future, advancements in more powerful mass spectrometry (MS) instruments are expected to enable the routine quantification of additional vitamin D metabolites further along the metabolic pathway. This will help provide a comprehensive set of meaningful markers for assessing vitamin D status and metabolic phenotypes (Herrmann, 2023). Future efforts should focus on developing new sample preparation methods that utilize innovative materials, eco-friendly solvents, and compact devices to enhance the sensitivity, reliability, and standardization of analytical techniques.

References

Abdel-Wareth, L., Haq, A., Turner, A., Khan, S., Salem, A., Mustafa, F., Hussein, N., Pallinalakam, F., Grundy, L., Patras, G., & Rajah, J. (2013). Total vitamin D assay comparison of the roche diagnostics "Vitamin D Total" electrochemiluminescence protein binding assay with the chromsystems HPLC method in a population with both D2 and D3 forms of Vitamin D. *Nutrients, 5*(3), 971–980. https://doi.org/10.3390/nu5030971.

Alonso, N., Zelzer, S., Eibinger, G., & Herrmann, M. (2023). Vitamin D metabolites: Analytical challenges and clinical relevance. *Calcified Tissue International, 112*(2), 158–177. https://doi.org/10.1007/s00223-022-00961-5.

Atef, S. H. (2018). Vitamin D assays in clinical laboratory: Past, present and future challenges. *Journal of Steroid Biochemistry and Molecular Biology, 175*, 136–137. https://doi.org/10.1016/j.jsbmb.2017.02.011, http://www.elsevier.com/locate/jsbmb.

Bedner, M., Bedner, M., LippaK., A., Tai, S.S., Burdette, C.Q. (2020). NIST/NIH Vitamin D metabolites quality assurance program (VitDQAP).

Belsey, R. E., Deluca, H. F., & Potts, J. T. (1974). A rapid assay for 25-OH-Vitamin D 3 Without Preparative Chromatography*. *The Journal of Clinical Endocrinology & Metabolism, 38*(6), 1046–1051. https://doi.org/10.1210/jcem-38-6-1046.

Bjorkhem, I., Holmberg, I., Kristiansen, T., & Pedersen, J. I. (1979). Assay of 1,25-dihydroxy vitamin D3 by isotope dilution-mass fragmentography. *Clinical Chemistry, 25*(4), 584–588. https://doi.org/10.1093/clinchem/25.4.584.

Bone Metabolism (C-BM). (2019),

Carlucci, L., Favero, G., Tortolini, C., Di Fusco, M., Romagnoli, E., Minisola, S., & Mazzei, F. (2013). Several approaches for vitamin D determination by surface plasmon resonance and electrochemical affinity biosensors. *Biosensors and Bioelectronics, 40*(1), 350–355. https://doi.org/10.1016/j.bios.2012.07.077.

Carter, G. D. (2009). 25-Hydroxyvitamin D assays: The quest for accuracy. *Clinical Chemistry, 55*(7). https://doi.org/10.1373/clinchem.2009.125906, http://www.clinchem.org/cgi/reprint/55/7/1300 United Kingdom.

Carter, G. D. (2012). *Are 25-hydroxyvitamin D assays fit for purpose? Advances in clinical chemistry and laboratory medicine*. United Kingdom: De Gruyter, 58–60. http://doi.org/10.1515/9783110224641.58, https://www.degruyter.com/document/doi/10.1515/9783110224641/html.

Cashman, K. D. (2020). Vitamin D deficiency: Defining, prevalence, causes, and strategies of addressing. *Calcified Tissue International, 106*(1), 14–29. https://doi.org/10.1007/s00223-019-00559-4, http://link.springer.de/link/service/journals/00223/index.htm.

Chen, X., Sun, S., Liu, Q., Ren, F., Bai, Z., & Wang, C. (2020). A rapid chemiluminescence immunoassay for total vitamin D status assessment in fingertip blood. *Clinical Laboratory, 66*(08/2020). https://doi.org/10.7754/clin.lab.2020.191034.

Clarke, W., Rhea, J. M., & Molinaro, R. (2013). Challenges in implementing clinical liquid chromatography-tandem mass spectrometry methods - Seeing the light at the end of the tunnel. *Journal of Mass Spectrometry, 48*(7), 755–767. https://doi.org/10.1002/jms.3214.

Di Maio, E., Iannace, S., & Mensitieri, G. (2021). *Supercritical fluids*. Elsevier BV, 55–68. http://doi.org/10.1016/b978-0-444-63724-6.00004-4.

Dirks, N. F., Ackermans, M. T., Lips, P., de Jongh, R. T., Vervloet, M. G., de Jonge, R., & Heijboer, A. C. (2018). The when, what & how of measuring vitamin D metabolism in clinical medicine. *Nutrients, 10*(4). https://doi.org/10.3390/nu10040482, http://www.mdpi.com/2072-6643/10/4/482/pdf.

Dorantes, L. M., Arnaud, S. B., Arnaud, C. D., & Kilgust, K. A. (1978). Importance of the isolation of 25-hydroxyvitamin D before assay. *Journal of Laboratory and Clinical Medicine, 91*(5), 791–796.

El-Khoury, J. M., Reineks, E. Z., & Wang, S. (2011). Progress of liquid chromatography-mass spectrometry in measurement of vitamin D metabolites and analogues. *Clinical Biochemistry, 44*(1), 66–76. https://doi.org/10.1016/j.clinbiochem.2010.05.007.

Elpa, D. P., Prabhu, G. R. D., Wu, S. P., Tay, K. S., & Urban, P. L. (2020). Automation of mass spectrometric detection of analytes and related workflows: A review. *Talanta, 208*. https://doi.org/10.1016/j.talanta.2019.120304, https://www.journals.elsevier.com/talanta.

Ersfeld, D. L., Rao, D. S., Body, J. J., Sackrison, J. L., Miller, A. B., Parikh, N., Eskridge, T. L., Polinske, A., Olson, G. T., & MacFarlane, G. D. (2004). Analytical and clinical validation of the 25 OH vitamin D assay for the LIAISON® automated analyzer. *Clinical Biochemistry, 37*(10), 867–874. https://doi.org/10.1016/j.clinbiochem.2004.06.006.

Farrell, C. J. L., Martin, S., McWhinney, B., Straub, I., Williams, P., & Herrmann, M. (2012). State-of-the-art vitamin D assays: A comparison of automated immunoassays with liquid chromatography-tandem mass spectrometry methods. *Clinical Chemistry, 58*(3), 531–542. https://doi.org/10.1373/clinchem.2011.172155 Australia, http://www.clinchem.org/content/58/3/531.full.pdf+html.

Greaves, R. F. (2024). LC-MS/MS random access automation - A game changer for the 24/7 clinical laboratory. *Clinical Chemistry and Laboratory Medicine, 62*(7), 1249–1251. https://doi.org/10.1515/cclm-2024-0501, https://www.degruyter.com/journal/key/cclm/html.

Haddad, J. G., & Chyu, K. J. (1971). Competitive protein-binding radioassay for 25-hydroxycholecalciferol. *Journal of Clinical Endocrinology and Metabolism, 33*(6), 992–995. https://doi.org/10.1210/jcem-33-6-992.

Haddad, J. G., & Walgate, J. (1976). Radioimmunoassay of the binding protein for vitamin D and its metabolites in human serum. Concentrations in normal subjects and patients with disorders of mineral homeostasis. *Journal of Clinical Investigation, 58*(5), 1217–1222. https://doi.org/10.1172/JCI108575.

Herrmann, M. (2023). Assessing vitamin D metabolism – Four decades of experience. *Clinical Chemistry and Laboratory Medicine (CCLM), 61*(5), 880–894. https://doi.org/10.1515/cclm-2022-1267.

Holick, M. F. (1996). Vitamin D and bone health. *The Journal of Nutrition, 126*(suppl_4), 1159S. https://doi.org/10.1093/jn/126.suppl_4.1159S.

Hollis, B. W., Kamerud, J. Q., Selvaag, S. R., Lorenz, J. D., & Napoli, J. L. (1993). Determination of vitamin D status by radioimmunoassay with an 125I-labeled tracer. *Clinical Chemistry, 39*(3), 529–533. https://doi.org/10.1093/clinchem/39.3.529.

Hollis, B. W., & Napoli, J. L. (1985). Improved radioimmunoassay for vitamin D and its use in assessing vitamin D status. *Clinical Chemistry, 31*(11), 1815–1819. https://doi.org/10.1093/clinchem/31.11.1815.

Hollis, B. W. (2004). Editorial: The determination of circulating 25-hydroxyvitamin D: No easy task. *Journal of Clinical Endocrinology and Metabolism, 89*(7), 3149–3151. https://doi.org/10.1210/jc.2004-0682.

Hollis, B. W. (2008). Measuring 25-hydroxyvitamin D in a clinical environment: Challenges and needs. *American Journal of Clinical Nutrition, 88*(2). https://doi.org/10.1093/ajcn/88.2.507s, http://www.ajcn.org/cgi/reprint/88/2/507S.

Horst, R. L., Reinhardt, T. A., & Hollis, B. W. (1981). Improved methodology for analysis of plasma vitamin D metabolites. *Analytical Biochemistry, 116*(1), 189–194.

Hunty, A.D.L., Wallace, A.M., Gibson, S., Viljakainen, H., Lamberg-Allardt, C., Ashwell, M. (2010) 8 28 2010/08/28 British Journal of Nutrition 10.1017/S000711451000214X 14752662 4 612 619 United Kingdom UK Food Standards Agency Workshop Consensus Report: The choice of method for measuring 25-hydroxyvitamin D to estimate vitamin D status for the UK National Diet and Nutrition Survey 104

Jenkinson, C., Taylor, A., Storbeck, K. H., & Hewison, M. (2018). Analysis of multiple vitamin D metabolites by ultra-performance supercritical fluid chromatography-tandem mass spectrometry (UPSFC-MS/MS). *Journal of Chromatography B: Analytical Technologies in the Biomedical and Life Sciences, 1087-1088*, 43–48. https://doi.org/10.1016/j.jchromb.2018.04.025, http://www.elsevier.com/inca/publications/store/5/0/2/6/8/9.

Jessome, L. L., & Volmer, D. A. (2006). Ion suppression: A major concern in mass spectrometry. *LCGC North America, 24*(5), 498–510. http://www.chromatographyonline.com/lcgc/issue/issueList.jsp?id=21.

Jiao, Z., Zhang, Y., & Fan, H. (2016). Ultrasonic-microwave method in preparation of polypyrrole-coated magnetic particles for vitamin D extraction in milk. *Journal of Chromatography. A, 1457*, 7–13. https://doi.org/10.1016/j.chroma.2016.06.041.

Jorgenson, J. W., & Lukacs, K. D. (1981). Free-zone in glass capillary. *Clinical Chemistry, 27*(9).

Jorgenson, J. W., & Lukacs, K. D. A. (1983). Capillary zone electrophoresis. *Science (New York, N.Y.), 222*(4621), 266–272. https://doi.org/10.1126/science.6623076.

Jumaah, F., Larsson, S., Essén, S., Cunico, L. P., Holm, C., Turner, C., & Sandahl, M. (2016). A rapid method for the separation of vitamin D and its metabolites by ultra-high performance supercritical fluid chromatography-mass spectrometry. *Journal of Chromatography. A, 1440*, 191–200. https://doi.org/10.1016/j.chroma.2016.02.043, www.elsevier.com/locate/chroma.

Kamankesh, M., Shahdoostkhany, M., Mohammadi, A., & Mollahosseini, A. (2018). Fast and sensitive low density solvent-based dispersive liquid–liquid microextraction method combined with high-performance liquid chromatography for determining cholecalciferol (vitamin D3) in milk and yogurt drink samples. *Analytical Methods, 10*(9), 975–982. https://doi.org/10.1039/C7AY02915B.

Lee, S., Oncescu, V., Mancuso, M., Mehta, S., & Erickson, D. (2014). A smartphone platform for the quantification of vitamin D levels. *Lab on a Chip, 14*(8), 1437–1442. https://doi.org/10.1039/c3lc51375k, http://pubs.rsc.org/en/journals/journal/lc.

Lensmeyer, G. L., Wiebe, D. A., Binkley, N., & Drezner, M. K. (2006). HPLC method for 25-hydroxyvitamin D measurement: Comparison with contemporary assays. *Clinical Chemistry, 52*(6), 1120–1126. https://doi.org/10.1373/clinchem.2005.064956.

Liel, Y., Ulmer, E., Shary, J., Hollis, B. W., & Bell, N. H. (1988). Low circulating vitamin D in obesity. *Calcified Tissue International, 43*(4), 199–201. https://doi.org/10.1007/BF02555135.

Liu, T. T., Cheong, L. Z., Man, Q. Q., Zheng, X., Zhang, J., & Song, S. (2019). Simultaneous profiling of vitamin D metabolites in serum by supercritical fluid chromatography-tandem mass spectrometry (SFC-MS/MS). *Journal of Chromatography B: Analytical Technologies in the Biomedical and Life Sciences, 1120*, 16–23. https://doi.org/10.1016/j.jchromb.2019.04.050, http://www.elsevier.com/inca/publications/store/5/0/2/6/8/9.

Matsuyama, N., Okano, T., Kakada, K., Takao, T., Terao, Y., Hashimoto, N., & Kobayashi, T. (1979). Assay of 25-hydroxyvitamin D3 in human plasma by high-performance liquid chromatography. *Journal of Nutritional Science and Vitaminology, 25*(6), 469–478. https://doi.org/10.3177/jnsv.25.469.

Müller, M. J., Stokes, C. S., & Volmer, D. A. (2017). Quantification of the 3α and 3β epimers of 25-hydroxyvitamin D3 in dried blood spots by LC-MS/MS using artificial whole blood calibration and chemical derivatization. *Talanta, 165*, 398–404. https://doi.org/10.1016/j.talanta.2016.12.081, https://www.journals.elsevier.com/talanta.

Oberson, J. M., Bénet, S., Redeuil, K., & Campos-Giménez, E. (2020). Quantitative analysis of vitamin D and its main metabolites in human milk by supercritical fluid chromatography coupled to tandem mass spectrometry. *Analytical and Bioanalytical Chemistry, 412*(2), 365–375. https://doi.org/10.1007/s00216-019-02248-5.

Palaiogiannis, D., Bekou, E., Pazaitou-Panayiotou, K., Samanidou, V., & Tsakalof, A. (2017). On-line SPE sample treatment as a tool for method automatization and detection limits reduction: Quantification of 25-hydroxyvitamin D3/D2. *Journal of Chromatography B, 1043*, 219–227. https://doi.org/10.1016/j.jchromb.2016.10.006.

Petruzziello, F., Grand-Guillaume Perrenoud, A., Thorimbert, A., Fogwill, M., & Rezzi, S. (2017 Jul). Quantitative profiling of endogenous fat-soluble vitamins and carotenoids in human plasma using an improved UHPSFC-ESI-MS interface. *Analytical Chemistry, 89*(14), 7615–7622.

Phinney, K. W., Sempos, C. T., Tai, S. S. C., Camara, J. E., Wise, S. A., Eckfeldt, J. H., Hoofnagle, A. N., Carter, G. D., Jones, J., Myers, G. L., Durazo-Arvizu, R., Miller, W. G., Bachmann, L. M., Young, I. S., Pettit, J., Caldwell, G., Liu, A., Brooks, S. P. J., Sarafin, K., ... Betz, J. M. (2017). Baseline assessment of 25-hydroxyvitamin d reference material and proficiency testing/external quality assurance material commutability: A Vitamin D Standardization Program Study. *Journal of AOAC International, 100*(5), 1288–1293. https://doi.org/10.5740/jaoacint.17-0291, http://docserver.ingentaconnect.com/deliver/connect/aoac/10603271/v100n5/s9.pdf?expires=1505834187&id=91429740&titleid=41000050&accname=Elsevier+BV&checksum=6D3FE9EDDE2CC60021407CC8D00D4939.

Rahme, M., Al-Shaar, L., Singh, R., Baddoura, R., Halaby, G., Arabi, A., Habib, R. H., Daher, R., Bassil, D., El-Ferkh, K., Hoteit, M., & El-Hajj Fuleihan, G. (2018). Limitations of platform assays to measure serum 25OHD level impact on guidelines and practice decision making. *Metabolism: Clinical and Experimental, 89*, 1–7. https://doi.org/10.1016/j.metabol.2018.09.003.

Saber-Tehrani, M., Aberoomand-Azar, P., & Raziee, M. (2014). Hollow fiber-based liquid phase microextraction coupled with high-performance liquid chromatography for extraction and determination of vitamin D3 in biological fluids. *Journal of Liquid Chromatography and Related Technologies, 37*(3), 404–419. https://doi.org/10.1080/10826076.2012.745144.

Schepdael, A. V. (2023). Capillary electrophoresis as a simple and low-cost analytical tool for use in money-constrained situations. *TrAC Trends in Analytical Chemistry, 160*.

Seger, C. (2012). Usage and limitations of liquid chromatography-tandem mass spectrometry (LC–MS/MS) in clinical routine laboratories. *Wiener Medizinische Wochenschrift, 162*(21-22), 499–504. https://doi.org/10.1007/s10354-012-0147-3.

Sempos, C. T., Betz, J. M., Camara, J. E., Carter, G. D., Cavalier, E., Clarke, M. W., Dowling, K. G., Durazo-Arvizu, R. A., Hoofnagle, A. N., Liu, A., Phinney, K. W., Sarafin, K., Wise, S. A., & Coates, P. M. (2017). General steps to standardize the laboratory measurement of serum total 25-hydroxyvitamin D. *Journal of AOAC International, 100*(5), 1230–1233. https://doi.org/10.5740/jaoacint.17-0259, http://docserver.ingentaconnect.com/deliver/connect/aoac/10603271/v100n5/s3.pdf?expires=1505834165&id=91429729&titleid=41000050&accname=Elsevier+BV&checksum=18FF0B30FB1EF91190BBCCB0E249030A.

Sempos, C. T., Carter, G. D., & Binkley, N. C. (2018). 25-Hydroxyvitamin D assays: Standardization guidelines, problems, and interpretation. *Vitamin D: Fourth Edition, 1*, 939–957. https://doi.org/10.1016/B978-0-12-809965-0.00052-5, http://www.sciencedirect.com/science/book/9780128099650.

Shahdousti, P., & Aghamohammadi, M. (2018). Flotation/ultrasound-assisted microextraction followed by HPLC for determination of fat-soluble vitamins in multivitamin pharmaceutical preparations. *Journal of Separation Science, 41*(8), 1821–1828. https://doi.org/10.1002/jssc.201701347.

Singh, R. J., Taylor, R. L., Reddy, G. S., & Grebe, S. K. G. (2006). C-3 epimers can account for a significant proportion of total circulating 25-hydroxyvitamin D in infants, complicating accurate measurement and interpretation of vitamin D status. *Journal of Clinical Endocrinology and Metabolism, 91*(8), 3055–3061. https://doi.org/10.1210/jc.2006-0710, http://jcem.endojournals.org/cgi/reprint/91/8/3055.

Stepman, H. C. M., Vanderroost, A., Van Uytfanghe, K., & Thienpont, L. M. (2011). Candidate reference measurement procedures for serum 25-hydroxyvitamin D3and 25-hydroxyvitamin D2by using isotope-dilution liquid chromatography-tandem mass spectrometry. *Clinical Chemistry, 57*(3), 441–448. http://doi.org/10.1373/clinchem.2010.152553Belgium, http://www.clinchem.org/cgi/reprint/57/3/441.

Stokes, C. S., Lammert, F., & Volmer, D. A. (2018). Analytical methods for quantification of Vitamin D and implications for research and clinical practice. *Anticancer Research, 38*(2), 1137–1144. https://doi.org/10.21873/anticanres.12332, http://ar.iiarjournals.org/content/38/2/1137.full.pdf.

Tai, S. S. C., Bedner, M., & Phinney, K. W. (2010). Development of a candidate reference measurement procedure for the determination of 25-hydroxyvitamin D3 and 25-hydroxyvitamin D 2 in human serum using isotope-dilution liquid chromatography tandem mass spectrometry. *Analytical Chemistry, 82*(5), 1942–1948. https://doi.org/10.1021/ac9026862.

Tripathi, A., Ansari, M. S., Dandekar, P., & Jain, R. (2022). Analytical methods for 25-hydroxyvitamin D: Advantages and limitations of the existing assays. *The Journal of Nutritional Biochemistry, 109*, 109123. https://doi.org/10.1016/j.jnutbio.2022.109123.

Xu, X., Mei, H., Wang, S., Zhou, Q., Wang, G., Broske, L., Pena, A., & Korfmacher, W. A. (2005). A study of common discovery dosing formulation components and their potential for causing time-dependent matrix effects in high-performance liquid chromatography tandem mass spectrometry assays. *Rapid Communications in Mass Spectrometry, 19*(18), 2643–2650. https://doi.org/10.1002/rcm.2102, http://onlinelibrary.wiley.com/journal/10.1002/(ISSN)1097-0231.

Yetley, E. A., Pfeiffer, C. M., Schleicher, R. L., Phinney, K. W., Lacher, D. A., Christakos, S., Eckfeldt, J. H., Fleet, J. C., Howard, G., Hoofnagle, A. N., Hui, S. L., Lensmeyer, G. L., Massaro, J., Peacock, M., Rosner, B., Wiebe, D., Bailey, R. L., Coates, P. M., Looker, A. C., & Picciano, M.F.(2010).NHANES monitoring of serum 25-hydroxyvitamin D: A roundtable summary, Journal of Nutrition, 10.3945/jn.110.121483 15416100 11 United States http://jn.nutrition.org/cgi/reprint/140/11/2030S 140

Yin, S., Yang, Y., Wu, L., Li, Y., & Sun, C. (2019). Recent advances in sample preparation and analysis methods for vitamin D and its analogues in different matrices. *TrAC Trends in Analytical Chemistry, 110*, 204–220. https://doi.org/10.1016/j.trac.2018.11.008.

Zerwekh, J. E. (2008). Blood biomarkers of vitamin D status. *The American Journal of Clinical Nutrition, 87*(4), 1087S. https://doi.org/10.1093/ajcn/87.4.1087s.

Zhang, Y. V., & Rockwood, A. (2015). Impact of automation on mass spectrometry. *Clinica Chimica Acta, 450*, 298–303. https://doi.org/10.1016/j.cca.2015.08.027, http://www.elsevier.com/locate/clinchim.

CHAPTER 28

Practical tips for maintaining optimal vitamin D levels

Lena Jafri[1], Hafsa Majid[2], and Nayab Afzal[2]

[1]*Section of Chemical Pathology, Department of Pathology and Laboratory Medicine, Aga Khan University, Karachi, Sindh, Pakistan* [2]*Pathology and Laboratory Medicine, Aga Khan University, Karachi, Sindh, Pakistan*

28.1 Introduction

Maintaining optimal vitamin D levels is crucial for overall health, particularly for bone strength, immune function, and well-being. Adequate sunlight exposure is one of the most effective ways to achieve this, with 5–30 minutes of daily sun exposure during mid-morning to early afternoon being ideal (Fact sheet for health professionals, 2017; Wacker & Holick, 2013). Additionally, incorporating vitamin D-rich foods into the diet, such as fatty fish, egg yolks, fortified foods, and UV-exposed mushrooms, is essential. Since vitamin D is fat-soluble, consuming it with healthy fats can enhance absorption (Dawson-Hughes et al., 2015; Dominguez et al., 2021).

Supplementation is recommended for individuals unable to meet their needs through sunlight and diet. Age-specific guidelines suggest 400 IU/day for infants, 600 IU/day for adults, and 800 IU/day for older adults, with vitamin D3 being the preferred form. High-risk groups, such as older adults, obese individuals, and those with chronic conditions, may require tailored supplementation plans and periodic monitoring of serum 25-hydroxyvitamin D [25(OH)D] levels to ensure they remain within the optimal range of 30–50 ng/mL (Grant et al., 2023). Public health measures, including food fortification and awareness campaigns, can further support vitamin D sufficiency on a broader scale, benefiting populations with widespread deficiency (Cashman and O'Neill, 2024).

This chapter explores the strategies, such as sunlight exposure, dietary sources, and supplementation, to achieve sufficiency. Tailored approaches for high-risk groups, periodic monitoring of serum 25(OH)D levels, and guidelines for preventing toxicity through safe dosing and regular testing were discussed in the chapter on vitamin D supplementation. Additionally, the role of public health measures, including food fortification and awareness campaigns, will be highlighted as essential strategies for addressing vitamin D deficiency on a population level.

The Impact of Vitamin D on Health and Disease. DOI: https://doi.org/10.1016/B978-0-443-34037-6.00002-9

28.2   Optimal levels of vitamin D

The determination of optimal vitamin D cutoffs is critical for diagnosing deficiency, guiding supplementation, and improving public health outcomes. This debate, particularly relevant to low-middle income countries (LMICs), including Pakistan, revolves around the interpretation of serum 25(OH)D levels, the best marker for assessing nutritional vitamin D status due to its longer half-life and role as the major circulating form of vitamin D (Hollis et al., 2007).

Vitamin D is pivotal in calcium absorption, bone metabolism, and muscle function. Deficiency can result in short-latency diseases like rickets in children and osteomalacia in adults, as well as long-latency conditions such as osteoporosis and cardiovascular disease (Janoušek et al., 2022). The increased demand for vitamin D testing is evident; data from the large lab networks associated with tertiary care centres showed a sharp rise in tests ordered over eight years, underscoring the clinical and public interest in assessing vitamin D levels (Majid et al., 2022). The guidelines on vitamin D sufficiency vary significantly between the Institute of Medicine (IOM) and the Endocrine Society, USA, creating challenges for clinicians and policymakers. The IOM recommends serum 25OHD levels for bone health outcomes (Demay et al., 2024; Ross et al., 2011). In contrast, the Endocrine Society advocates for a higher threshold to optimize bone, calcium, and muscle metabolism, as shown in Table 28.1 So the safe recommended therapeutic range for serum 25(OH)D levels is 20–50 ng/mL (Rosen et al., 2012).

This lack of consensus impacts how deficiency is diagnosed and managed globally and highlights the need for context-specific thresholds, especially in LMICs, where no standardized guidelines exist. These countries face unique challenges related to vitamin D status, influenced by cultural and geographical factors such as limited sun exposure due to clothing, hijab or covering bodies in Muslim countries and urban lifestyles, with emphasis on using sunscreens and avoiding sun exposure (Mohamed et al., 2021; Roth et al., 2018). Studies indicate widespread deficiency, with large segments of the population showing levels below both IOM and Endocrine Society cutoffs (Javed & Ghafoor, 2016). Lack of local guidelines leaves clinicians to rely on international recommendations, which may not fully

Table 28.1 Comparison of vitamin D guidelines.

Organization	Deficient level (ng/mL)	Sufficient level (ng/mL)	Upper limit for toxicity (ng/mL)	Target outcome
IOM Ströhle (2011)	< 12	≥20	< 50	Bone health (e.g., rickets prevention)
Endocrine Society	< 20	≥30	< 150	Calcium, bone, and muscle health

IOM, Institute of Medicine.

account for local contexts. Defining a range that balances sufficiency and toxicity is essential to avoid toxicity and achieve optimal health outcomes, as excessive supplementation leading to hypercalcemia is as concerning as deficiency. Tailored guidelines could help ensure safe and effective management, optimizing outcomes for bone health while mitigating risks. Ensuring standardized practices will help bridge the gap between deficiency and toxicity, improving population health outcomes effectively.

28.3 Sources of vitamin D

Vitamin D, essential for calcium absorption and bone health, is obtained primarily through sunlight exposure, with dietary sources and supplementation playing a secondary role (Benedik, 2022). It is an essential nutrient that plays a key role in bone health, immune function, and overall health of humans. The primary source of vitamin D is sunlight, as the skin produces it when exposed to UV rays. Fatty fish like salmon, mackerel, and sardines, as well as fortified foods like milk, cereals, and orange juice, are examples of dietary sources. Vitamin D is also found in trace amounts in beef liver and egg yolks. Some people, particularly those with limited sun exposure or certain dietary limitations, may take supplements to meet their vitamin D needs. However, the modern environment, cultural practices, and dietary habits contribute to widespread vitamin D deficiency, creating a global health concern (Charoenngam et al., 2019). Addressing vitamin D deficiency requires careful management to prevent both deficiency-related complications and the risks associated with hypervitaminosis D.

28.4 Sun exposure

The amount of sun exposure necessary to maintain adequate vitamin D levels varies widely and depends on multiple factors, including skin type, geographical location, time of day, and season (Charoenngam et al., 2019). For most individuals, 5–30 minutes of sunlight exposure, at least two times a week, is generally sufficient to meet vitamin D needs. However, this is not universal and should be adjusted based on individual circumstances ("Fact sheet for health professionals," 2017; Wacker & Holick, 2013).

28.5 Skin tone and sunscreens

Skin type plays a crucial role in determining the duration of sun exposure. People with darker skin tones have higher levels of melanin, which reduces the skin's ability to synthesize vitamin D from sunlight. As a result, they may require longer exposure compared to individuals with lighter skin. Melanin, the pigment responsible for skin color, acts as a natural sunscreen, reducing the skin's ability to synthesize vitamin D (Solano, 2020). Research on volunteers with different skin tones showed that fair-skinned individuals experienced significant increases in 25(OH)D levels after sun exposure, while dark-skinned individuals did not show significant changes over the same period (Al-Daghri et al., 2016). Sunscreens offering a sun protection factor (SPF) of 30 or more can diminish the skin's ability to produce vitamin D by as much as 95%–98%. Although sunscreen is crucial for skin cancer prevention, those who frequently apply high-SPF sunscreen might need to seek out other vitamin D sources, like fortified foods or supplements, to fulfill their requirements (Holick, 2007; Holick, 2014; Passeron et al., 2019).

28.6   Geographical location and latitude

Geographical location and latitude also significantly influence vitamin D synthesis, with people living in higher latitudes receiving less UVB radiation, particularly during winter months when the sun's rays are weaker (Kift & Webb, 2024). Populations living at higher altitudes or latitudes are often at risk of lower vitamin D levels due to reduced solar intensity (Mendes et al., 2019). A study by Mata-Greenwood et al. reported that people residing at a high altitude (3600 m) had significantly lower levels of 25(OH)D compared to their low-altitude counterparts (Mata-Greenwood et al., 2023). These findings highlight the need for tailored vitamin D supplementation strategies in high-latitude and high-altitude regions.

28.7   Time of day, season, and body surface area

The duration of sunlight exposure and the area of the body exposed are crucial for vitamin D synthesis (Ladizesky et al., 1995). Research indicates that exposure between 10:00 AM and 3:00 PM is the most efficient time for UVB radiation (Alamri, 2015; Alshahrani et al., 2013). According to Patwardhan et al., 15 minutes of sunlight exposure on one-fourth of the body surface area (e.g., arms, hands, and face) is adequate for vitamin D production in light-skinned populations (Patwardhan et al., 2018). However, darker-skinned individuals or those exposing smaller body areas may require longer exposure times. For optimal vitamin D synthesis, the face, arms, and legs are commonly recommended areas to be expose to sunlight, as they can efficiently absorb UVB rays. However, research suggests that the duration of exposure is more critical than the specific area exposed. Larger areas like the back or torso can increase vitamin D production, but even smaller exposed areas can be effective if the exposure duration is adequate (Holick & Slominski, 2024).

Seasonal changes significantly impact vitamin D synthesis. During winter months, the intensity of UVB radiation is substantially reduced, leading to lower serum 25(OH)D levels (Brustad et al., 2007). Studies confirm that vitamin D status decreases in winter and increases during summer due to seasonal variations in sunlight intensity. This necessitates increased reliance on dietary sources or supplements during the colder months to maintain adequate vitamin D levels (Table 28.2).

Table 28.2 Summary of sunlight requirements for vitamin D synthesis.

Factor	Effect on vitamin D synthesis
Skin tone	Darker skin requires longer exposure due to higher melanin levels
Sunscreen use Chesney (2012)	SPF > 30 blocks 95%–98% of ultra violet B radiation (UVB), limiting vitamin D production
Geographical location	Higher latitudes have reduced UVB availability, especially in winter
Time of day	Midday sun is most effective for UVB exposure
Season Holick (2014)	Winter reduces UVB intensity, lowering vitamin D levels
	Winter months require longer exposure or supplementation
Duration vs. area exposed	Longer exposure is more critical than the specific body area exposed
	15 minutes on 25% of the body area is adequate for light skin; more is needed for dark skin

It is important to balance sun exposure with the risk of skin damage from excessive UV radiation. Using sunscreen or protective clothing after the recommended exposure time can help prevent harmful effects like sunburn or an increased risk of skin cancer. For individuals unable to get sufficient sunlight, such as those in high-latitude regions, during winter months, or with limited outdoor activity, dietary intake and supplementation become essential alternatives to maintain adequate vitamin D levels. Incorporating these considerations into daily routines can help optimize vitamin D production from sunlight while minimizing risks associated with overexposure.

28.8   Diet and D-absorption

A diet rich in vitamin D is essential, particularly for individuals with limited sun exposure. Vitamin D is naturally found in very few foods. However, some common dietary sources include fatty fish such as salmon, mackerel, and tuna, which are among the richest sources of vitamin D (Dominguez et al., 2021; Pfotenhauer & Shubrook, 2017).

For example, wild salmon provides approximately 988 IU of vitamin D per 3.5 ounces, while farmed salmon offers about 250 IU (Lu et al., 2007). Other excellent sources include cod liver oil, which contains around 1360 IU per tablespoon, and egg yolks, which provide approximately 37 IU per yolk. Ultraviolet (UV) light-treated mushrooms also serve as an excellent source of vitamin D (Dominguez et al., 2021; Nölle et al., 2017).

Maximizing vitamin D absorption is critical to ensuring its effectiveness, as it is a fat-soluble vitamin absorbed in the small intestine. Consuming vitamin D-rich foods or supplements with healthy fats, such as olive oil, avocados, or nuts, significantly enhances absorption (Shahsavani et al., 2021). Magnesium, a vital cofactor for activating vitamin D, should also be included in the diet. Foods like spinach, almonds, and pumpkin seeds are excellent magnesium sources that support better metabolism of vitamin D. Vitamin D is a fat-soluble vitamin, meaning it is better absorbed in the presence of dietary fat. Consuming vitamin D-rich foods with healthy fats (e.g., avocados, nuts, olive oil) can improve absorption (Dawson-Hughes et al., 2015; Ravisankar et al., 2015).

Maintaining gut health is equally important, as a healthy gut microbiome aids nutrient absorption. Incorporating probiotics, found in yogurt and kefir, alongside prebiotics like bananas and garlic, can improve gut health and enhance vitamin D uptake. Individuals should avoid excessive intake of fiber or phytates, which can bind to vitamin D and reduce its absorption (Maurya & Aggarwal, 2017). Similarly, staggering high doses of calcium or iron supplements are not recommended, as these nutrients can compete with vitamin D for absorption.

28.9   *Food fortification*

Fortified foods play a crucial role in ensuring adequate vitamin D intake, especially in regions where natural sources are limited. It is a proven, cost-effective strategy to address micronutrient deficiencies. It involves adding vitamins and minerals to staple foods to improve their nutritional value without requiring significant changes in consumer behavior (Nyakundi et al., 2023). In Pakistan, edible oil and ghee are ideal vehicles for fortification due to their high per capita consumption (20–22 kg/year), and the stability of vitamins D in these products makes these foods an ideal product for fortification (Osendarp et al., 2018).

Common fortified options include dairy products such as milk (120–180 IU per cup) (Roth et al., 2018) as well as plant-based alternatives like soy, almond, and oat milk (Cashman & Kiely, 2023; Walia & Chen, 2020). Fortified breakfast cereals and orange juice can add an additional 40–100 IU per serving. Margarine and butter are also fortified with about 60 IU per tablespoon in many countries, making them another convenient dietary source. Many foods are fortified with vitamin D, including milk, orange juice, and cereals. These typically contain either vitamin D2 or D3, depending on the product and manufacturer (Cashman et al., 2021). In Pakistan, the Food Fortification Program (FFP) was funded by the Department for International Development (DFID) and was then implemented between 2016 and 2021. The program's key components, shown in Table 28.3, included technical assistance to governments and industries, public advocacy, and targeted research to inform fortification strategies.

Table 28.3 Key components of the food fortification program.

Component	Description
Technical assistance	Support to federal/provincial governments and industries
Technical assistance	For the wheat flour and edible oil/ghee industries
Public advocacy	Awareness campaigns targeting policymakers and the public
Research and development	Studies on fortification effectiveness and consumer behavior

The Food Fortification Program represents a scalable, sustainable solution to combat micronutrient deficiencies in Pakistan (Evaluation of the Supporting Nutrition in Pakistan Food Fortification Programme Endline Evaluation Report, 2021). By leveraging widespread consumption patterns of edible oil and ghee, this initiative offers a practical approach to improving population health and reducing the socioeconomic burden of malnutrition (Evaluation of the Supporting Nutrition in Pakistan Food Fortification Programme Endline Evaluation Report, 2021). Further expansion, public engagement, and legislative support are vital to achieving comprehensive national coverage. By combining a diet rich in natural and fortified vitamin D sources with strategies to enhance absorption, individuals can maintain optimal vitamin D levels, supporting bone health, immunity, and overall well-being. Regular dietary planning and mindful supplementation can effectively address the body's vitamin D needs.

28.10   Special consideration for high-risk populations

Certain populations are at higher risk for vitamin D deficiency due to underlying medical conditions, lifestyle factors, or physiological changes. For example, individuals with dark complexions, who may have reduced synthesis of vitamin D due to higher melanin levels (Wolf et al., 2022), especially in northern latitudes or resource-poor settings; pregnant individuals, who have increased nutritional needs for both themselves and their developing fetus; older adults, particularly those aged 75 years and older, who may have decreased skin synthesis and dietary intake of vitamin D; individuals with obesity, as they often have lower serum 25(OH)D levels due to factors such as reduced sun exposure and altered metabolism (Holick, 2014; Migliaccio et al., 2019; Wortsman et al., 2000). For high-risk populations, the panel suggests empiric vitamin D supplementation to prevent deficiency (Siddiqee et al., 2022). This includes daily supplementation rather than intermittent high doses, as daily dosing may be more effective in maintaining adequate serum levels; specific attention to those with low baseline 25OHD levels, as they may require higher doses to achieve optimal levels. Regular monitoring of serum 25OHD levels is crucial for high-risk populations to ensure that supplementation is effective and to adjust dosages as needed. This is particularly important for individuals with malabsorption issues or those on medications that may affect vitamin D metabolism. Increasing awareness about the importance of vitamin D and its sources among high-risk populations can help encourage dietary changes and adherence to supplementation guidelines. This includes educating about the benefits of sun exposure, dietary sources of vitamin D, and the importance of regular health check-ups. Table 28.4 shows an overview of high-risk groups and strategies to maintain vitamin D levels in these groups.

Table 28.4 High-risk populations and strategies for optimal vitamin D levels.

Population type	Cause	Strategies for optimal vitamin D levels
Rickets and osteomalacia	Due to severe vitamin D deficiency	• Regular supplementation with vitamin D, along with calcium • Ensuring adequate dietary intake and sun exposure in children, for adults, tailored supplementation regimens
Osteoporosis	Condition with low bone density, more prone to fractures	
CKD	Impaired activation of vitamin D due to reduced kidney function	• Supplementation with active forms of vitamin D, such as calcitriol • Regular monitoring of calcium and phosphate levels
Chronic liver disease	Impaired vitamin D metabolism in liver	• May require higher doses of supplementation, including both inactive and active forms of vitamin D
Hyperparathyroidism	Condition is associated with abnormal calcium and vitamin D metabolism	• Vitamin D supplementation
Medications impacting vitamin D	Drugs, such as anticonvulsants, glucocorticoids, antiretroviral medications, antifungals (e.g., ketoconazole), cholestyramine, and proton pump inhibitors, can interfere with vitamin D metabolism or absorption	• Switch to another drug • May require higher doses of supplementation • Frequent monitoring of vitamin D levels
Older adults and fall risk	Needed for reducing fall risk and improving muscle function in older adults	• Combined vitamin D and calcium supplementation
Obesity (BMI > 30 kg/m²)	Vitamin D is sequestered in adipose tissue, reducing its bioavailability in obese individuals	• Require higher doses of supplementation
Granuloma-forming disorders and lymphomas (sarcoidosis, tuberculosis, histoplasmosis, coccidioidomycosis, berylliosis, and lymphomas)	Increased conversion of vitamin D to its active form, raising the risk of hypercalcemia	• Frequent monitoring of 25OHD levels when supplementing vitamin D
Pregnant and lactating women	Increased requirements to support maternal health and fetal development	• Supplementation with 1000–2000 IU/day of vitamin D • Routine monitoring of 25OHD d

CKD, Chronic kidney disease.

AI disclosure

During the preparation of this work, the authors used ChatGPT for English editing of the document. After using this tool/service, the authors reviewed and edited the content as needed and took full responsibility for the content of the publication.

References

Al-Daghri, N. M., Al-Saleh, Y., Khan, N., Sabico, S., Aljohani, N., Alfawaz, H., Alsulaimani, M., Al-Othman, A. M., & Alokail, M. S. (2016). Sun exposure, skin color and vitamin D status in Arab children and adults. *Journal of Steroid Biochemistry and Molecular Biology, 164*, 235–238. https://doi.org/10.1016/j.jsbmb.2016.05.012, http://www.elsevier.com/locate/jsbmb.

Alamri, F. (2015). Optimum sun exposure times for vitamin D status correction in Saudi Arabia. *European Journal of Preventive Medicine, 3*(5), 147. https://doi.org/10.11648/j.ejpm.20150305.14.

Alshahrani, F. M., Almalki, M. H., Aljohani, N., Alzahrani, A., Alsaleh, Y., & Holick, M. F. (2013). Vitamin D: Light side and best time of sunshine in Riyadh, Saudi Arabia. *Dermato-Endocrinology, 5*(1), 177–180. https://doi.org/10.4161/derm.23351, http://www.landesbioscience.com/journals/dermatoendocrinology/2012DE0209.pdf.

Benedik, E. (2022). Sources of vitamin D for humans. *International Journal for Vitamin and Nutrition Research, 92*(2), 118–125. https://doi.org/10.1024/0300-9831/a000733, https://econtent.hogrefe.com/loi/vit.

Brustad, M., Edvardsen, K., Wilsgaard, T., Engelsen, O., Aksnes, L., & Lund, E. (2007). Seasonality of UV-radiation and vitamin D status at 69 degrees north. *Photochemical & Photobiological Sciences, 6*(8), 903–908. https://doi.org/10.1039/b702947k.

Cashman, K. D., & Kiely, M. (2023). Vitamin D and food fortification. In *Feldman and Pike's vitamin D: Volume two: Disease and therapeutics*. Ireland: Elsevier, 135–160. https://www.sciencedirect.com/book/9780323913386, https://doi.org/10.1016/B978-0-323-91338-6.00008-2.

Cashman, K. D., & O'Neill, C. M. (2024). Strategic food vehicles for vitamin D fortification and effects on vitamin D status: A systematic review and meta-analysis of randomised controlled trials. *Journal of Steroid Biochemistry and Molecular Biology, 238*. https://doi.org/10.1016/j.jsbmb.2023.106448, https://www.sciencedirect.com/science/journal/09600760.

Cashman, K. D., Kiely, M. E., Andersen, R., Grønborg, I. M., Madsen, K. H., Nissen, J., Tetens, I., Tripkovic, L., Lanham-New, S. A., Toxqui, L., Vaquero, M. P., Trautvetter, U., Jahreis, G., Mistry, V. V., Specker, B. L., Hower, J., Knoll, A., Wagner, D., Vieth, R., ... Ritz, C. (2021). Individual participant data (IPD)-level meta-analysis of randomised controlled trials with vitamin D-fortified foods to estimate dietary reference values for vitamin D. *European Journal of Nutrition, 60*(2), 939–959. https://doi.org/10.1007/s00394-020-02298-x, https://www.springer.com/journal/394.

Charoenngam, N., Shirvani, A., & Holick, M. F. (2019). Vitamin D for skeletal and non-skeletal health: What we should know. *Journal of Clinical Orthopaedics and Trauma, 10*(6), 1082–1093. https://doi.org/10.1016/j.jcot.2019.07.004, http://www.elsevier.com/wps/find/journaldescription.cws_home/724754/description#description.

Chesney, R. W. (2012). The five paradoxes of vitamin D and the importance of sunscreen protection. *Clinical Pediatrics, 51*(9), 819–827. https://doi.org/10.1177/0009922811431161.

Dawson-Hughes, B., Harris, S. S., Lichtenstein, A. H., Dolnikowski, G., Palermo, N. J., & Rasmussen, H. (2015). Dietary fat increases vitamin D-3 absorption. *Journal of the Academy of Nutrition and Dietetics, 115*(2), 225–230. https://doi.org/10.1016/j.jand.2014.09.014, http://www.elsevier.com/wps/find/journaldescription.cws_home/727057/description#description.

Demay, M. B., Pittas, A. G., Bikle, D. D., Diab, D. L., Kiely, M. E., Lazaretti-Castro, M., Lips, P., Mitchell, D. M., Murad, M. H., Powers, S., Rao, S. D., Scragg, R., Tayek, J. A., Valent, A. M., Walsh, J. M. E., & McCartney, C. R. (2024). Vitamin D for the prevention of disease: An endocrine society clinical practice guideline. *Journal of Clinical Endocrinology and Metabolism, 109*(8), 1907–1947. https://doi.org/10.1210/clinem/dgae290, https://academic.oup.com/jcem.

Dominguez, L. J., Farruggia, M., Veronese, N., & Barbagallo, M. (2021). Vitamin D sources, metabolism, and deficiency: Available compounds and guidelines for its treatment. *Metabolites, 11*(4), 255. https://doi.org/10.3390/metabo11040255.

Evaluation of the Supporting Nutrition in Pakistan Food Fortification Programme Endline Evaluation Report. (2021).

Fact sheet for health professionals. Natl. Institutes Heal. Off. Diet. Suppl. (2017).

Grant, W. B., Al Anouti, F., Boucher, B. J., Fakhoury, H. M. A., Moukayed, M., Pilz, S., & Al-Daghri, N. M. (2023). Evidence that increasing serum 25(OH)D concentrations to 30 ng/mL in the Kingdom of Saudi Arabia and the United Arab Emirates could greatly improve health outcomes. *Biomedicines, 11*(4). https://doi.org/10.3390/biomedicines11040994, http://www.mdpi.com/journal/biomedicines.

Holick, M. F. (2007). Vitamin D deficiency. *New England Journal of Medicine, 357*(3), 266–281. https://doi.org/10.1056/nejmra070553.

Holick, M. F. (2014). Sunlight, ultraviolet radiation, vitamin D and skin cancer: How much sunlight do we need? In *Advances in Experimental Medicine and Biology, 810*, 1–16. http://www.springer.com/series/5584.

Holick, M. F., & Slominski, A. T. (2024). *Photobiology of vitamin D*. Elsevier BV, 27–45. https://doi.org/10.1016/b978-0-323-91386-7.00006-4.

Hollis, B. W., Wagner, C. L., Drezner, M. K., & Binkley, N. C. (2007). Circulating vitamin D3 and 25-hydroxyvitamin D in humans: An important tool to define adequate nutritional vitamin D status. *Journal of Steroid Biochemistry and Molecular Biology, 103*(3-5), 631–634. https://doi.org/10.1016/j.jsbmb.2006.12.066.

Janoušek, J., Pilařová, V., Macáková, K., Nomura, A., Veiga-Matos, J., Silva, D. Dd, Remião, F., Saso, L., Malá-Ládová, K., Malý, J., Nováková, L., & Mladěnka, P. (2022). Vitamin D: Sources, physiological role, biokinetics, deficiency, therapeutic use, toxicity, and overview of analytical methods for detection of vitamin D and its metabolites. *Critical Reviews in Clinical Laboratory Sciences, 59*(8), 517–554. https://doi.org/10.1080/10408363.2022.2070595, http://www.tandfonline.com/loi/ilab20.

Javed, R., & Ghafoor, F. (2016). A review of vitamin D in Pakistani population. *Pakistan Journal of Medical Research, 55*(2).

Kift, R. C., & Webb, A. R. (2024). Globally estimated UVB exposure times required to maintain sufficiency in vitamin D levels. *Nutrients, 16*(10). https://doi.org/10.3390/nu16101489.

Ladizesky, M., Lu, Z., Oliveri, B., Roman, N. S., Diaz, S., Holick, M. F., & Mautalen, C. (1995). Solar ultraviolet B radiation and photoproduction of vitamin D3 in central and southern areas of argentina. *Journal of Bone and Mineral Research, 10*(4), 545–549. https://doi.org/10.1002/jbmr.5650100406.

Lu, Z., Chen, T. C., Zhang, A., Persons, K. S., Kohn, N., Berkowitz, R., Martinello, S., & Holick, M. F. (2007). An evaluation of the vitamin D3 content in fish: Is the vitamin D content adequate to satisfy the dietary requirement for vitamin D? *The Journal of Steroid Biochemistry and Molecular Biology, 103*(3-5), 642–644. https://doi.org/10.1016/j.jsbmb.2006.12.010.

Majid, H., Abid, M. A., Zehra, N., Muneer, S., Jafri, L., & Khan, A. H. (2022). Paradigm shifts in vitamin D testing and diagnosis: A decade-long observational study. *Pakistan Journal of Pathology, 33*(1), 1–4. https://doi.org/10.55629/pakjpathol.v33i1.690.

Mata-Greenwood, E., Westenburg, H. C., Zamudio, S., Illsley, N. P., & Zhang, L. (2023). Decreased vitamin D levels and altered placental vitamin D gene expression at high altitude: role of genetic ancestry. *International Journal of Molecular Sciences, 24*(4), 3389.

Maurya, V. K., & Aggarwal, M. (2017). Factors influencing the absorption of vitamin D in GIT: An overview. *Journal of Food Science and Technology, 54*(12). https://doi.org/10.1007/s13197-017-2840-0, http://www.springerlink.com/content/121580/.

Mendes, M. M., Darling, A. L., Hart, K. H., Morse, S., Murphy, R. J., & Lanham-New, S. A. (2019). Impact of high latitude, urban living and ethnicity on 25-hydroxyvitamin D status: A need for multidisciplinary action? *Journal of Steroid Biochemistry and Molecular Biology, 188*, 95–102. https://doi.org/10.1016/j.jsbmb.2018.12.012, http://www.elsevier.com/locate/jsbmb.

Migliaccio, S., Di Nisio, A., Mele, C., Scappaticcio, L., Savastano, S., & Colao, A. (2019). Obesity and hypovitaminosis D: Causality or casualty? *International Journal of Obesity Supplements, 9*(1), 20–31. https://doi.org/10.1038/s41367-019-0010-8.

Mohamed, S. H., Alizadeh, S., Tessema, M., Samuel, A., Petros, A., & Hussen, A. (2021). *Clothing type and vitamin D status: A systematic review and meta-analysis. Research Square.* Ethiopia Research Square. https://www.researchsquare.com/browse, https://doi.org/10.21203/rs.3.rs-376562/v1.

Nölle, N., Argyropoulos, D., Ambacher, S., Müller, J., & Biesalski, H. K. (2017). Vitamin D2 enrichment in mushrooms by natural or artificial UV-light during drying. *LWT - Food Science and Technology, 85,* 400–404. https://doi.org/10.1016/j.lwt.2016.11.072.

Nyakundi, P. N., Némethné Kontár, Z., Kovács, A., Járomi, L., Zand, A., & Lohner, S. (2023). Fortification of staple foods for household use with vitamin D: An overview of systematic reviews. *Nutrients, 15*(17), 3742. https://doi.org/10.3390/nu15173742.

Osendarp, S. J. M., Martinez, H., Garrett, G. S., Neufeld, L. M., De-Regil, L. M., Vossenaar, M., & Darnton-Hill, I. (2018). Large-scale food fortification and biofortification in low- and middle-income countries: a review of programs, trends, challenges, and evidence gaps. *Food and Nutrition Bulletin, 39*(2), 315–331. https://doi.org/10.1177/0379572118774229.

Patwardhan, V. G., Mughal, Z. M., Chiplonkar, S. A., Webb, A. R., Kift, R., Khadilkar, V. V., Padidela, R., & Khadilkar, A. V. (2018). Duration of casual sunlight exposure necessary for adequate Vitamin D status in Indian Men. *Indian Journal of Endocrinology and Metabolism, 22*(2), 249–255.

Passeron, T., Bouillon, R., Callender, V., Cestari, T., Diepgen, T. L., Green, A. C., van der Pols, J. C., Bernard, B. A., Ly, F., Bernerd, F., Marrot, L., Nielsen, M., Verschoore, M., Jablonski, N. G., & Young, A. R. (2019). Sunscreen photoprotection and vitamin D status. *British Journal of Dermatology, 181*(5), 916–931. https://doi.org/10.1111/bjd.17992.

Pfotenhauer, K. M., & Shubrook, J. H. (2017). Vitamin D deficiency, its role in health and disease, and current supplementation recommendations. *Journal of Osteopathic Medicine, 117*(5), 301–305. https://doi.org/10.7556/jaoa.2017.055.

Ravisankar, P., Reddy, A. A., Nagalakshmi, B., Koushik, O. S., Kumar, B. V., & Anvith, P. S. (2015). The comprehensive review on fat soluble vitamins. *IOSR Journal of Pharmacy, 5*(11), 12–28.

Rosen, C. J., Abrams, S. A., Aloia, J. F., Brannon, P. M., Clinton, S. K., Durazo-Arvizu, R. A., Gallagher, J. C., Gallo, R. L., Jones, G., Kovacs, C. S., Manson, J. A. E., Mayne, S. T., Ross, A. C., Shapses, S. A., & Taylor, C. L. (2012). IOM committee members respond to endocrine society vitamin D guideline. *Journal of Clinical Endocrinology and Metabolism, 97*(4), 1146–1152. https://doi.org/10.1210/jc.2011-2218, http://jcem.endojournals.org/content/97/4/1146.full.pdf+html United States.

Ross, A. C., Manson, J. A. E., Abrams, S. A., Aloia, J. F., Brannon, P. M., Clinton, S. K., Durazo-Arvizu, R. A., Gallagher, J. C., Gallo, R. L., Jones, G., Kovacs, C. S., Mayne, S. T., Rosen, C. J., & Shapses, S. A. (2011). The 2011 report on dietary reference intakes for calcium and vitamin D from the Institute of Medicine: What clinicians need to know. *Journal of Clinical Endocrinology and Metabolism, 96*(1), 53–58. https://doi.org/10.1210/jc.2010-2704, http://jcem.endojournals.org/cgi/reprint/96/1/53.

Roth, D. E., Abrams, S. A., Aloia, J., Bergeron, G., Bourassa, M. W., Brown, K. H., Calvo, M. S., Cashman, K. D., Combs, G., De-Regil, L. M., Jefferds, M. E., Jones, K. S., Kapner, H., Martineau, A. R., Neufeld, L. M., Schleicher, R. L., Thacher, T. D., & Whiting, S. J. (2018). Global prevalence and disease burden of vitamin D deficiency: A roadmap for action in low-and middle-income countries. John Wiley and Sons Inc, Canada. *Annals of the New York Academy of Sciences, 1430*(1), 44–79. https://doi.org/10.1111/nyas.13968, http://onlinelibrary.wiley.com/journal/10.1111/(ISSN)1749-6632.

Shahsavani, Z., Asadi, A., Shamshirgardi, E., Akbarzadeh, M., & Vitamin, D. (2021). Magnesium and their interactions: A review. *International Journal of Nutrition Sciences, 6*(3), 113–118. https://doi.org/10.30476/IJNS.2021.91766.1144, https://ijns.sums.ac.ir/article_47789_d57ff3f9dd0ed84f0bb26798b73516c9.pdf.

Siddiqee, M. H., Bhattacharjee, B., Siddiqi, U. R., & Rahman, M. M. (2022). High burden of hypovitaminosis D among the children and adolescents in South Asia: A systematic review and meta-analysis. *Journal of Health, Population, and Nutrition, 41*(1). https://doi.org/10.1186/s41043-022-00287-w, https://jhpn.biomedcentral.com/.

Solano, F. (2020). Photoprotection and skin pigmentation: Melanin-related molecules and some other new agents obtained from natural sources. *Molecules, 25*(7), 1537. https://doi.org/10.3390/molecules25071537.

Ströhle (2011). The updated recommendations of the US Institute of Medicine (IOM) on the intake of vitamin D. A critical appraisal. *Medizinische Monatsschrift fur Pharmazeuten, 34*(8), 291–298.

Wacker, M., & Holick, M. F. (2013). Sunlight and vitamin D: A global perspective for health. *Dermato-Endocrinology, 5*(1), 51–108. https://doi.org/10.4161/derm.24494, http://www.landesbioscience.com/journals/dermatoendocrinology/2013DE0239.pdf.

Walia, N., & Chen, L. (2020). Pea protein based vitamin D nanoemulsions: Fabrication, stability and in vitro study using Caco-2 cells. *Food chemistry, 305*, 125475. https://doi.org/10.1016/j.foodchem.2019.125475.

Wolf, S. T., Dillon, G. A., Alexander, L. M., Jablonski, N. G., & Kenney, W. L. (2022). Integrative cardiovascular physiology and pathophysiology: Skin pigmentation is negatively associated with circulating vitamin D concentration and cutaneous microvascular endothelial function. *American Journal of Physiology-Heart and Circulatory Physiology, 323*(3).

Wortsman, J., Matsuoka, L. Y., Chen, T. C., Lu, Z., & Holick, M. F. (2000). Decreased bioavailability of vitamin D in obesity. *American Journal of Clinical Nutrition, 72*(3), 690–693. https://doi.org/10.1093/ajcn/72.3.690, http://www.ajcn.org/contents-by-date.2005.shtml.

CHAPTER 29

The Vitamin D supplementation protocols

Lena Jafri[1], Hafsa Majid[2], and Nayab Afzal[2]

[1]Section of Chemical Pathology, Department of Pathology and Laboratory Medicine, Aga Khan University, Karachi, Sindh, Pakistan [2]Pathology and Laboratory Medicine, Aga Khan University, Karachi, Sindh, Pakistan

29.1 Introduction

Global literature highlights widespread vitamin D deficiency, despite its availability from various sources such as sunlight exposure and diet (Benedik, 2022; Cui et al., 2023). However, modern lifestyle changes have reduced the effectiveness of these sources in meeting daily requirements. Many individuals now avoid sunlight due to medical or aesthetic concerns, and the increased use of sunscreens further limits the skin's ability to synthesize vitamin D naturally (Passeron et al., 2019; Skaaby et al., 2016) Additionally, as a fat-soluble vitamin, vitamin D is commonly added to fatty foods like oil, ghee, and butter. However, growing awareness of cardiometabolic risks, combined with increased focus on weight manage mental and physical appearance has led many to limited intake of such foods, further contributing to vitamin D insufficiency (Lips et al., 2014).

Vitamin D supplementation is a key component of preventive and therapeutic healthcare, but its efficacy relies on appropriate dosing and strict adherence to established protocols (Bouillon et al., 2022). As awareness of vitamin D's role in managing various diseases grows, there has been a corresponding increase in its prescription by physicians (Rebelos et al., 2023). According to a survey conducted to analyze changes in prescription patterns of vitamin D supplements in the adult population of Tuscany, Italy, over an 8 year period (2006–13), showed a significant increase in vitamin D prescriptions across all age groups and genders, particularly for cholecalciferol, which showed a 75.3 fold rise. While only a modest rise was noted in the use of calcium salts combined with cholecalciferol and calcium alone. The total reimbursement costs for vitamin D-related compounds rose substantially, from €3.24 million in 2006 to €8.16 million in 2013 (Cianferotti et al., 2015). This trend highlights growing awareness of the potential consequences of poor vitamin D status.

The increasing trend in vitamin D prescriptions has raised concerns about toxicity, particularly due to the wide therapeutic index of the vitamin. There is also a growing use of over-the-counter (OTC) vitamin D supplements for extended periods, which can result in excessive dosing and serious health complications . The ease of access to OTC vitamin D supplements has heightened the risk of

The Impact of Vitamin D on Health and Disease. DOI: https://doi.org/10.1016/B978-0-443-34037-6.00023-6

self-medication, unintentional overdosing, and potential toxicity (Marcinowska-Suchowierska et al., 2018). Early detection and effective management of vitamin D toxicity are therefore essential to prevent severe outcomes (Galior et al., 2018). Current practices among physicians vary widely, ranging from low-dose to mega-dose supplementation, differing routes of administration, and inconsistent treatment durations and monitoring practices (Bilezikian et al., 2021; Romagnoli et al., 2008; Takács et al., 2017). Addressing these concerns requires raising awareness among healthcare providers about appropriate supplementation protocols, the toxic potential of high-dose vitamin D, and the importance of careful use and consistent monitoring. This chapter will provide guidance on evidence-based vitamin D supplementation protocols designed to treat deficiency effectively and improve treatment outcomes for this critical clinical challenge.

29.2   Daily requirements of vitamin D

The maintenance doses of vitamin D, commonly referred to as the recommended dietary allowance (RDA), and treatment doses serve distinct purposes and differ significantly in their application. The maintenance RDA aims to prevent deficiency and promote overall health in healthy individuals, whereas treatment doses are designed to address existing deficiencies or specific medical conditions more aggressively (Holick et al., 2007; National Institutes of Health NIH, 2021). The maintenance RDA for vitamin D varies by age, gender, and life stage, shown in Table 29.1.

These doses are intended for long-term use to sustain serum 25-hydroxyvitamin D [25(OH)D] levels of at least 20 ng/mL (50 nmol/L), which is considered adequate for bone health and general wellbeing. Maintenance RDAs are targeted toward healthy individuals without significant deficiencies or underlying medical conditions. In contrast, treatment doses of vitamin D are prescribed to correct deficiency, typically identified by serum 25(OH)D levels below 20 ng/mL (50 nmol/L) or according to the Institute of Medicine's (IOM) recommendation below 12 ng/mL (30 nmol/L). Vitamin D deficiency treatment regimens are considerably higher than maintenance doses, but once optimal serum levels, generally within the range of 30–50 ng/mL (75–125 nmol/L), are achieved, a maintenance dose or RDA is initiated to sustain these levels. Adequate vitamin D levels (30–50 ng/mL or 75–125 nmol/L) can often be maintained through appropriate sun exposure, dietary intake, and supplementation when necessary. The most followed recommendations for RDA and TUI for vitamins are by the Institute of Medicine's (IOM), now known as the National Academy of Medicine, and represent a baseline standard for all individuals (Ströhle, 2011).

29.3   Vitamin D deficiency management

29.3.1   When to treat?

Individuals with confirmed vitamin D deficiency, defined as serum 25(OH)D concentrations below 20 ng/mL (50 nmol/L), should receive treatment (de la Guía-Galipienso et al., 2021).

Table 29.1 Recommended daily allowance and tolerable upper intake values for vitamin D.

Age (RDA)	All genders			Pregnancy and lactation		
	TUI		**RDA**	**TUI**		**RDA**
	IOM (Ströhle, 2011)	**Endocrine society (Holick et al., 2011)**		**IOM (Ströhle, 2011)**	**Endocrine society (Holick et al., 2011)**	
0–6 months[a]	400 IU (10 µg)	1000 IU (25 µg)	2000 IU (50 µg)			
7–12 months[a]		1500 IU (38 µg)				
1–3 years	600 IU (15 µg)	2500 IU (63 µg)	4000 IU (100 µg)			
4–8 years		3000 IU (75 µg)				
9–13 years		4000 IU (100 µg)				
14–18 years				600 IU (15 µg)	4000 IU (100 µg)	5000 IU (125 µg)
19–50 years				–	–	10,000 IU (250 µg)
51–70 years				–	–	
71+ years					800 IU (20 µg)	

1 international unit (IU) of vitamin D is equal to 0.025 µg.

[a] Adequate Intake (AI). Ref: NIH (National Institute of Health). Vitamin D. Fact sheet for health professionals. Natl. Institutes. Heal. Off. Diet. Suppl. Available online https://ods.od.nih.gov/factsheets/VitaminC-HealthProfessional. 2017., IOM: Institute of Medicine.

Certain populations are at higher risk of deficiency, including the elderly, pregnant and lactating women, infants, children, individuals with obesity, and those with chronic diseases such as kidney or liver disease (Giustina et al., 2023; Franca Gois et al., 2018; Mulligan et al., 2010; Vranić, Mikolašević and Milić, 2019; Chen et al., 2020). Regular screening for vitamin D levels is recommended for these at-risk groups to facilitate early identification of deficiency and timely initiation of treatment. While the general population need not be screened to identify vitamin D deficiency.

The primary goal of treatment is to achieve serum 25(OH)D levels above 50 nmol/L (20 ng/mL), as severe deficiency (serum levels below 30 nmol/L or 12 ng/mL) is associated with increased risks of mortality, infections, and other health complications. Prompt treatment is essential for individuals with severe deficiencies to mitigate these risks. Additionally, symptoms such as bone pain, muscle weakness, or other signs indicative of deficiency should prompt evaluation and appropriate intervention (Amrein et al., 2020).

Vitamin D supplementation is also advised for individuals who may not have established indications for treatment or routine 25(OH)D testing but are at risk of deficiency. While those with lower baseline 25(OH)D levels are likely to benefit most from supplementation, there is a lack of robust evidence regarding the efficacy and safety of supplementation in such populations. Addressing these gaps in evidence and tailoring interventions to individual needs are critical for improving health outcomes related to vitamin D deficiency.

29.4   Choosing the route of administration

Oral supplementation is the most commonly used and preferred route for vitamin D administration. It is convenient, effective, and widely accepted for maintaining or correcting vitamin D levels in most individuals (Pludowski et al., 2018). Oral doses can be tailored to individual needs and severity of deficiency, with regimens ranging from daily, weekly, or even monthly administrations. Vitamin D is available in various forms, and most multivitamin preparations contain 800 to 1000 IU (20–25 µg) per dose (Nair & Maseeh, 2012). These doses are sufficient for the general population and mild deficiencies, making oral supplementation the primary approach in most clinical scenarios (Giustina et al., 2024; "Doses and Schemes for Correcting Vitamin D Deficiency: An Update, 2024; Holick et al., 2007; Nair & Maseeh, 2012). On the other hand, injectable vitamin D offers distinct advantages, particularly for patients with malabsorption syndromes or bariatric surgeries (Gupta et al., 2017). For individuals with malabsorption issues, such as those with gastrointestinal disorders, achieving adequate serum levels of vitamin D through oral supplements alone may not be effective (Hultin et al., 2018).

In such cases, higher oral doses or alternative routes of administration, such as intramuscular injections, may be necessary. Intramuscular administration offers a feasible and effective solution for patients who cannot absorb vitamin D adequately through the gastrointestinal tract. By bypassing the gastrointestinal tract, injections ensure effective delivery of vitamin D, even in cases where oral absorption is impaired. Injectable forms also allow for rapid correction of vitamin D levels, making them suitable for patients with severe deficiency or those requiring immediate replenishment. A single intramuscular injection can provide long-lasting effects, often for several months, improving adherence in patients who struggle with daily or weekly oral doses. However, injections are more invasive, typically require administration by healthcare professionals, and are generally more expensive. Moreover, there is a risk of overdosing with high-dose injections if not carefully monitored. This route is particularly useful in cases of severe deficiency or when compliance with frequent oral dosing is a challenge (Bilezikian et al., 2021).

Vitamin D supplements are also available in various delivery forms, including capsules, softgels, tablets, and liquid drops (Helde Frankling et al., 2020). Liquid formulations are especially useful for infants and individuals who have difficulty swallowing pills. These delivery options make vitamin D supplementation accessible to people across different age groups and health conditions. Oral supplementation remains the most acceptable and feasible intervention for the majority of patients. However, intramuscular or intravenous administration should be considered in specific cases where oral supplementation is ineffective or impractical. By tailoring the mode of administration to the individual's needs, vitamin D levels can be effectively managed to optimize health outcomes (Chauhan et al., 2023).

29.5 Types, forms, and choices of vitamin D supplements

Several types of vitamin D supplements are available, each catering to diverse needs and preferences. Vitamin D2 (ergocalciferol) is derived from plant sources such as yeast and fungi and is often used in prescription supplements and fortified foods. While it effectively raises serum 25(OH)D levels, it is generally considered less potent and has a shorter duration of action compared to vitamin D3. Being plant-based, vitamin D2 is widely available and suitable for individuals with dietary restrictions, such as vegans (Bikle, 2014).

Vitamin D3 (cholecalciferol) is a commonly recommended form of supplementation due to its superior efficacy in raising and maintaining serum 25(OH)D levels. It is typically derived from animal sources, including lanolin (from sheep's wool) or fish liver oil. Vegan-friendly options made from lichen are also available. Vitamin D3 is naturally synthesized in the skin in response to sunlight exposure, further supporting its preference in supplementation (Dominguez et al., 2021). Some supplements combine vitamin D with other nutrients, such as calcium, to support bone health. These combination products are particularly beneficial for populations with specific nutritional needs, such as the elderly or postmenopausal women (Bolland et al., 2018).

Among the available options, vitamin D3 is generally preferred over vitamin D2 due to its greater potency and ability to maintain serum 25(OH)D levels for longer periods. While most vitamin D3 is derived from animal sources, vegan options from lichen cater to those with specific dietary preferences. Vitamin D2, being plant-based, is an alternative for those avoiding animal products, although it is less effective than D3 in maintaining optimal levels (van den Heuvel et al., 2024). Vitamin D supplements are available in various forms and combinations to suit the needs of different populations. While both vitamin D2 and D3 are effective, D3 is preferred for its superior efficacy. Combined formulations and diverse delivery options enhance the flexibility of supplementation, making it easier to address individual preferences and medical requirements. Selecting the appropriate vitamin D supplement requires consideration of dietary restrictions, health needs, and convenience, with regular monitoring to ensure optimal health outcomes (Bolland et al., 2018).

29.6 Low-dose versus megadose supplements

Recommendation is to use daily, lower-dose vitamin D supplementation rather than higher-dose regimens for treatment. The recommendation emphasizes the potential benefits of daily dosing in maintaining consistent and adequate vitamin D levels (Pludowski et al., 2018). For individuals needing maintenance supplementation, lower daily doses ranging from 400 to 2000 IU are commonly advised (Pludowski et al., 2018; Haines & Park, 2012). These doses are sufficient to maintain adequate vitamin D levels, particularly for those who are not severely deficient. OTC supplements in these dosage ranges are widely available, offering flexibility for individuals to select the appropriate level based on their needs.

In cases of severe deficiency (serum 25OHD levels < 12 ng/ml or 20 nmol/L), high-dose vitamin D supplementation, often referred to as megadoses (doses higher than 100,000 IU of vitamin D) may be necessary to rapidly correct serum 25(OH)D levels (Narvaez et al., 2020). A typical protocol involves a loading dose of 50,000 IU weekly for several weeks, followed by a maintenance dose to sustain adequate levels (van Groningen et al., 2010). These high-dose supplements are generally prescribed and require close monitoring by a healthcare professional to avoid the risk of toxicity. While effective for correcting deficiencies, megadose should be used cautiously, as prolonged or excessive dosing can lead to adverse effects such as hypercalcemia (Ataide et al., 2021; Haines & Park, 2012).

Prescription formulations of vitamin D, available in higher concentrations, are often necessary for individuals with significant deficiencies or specific medical conditions (Baeke et al., 2010). These formulations may contain either vitamin D2 or D3 and are typically used for short-term correction under medical supervision (Bolland et al., 2018). In contrast, OTC vitamin D supplements are widely accessible in various dosages, ranging from 400 IU to 2000 IU, and are suitable for individuals requiring maintenance supplementation. These options allow flexibility and ease of access for those without severe deficiencies or complex medical needs (Demay et al., 2024).

Treatment of vitamin D deficiency should be tailored to the individual, focusing on high-risk populations and those with severe deficiency (Jacot et al., 2016). Oral vitamin D3 is the preferred form due to its superior efficacy, and the choice between low-dose daily supplementation and high-dose regimens depends on the severity of deficiency and the patient's clinical circumstances. Regular monitoring of serum vitamin D levels is essential to ensure the safety and effectiveness of treatment. A tailored approach that promotes daily lower-dose supplementation, while addressing individual baseline levels and health conditions, is a preferred strategy for achieving and maintaining optimal vitamin D status.

29.7   Vitamin D replacement protocols

The growing awareness of the beneficial effects of vitamin D in various diseases has led to increased prescriptions by physicians, which can lead to toxicity. Due to a wide therapeutic index, it may happen at excessively high doses, and if the supplements are taken for prolonged periods. The primary treatment goal is to achieve a serum 25(OH)D level of > 50 nmol/L (or 20 ng/ml), and severe deficiency should be avoided due to its association with increased risks of mortality and other health issues (Demay et al., 2024).

29.8   D-dosage and frequency

Significant variation exists in physicians' practices regarding the use of mega-dose vitamin D preparations. A common approach involves administering 600,000 IU intramuscularly every three months, while others recommend a second injection after 1 month in cases of severe deficiency. Some physicians prescribe three injections of vitamin D at 2-week intervals, followed by a repeat regimen after 3 months if required. In clinical trials, such as the VITDALIZE study, a loading dose of 540,000 IU oral/enteral vitamin D3 was administered to patients with severe deficiency (serum 25OHD < 30 nmol/L or 12 ng/mL). These wide-ranging practices highlight the need for standardized protocols, as summarized in Table 29.2, which outlines recommendations from different professional societies.

Recent research has explored various dosing regimens, routes of administration, and intervals for vitamin D supplementation. In a prospective intervention study by Masood et al., 100 patients with vitamin D deficiency (VDD) were randomised to receive either 600,000 IU or 200,000 IU of cholecalciferol through oral or intramuscular routes (Masood et al., 2015). Serum 25OHD levels were measured at 2, 4, and 6 months, revealing that VDD was corrected in 70.6% to 93.85% of participants. All groups demonstrated sustained, significantly elevated vitamin D levels during the 6-month follow-up (Masood et al., 2015). Similarly, Basit et al. reported a significant increase in vitamin D and calcium levels following a single intramuscular dose of 600,000 IU of vitamin D3 for the treatment of painful diabetic neuropathy, with benefits observed up to 20 weeks (Basit et al., 2016).

Table 29.2 Treatment protocols for correction of vitamin D deficiency.

Guidelines/recommendations by	Recognition of vitamin D deficiency	Replacement protocol
Endocrine Society (Holick et al., 2011)	25(OH)D below 20 ng/ml (50 nmol/liter)	• 0–18 years—50,000 IU of D2 or D3 once weekly for 6 weeks 400–1000 IU/day or 2000 IU/day for 6 weeks • > 18 years—50,000 IU of D2 or vitamin D3 once a week for 8 weeks or its equivalent of 6000 IU of vitamin D2 or vitamin D3 daily to achieve a blood level of 25(OH)D above 30 ng/ml, followed by maintenance therapy of IU/day
American Family Physician (LeFevre & LeFevre, 2018)	Below 12 ng/mL (30 nmol/ L)	D_2 at 50,000 IU per week for 8 weeks
Royal Children's Hospital, Melbourne, Australia (Vitamin D deficiency. Royal Children's Hospital Melbourne, 2025)	25(OH)D below 20 ng/ml (50 nmol/liter)	• Preterm—800 IU/Day, review after 1 month 0–3 months—1000 IU/day for 3 months 3–12 months—1000 IU/day for 3 months OR 50,000 IU once and review after 1 month • 1–18 years—1000–2000 IU/day for 6 months OR 3000–4000 IU/day for 3 months OR 150,000 stat and repeat at 6 weeks

For individuals with vitamin D deficiency, a common approach is to initiate high-dose vitamin D3 (cholecalciferol) supplementation. This may involve a loading dose (e.g., 50,000 IU weekly for several weeks), followed by a maintenance dose (e.g., 800–2000 IU daily) based on individual needs and response. The Global Consensus Group provides specific recommendations for treating nutritional rickets and vitamin D-deficient rickets. They recommend a 3-month regimen of vitamin D2 or D3 with daily doses of 2000 IU for children under 12 months; 3000–6000 IU for children aged 12 months to 12 years, and 6000 IU for individuals older than 12 years. In resource-limited settings, single high-dose or Stoss therapy may be employed, such as 50,000 IU for infants (3–12 months), 150,000 IU for children (12 months to 12 years), and 300,000 IU for individuals older than 12 years. The oral route is preferred for its more rapid correction of 25OHD levels. Additionally, 500 mg/day of calcium, either through diet or supplements, is advised to support bone health during treatment (Munns et al., 2016).

29.9   Availability and risks of high-dose vitamin D

Until recently, nonprescription vitamin D supplements were predominantly available as multivitamin formulations or single-nutrient tablets containing 800–1000 IU per dose.[28]

However, new products now offer high-dose options, such as 5000, 25,000, or 50,000 IU, predominantly in the form of cholecalciferol. Mega-dose supplements ranging from 200,000 to 600,000 IU are also available, although their accessibility varies by country. The inadvertent use of these high-dose formulations has been associated with toxicity, including hypercalcemia and complications like nephrocalcinosis (Letavernier & Daudon, 2018).

To minimize risks, it is critical to evaluate patients both clinically and biochemically before prescribing vitamin D supplements. While numerous types of vitamin D supplements are available in oral and injectable forms, they differ in efficacy and therapeutic applications based on their chemical composition. Careful consideration of these factors and adherence to recommended guidelines can help avoid vitamin D toxicity while ensuring effective treatment of deficiencies (Ataide et al., 2021).

29.10 Follow-up and monitoring of D deficiency

Monitoring serum 25(OH)D levels is an essential component of assessing the effectiveness of vitamin D supplementation and prevent toxicity (Holick, 2007). This is particularly critical for individuals at risk of deficiency or those diagnosed with low vitamin D levels prior to treatment. Regular follow-up allows healthcare providers to ensure that serum levels remain within the desired range and make necessary adjustments to supplementation regimens.

Follow-up testing of serum 25(OH)D levels is recommended approximately 8–12 weeks after initiating treatment. This timeframe allows for the body to adequately respond to supplementation and for levels to stabilize. The goal of treatment is to achieve and maintain serum 25(OH)D concentrations of at least 20 ng/mL (50 nmol/L) (Ströhle, 2011). However, many studies suggest aiming for higher levels, typically in the range of 30–50 ng/mL (75–125 nmol/L), for optimal health benefits (Bischoff-Ferrari, 2014). Based on follow-up serum levels, vitamin D dosages may need adjustment. If levels remain below the target range after the initial treatment period, higher doses or alternative formulations may be required. Conversely, if levels exceed the desired range, dosages should be reduced to avoid potential toxicity. Adjustments should account for individual factors such as age, body weight, health status, and coexisting medical conditions that may affect vitamin D metabolism.

For individuals on long-term vitamin D supplementation, periodic monitoring is essential to maintain levels within the target range and to prevent toxicity. Testing every 6–12 months is typically recommended, particularly for individuals with chronic conditions like malabsorption syndromes, chronic kidney disease, or limited sun exposure (Kidney Disease - Improving Global Outcomes KDIGO, 2017). For such patients, ongoing low-dose supplementation may be necessary. Patients should also be educated about dietary sources of vitamin D and safe sun exposure practices to naturally support their vitamin D levels (Khundmiri et al., 2016).

While vitamin D supplementation is generally safe, high-dose regimens carry the risk of toxicity. Some of the symptoms of vitamin D toxicity include hypercalcemia, hypercalciuria, nausea, vomiting, and weakness. Monitoring serum calcium levels may be warranted, especially for individuals receiving high doses or those at higher risk for hypercalcemia. Patient education on recognizing symptoms of toxicity is critical to mitigate risks (Majid et al., 2022). Monitoring should extend beyond serum levels to assess broader health outcomes, such as bone health, muscle function, and overall well-being. This holistic approach ensures the effectiveness of vitamin D treatment in improving quality of life and addressing patient-specific health concerns (Marcinowska-Suchowierska et al., 2018).

Follow-up results may necessitate adjustments in treatment plans. For persistent deficiencies, higher doses or alternative forms of vitamin D supplementation may be required. If serum levels are adequate, a maintenance dose can be continued or tailored to the patient's needs. In cases of toxicity or excessively high levels, discontinuing or reducing supplementation may be necessary. Monitoring and follow-up in vitamin D treatment are vital for achieving and maintaining optimal serum 25(OH)D levels. Regular testing, dosage adjustments, and attention to individual factors and health outcomes ensure effective management while minimizing risks. This approach not only addresses deficiencies but also supports long-term health and well-being.

References

Amrein, K., Scherkl, M., Hoffmann, M., Neuwersch-Sommeregger, S., Köstenberger, M., Tmava Berisha, A., Martucci, G., Pilz, S., & Malle, O. (2020). Vitamin D deficiency 2.0: An update on the current status worldwide. *European Journal of Clinical Nutrition, 74*(11), 1498–1513. https://doi.org/10.1038/s41430-020-0558-y.

Ataide, F. L., Carvalho Bastos, L. M., Vicente Matias, M. F., Skare, T. L., & Freire de Carvalho, J. (2021). Safety and effectiveness of vitamin D mega-dose: A systematic review. *Clinical Nutrition ESPEN, 46*, 115–120. https://doi.org/10.1016/j.clnesp.2021.09.010, http://www.journals.elsevier.com/clinical-nutrition-espen.

Baeke, F., Takiishi, T., Korf, H., Gysemans, C., & Mathieu, C. (2010). Vitamin D: modulator of the immune system. *Current Opinion in Pharmacology, 10*(4), 482–496. https://doi.org/10.1016/j.coph.2010.04.001.

Basit, A., Basit, K. A., Fawwad, A., Shaheen, F., Fatima, N., Petropoulos, I. N., Alam, U., & Malik, R. A. (2016). Vitamin D for the treatment of painful diabetic neuropathy. *BMJ Open Diabetes Research and Care, 4*(1). https://doi.org/10.1136/bmjdrc-2015-000148, http://drc.bmj.com/content/4/1/e000148.full.pdf.

Benedik, E. (2022). Sources of vitamin D for humans. *International Journal for Vitamin and Nutrition Research, 92*(2), 118–125. https://doi.org/10.1024/0300-9831/a000733.

Bikle, D. D. (2014). Vitamin D metabolism, mechanism of action, and clinical applications. *Chemistry and Biology, 21*(3), 319–329. https://doi.org/10.1016/j.chembiol.2013.12.016, www.elsevier.com/inca/publications/store/6/0/1/2/8/1/index.htt.

Bilezikian, J. P., Formenti, A. M., Adler, R. A., Binkley, N., Bouillon, R., Lazaretti-Castro, M., Marcocci, C., Napoli, N., Rizzoli, R., & Giustina, A. (2021). Vitamin D: Dosing, levels, form, and route of administration: Does one approach fit all? *Reviews in Endocrine and Metabolic Disorders, 22*(4), 1201–1218. https://doi.org/10.1007/s11154-021-09693-7, https://link.springer.com/journal/11154.

Bischoff-Ferrari, H. A. (2014). Optimal serum 25-hydroxyvitamin D levels for multiple health outcomes. *Advances in Experimental Medicine and Biology, 810*, 500–525. https://doi.org/10.1007/978-1-4939-0437-2_28.

Bolland, M. J., Grey, A., & Avenell, A. (2018). Effects of vitamin D supplementation on musculoskeletal health: a systematic review, meta-analysis, and trial sequential analysis. *The Lancet Diabetes and Endocrinology,*

6(11), 847–858. https://doi.org/10.1016/S2213-8587(18)30265-1, http://www.journals.elsevier.com/the-lancet-diabetes-and-endocrinology.

Bouillon, R., Manousaki, D., Rosen, C., Trajanoska, K., Rivadeneira, F., & Richards, J. B. (2022). The health effects of vitamin D supplementation: Evidence from human studies. *Nature Reviews Endocrinology, 18*(2), 96–110. https://doi.org/10.1038/s41574-021-00593-z, http://www.nature.com/nrendo/index.html.

Chauhan, S., Huecker, M. R., & Vitamin, D. (2023). *Treasure Island (FL)*. StatPearls Publishing 2025 Jan.

Chen, T., Zuo, X., Wang, S., Yu, P., Yuan, J., Wei, S., Chen, J., Sun, Y., Gao, Y., & Li, X. (2020). The effect of vitamin D supplementation on the progression of fibrosis in patients with chronic liver disease: A protocol for a systematic review and meta-analysis. *Medicine (United States), 99*(19). https://doi.org/10.1097/MD.0000000000020296, https://journals.lww.com/md-journal/pages/default.aspx.

Cianferotti, L., Parri, S., Gronchi, G., Rizzuti, C., Fossi, C., Black, D. M., & Brandi, M. L. (2015). Changing patterns of prescription in vitamin D supplementation in adults: analysis of a regional dataset. *Osteoporosis International, 26*(11), 2695–2702. https://doi.org/10.1007/s00198-015-3187-x, link.springer.de/link/service/journals/00198/index.htm.

Cui, A., Zhang, T., Xiao, P., Fan, Z., Wang, H., & Zhuang, Y. (2023). Global and regional prevalence of vitamin D deficiency in population-based studies from 2000 to 2022: A pooled analysis of 7.9 million participants. *Frontiers in Nutrition, 10*. https://doi.org/10.3389/fnut.2023.1070808.

Demay, M. B., Pittas, A. G., Bikle, D. D., Diab, D. L., Kiely, M. E., Lazaretti-Castro, M., Lips, P., Mitchell, D. M., Murad, M. H., Powers, S., Rao, S. D., Scragg, R., Tayek, J. A., Valent, A. M., Walsh, J. M. E., & McCartney, C. R. (2024). Vitamin D for the prevention of disease: An endocrine society clinical practice guideline. *Journal of Clinical Endocrinology and Metabolism, 109*(8), 1907–1947. https://doi.org/10.1210/clinem/dgae290, https://academic.oup.com/jcem.

Dominguez, L. J., Farruggia, M., Veronese, N., & Barbagallo, M. (2021). Vitamin D sources, metabolism, and deficiency: Available compounds and guidelines for its treatment. *Metabolites, 11*(4), 255. https://doi.org/10.3390/metabo11040255.

Doses and Schemes for Correcting Vitamin D Deficiency: An Update. (2024). *Food & Nutrition Journal, 9*(1). https://doi.org/10.29011/2575-7091.100190.

Franca Gois, P. H., Wolley, M., Ranganathan, D., & Seguro, A. C. (2018). Vitamin D deficiency in chronic kidney disease: Recent evidence and controversies. *International Journal of Environmental Research and Public Health, 15*(8), 1773. https://doi.org/10.3390/ijerph15081773.

Galior, K., Grebe, S., & Singh, R. (2018). Development of vitamin D toxicity from overcorrection of vitamin D deficiency: A review of case reports. *Nutrients, 10*(8), 953. https://doi.org/10.3390/nu10080953.

Giustina, A., Bilezikian, J. P., Adler, R. A., Banfi, G., Bikle, D. D., Binkley, N. C., Bollerslev, J., Bouillon, R., Brandi, M. L., Casanueva, F. F., Di Filippo, L., Donini, L. M., Ebeling, P. R., Fuleihan, G. E. H., Fassio, A., Frara, S., Jones, G., Marcocci, C., Martineau, A. R., ... Virtanen, J. K. (2024). Consensus statement on vitamin D status assessment and supplementation: Whys, whens, and hows. *Endocrine Reviews, 45*(5), 625–654. https://doi.org/10.1210/endrev/bnae009, https://academic.oup.com/edrv/issue.

Giustina, A., Bouillon, R., Dawson-Hughes, B., Ebeling, P. R., Lazaretti-Castro, M., Lips, P., Marcocci, C., & Bilezikian, J. P. (2023). Vitamin D in the older population: A consensus statement. *Endocrine, 79*(1), 31–44. https://doi.org/10.1007/s12020-022-03208-3.

van Groningen, L., Opdenoordt, S., van Sorge, A., Telting, D., Giesen, A., & de Boer, H. (2010). Cholecalciferol loading dose guideline for vitamin D-deficient adults. *European Journal of Endocrinology, 162*(4), 805–811. https://doi.org/10.1530/eje-09-0932.

de la Guía-Galipienso, F., Martínez-Ferran, M., Vallecillo, N., Lavie, C. J., Sanchis-Gomar, F., & Pareja-Galeano, H. (2021). Vitamin D and cardiovascular health. *Clinical Nutrition, 40*(5), 2946–2957. https://doi.org/10.1016/j.clnu.2020.12.025, http://www.elsevier-international.com/journals/clnu/.

Gupta, N., Farooqui, K., Batra, C., Marwaha, R., & Mithal, A. (2017). Effect of oral versus intramuscular Vitamin D replacement in apparently healthy adults with Vitamin D deficiency. *Indian Journal of Endocrinology and Metabolism, 21*(1), 131–136. https://doi.org/10.4103/2230-8210.196007, www.ijem.in/.

Haines, S. T., & Park, S. K. (2012). Vitamin D supplementation: What's known, what to do, and what's needed. *Pharmacotherapy, 32*(4), 354–382. https://doi.org/10.1002/phar.1037.

Helde Frankling, M., Norlin, A. C., Hansen, S., Wahren Borgström, E., Bergman, P., & Björkhem-Bergman, L. (2020). Are vitamin D3 tablets and oil drops equally effective in raising S-25-hydroxyvitamin D concentrations? A post-hoc analysis of an observational study on immunodeficient patients. *Nutrients, 12*(5). https://doi.org/10.3390/nu12051230.

van den Heuvel, E. G., Lips, P., Schoonmade, L. J., Lanham-New, S. A., & van Schoor, N. M. (2024). Comparison of the effect of daily vitamin D2 and vitamin D3 supplementation on serum 25-hydroxyvitamin D concentration (Total 25(OH)D, 25(OH)D2, and 25(OH)D3) and importance of body mass index: A systematic review and meta-analysis. *Advances in Nutrition, 15*(1). https://doi.org/10.1016/j.advnut.2023.09.016, https://www.sciencedirect.com/science/journal/21618313.

Holick, M. F., Vitamin, Vidal, F., Vidal, M., Lane, Keen, & Alba, R. (2007). Doses and schemes for correcting vitamin D deficiency: An update. *The New England Journal of Medicine, 357*. https://doi.org/10.1056/NEJMra070553.

Holick, M. F., Binkley, N. C., Bischoff-Ferrari, H. A., Gordon, C. M., Hanley, D. A., Heaney, R. P., Murad, M. H., & Weaver, C. M. (2011). Evaluation, treatment, and prevention of vitamin D deficiency: An endocrine society clinical practice guideline. *Journal of Clinical Endocrinology and Metabolism, 96*(7), 1911–1930. https://doi.org/10.1210/jc.2011-0385, http://jcem.endojournals.org/content/96/7/1911.full.pdf+html.

Holick, M. F. (2007). Vitamin D deficiency. *New England Journal of Medicine, 357*(3), 266–281. https://doi.org/10.1056/nejmra070553.

Hultin, H., Stevens, K., & Sundbom, M. (2018). Cholecalciferol injections are effective in hypovitaminosis D after duodenal switch: A randomized controlled study. *Obesity Surgery, 28*(10), 3007–3011. https://doi.org/10.1007/s11695-018-3307-8.

Jacot, W., Firmin, N., Roca, L., Topart, D., Gallet, S., Durigova, A., Mirr, S., Abach, L., Pouderoux, S., D'Hondt, V., Bleuse, J. P., Lamy, P. J., & Romieu, G. (2016). Impact of a tailored oral vitamin D supplementation regimen on serum 25-hydroxyvitamin D levels in early breast cancer patients: A randomized phase III study. *Annals of Oncology, 27*(7), 1235–1241. https://doi.org/10.1093/annonc/mdw145.

Khundmiri, S. J., Murray, R. D., & Lederer, E. (2016). PTH and vitamin D. *Comprehensive Physiology, 6*(2), 561–601. https://doi.org/10.1002/cphy.c140071, http://onlinelibrary.wiley.com/store/10.1002/cphy.c140071/asset/c140071.pdf?v=1&t=j4ayhzaq&s=890f801158164fcbd3f0378cef4397cebfd0222c.

Kidney Disease - Improving Global Outcomes (KDIGO) (2017). KDIGO 2017 Clinical Practice Guideline Update for the Diagnosis, Evaluation, Prevention, and Treatment of Chronic Kidney Disease-Mineral and Bone Disorder (CKD-MBD). Kidney International Supplements, 7(3), 1-59. https://doi.org/10.1016/j.kisu.2017.04.001. Erratum in: Kidney International Supplements (2011). 2017 Dec; 7(3), e1. https://doi.org/10.1016/j.kisu.2017.10.001.

LeFevre, M. L., & LeFevre, N. M. (2018). Vitamin D screening and supplementation in community-dwelling adults: Common questions and answers. *American Family Physician, 97*(4), 254–260.

Letavernier, E., & Daudon, M. (2018). Vitamin D, hypercalciuria and kidney stones. *Nutrients, 10*(3). https://doi.org/10.3390/nu10030366, http://www.mdpi.com/2072-6643/10/3/366/pdf.

Lips, P., van Schoor, N. M., & de Jongh, R. T. (2014). Diet, sun, and lifestyle as determinants of vitamin D status. *Annals of the New York Academy of Sciences, 1317*(1), 92–98. https://doi.org/10.1111/nyas.12443, http://www.blackwellpublishing.com/0077-8923.

Majid, H., Abid, M. A., Zehra, N., Muneer, S., Jafri, L., & Khan, A. H. (2022). Paradigm shifts in vitamin D testing and diagnosis: A decade-long observational study. *Pakistan Journal of Pathology, 33*(1), 1–4. https://doi.org/10.55629/pakjpathol.v33i1.690.

Marcinowska-Suchowierska, E., Kupisz-Urbańska, M., Łukaszkiewicz, J., Płudowski, P., & Jones, G. (2018). Vitamin D toxicity—A clinical perspective. *Frontiers in Endocrinology, 9*. https://doi.org/10.3389/fendo.2018.00550.

Masood, M. Q., Khan, A., Awan, S., Dar, F., Naz, S., Naureen, G., Saghir, S., & Jabbar, A. (2015). Comparison of vitamin D replacement strategies with high-dose intramuscular or oral cholecalciferol: A prospective intervention study. *Endocrine Practice, 21*(10), 1125–1133. https://doi.org/10.4158/ep15680.or.

Mulligan, M. L., Felton, S. K., Riek, A. E., & Bernal-Mizrachi, C. (2010). Implications of vitamin D deficiency in pregnancy and lactation. *American Journal of Obstetrics and Gynecology, 202*(5), 429. https://doi.org/10.1016/j.ajog.2009.09.002 e1.

Munns, C. F., Shaw, N., Kiely, M., Specker, B. L., Thacher, T. D., Ozono, K., Michigami, T., Tiosano, D., Mughal, M. Z., Mäkitie, O., Ramos-Abad, L., Ward, L., DiMeglio, L. A., Atapattu, N., Cassinelli, H., Braegger, C., Pettifor, J. M., Seth, A., Idris, H. W., ... Högler, W. (2016). Global consensus recommendations on prevention and management of nutritional rickets. *The Journal of Clinical Endocrinology & Metabolism, 101*(2), 394–415. https://doi.org/10.1210/jc.2015-2175.

Nair, R., & Maseeh, A. (2012). Vitamin D: The sunshine vitamin. *Journal of Pharmacology and Pharmacotherapeutics, 3*(2), 118–126. https://doi.org/10.4103/0976-500X.95506.

National Institutes of Health (NIH). (2021). Vitamin D: Fact Sheet for Health Professionals. Office of Dietary Supplements. Retrieved July 30, 2025, from National Institutes of Health (NIH) | (.gov).

Narvaez, J., Maldonado, G., Guerrero, R., Messina, O. D., & Rios, C. (2020 Jun). Vitamin D megadose: Definition, efficacy in bone metabolism, risk of falls and fractures. *Open Access Rheumatology: Research and Reviews, 11*, 105–115.

Passeron, T., Bouillon, R., Callender, V., Cestari, T., Diepgen, T. L., Green, A. C., van der Pols, J. C., Bernard, B. A., Ly, F., Bernerd, F., Marrot, L., Nielsen, M., Verschoore, M., Jablonski, N. G., & Young, A. R. (2019). Sunscreen photoprotection and vitamin D status. *British Journal of Dermatology, 181*(5), 916–931. https://doi.org/10.1111/bjd.17992.

Pludowski, P., Holick, M. F., Grant, W. B., Konstantynowicz, J., Mascarenhas, M. R., Haq, A., Povoroznyuk, V., Balatska, N., Barbosa, A. P., Karonova, T., Rudenka, E., Misiorowski, W., Zakharova, I., Rudenka, A., Łukaszkiewicz, J., Marcinowska-Suchowierska, E., Łaszcz, N., Abramowicz, P., Bhattoa, H. P., & Wimalawansa, S. J. (2018). Vitamin D supplementation guidelines. *Journal of Steroid Biochemistry and Molecular Biology, 175*, 125–135. https://doi.org/10.1016/j.jsbmb.2017.01.021, www.elsevier.com/locate/jsbmb.

Rebelos, E., Tentolouris, N., & Jude, E. (2023). The role of vitamin D in health and disease: A narrative review on the mechanisms linking vitamin D with disease and the effects of supplementation. *Drugs, 83*(8), 665–685. https://doi.org/10.1007/s40265-023-01875-8.

Romagnoli, E., Mascia, M. L., Cipriani, C., Fassino, V., Mazzei, F., D'Erasmo, E., Carnevale, V., Scillitani, A., & Minisola, S. (2008). Short and long-term variations in serum calciotropic hormones after a single very large dose of ergocalciferol (vitamin D2) or cholecalciferol (vitamin D3) in the elderly. *Journal of Clinical Endocrinology and Metabolism, 93*(8), 3015–3020. https://doi.org/10.1210/jc.2008-0350, http://jcem.endojournals.org/cgi/reprint/93/8/3015.

Skaaby, T., Husemoen, L. L. N., Thuesen, B. H., Pisinger, C., Hannemann, A., Jørgensen, T., & Linneberg, A. (2016). Longitudinal associations between lifestyle and vitamin D: A general population study with repeated vitamin D measurements. *Endocrine, 51*(2), 342–350. https://doi.org/10.1007/s12020-015-0641-7, http://www.springer.com/humana+press/journal/12020.

Ströhle, A. (2011). Die aktuellen empfehlungen des US-amerikanischen Institute of Medicine (IOM) für die vitamin-D-zufuhr: Eine kritische würdigung. *Medizinische Monatsschrift fur Pharmazeuten, 34*(8). http://www.justscience.de/en/drugbase/medizinische-monatsschrift-fuer-pharmazeuten/artikel.html?tx_crondavdbmmp_pi%5Buid%5D=1739&cHash=17b75cd3fc Germany.

Takács, I., Tóth, B. E., Szekeres, L., Szabó, B., Bakos, B., & Lakatos, P. (2017). Randomized clinical trial to comparing efficacy of daily, weekly and monthly administration of vitamin D3. *Endocrine, 55*(1), 60–65. https://doi.org/10.1007/s12020-016-1137-9, http://www.springer.com/humana+press/journal/12020.

Vitamin D deficiency. (2025). *Royal Children's Hospital Melbourne*. Royal Children's Hospital.

Vranić, L., Mikolašević, I., & Milić, S. (2019). Vitamin D Deficiency: Consequence or Cause of Obesity? *Medicina, 55*(9), 541. https://doi.org/10.3390/medicina55090541.

CHAPTER 30

Vitamin D therapy: a promising appraoch for subfertility

Chaman Nasrullah[1], Fatima Syed[2], and Rehana Rehman[3]

[1]University College of Medicine & Dentistry, The University of Lahore, Lahore, Pakistan [2]Department of Pathology, Fazaia Ruth Pfau Medical College, Karachi, Pakistan [3]Department of Biological & Biomedical Sciences, Aga Khan University, Karachi, Pakistan

30.1 Introduction: vitamin D and subfertility

The increase in prevalence of subfertility has resulted in an increase in patients utilizing assisted reproductive technology (ART) for treatment (Alam, 2020). Research suggests that hypovitaminosis D (serum levels < 20 ng/dL) is one of the major causes of subfertility, with its deficiencies contributing to insulin resistance (IR), metabolic dysfunction, and polycystic ovary syndrome (PCOS) (Rehman et al., 2021). Patients with PCOS who are also vitamin D–deficient are found to have decreased ovulation by induction. These conditions of vitamin deficiency (VD) are closely linked to poor ovarian responsiveness to ART, which makes the treatment less effective. Paying attention to these factors increases clinical effectiveness while reducing the financial load on the healthcare systems caused by extensive or excessive ART cycles (Rehman et al., 2024).

30.1.1 Overview of vitamin D's potential in polycystic ovary syndrome

30.1.1.1 Polycystic ovary syndrome

Polycystic ovary syndrome is characterized by the presence of at least two of the following three criteria: chronic anovulation, clinical or biological hyperandrogenism, and polycystic ovaries (Goodman et al., 2015; Samma et al., 2024). Most PCOS-afflicted women have low levels of vitamin D (< 20 ng/mL) (Azhar et al., 2020). The metabolic disorders that are common in PCOS, such as obesity, IR, and hyperlipidemia, are made worse by VD insufficiency.

30.1.1.2 Therapeutic role of vitamin D: evidence from animal models

30.1.1.2.1 Reduction in weight

In a study, DHEA was used for 30 days to create an animal model of PCOS that resembled human PCOS. Thirty female Sprague–Dawley rats were split into three groups: VD-treated

PCOS (DHEA + 25 (OH)2D3 weekly), PCOS (DHEA daily), and a control group (sesame oil). While the VD-treated group showed better ovarian morphology, decreased weight, and improved menstrual cycle features, the PCOS group displayed considerable weight gain, obesity, and irregular estrogenic cycles. These results imply that VD may aid in reversing the metabolic and reproductive abnormalities associated with PCOS (Azhar et al., 2021).

30.1.1.2.2 Histological improvements

VD supplementation in PCOS rat models showed no significant changes in uterine histomorphometry but normalized the biochemical composition of gland secretions, restoring them to normal levels (Kamińska et al., 2024).

- *Insulin sensitivity*: VD treatment reduced IR in PCOS rats by activating the PI3K/Akt signaling pathway, enhancing glucose metabolism (Kamińska et al., 2024).
- *Follicle development*: Retinoic acid (RA) and fibroblast growth factor-2 (FGF2) improved follicle maturation and embryo development in PCOS mouse models, suggesting a synergistic effect with VD (Rustamzadeh et al., 2024).

30.1.1.3 Therapeutic role of vitamin D: evidence from human studies

Clinical studies in women with PCOS show that using VD supplements enhances ovulation, hormonal balance, and menstrual regularity.

LH/FSH ratio: In a randomized controlled study (RCT), 180 women with PCOS and 150 women without PCOS who had low VD levels were recruited at the Medical University of Graz in Austria. For 24 weeks, participants were given a placebo or 20,000 IU of vitamin D3 weekly. The findings indicated possible advantages for reproductive function as VD administration dramatically raised follicle-stimulating hormone (FSH) levels and decreased the luteinizing hormone (LH)/FSH ratio in PCOS women. However, neither anti-Müllerian hormone (AMH) levels nor non-PCOS women showed any discernible change. The results emphasize how VD affects hormonal balance in PCOS (Lerchbaum et al., 2021).

Testosterone levels: Most PCOS-afflicted women have low levels of VD (< 20 ng/mL). The metabolic disorders that are common in PCOS, including obesity, IR, and hyperlipidemia, are made worse by VD insufficiency. The supplementation has a mixed effect on testosterone levels, although it improves lipid profiles, insulin production, and irregular menstruation (Nandi et al., 2016).

Ovarian morphology: In a randomized, placebo-controlled prospective clinical trial VD treatment in a dose of 50,000 IU/week for 12 weeks improved ovarian morphology and menstrual regularity, significantly decreased total testosterone, free androgen index, and hirsutism score and increased dehydroepiandrosterone (DHEA) and sex hormone binding globulin (SHBG) whereas the placebo group did not show any improvement. According to these results, VD may help PCOS women's fertility and reproductive health (Al-Bayyari et al., 2021).

Anthropometric measurements: In another study, sixty PCOS women with VD deficiency or insufficiency were randomly assigned to receive 2000 IU/day of VD or a placebo. After 12 weeks, the VD group showed significantly higher serum 25 (OH)D levels and improvements in body mass index (BMI), waist-to-hip ratio (WHR), IR (HOMA-IR), and lipid metabolism, including lower triglycerides (TG), total cholesterol (TC), and low-density lipoprotein cholesterol (LDL-C) (Wen et al., 2024).

Lipid profile: In our population, the association of decreased VD levels in females with PCOS with abnormal lipid profile; rise in cholesterol, triglycerides, and low-density lipoproteins points towards susceptibility to metabolic abnormalities (Arfa JCPS). A comprehensive metaanalysis of randomized controlled trials discovered that VD significantly decreased DHEA, total testosterone (TT), low-density lipoprotein cholesterol (LDL-C), total cholesterol (TC), and triglycerides (TG). However, there were no discernible changes in body mass index (BMI), insulin levels, or high-density lipoprotein cholesterol (HDL-C), reflecting that VD has no effect on weight or insulin management; it may aid PCOS patients' lipid profiles and hormonal balance (Yin et al., 2024). At Aga Khan University Karachi, Pakistan, an RCT is being conducted to compare and report the effect of VD on total antioxidant capacity in females with PCOS (Khan et al., 2024). In another trial, the effect of VD therapy on follicular size and endometrial thickness is being compared with the routine metformin therapy in infertile females with PCOS (Rehman et al., 2023) (Fig. 30.1).

30.1.2 Overview of vitamin D's potential in endometriosis

30.1.2.1 Endometriosis

It is a prevalent gynecological condition and 10% of women during their reproductive life are affected by it and accounting for 5% of female infertility and are characterized by peritoneal lesions, adhesions, and cysts (Alam, 2020). It is considered to be an inflammatory condition in which inflammatory pathways like NF-κB are unchecked, and there is more production of prostaglandins and cytokines, which in turn support the invasion and survival of ectopic endometrial cells. The pathogenesis of endometriosis involves overexpression of estrogen receptor β (ERβ) that accelerates the progression of lesions by preventing TNF-α-induced apoptosis, raising IL-1β levels, and accelerating the epithelial-mesenchymal transition (EMT) pathways (Xu et al., 2021). Overactivation of the AKT signaling pathway promotes lesion formation and invasiveness (Farhangnia et al., 2024). Proinflammatory mediators like TNF, VEGF, and MMP-9 are secreted by activated macrophages in peritoneal fluid, and they encourage the formation of lesions. ROS formation from iron deposition during in situ menstruation further activates NF-κB in endometriotic cells (Farhangnia et al., 2024). Ectopic growth is made possible by endometrial cells' decreased apoptosis. Immune-mediated cell clearance is also disturbed. Immune cells expressing the Fas molecule interact with cells expressing the Fas ligand to induce the process of apoptosis (Burjiah et al., 2022). However,

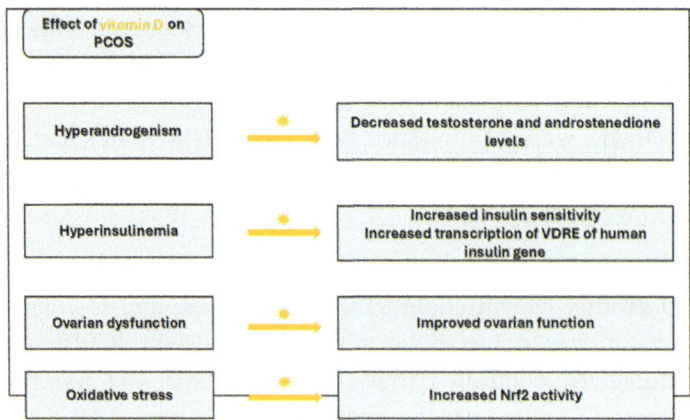

Figure 30.1

Effect of vitamin D supplementation on pathophysiological hallmarks of polycystic ovarian syndrome.

metalloprotease may break FasL and generate soluble FasL. Immune cells with Fas have to undergo apoptosis when they face FasL in the peritoneal fluid of patients with endometriosis (Farhangnia et al., 2024).

30.1.2.2   Vitamin D's potential for treating endometriosis

Recent research demonstrates how VD's impact on inflammation, proliferation, and angiogenesis can be used therapeutically to manage endometriosis. In peripheral blood mononuclear cells (PBMCs), peritoneal fluid mononuclear cells (PFMCs), and both ectopic (EESCs) and eutopic (EuESCs) endometrial stromal cells, VD therapy decreases the expression of MCP-1 (monocyte chemoattractant protein-1 that causes the recruitment of monocytes at the site of inflammation), HGF (hepatocyte growth factor, involved in the process of neovascularization, regeneration and growth of the cells), and IGF-1 (insulin like growth factor-1 [Heidari et al., 2021] involved in the process of proliferation and survival of cells) both at the gene and protein levels. By downregulating VEGF-α (vascular endothelial growth factor-alpha), Bcl-2, Bcl-xL (antiapoptotic proteins), and IL-6, it also improves cell adherence while preventing ESC invasion and proliferation. VD dramatically lowers the expression of PDGFB (platelet-derived growth factor) and EGF (epidermal growth factor), proving its ability to inhibit angiogenesis and cellular invasion.

30.1.2.3   Antiendometriotic effects of vitamin D: molecular mechanisms

VD follows multiple routes: It suppresses NF-κB activation, a major contributor to inflammation, by stabilizing the inhibitor of kappa B alpha (IkBα) protein. Additionally, it suppresses the synthesis of proinflammatory cytokines by upregulating MKP-1 (mitogen-activated protein kinase phosphatase-1) and lowers IGF-1 expression by interfering with the IGF-1R/PI3K/AKT signaling pathway. By controlling cyclins and (cyclin-dependent kinase) CDKs, upregulating inhibitors of CDK (P21 and P27), and downregulating cyclin D and CDKs 4 and 5, vitamin D induces arrest of the cell cycle in G0/G1 (Burjiah et al., 2022). All these processes work together to prevent ESC migration, angiogenesis, and proliferation (Farhangnia et al., 2024).

30.1.2.4 Therapeutic role of vitamin D: evidence from animal models

VD therapy caused the endometriotic implants to regress in rat experiments by enhancing the expression of TIMP-2 (tissue inhibitor of metalloproteinase-2), inhibiting neovascularization, and modifying MMP-9 (matrix metalloproteinase-9, a protein involved in remodeling extracellular matrix) and VEGF levels. Similar results were found in another study where VD controlled interleukin-17 levels to decrease endometrial implants and stop the development of endometriosis in mice (Burjiah et al., 2022).

- VD treatment has been shown to significantly decrease inflammatory markers such as interleukin-6 (IL-6) and tumor necrosis factor-alpha (TNFα) in rat models, indicating a reduction in inflammation associated with endometriosis (Shiravani et al., 2024).
- In mice, higher doses of VD (16 IU and 24 IU) resulted in a notable decrease in IL-17 expression, which correlates with reduced endometriotic lesion size (Burjiah et al., 2022).

30.1.2.5 Therapeutic role of vitamin D: evidence from human studies

Agonists for VDR are now part of therapeutic strategies. The potential of VDR-targeted treatments in the management of endometriosis is further supported by the notable observation that elocalcitol, a selective VDR agonist, inhibits macrophage recruitment and reduces peritoneal inflammation, thereby preventing the formation and progression of endometriosis in mice (Farhangnia et al., 2024). There is debate over the relationship between VD levels and the likelihood or severity of endometriosis in women. Endometriosis-affected women frequently have lower VD levels compared to healthy controls, which may indicate that hypovitaminosis D is a risk factor. On the other hand, another research indicates that VD levels are higher in endometriosis patients or that there is no discernible difference between those who have the disease and those who do not. Differences in study methodologies, population variables, and sample sizes can all lead to inconsistent results. Furthermore, women with endometriosis who have not had treatment have been found to have lower levels of vitamin D-binding protein (DBP) in peritoneal fluid but not in plasma.

Results from clinical studies on VD supplementation in endometriosis are not entirely consistent. Some studies reveal no statistically significant difference in pelvic pain relief when compared to a placebo, while others demonstrate a considerable reduction in pain in women with primary dysmenorrhea. To determine its effectiveness and methods of action, further extensive clinical trials are required to fully explore vitamin D's therapeutic role in the treatment of endometriosis (Farhangnia et al., 2024).

There are conflicting results regarding the involvement of DBP and VDR gene polymorphisms in endometriosis-related infertility. While some studies revealed no significant link, others suggest that these polymorphisms are risk factors for endometriosis and infertility. Different ethnic populations may cause variations in the results, which calls for more investigation (Fig. 30.2).

30.1.3   Overview of vitamin D's potential in assisted reproductive technologies

30.1.3.1   Assisted reproductive technologies

The American Center for Disease Control defines assisted reproductive technologies (ART) as fertility therapies that involve the manipulation of eggs or embryos, excluding the techniques that merely modify sperm (such as intrauterine insemination) or involve ovarian stimulation without planned egg retrieval.

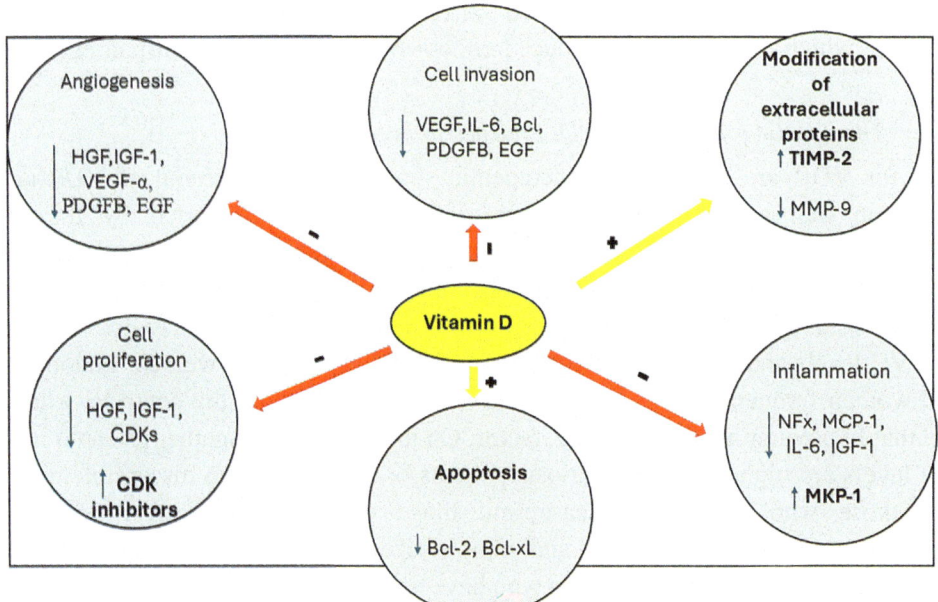

Figure 30.2
Role of vitamin D to prevent endometriosis: Yellow arrows indicate facilitation, red arrows indicate inhibition.

The term "Assisted Reproductive Technology" (ART) refers to a broad range of medical procedures and methods used to help women conceive, including in vitro fertilization (IVF), intracytoplasmic sperm injection (ICSI), intrauterine insemination (IUI), gestational surrogacy, sperm and egg donation, freezing of eggs and embryos, and drugs like ovulation-inducing hormones (Carson et al., 2021).

One in 20 births in developed countries now involve ARTs, such as IVF and ICSI; nevertheless, access is still an issue in developing countries with greater rates of infertility. With only one in five cycles ending in a live birth, success rates are low despite technological breakthroughs, placing a heavy financial and emotional burden on patients. Impact of dietary intake on infertility and ART outcomes has drawn attention in recent years, especially in relation to polycystic ovarian syndrome (PCOS) (Winter et al., 2023).

Numerous studies have examined the impact of VD on ART outcomes, including in vitro fertilization (IVF). The quantity of mature oocytes recovered, fertilization rates, and embryo quality are all favorably correlated with serum VD levels. Contradictory results, however, highlight the necessity of standardized procedures, such as the assessment of bioavailable VD and VDR expression in follicular cells (Xu et al., 2021).

30.1.3.2 Impact of vitamin D on hormone levels in ART

In a study conducted on women undergoing IVF, VD supplementation did not change the levels of progesterone (P4) or estradiol (E2), but it did dramatically raise follicular fluid 25-hydroxyvitamin D levels (2.8 times higher in the VD group compared to placebo). Granulosa cell cultures produced more progesterone and estrogen when VD was supplemented in patients undergoing IVF treatment (Makieva et al., 2021).

RNA-sequencing revealed 44 genes that were expressed differently in GCs from the VD group than in the placebo group. Important alterations included the downregulation of genes like PTGS2 (prostaglandin-endoperoxide synthase 2), VEGF (vascular endothelial growth factor), and the overexpression of genes involved in antioxidant defense, such as VDR (VD receptor) and GSTA3 (glutathione S-transferase A3) in these patients (Makieva et al., 2021).

30.1.3.2.1 Stage-specific success rates

Ovarian response/ovulation rate: The effects of VD supplementation on ovulation rates in overweight, subfertile women with PCOS receiving clomiphene citrate ovulation induction were examined in an experimental trial. For 4 cycles, 186 women received either a placebo with calcium or VD (10,000 IU twice weekly). The VD group had a considerably greater ovulation rate (92.5%) than the control group. The groups' biochemical and clinical pregnancy rates did not, however, differ significantly (Rasheedy et al., 2020).

Calcitriol supplementation has been demonstrated to enhance IVF results and encourage spontaneous ovulation in PCOS patients with VD deficiency (Heidari et al., 2021; Xu et al., 2021).

Cleavage/embryo development rate: In women with PCOS, vitamin D administration dramatically lowered androgen levels, LH, FSH, early miscarriage, and premature delivery rates while increasing the rate of ovulation and pregnancy. It had no discernible impact on cleavage rate, fertilization rate, or other hormonal markers, though. The results point to possible advantages for reproductive outcomes, but these need to be confirmed by better RCTs (Yang et al., 2023). The study discovered that while VD had no significant impact on clinical pregnancy rate, fertilization rate, embryo quality, ongoing pregnancy, or miscarriage, it dramatically increased the chemical pregnancy rate. Sequential analysis of the trials showed that further investigation is required to validate these results (Nandi et al., 2016; Zhou et al., 2022).

Implantation rate: VD supplementation significantly enhanced embryo implantation rates in the treatment group (53.2% vs. 46.7%) in comparison to the nontreatment group, supporting the role of VD levels in improving implantation outcomes after intracytoplasmic sperm injection procedures.

Clinical pregnancy rate: In a metaanalysis, 20 randomised controlled trials with 1961 participants were evaluated to assess the effect of VD supplementation on ovulation and pregnancy outcomes in women with polycystic ovarian syndrome (PCOS) (Makieva et al., 2021). It was found that VD supplementation significantly decreased the rates of early miscarriage, androgen levels, luteinizing hormone (LH), follicle-stimulating hormone (FSH), and premature delivery while increasing the rates of pregnancy, ovulation, and matured oocytes. Biochemical pregnancy rates, fertilization rates, cleavage rates, and embryo quality, however, did not show any discernible changes (Yang et al., 2023). VD treatment affected the results of IVF in infertile women with VD insufficiency.

IVF success rates: The effects of VD and probiotic supplementation on anti-Mullerian hormone AMH, glycaemic management, inflammation, and IVF success were evaluated in a randomised, double-blind, placebo-controlled trial with 120 PCOS-afflicted women. For eight weeks, participants were split into four groups and given either a placebo, probiotics (1.8×10^9 CFU), vitamin D (4000 IU), or a combination of the two. When compared to other groups, the combination group's insulin levels, IR, and insulin sensitivity all significantly improved ($P < .05$). Additionally, it resulted in a significant decrease in TNF-α gene expression ($P = .007$) and hs-CRP, indicating less inflammation. However, there were no discernible alterations in the levels of plasma total nitrite, fasting glucose, or AMH. According to these results, probiotic and vitamin D supplements together improve insulin function and lower inflammation in PCOS women undergoing IVF, but they have no effect on AMH or glucose metabolism (Farhangnia et al., 2024).

Live birth rates: The effect of VD fortification on reproductive outcomes was evaluated in Danish population-based cohort research. Using Denmark's mandatory VD fortification of margarine, which was abruptly terminated in 1985, researchers examined data from 16,212 women who were diagnosed with infertility between 1980 and 1991. According to the study, women who were exposed to VD fortification had a noticeably better chance of giving birth alive than women who were diagnosed after the fortification was discontinued. In particular, the live birth rate was only 8.7% in the nonexposed group, 14.5% in the VD-exposed group, and 12.4% during the wash-out phase. When comparing VD-exposed women to nonexposed women, the odds ratio (OR) for a live birth within 12 months was 1.87 (95% CI: 1.68–2.08, $P < .05$), showing substantial statistical significance. There was little seasonal change in the outcomes, which held true for anovulatory infertility cases and various follow-up periods. These results highlight the significance of dietary fortification or supplementation of vitamin D for women experiencing infertility (Jensen et al., 2020).

30.2   Conclusion: vitamin D as a supportive therapy

VD has a great deal of promise as a supportive treatment for diseases linked to infertility, especially PCOS and endometriosis. Its therapeutic value is highlighted by its ability to improve hormonal balance, modulate ovarian function, and improve reproductive outcomes. More carefully planned clinical trials are required to fine-tune dosage recommendations and completely comprehend its long-term effects, even if the available data support its advantages in enhancing ovulation and conception rates, as well as lowering inflammation and metabolic disorders. Optimizing fertility therapies and general reproductive well-being may be possible with the straightforward but efficient integration of VD evaluation and supplementation into reproductive health plans. Further high-quality trials are required for understanding the mechanisms behind the effects of VD supplementation on hormonal, metabolic, and reproductive outcomes in PCOS, endometriosis, and other causes (Rehman et al., 2021) of subfertility.

AI disclosure

During the preparation of this work, the author(s) used ChatGPT, and DeepSeek was used as a supplementary tool to improve the grammar and structure of the sentences. After using this tool/service, the author(s) reviewed and edited the content as needed and take(s) full responsibility for the content of the publication.

References

Alam, F. (2020). *Introduction to subfertility subfertility: Recent advances in management and prevention*. Brunei Darussalam: Elsevier, 97–106. https://doi.org/10.1016/B978-0-323-75945-8.00005-0, https://www.elsevier.com/books/subfertility/978-0-323-75945-8.

Al-Bayyari, N., Al-Domi, H., Zayed, F., Hailat, R., & Eaton, A. (2021). Androgens and hirsutism score of overweight women with polycystic ovary syndrome improved after vitamin D treatment: A randomized placebo controlled clinical trial. *Clinical Nutrition, 40*(3), 870–878. https://doi.org/10.1016/j.clnu.2020.09. 024, http://www.elsevier-international.com/journals/clnu/.

Azhar, A., Haider, G., Naseem, Z., Farooqui, N., Farooqui, M. U., & Rehman, R. (2021). Morphological changes in the experimental model of polycystic ovary syndrome and effects of vitamin D treatment. *Journal of Obstetrics and Gynaecology Research, 47*(3), 1164–1171. https://doi.org/10.1111/jog.14671, http://obgyn. onlinelibrary.wiley.com/hub/journal/10.1111/(ISSN)1447-0756/.

Azhar, A., Abid, F., & Rehman, R. (2020). Polycystic ovary syndrome, subfertility and vitamin D deficiency. *Pakistan Journal of the College of Physicians and Surgeons Pakistan, 30*(5), 545–546. https://doi.org/10.29271/jcpsp.2020. 5.545, http://www.jcpsp.pk/index.php?code=SkNQU1B8QXJ0aWNsZXxhcmNoaXZlcy5waHB8MHwwfDA=.

Burjiah, A. R., Sa'adi, A., & Widjiati, W. (2022). Vitamin D inhibited endometriosis development in mice model through interleukin-17 modulation. *Open Veterinary Journal, 12*(6), 956–964. https://doi.org/10.5455/OVJ. 2022.v12.i6.23, https://www.openveterinaryjournal.com/?sec=cissue.

Carson, A., Webster, F., Polzer, J., & Bamford, S. (2021). The power of potential: Assisted reproduction and the counterstories of women who discontinue fertility treatment. *Social Science & Medicine, 282*, 114153. https:// doi.org/10.1016/j.socscimed.2021.114153.

Farhangnia, P., Noormohammadi, M., & Delbandi, A.-A. (2024). Vitamin D and reproductive disorders: A comprehensive review with a focus on endometriosis. *Reproductive Health, 21*(1). https://doi.org/10.1186/ s12978-024-01797-y.

Goodman, N. F., Cobin, R. H., Futterweit, W., Glueck, J. S., Legro, R. S., & Carmina, E. (2015). American association of clinical endocrinologists, American college of endocrinology, and androgen excess and pcos society disease state clinical review: Guide to the best practices in the evaluation and treatment of polycystic ovary syndrome - Part 1. *Endocrine Practice, 21*(11), 1291–1300. https://doi.org/10.4158/EP15748.DSC, http://journals.aace.com/loi/endp.

Heidari, S., Kolahdouz-Mohammadi, R., Khodaverdi, S., Tajik, N., & Delbandi, A.-A. (2021). Expression levels of MCP-1, HGF, and IGF-1 in endometriotic patients compared with non-endometriotic controls. *BMC Women's Health, 21*(1). https://doi.org/10.1186/s12905-021-01560-6.

Jensen, A., Nielsen, M. L., Guleria, S., Kjaer, S. K., Heitmann, B. L., & Kesmodel, U. S. (2020). Chances of live birth after exposure to vitamin D–fortified margarine in women with fertility problems: Results from a Danish population-based cohort study. *Elsevier Inc., Denmark Fertility and Sterility, 113*(2), 383–391. https://doi.org/ 10.1016/j.fertnstert.2019.09.017, http://www.elsevier.com/locate/fertnstert.

Kamińska, K., Tchurzyk, M., Fraczek, O., Szlaga, A., Sambak, P., Tott, S., Małek, K., Knapczyk-Stwora, K., Błasiak, A., Rak, A., & Grzesiak, M. (2024). Effect of vitamin D3 on uterine morphology and insulin signaling in a polycystic ovary syndrome (PCOS) rat model. *Annals of Animal Science, 24*(4), 1197–1209. https://doi.org/10.2478/aoas-2024-0038, https://sciendo.com/journal/aoas.

Khan., H., Khan, U., Khan, H. N., Zahid, N., & Rehman, R. (2024). Vitamin D supplementation in polycystic ovary syndrome: Aa randomized open label delayed-start design: Sstudy protocol. https://doi.org/10.21203/rs. 3.pex-2558/v1.

Lerchbaum, E., Theiler-Schwetz, V., Kollmann, M., Wölfler, M., Pilz, S., Obermayer-Pietsch, B., & Trummer, C. (2021). Effects of vitamin D supplementation on surrogate markers of fertility in PCOS women: A randomized controlled trial. *Nutrients, 13*(2), 547. https://doi.org/10.3390/nu13020547.

Makieva, S., Reschini, M., Ferrari, S., Bonesi, F., Polledri, E., Fustinoni, S., Restelli, L., Sarais, V., Somigliana, E., & Viganò, P. (2021). Oral vitamin D supplementation impacts gene expression in granulosa cells in women undergoing IVF. *Human Reproduction, 36*(1), 130–144. https://doi.org/10.1093/humrep/deaa262.

Nandi, A., Sinha, N., Ong, E., Sonmez, H., & Poretsky, L. (2016). Is there a role for vitamin D in human reproduction? *Hormone Molecular Biology and Clinical Investigation, 25*(1), 15–28. https://doi.org/10.1515/ hmbci-2015-0051.

Rasheedy, R., Sammour, H., Elkholy, A., & Salim, Y. (2020). The efficacy of vitamin D combined with clomiphene citrate in ovulation induction in overweight women with polycystic ovary syndrome: A double blind, randomized clinical trial. *Endocrine, 69*(2), 393–401. https://doi.org/10.1007/s12020-020-02315-3, http://www.springer.com/humana+press/journal/12020.

Rehman, N., Khan, H. N., Sheikh, A., Azhar, A., Ashraf, M., Afzal, S., & Khan, A. H. (2023). *Efficacy of vitamin D supplementation and metformin compared to metformin alone in infertile females with polycystic ovary syndrome: A randomized open label trial.* https://doi.org/10.21203/rs.3.pex-2199/v1.

Rehman, R., Alam, F., Baig, M., Khan, A. H., & Ahmed, N. (2021). Editorial: Vitamin D deficiency and sufficiency in reproduction and bone metabolism. *Frontiers in Endocrinology, 12.* https://doi.org/10.3389/fendo.2021.740021.

Rehman, R., Alam, F., & Khan, R. (2024). Situation analysis of polycystic ovary syndrome in Central and East Asia. In *Polycystic ovary syndrome* (pp. 191–199). Elsevier. https://doi.org/10.1016/B978-0-323-87932-3.00035-9.

Rustamzadeh, A., Anjomshoa, M., Bahreini, N., Darabi, S., Rezaie, M. J., Rezaei, S., Rahimi-Madiseh, M., Deris, F., & Zamani, S. (2024). All-trans retinoic acid and fibroblast growth factor-2 enhance the fertility rate and embryo development in polycystic ovary syndrome mouse model. *Iranian Journal of Basic Medical Sciences, 27*(4), 418–424. https://doi.org/10.22038/IJBMS.2024.70509.15328, https://ijbms.mums.ac.ir/article_23649_11df8326bdb2e44d9e261fa4c07a9fc2.pdf.

Samma, Z. H., Khan, H. N., Riffat, S., Ashraf, M., & Rehman, R. (2024). Unraveling the genetic associations of DENND1A (rs9696009) and ERBB4 (rs2178575) with infertile polycystic ovary syndrome females in Pakistan. *Biochemical Genetics, 62*(3), 2148–2165. https://doi.org/10.1007/s10528-023-10537-z, https://www.springer.com/journal/10528.

Shiravani, Z., Najib, F. S., Alirahimi, M., Askary, E., Poordast, T., Tanideh, N., Roozmeh, S., Shekarkhar, G., Atbaei, S., Porro, D., Sabetian, S., & Cava, C. (2024). The supplemental effect of vitamin-D3 and omega-3 on induced endometriosis in rat model to investigate the inflammatory response. *Journal of Obstetrics, Gynecology and Cancer Research, 9*(5), 498–506. https://doi.org/10.30699/jogcr.9.5.498, https://www.jogcr.com/article_707363.html.

Wen, X., Wang, L., Li, F., & Yu, X. (2024). Effects of vitamin D supplementation on metabolic parameters in women with polycystic ovary syndrome: A randomized controlled trial. *Journal of Ovarian Research, 17*(1). https://doi.org/10.1186/s13048-024-01473-6.

Winter, H. G., Rolnik, D. L., Mol, B. W. J., Torkel, S., Alesi, S., Mousa, A., Habibi, N., Silva, T. R., Oi Cheung, T., Thien Tay, C., Quinteros, A., Grieger, J. A., & Moran, L. J. (2023). Can dietary patterns impact fertility outcomes? A systematic review and meta-analysis. *Nutrients, 15*(11). https://doi.org/10.3390/nu15112589, http://www.mdpi.com/journal/nutrients/.

Xu, F., Wolf, S., Green, O.', & Xu, J. (2021). Vitamin D in follicular development and oocyte maturation. *Reproduction, 161*(6). https://doi.org/10.1530/REP-20-0608.

Yang, M., Shen, X., Lu, D., Peng, J., Zhou, S., Xu, L., & Zhang, J. (2023). Effects of vitamin D supplementation on ovulation and pregnancy in women with polycystic ovary syndrome: A systematic review and meta-analysis. *Frontiers in Endocrinology, 14.* https://doi.org/10.3389/fendo.2023.1148556.

Yin, T., Lin, W., Ming, K., Lv, H., Wang, Y., Yuanchao, L. I., Zhen, H., Yuan, J., & Asadi, H. (2024). Effect of vitamin D supplementation on lipid profile, and hormonal functions in polycystic ovary syndrome: An umbrella systematic review and meta-analysis. *Prostaglandins & Other Lipid Mediators, 175*, 106913. https://doi.org/10.1016/j.prostaglandins.2024.106913.

Zhou, X., Wu, X., Luo, X., Shao, J., Guo, D., Deng, B., & Wu, Z. (2022). Effect of vitamin D supplementation on in vitro fertilization outcomes: A trial sequential meta-analysis of 5 randomized controlled trials. *Frontiers in Endocrinology, 13.* https://doi.org/10.3389/fendo.2022.852428, https://www.frontiersin.org/journals/endocrinology#.

CHAPTER 31

Public health initiatives in promoting awareness and vitamin D supplement use in low- and middle-income countries

Kiran Fatima[1], Shiza Batool[2], Irum Fatima[3], and Nighat Nisar Khan[4]

[1]Department of Community Medicine, Sindh Medical College, Jinnah Sindh Medical University, Karachi, Pakistan [2]Instit fuer Didaktik und Ausbildungsforschung in der Medizin, Ludwig Maximilian University, Munich, Germany [3]Department of Education, Sindh Madrasatul Islam University, Karachi, Pakistan [4]Community Health Sciences, Dow Medical College, Dow University of Health Sciences, Karachi, Pakistan

31.1 Introduction: vitamin D and population health

Vitamin D is frequently designated as the "sunshine vitamin" due to the fact that its endogenous synthesis in the human body commences when exposed to ultraviolet B (UVB) radiation from sunlight (Wacker & Holick, 2013). In the early 20th century, the researchers linked vitamin D deficiency to the development of rickets, a debilitating bone disease affecting children (Jones, 2022). Vitamin D is a fat-soluble vitamin that exists in two main forms: vitamin D2 (ergocalciferol) and vitamin D3 (cholecalciferol) (Balachandar et al., 2021). These forms differ in their chemical structure and sources. Vitamin D3 is more potent than vitamin D2 with a longer duration of action, more effective in raising and maintaining vitamin D levels in bloodstream. Vitamin D3 is more efficiently absorbed and utilized by the human body. The two forms of vitamin D are converted in the human body to the active form, 1,25-dihydroxyvitamin D, which is responsible for vitamin D physiological effects (van den Heuvel et al., 2024). The main sources of vitamin D3 are: animal red meat, liver, fatty fish, fish oil, egg yolk, and dietary supplements. The sources of vitamin D2 are plants, such as irradiated mushrooms (grown in UV light), dietary supplements, and fortified foods (Benedik, 2022). A considerable attention has been focused on vitamin D due to its pivotal role in sustaining optimal bone health, immune system function, and overall physiological well-being (Paul et al., 2024). Vitamin D status is an important public health indicator reflecting overall nutritional and environmental conditions of a population (Hilger et al., 2014; Oskarsson et al., 2022). Vitamin D deficiency can lead to a number of health problems, including rickets in children, osteoporosis, osteopenia, and fractures in adults. Furthermore, it is linked to other health problems, including hypertension, diabetes, metabolic syndrome, cancer, immune

The Impact of Vitamin D on Health and Disease. DOI: https://doi.org/10.1016/B978-0-443-34037-6.00022-4

system regulation, cardiovascular health, neurological function, autoimmune, and infectious diseases. Vitamin D plays a crucial role in human health, extending beyond its traditional function in bone health (Daryabor et al., 2023; Henn et al., 2022; Sanlier & Guney-Coskun, 2022; Sultan et al., 2020; Trimarco et al., 2022).

Vitamin D deficiency is a multifactorial health issue that affects nearly half of the world's population (Palacios & Gonzalez, 2014). A research reported data from the year 2000 to 2022, showing the global prevalence of the serum 25(OH) D < 30 nmol/L as 15.7% (Cui et al., 2023). Numerous determinants are responsible for this deficiency, like genetic, environmental, and lifestyle. Reduced exposure to sunshine, poor dietary intake, restricted availability of fortified foods, and supplements are the primary causes that act synergistically to influence the vitamin D status of an individual (Amrein et al., 2020; Calvo & Lamberg-Allardt, 2017; El Hoss et al., 2023; Hatchell et al., 2020; Shraim et al., 2022). Geographical differences brought about by latitude, solar exposure, dietary practices, and socioeconomic status results in variations in vitamin D levels among the world's population (Cashman, 2022). Pregnant women, young children, and the elderly are at high risk. Insufficient vitamin D during pregnancy poses detrimental effects on fetal growth and early childhood development (Chien et al., 2024). Furthermore, those who don't get enough vitamin D are more susceptible to falls, have weaker muscles, and develop neurodegenerative disorders and cognitive decline later in life (Kupisz-Urbańska et al., 2021; Terock et al., 2022). Additionally, a person's vitamin D levels can affect the prognosis of a number of chronic illnesses, such as autoimmune diseases and cancer (Berretta et al., 2022; Wang et al., 2017). This chapter explains the significance of vitamin D in population health with a focus on developing and implementing interventions to improve food fortification, community involvement, supplementation, and educational campaigns in low- and middle-income countries (LMICs). Nonetheless, it highlights important areas for evidence-based research, epidemiological developments, demographic analysis, and emphasizes collaborative efforts among stakeholders to address the deficiency of vitamin D in LMICs.

31.2   Epidemiology and prevalence: vitamin D deficiency in low- and middle-income countries

Vitamin D deficiency is a global public health concern. Nearly 1 billion people have vitamin D deficiency, while 50% of the population has been reported as having vitamin D insufficiency (Nair & Maseeh, 2012). The World Bank classifies countries according to their level of development measured by Gross National Income (GNI) per capita in United States Dollar (US$). According to this distribution for the fiscal year 2024 (FY24), the reported GNI per capita in US$, for low-income countries < 1145$, low- and middle-income countries 1146$ to 4515$, upper middle-income countries 4516$ to 14,005$, and high-income countries > 14,005$, as shown in Fig. 31.1 and Table 31.1.

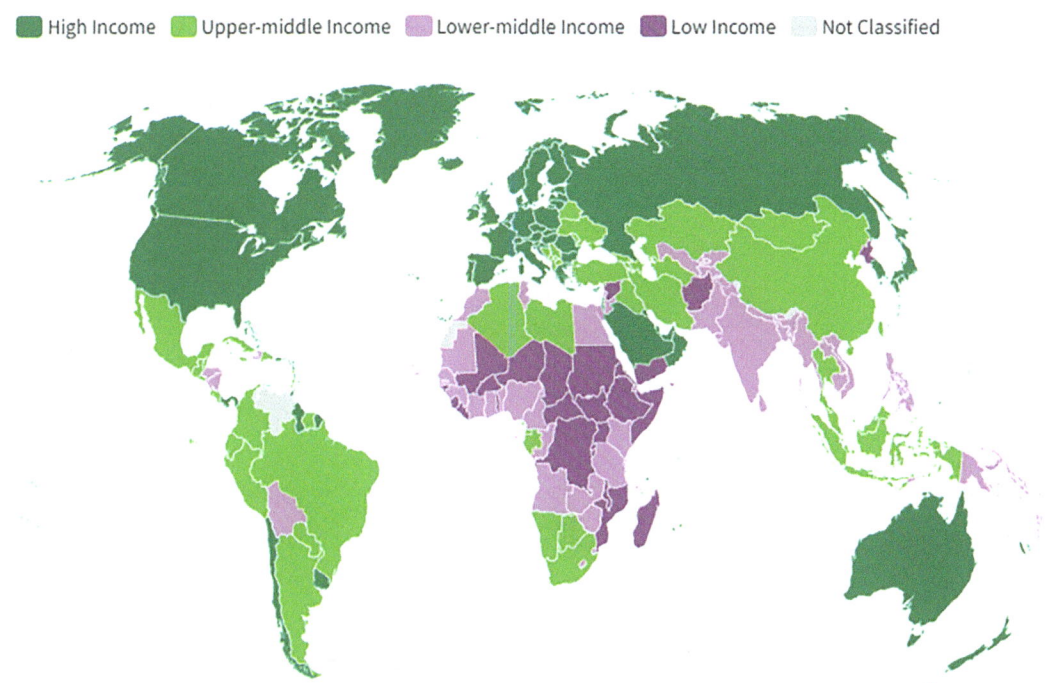

Figure 31.1

World Bank Group country classification by income level for the year 2024–2025. World Bank classify countries according to their level of development measured by Gross National Income (GNI) per capita in United States Dollar (US $), for the fiscal year 2024–25 (low-income countries < 1145, low- and middle-income countries 1,146 to 4,515, upper-middle-income countries 4516 to 14,005 and, high-income countries > 14,005). Map lines delineate study areas and do not necessarily depict accepted national boundaries. *Source: From Metreau, E., Young, K. E., & Eapen, S. G. (2024).* World Bank country classifications by income level for 2024–2025. *World Bank Blogs.*

The countries grouped as low-income and low-middle-income economies are 77 in total, out of which 51 countries are grouped as low-middle-income countries (Metreau et al., 2024). The existing literature highlighted a significant paucity of data reporting vitamin D deficiency prevalence in all 51 LMICs, spread across six world regions (Cashman & O'Dea, 2019; Hilger et al., 2014; Palacios & Gonzalez, 2014; Metreau et al., 2024). Research studies conducted on vitamin D deficiency prevalence in LMICs have limitations of sample size, not stemmed on large population-based surveys. The following statistics demonstrate that there is a significant risk of vitamin D deficiency in populations living in LMICs. The prevalence of vitamin D deficiency is highest in Asia, the Middle East, and Africa; and subsequently more prevalent among immigrants from these regions living at higher latitudes (Munns et al., 2012). The South Asian region showed the highest number of "hot spot" countries, including Afghanistan children had a deficiency of vitamin between 16.8% and 73% (Azizi & Tariq, 2019).

Table 31.1 Low-income countries and low-middle-income countries list 2024–25; number of low-income countries (LICs): 26; number of low-middle-income countries (LIMCs): 51. The countries grouped as low income and, low-middle income economies are 77, out of which 51 countries grouped as low-middle-income countries, and 26 are countries grouped as low-income countries.

Afghanistan	LIC	Malawi	LIC
Angola	LMIC	Mali	LIC
Bangladesh	LMIC	Mauritania	LMIC
Benin	LMIC	Micronesia, Fed. Sts.	LMIC
Bhutan	LMIC	Morocco	LMIC
Bolivia	LMIC	Mozambique	LIC
Burkina Faso	LIC	Myanmar	LMIC
Burundi	LIC	Nepal	LMIC
Cabo Verde	LMIC	Nicaragua	LMIC
Cambodia	LMIC	Niger	LIC
Cameroon	LMIC	Nigeria	LMIC
Central African Republic	LIC	Pakistan	LMIC
Chad	LIC	Papua New Guinea	LMIC
Comoros	LMIC	Philippines	LMIC
Congo, Dem. Rep.	LIC	Rwanda	LIC
Congo, Rep.	LMIC	Samoa	LMIC
Côte d'Ivoire	LMIC	São Tomé and Príncipe	LMIC
Djibouti	LMIC	Senegal	LMIC
Egypt, Arab Rep.	LMIC	Sierra Leone	LIC
Eritrea	LIC	Solomon Islands	LMIC
Eswatini	LMIC	Somalia	LIC
Ethiopia	LIC	South Sudan	LIC
Gambia, The	LIC	Sri Lanka	LMIC
Ghana	LMIC	Sudan	LIC
Guinea	LMIC	Syrian Arab Republic	LIC
Guinea-Bissau	LIC	Tajikistan	LMIC
Haiti	LMIC	Tanzania	LMIC
Honduras	LMIC	Timor-Leste	LMIC
India	LMIC	Togo	LIC
Jordan	LMIC	Tunisia	LMIC
Kenya	LMIC	Uganda	LIC
Kiribati	LMIC	Uzbekistan	LMIC
Korea, Dem. People's Rep.	LIC	Vanuatu	LMIC
Kyrgyz Republic	LMIC	Vietnam	LMIC
Lao PDR	LMIC	West Bank and Gaza	LMIC
Lebanon	LMIC	Yemen, Rep.	LIC
Lesotho	LMIC	Zambia	LMIC
Liberia	LIC	Zimbabwe	LMIC
Madagascar	LIC		

Source: From World Bank Country and Lending Groups. (2024). The World Bank. www.worldbank.org.

Similarly, India reported 19.7% among children and adolescents; and 19.4%–87% for adults Bangladesh and Nepal reported 0%–6.3%, a low prevalence of vitamin D deficiency in children and adults. In Sri Lanka, the prevalence of vitamin D among infants was as low as 0.6%–6% (Cashman and O'Dea, 2019). The prevalence of vitamin D deficiency in the Eastern Mediterranean Region is reported as 30%–90% particularly high in Middle Eastern countries. The research findings vary with the type of studies, age group, ethnicity, country, and analytical methods used to report study results (The World Bank, 2024). Vitamin D deficiency as reported in Pakistani neonates was 46.7%–75.3%, whereas, between 26.5% and 91.3% in pregnant women, and 25.3% in nonpregnant women (Cashman and O'Dea, 2019). Another study of the adult population in Pakistan, India, and Bangladesh reveals that more than 80% of adults in these countries are deficient in vitamin D (Kaur et al., 2025). Research studies from Asia reported vitamin D deficiency among infants; 51% in Turkey, 86% in Iran, 61% in India, and 61% infants in Pakistan (Palacios and Gonzalez, 2014). Studies conducted on pregnant and lactating women in Asia and the Middle East demonstrated a significant risk of vitamin D deficiency, with prevalence rates of 50% in Turkey, 60% in India, and 45% in Pakistan (Palacios and Gonzalez, 2014). It is reported that 20% of the population in Afghanistan, Pakistan, India, Mongolia, and Tunisia is vitamin D deficient, with serum vitamin D level 25-hydroxy below 30 nmol/L (Cashman & O'Dea, 2019; Roth et al., 2018; Siddiqee et al., 2021). Particularly Tunisian pregnant women, infants, and children had a high prevalence of 40.9%–90%; while in adults it was 17.2%–61%. Deficiency of vitamin D among women of child-bearing age in the West Bank and Gaza was reported as 56%–70%, whereas children had 5%–13% vitamin D inadequacy. Girls in Yemen had 61%, while adults in Syria had 58.2%. Morocco has alarming statistics with a high prevalence of > 90% in infants and women, while between 7.1% and 51.6% in adults. Studies in Egypt report vitamin D inadequacy as 11.5% and 45% among infants, adolescents, and women (Cashman and O'Dea, 2019). In Africa, vitamin D deficiency is also widespread, with significant variations across regions and higher prevalence in urban areas compared to rural ones. Sub-Saharan Africa exhibits a prevalence of approximately one in five individuals experiencing vitamin D deficiency. In Sub-Saharan Africa, vitamin deficiency is particularly pronounced among newborns and women (Mogire et al., 2020). In Uganda children 2.5%, whereas women 25% and 36% had vitamin D deficiency. In Ethiopia, the prevalence of vitamin D among the adult population varies between 14.8% and 77%. Tanzania reported a low prevalence of vitamin D inadequacy in pregnant women, adolescents, and adults. Similarly, Malawi and Zimbabwe had a low prevalence of inadequate vitamin D in adults. Cameroon also shows less prevalence of vitamin D insufficiency among older adults. However, interestingly, in Nigeria, older adults showed 51.4% prevalence of vitamin D deficiency, while adults 0%, and children in Nigeria and adults in Guinea-Bissau showed 0%–4.9% prevalence. Likewise, children in Gambia had 0.5% vitamin D deficiency (Cashman and O'Dea, 2019). Certain groups are more vulnerable to vitamin D deficiency. It has been reported that breastfed infants, children, and women of child-bearing age, pregnant and lactating women, dark-skinned, elderly, and people with limited sun exposure are at high risk for vitamin D deficiency (Heo et al., 2022; Khadilkar et al., 2017; Lips, 2010; Lips et al., 2021). These groups are vulnerable due to factors like limited sun exposure, cultural practices, and dietary habits (Cashman, 2017; Lips et al., 2019; Roth et al., 2018). Despite the abundance of sunlight in many LMICs, the population often exhibits suboptimal vitamin D levels. Low vitamin D status is a multifactorial complex phenomenon that is caused by various factors, including biological, genetic, including skin pigmentation, socio-demographical factors, like air pollution, high-latitude, sunlight exposure, and cultural customs (Cashman, 2017; Mogire et al., 2020). Compared to people with lighter complexion, the dark skinned individuals need more exposure to UVB radiation to preserve vitamin D (Armas et al., 2007; Kimball et al., 2017). Low vitamin D levels are found in those who wear clothing that covers much of their skin or use sunscreen. Similarly, limited mobility is common in the elderly population, which leads to extended periods of indoor activity; they barely get exposure to direct sunlight, resulting in a high prevalence of vitamin D deficiency (Dawson-Hughes, 2024; Houston et al., 2023; Kalyani et al., 2010; Libon et al., 2017; Toffanello et al., 2012). The dietary intake lacking in vitamin D-rich food, for example: fatty fish, eggs, and fortified dairy, is a contributing factor to large number of the underserved population. The prevalence of nutritional rickets is reported to be the highest in Asia, the Middle East, and Africa, ranging from 1% to 24% among children (Bener & Hoffmann, 2010; Creo et al., 2017; Karim et al., 2003; Strand et al., 2007). Few studies reported the prevalence of acute life-threatening complications of nutritional rickets, for example, seizures due to hypocalcemia and cardiomyopathy (Bansal et al., 2014; Basatemur & Sutcliffe, 2015; Brown et al., 2009). In LMICs, rickets surveillance programs are supposed to significantly improve these threats, enable early identification in communities at high risk and in need of vitamin D interventions. The vitamin D status of infants depends on the mother's vitamin D status, and the breast milk vitamin D content. The mothers should have adequate intake of vitamin D during lactation period and good sunlight exposure to maintain vitamin D levels (Heo et al., 2022; Khadilkar et al., 2017). A gender disparity is observed in LMICs' vitamin D levels; Jordan, Sri Lanka, Vietnam, Mexico, Nigeria, and Malaysia have reported lower vitamin D levels in women and girls as compared to men and boys. This is related to occupation, clothing, and cultural practices in these countries for low vitamin D status, not due to the biological difference between men and women (Jabbour et al., 2023; Palacios & Gonzalez, 2014). All age groups are at highest risk of vitamin D deficiency worldwide; however, diet, supplement use, age, gender, geographic latitude, cultural and lifestyle factors, skin pigmentation, and individual vitamin D metabolism can increase or decrease the risk of vitamin D deficiency (Cashman, 2022; Goswami et al., 2000). The health systems of many LMICs did not support diagnostic and treatment facilities to combat with vitamin D deficiency disorders. The vitamin D deficiency is linked to increased risk of rickets, osteomalacia, noncommunicable diseases like cardiovascular diseases, and diabetes. Early and effective interventions of vitamin D supplementation, food fortification, and public awareness campaigns are required to address the growing concern in LMICs.

31.3 Public health initiatives: vitamin D awareness in low- and middle-income countries

"Alone, we can do so little; together, we can do so much" (Helen Keller). Holistically, public health engages multiple sectors for taking an impactful initiative that includes empowering healthcare workers, including physicians, nurses, and community health workers, with proper training, knowledge and skills in vitamin D health promotion; which is crucial for scaling up global awareness efforts (Cashman, 2022; El Hoss et al., 2023). Global capacity building for vitamin D awareness requires comprehensive training programs that can equip these front-line providers to collect and disseminate data, educate patients, screen for deficiency, and support vitamin D supplementation. Fostering a global network of vitamin D researchers, public health experts, and community advocates to facilitate the exchange of knowledge, best practices, and innovative approaches (Hassan Ali et al., 2021). This collaborative platform can strengthen the capacity for vitamin D awareness, research, and advocacy worldwide. Encouraging the transfer of knowledge, resources, and expertise between high-income countries (HICs) and LMICs can help address global disparities in vitamin D awareness and access to supplementation (Cashman, 2020; Cashman, 2022). LMICs can share their distinct perspective, challenges, creative and innovative approaches with partner high-income countries (HICs), to spread vitamin D awareness. In resource-constrained settings, cooperative efforts like twinning programs or technical assistance can help to develop and implement successful strategies to mitigate vitamin D deficiency (Cashman, 2020; Cashman, 2022). This mutual knowledge sharing can promote cooperative problem-solving and the creation of more successful and internationally applicable vitamin D initiatives by stakeholders. For instance, researchers and public health specialists from HICs can provide training and offer technical support to their colleagues in LMICs. The holistic approach might involve integrating research techniques, best practices, and instructional resources about vitamin D awareness campaigns, supplementation plans, and monitoring systems. The transfer of knowledge and expertise will allow local capacity building and empower stakeholders to formulate initiatives and carry out context-appropriate vitamin D programs in LMICs (Cashman, 2020).

31.3.1 Community engagement

Public health initiatives for vitamin D awareness can be done in various ways. Community engagement is the foundation upon which sustainable public health programs are built (World Health Organization, 2020) . It is one of the most effective methods, especially in LMICs, to actively involve and empower local communities (Unicef.org, 2018). Community engagement starts with the identification of the target community, and then needs assessment is crucial for understanding the unique challenges, barriers, and opportunities within a community. By gathering data through surveys, focus groups, and interviews, we gain valuable insights into the community's knowledge, attitudes, and practices related to vitamin D (George et al., 2015;

Unicef.org, 2018). This information will inform the development of tailored educational materials and engagement strategies. Within every community, some individuals and organizations hold significant influence. Early engagement with these important stakeholders in communities can help to prioritize the objectives of the program. Furthermore, it reflects to foster confidence, builds trust, establishes credibility, and ensures that the vitamin D initiatives are aligned with the values of the community (Maryam et al., 2022). It is critical to acknowledge the cultural norms, attitudes, and practices that can significantly influence people's acceptance and awareness of vitamin D. For example, dietary habits may influence the consumption of foods high in vitamin D, and cultural or societal conventions may restrict sun exposure in some populations. Understanding these subtleties will help to develop culturally sensitive educational materials, instructional resources, and engagement tactics and strategies. The instructional materials must be according to the target community that connects with the audience and effectively communicates the significance of vitamin D. Even those with low literacy levels should find the instructional materials visually appealing, captivating, and simple to understand. Using relatable examples, straightforward language, and unambiguous pictures to explain concepts related to vitamin D (Maryam et al., 2022). Creating educational resources in the community's local languages and dialects is essential. This shows respect for the community's cultural identity in addition to ensuring optimum accessibility and understanding of the disseminated information. Consequently, absorption and retention of information are augmented in the community (World Health Organization, 2024). Misconceptions or myths regarding vitamin D and its sources related to health advantages/disadvantages may exist in many communities. Thus, the disseminated educational materials should proactively address these common misunderstandings and provide clear, evidence-based information to dispel any inaccurate beliefs. Community engagement requires a holistic, multifaceted approach that makes use of both conventional and contemporary communication channels to engage communities in vitamin D education and awareness-raising. In the current digital era, social media and mobile technologies, such as Facebook, WhatsApp, Instagram, local messaging apps, and other social media platforms, can provide effective channels for connecting and interacting with communities. These platforms promote sharing educational materials, interactive conversations, and spreading knowledge about vitamin D at faster pace (World Health Organization, 2020; World Health Organization, 2024). Community meetings and in-person contacts can be quite successful in raising awareness of vitamin D. Consider about planning activities where people may learn about vitamin D, take part in interactive activities, and interact with medical professionals, including health fairs, cookery demos, or community discussions (Chandaria et al., 2011). The reach and credibility of vitamin D programs can be greatly increased by forming collaborations with respected community leaders, such as community elders, religious leaders, or local government representatives (World Health Organization, 2020; World Health Organization, 2024). These powerful people have the ability to mobilize their communities, spread the right information, and support group initiatives. A long-lasting network of vitamin D advocates may be established in the community by giving these front-line employees the skills and resources they need to inform their colleagues. To educate and engage community members, give them useful tools to aid in their outreach activities, as well as effective educational materials and communication skills. Establish a network of support for community health workers (CHWs) and provide them with the resources and tools they need to carry out successful community outreach. These could include mobile devices for data collecting and reporting, vitamin D screening kits, supplemental samples, and educational brochures. This will guarantee the continuing effectiveness of vitamin D programs and keep them motivated (Chandaria et al., 2011; World Health Organization, 2020; World Health Organization, 2024). Public Health strategies may also include various other approaches for effective awareness campaigns, as discussed below:

31.3.1.1 Participatory learning approaches

According to the World Health Organization (WHO), effective vitamin D education involves more than just spreading knowledge; it also entails involving community members in interactive, participatory learning activities that improve memory retention and encourage behavioral change (World Health Organization, 2024).

31.3.1.1.1 Interactive workshops and group discussions

Develop interactive workshops and roundtable discussions that inspire community members to take an active role, contribute their viewpoints, and work through vitamin D-related difficulties. Participants gain a better understanding of the subject and a sense of ownership as a result of this method (Unicef.org, 2018).

31.3.1.1.2 Hands-on activities for vitamin D-rich food preparation

Plan interactive events and cooking demos to teach locals how to include foods high in vitamin D in their everyday diets. These practical, experiential learning approaches can be extremely impactful in removing barriers related to dietary habits and food preferences (Unicef.org, 2018).

31.3.1.1.3 Addressing economic constraints in low-income communities

In low-income communities, a major deterrent to access vitamin D supplements could be the high cost. Reducing the cost of supplements, by distributing them at a discounted rate or subsidizing them through partnerships with nonprofit organizations or local governments, will provide relief to the people (Oktaria et al., 2020) Global Alliance for Improved Nutrition GAIN.

31.3.1.1.4 Developing strategies for hard-to-reach populations

Accessing information regarding vitamin D deficiency/insufficiency, treatment and supplements could be a hard task for certain groups of population, especially elderly, those who are housebound, females who stay in house due to religious or cultural restrictions, disabled people or marginalized population (World Health Organization, 2024). Develop focused outreach plans, such as house calls, spread the words via social media, home visits, pamphlets/pictorial flyers distribution initiatives, to ensure the difficult-to-reach groups do not get neglected.

31.3.1.1.5   Develop community-led awareness projects for vitamin D

Providing community members the chance to take the lead in creating and carrying out vitamin D awareness initiatives, including a range of stakeholders, such as healthcare professionals, community leaders, and the people of community (World Health Organization, 2024). This could entail starting community-based supplementation programs, producing instructional materials, or planning regional events. Encourage community members to share their expertise and experiences with their colleagues as educators and ambassadors for vitamin D. This peer-to-peer method can be very successful in fostering behavioral change, boosting credibility, and fostering trust. The long-term viability of these initiatives can be ensured by cultivating this sense of ownership (World Health Organization, 2024).

31.3.1.1.6   Evaluate the impact of community engagement and community feedback

Monitoring, surveillance, and evaluation of the launched programs are vital for achieving the desired objectives propitiously. Evaluating the performance of community engagement tactics is essential for ongoing development and the long-term viability of vitamin D programs. Create a thorough assessment system that incorporates both qualitative and quantitative indicators. This could involve assessments of vitamin D-related knowledge, attitudes, and behaviors in addition to the scope and results of community involvement initiatives (Unicef.org, 2018; World Health Organization, 2024). Assessing the response of the community, medical professionals, and other stakeholders regarding the usefulness and applicability of the vitamin D programs, to get their input and feedback, is an integral part of community-based programs. This feedback can be used to improve the strategies being used and deal with any new issues that may arise (Unicef.org, 2018). To find areas for improvement and guide the development of the community involvement strategies, continuously evaluate the data and gather input. According to the (The World Bank, 2024), this iterative method will guarantee that the vitamin D programs continue to be sensitive to community needs and efficiently promote a lasting improvement.

Vitamin D: Collaboration of Government and Non-governmental Organizations (NGOs) To address the worldwide burden of vitamin D deficiency, it is crucial to working with international, national, local health authorities and nongovernmental organizations (NGOs) for incorporating the recent scientific evidences into public health strategies and policies. This collaboration entails creating regional or national vitamin D fortification initiatives, launching public awareness campaigns, and implementations screening and supplementation programs in low- and middle-income countries. Globally established international organization, WHO recommended standard guidelines serve as a crucial reference for national governments and healthcare providers (Oktaria et al., 2020; World Health Organization, 2024). The World Health Organization (WHO) reports, technical documents, and recommended guidelines for vitamin D status, supplementations, and treatment methods delineate the significance of vitamin D deficiency. The United Nations Children's Fund (UNICEF) recognized the significance of vitamin D for the health and development of children. UNICEF incorporates vitamin D supplementation initiatives for maternal and children health programs, especially in regions where vitamin D deficiency prevails. The UNICEF aims to enhance the nutritional status, health, and general well-being of children worldwide by incorporating vitamin D supplementation into current existing maternal and child health programs (Unicef.org, 2018). The NGOs have also been instrumental in driving global vitamin D awareness by reaching underprivileged groups worldwide. These NGOs often collaborate and work with people and influential individuals who have significant impacts on the local communities. They approach religious leaders, healthcare providers, government representatives, policymakers and elders in the community to advocate for policy changes and promote legislative reforms by distributing supplements and implementing targeted vitamin D awareness campaigns (Oktaria et al., 2020; World Health Organization, 2024). Integrating vitamin D awareness and supplementation into broader global health initiatives, such as the sustainable development goals (SDGs), can amplify the impact and sustainability of vitamin D programs. By aligning with existing frameworks and collaborating across sectors, vitamin D can be positioned as a key contributor to achieving universal health coverage and improving overall population health. Global coordination and collaboration among international organizations, national governments, and local stakeholders are crucial for driving vitamin D awareness worldwide (Oktaria et al., 2020; World Health Organization, 2024).

31.3.1.1.7 Vitamin D supplementation strategies in low- and middle-income countries

Vitamin D deficiency is considered a major public health issue; statistics defined it as a global pandemic, particularly pervasive in LMICs. Maintaining adequate vitamin D levels is imperative for ensuring good bone health, immunological function, and general well-being. The low- and middle-income nations with limited resources need proper strategies with effective methods for fortification, supplementation, and treatment to overcome the burden of vitamin D deficiency (Cashman et al., 2016; Cashman, 2022).

Optimized supplementation for specific populations Different populations have distinct requirements that indicate the need for customized and personalized supplementation programs to get a significant and long-lasting impact. Understanding the unique conditions and challenges faced by high-risk populations allows us to develop focused strategies to get optimize the benefits of vitamin D supplementation. Public health interventions must be applied with precision, tailored to specific communities, as any standard strategy does not always take into account the needs and situations of various population groups (Cashman, 2022; Cashman et al., 2016).

31.3.1.2 Identifying high-risk populations

31.3.1.2.1 Pregnant women and infants

Research has shown that vitamin D deficiency poses adverse effects on maternal health and fetal growth. It has been revealed that pregnant women and infants both are at risk of developing bone deformities and other systemic illnesses. Screening tests can help to identify these high-risk individuals; regular check-ups and monitoring during and after treatment will be of utmost benefit to prevent future complications and diseases (Özdemir et al., 2018).

31.3.1.2.2 Elderly population

Elderly gets less exposure to sunlight, mostly due to less activity and indoor activities, hence skin synthesizes less vitamin D. In this population, targeted vitamin D supplementation, balanced dietary intake, and good self-care can help maintain strong healthy bones, reducing the risk of fractures and fall (Giustina et al., 2023).

31.3.1.2.3 People with limited sun exposure

Certain groups of the population have limited sun exposure. These include individuals living in urban areas, working indoors, or wearing clothes that cover the full body, hence hindering exposure to direct sunlight. They are susceptible to developing vitamin D deficiency. The development of customized supplementation strategies is imperative to address their distinct requirements (Lips et al., 2021).

31.3.1.2.4 Tailoring supplement dosages for diverse populations

Determining the optimal vitamin D dosage necessitates an understanding of the target population. To illustrate, during pregnancy, a higher dosage may be required to meet the augmented physiological demands; conversely, infants may require lower, age-appropriate doses to avert the potential for toxicity. It is imperative to take these factors into careful consideration when formulating supplementation programs (Amrein et al., 2020; Cashman, 2022).

31.3.2 Vitamin D food fortification strategies

The World Health Organization defines food fortification as the aim to provide 97.5% of people who are at risk of micronutrient deficiencies with their daily intake, and to prevent excessive intake and toxicity in this group and in other groups. Nonetheless, as reaching out 97.5% population with the recommended dietary allowance (RDA) of vitamin D, which is 50 nmol/L, is practically not possible. Therefore, many countries recommended fortification of staple foods (rice, corn, wheat, potatoes, bread) with vitamin D, where the chosen food vehicle must be part of people's daily dietary pattern; easily available and affordable to all people with different socioeconomic levels (El Hoss et al., 2023). The food fortification techniques depend upon various factors. These include the extent of micronutrient deficiencies, influenced by the nation's dominant eating habits, and the general availability of technologies for food fortification. Additionally, the existing national food fortification legislations also play an important role in this process (Wang et al., 2017). Food-based remedies to improve low vitamin D levels are more effective than greater sun exposure to curtail the risk of skin cancer. Food sources provide a more reliable and accessible form of vitamin D in areas with longer duration of winters, which reduces certain risks of supplementation, including possible toxicity (Dunlop et al., 2021; Pilz et al., 2018). Prospective methods to improve vitamin D status at the population level includes "Fortification," direct addition of vitamin D to food items; and "Bio-fortification," the introduction of vitamin D to animal feed or ultraviolet B (UVB) irradiance of animals (Jääskeläinen et al., 2017; Kiely & Cashman, 2018).

31.3.2.1 History of vitamin D fortification

The practice of fortifying food with vitamin D originated in the 1930s, initially targeting milk products. However, in 1950, the European Union implemented a ban on vitamin D fortification, citing instances of hypercalcemia caused by excessive vitamin D absorption (Zittermann, 2017).

31.3.2.2 Suitable food vehicles for vitamin D fortification

Food vehicles encompass a diverse range of products, from fundamental commodities that are readily available on the retail market for consumer use to processed foods that are fortified at the manufacturing stage. A review of the literature reveals a multitude of suitable animal and plant-based food vehicles, encompassing both lipid and nonlipid food items. These include fluid milk, powdered milk, egg, edible oils, bread, biscuits or breakfast cereal, yogurt, cheese, UV (ultraviolet)-mushrooms, and orange juice (Alnafisah et al., 2024; Cashman & O'Dea, 2019; Cashman & O'Neill, 2024; Lavelli, D'Incecco, & Pellegrino, 2021; Nyakundi et al., 2023). Of the various food vehicles, the most frequently utilized are oil, rice, wheat flour, maize flour, and salt. In LMICs, oil is the most prevalent food vehicle, while wheat flour is the least common. This is in contrast to high-income and upper-middle-income countries, where oil, wheat flour, maize flour, and rice are highlighted almost with equal occurrence (Cashman & O'Neill, 2024; Lips et al., 2021).

31.3.2.3 Effects of fortification on circulatory vitamin D levels

Vitamin D food fortification has been demonstrated as safe and effective in improving circulating 25(OH)D concentrations. This has been notably observed in Finland that through fortification of fluid milk products and fat spreads, the prevalence of 25(OH)D < 30 nmol/L has been reduced to almost zero through mandatory fortification (Dunlop et al., 2021; Jääskeläinen et al., 2017).

31.3.2.4   WHO recommendations

The World Health Organization–Food and Agriculture Organization (WHO–FAO) recommended that the inadequacy of micronutrients can be addressed by increasing the diversity of foods consumed, food fortification, and/or food supplementation. However, each strategy has its merits and challenges. The WHO-FAO suggested food fortification because of its wide and more sustained impact, as well as being one of the most cost-effective and beneficial public health nutrition interventions (Allen et al., 2006; Cashman & O'Neill, 2024).

31.3.2.5   Challenges associated with food fortification

Implementing successful food fortification programs in LMICs can be challenging due to multiple factors, like limited resources, lack of infrastructure, inappropriate facilities for quality control, and potential concerns about affordability. Additional factors that contribute to substandard program implementation include insufficient supervision and enforcement, and industry noncompliance with established standards (Osendarp et al., 2018).

31.3.2.6   Strategies to overcome barriers in food fortification

There are opportunities to influence existing food distribution channels and leverage public–private partnerships to overcome above-described barriers. To ensure the efficacy of fortification strategies, it is imperative to consider the necessity for "in-field" cost data, which is indispensable for the development of models (Uauy et al., 2002). Moreover, the implementation of supportive food legislation is crucial, as is the cultivation of enhanced consumer and health professional awareness regarding the significance of vitamin D (Orriss, 1998). Additionally, it is essential to emphasize the clinical ramifications of inadequate vitamin D status and the consistent dissemination of government counsel across health and social care professions, as well as via the food industry (Buttriss et al., 2022). These domains necessitate the initiation of additional research promptly to facilitate the universal enhancement of vitamin D intake. It is essential to engage with community leaders and stakeholders to understand cultural and religious barriers and develop strategies to address them sensitively and respectfully (Julies et al., 2020; McAree et al., 2013; Yu et al., 2009; World Health Organization, 2024).

31.3.2.7   Vitamin D food fortification case studies

The following few real-world examples from LMIC will help to demonstrate the role of food fortification and community engagement in improving vitamin D status. In India, the underprivileged toddlers, fed with fortified laddoos (cereal–legume snack) with a very low cost of Indian Rupee (INR) 20 per laddoo, evident with a significant increase in serum calcium and vitamin D levels and also in total body less head (TBLH) bone mineral content (BMC) (Ekbote et al., 2011). Another study conducted in India, reported 776 subjects (boys and girls) who were given fortified milk, which resulted in a significant improvement in their vitamin D status (Khadgawat et al., 2013). These results support the strategy of fortification of foods for a remediation of malnutrition problems in India. These case studies demonstrate the importance of tailoring vitamin D initiatives to the unique needs of local communities, as well as the transformative impact that can be achieved through meaningful community engagement and ownership.

31.3.3 Approaches to delivering vitamin D supplements

Oral vitamin D supplements are the most common and extensively available delivery method. These supplements include various forms, such as tablets, capsules, and liquid drops (Wyon et al., 2021). Injectable vitamin D supplements are the preferred choice for individuals with malabsorption diseases (Gupta et al., 2017; Yu et al., 2020). Another effective method of administration of vitamin D is via topical application. The lipophilicity of this fat-soluble vitamin assists its penetration through the skin barrier (Alnafisah et al., 2024; Wyon et al., 2021). It is crucial to explore innovative approaches for vitamin D delivery, especially in remote or resource-constrained regions. This includes the fortification of cooking oils or the development of biofortified crops, which can assist in a more sustainable and accessible manner, and vitamin D delivery (Naik et al., 2024; Ofori et al., 2022). In addition, recent advances in delivery mechanisms include solid lipid nanoparticles, nanoemulsions, self-emulsifying drug delivery systems, polymeric nanoparticles, and solid dispersion techniques. These approaches have exhibited efficacy in the efficient delivery of vitamin D and simultaneously shown promising opportunities for further research and clinical applications (Gupta et al., 2019).

31.3.4 Integration of vitamin D supplementation with existing health programs

Vitamin D supplementation is important to be included as a supplement during pregnancy. Women visiting for antenatal care, postnatal visits, and children during the early years of life should be provided with vitamin D supplements with regular monitoring and follow-up. Approaching these high-risk groups and improving the existing healthcare facilities ultimately leads to mitigate the burden of vitamin D deficiency (Singleton et al., 2022). The routine immunization programs should include vitamin D supplementation. This is especially useful in "hot spot" regions with high prevalence of vitamin D deficiency and limited access to healthcare services (Anderson, 2014; Ekezie et al., 2022).

31.3.5 Targeting obstacles to vitamin D supplementation

Cultural and religious competency is an indispensable factor of health promotion. For initiating any program regarding vitamin D supplementation, it is vital to acknowledge and address any cultural or religious beliefs that may hinder acceptance and uptake of vitamin D supplementation. One effective strategy is to engage with local communities and include their perspectives with dignity and mindfulness. The objective may be achieved through the implementation of strategies, including the utilization of existing distribution networks, provision of cost-effective supplements, and subsidies to mitigate the costs (Lee et al., 2019; Tanna et al., 2021; Floreskul et al., 2020).

31.3.6 Enhancing quality assurance of vitamin D supplements in resource-limited settings: a comprehensive overview

The maintenance of the quality and safety of vitamin D supplements is crucial, particularly in resource-constrained settings. This is due to compromised regulatory oversight and quality control measures in these settings. The implementation of rigorous quality assurance protocols is vital (De Paula & Rosen, 2012; Shuck, 2017). Robust quality assurance protocols refer to the application of a comprehensive set of measures and procedures to ensure the consistent quality, purity, and safety of vitamin D supplements. Authenticating the identity, purity, and potency of the active vitamin D ingredient in the supplement formulation (dos Santos Ribeiro et al., 2021; National Institutes of Health, 2020). The establishment of rigorous controls and comprehensive monitoring throughout the manufacturing process is essential. This assists in achieving consistency and ensuring adherence to good manufacturing practices (GMPs) (EMA, 2024; FDA, 2024; Long, 2024). A laborious testing protocol must be executed to ensure that the final vitamin D supplement product meets all quality standards, including content, dissolution, and microbiological specifications (Bailey, 2020). The assessment of the shelf-life of the vitamin D supplement is vital to ensure the maintenance of its quality and potency throughout the proposed storage period. This objective can be achieved by implementing stability testing programs (Temova Rakuša et al., 2021; Zareie et al., 2021). The development of a well-structured traceability system assists in effective monitoring of vitamin D supplements from the manufacturing process to the distribution stage. This can facilitate the identification and removal of any products that may be substandard or contaminated. This ensuring the safety and quality of the supplements (Shurson & Urriola, 2019). The implementation of periodic audits and inspections of manufacturing facilities, suppliers, and distribution channels is mandatory to ensure adherence to quality standards (Long, 2024). In resource-constrained settings, these rigorous quality assurance protocols execution can establish the consistent quality, safety, and efficacy of vitamin D supplementation programs. This may contribute to the protection of the health and well-being of the target populations.

31.3.7 Sustainable approaches to vitamin D supplementation

The efforts to develop local capacity for vitamin D supplement production can increase the long-term sustainability of supplementation programs. This objective may be achieved through the provision of training and technical assistance to local manufacturers, as well as the establishment of public–private partnerships. Cooperation between the public and private sectors can facilitate in providing resources to enhance the reach, affordability, and sustainability of vitamin D supplementation initiatives (Hoddinott et al., 2015; Sablah et al., 2011). During vitamin D supplementation program, it is crucial to monitor for potential risks of toxicity or overdosing, which can cause hypercalcemia. Follow the international or national guidelines and protocols to prevent the risks, and for safe delivery of the recommended dose of supplements (Lim & Thadhani, 2020; Pludowski et al., 2018).

31.4 Future directions in vitamin D public health initiatives for low- and middle-income countries

31.4.1 Tailored nutrition: personalized approaches to vitamin D supplementation and delivery

A one-size-fits-all approach to healthcare is almost impossible to tackle the complex needs of individuals. The personalized medicine paradigm emerges as a potential solution. Advances in the health field, particularly influence by our understanding of genetic and metabolic factors that influence vitamin D status, foreshadow a shift towards a more personalized approach to public health initiatives (Mavar et al., 2024). The future of vitamin D research and policy is poised to become increasingly customized. The integration of cutting-edge technologies, such as nutrigenomics and big data analytics, holds promise for the progress in vitamin D recommendations. These recommendations would be informed by an individual's unique characteristics, including skin pigmentation, gut microbiome, and vitamin D receptor genotype. This precision nutrition approach holds great prospective in optimizing vitamin D supplementation and fortification strategies for diverse populations (Yoon et al., 2024). Conventional oral vitamin D supplements may not be the most efficacious or accessible option for all demographics. Consequently, future vitamin D initiatives may develop innovative delivery systems, such as transdermal patches, sublingual sprays, or even vitamin D-fortified edible products. These alternative approaches may improve bioavailability, enhance patient compliance, and more effective reach to underserved communities (Aggeletopoulou et al., 2024). The body's unique genetic composition exerts a significant effect on its capacity to absorb, metabolize, and utilize vitamin D. Certain genetic variants have been documented to affect the functionality of vitamin D receptors or enzymes involved in vitamin D metabolism. By understanding an individual's distinct genetic profile, vitamin D recommendations can be customized to enhance their vitamin D status and health outcomes (Trefilio et al., 2024). Nutrigenomics is the scientific study of how an individual's genetic makeup interacts with nutrients consumed. In the context of public health initiatives promoting vitamin D, the field of nutrigenomics holds significant importance. It empowers researchers and public health professionals to design more personalized vitamin D recommendations (Carlberg et al., 2023; Carlberg, 2019). Nutrigenomics-informed vitamin

D programs have the potential to integrate genetic testing to identify these individual differences. Utilizing these insights, recommendations can be tailored to address the supplementation, food fortification, and lifestyle of the individuals, with the target to impact vitamin D levels. Adopting a precision nutrition approach permits the optimization of vitamin D interventions for diverse populations, guaranteeing their effectiveness and relevance to individual needs (Yang, 2023). The merging of nutrigenomics with vitamin D public health initiatives signifies a substantial progression, as it transcends a one-size-fits-all methodology. Thus, facilitating more customized and efficacious vitamin D strategies to correct insufficiency and enhance population health (Carlberg et al., 2023).

31.4.2 New frontiers in vitamin D research and exploration

Recent findings have indicated a complicated relationship between the gut microbiome, the brain, and vitamin D. This has strong implications for mental health, cognitive function, and neurological disorders. Future research on vitamin D will involve the bidirectional communication between the gut and the brain to a greater extent, investigating the mechanisms by which vitamin D influences this communication. A more insightful comprehension of these mechanisms could inform the development of vitamin D-based interventions for a range of neuropsychiatric conditions (Ogbu et al., 2020). Recent studies have begun to explain the epigenetic mechanisms through which vitamin D exerts its influence on gene expression. Vitamin D initiatives might scrutinize the long-term, multigenerational consequences of vitamin D status. This examination would be particularly relevant within the context of maternal and child health. Moreover, it would explore the potential for vitamin D interventions to ameliorate the epigenetic consequences of environmental and lifestyle factors (Voltan et al., 2023). Artificial intelligence and machine learning algorithms can assist researchers to identify complex patterns, predict vitamin D deficiency risk, and develop personalized interventions with greater efficacy (Guo et al., 2024). The incorporation of these technologies with vitamin D research might accelerate the translation of scientific findings into practical public health applications (Polonowita & Wimalawansa, 2023).

31.4.3 Integrating vitamin D initiatives and public health approaches

Future public health initiatives should aim to integrate vitamin D status assessment as a standard component of routine health screening. This may aid in the normalization of vitamin D screening, the timely detection of deficiency, and the prompt implementation of appropriate vitamin D supplementation or fortification strategies (Płudowski et al., 2023). Vitamin D plays a critical role in maternal and child health. It helps in fetal development, prevents adverse pregnancy outcomes, and enhances child growth and immunity. Therefore, vitamin D initiatives should be closely linked with existing maternal and child health programs to optimize the health of mothers and their children (Chien et al., 2024; Moon et al., 2020).

Research evidence demonstrates that low vitamin D status is associated with the risk and prognosis of several noncommunicable diseases, such as cardiovascular disease, type 2 diabetes, and certain specific cancers. Therefore, vitamin D public health initiatives should explore try to synergistically integrate vitamin D interventions with broader noncommunicable disease prevention strategies to achieve a more holistic approach to population health (Martin-Gorgojo & Martin-Moreno, 2024).

31.5 Conclusion

In LMICs, the role of community engagement in vitamin D awareness and supplementation initiatives will continue to propagate in the future. Community health workers have the potential to fulfil a pivotal function in the context of future vitamin D initiatives, given their frequent role as conduits between the health care system and local communities. The education and interventions related to vitamin D can be more efficaciously disseminated and perpetuated at the grassroots level by equipping these frontline workers with the necessary training and empowering them to assume the role of vitamin D advocates. The virtual and augmented reality technologies can be used to engage and educate diverse groups about the importance of vitamin D. Through these interactive educational approaches, individuals will be able to comprehend the sources, functions, and health implications of vitamin D. This will eventually lead to behavioral change and increased vitamin D awareness among the population on large scale. Robust evolving trends, such as the increased use of digital technologies, the rise of community-led health programs, and the growing recognition of the social determinants of health, exhibit the critical need for a community-centric approach to public health. By empowering communities to take an active role in vitamin D education and supplementation, sustainable, scalable, and equitable programs can be created that can address the unique needs and challenges faced by populations in low- and middle-income countries. The success of these collective efforts can facilitate in the identification of effective strategies to overcome barriers, promote sustainable approaches, and seamlessly incorporate vitamin D supplementation into existing health programs. With the help of exploration of innovative solutions and the utilization of emerging technologies, the future of vitamin D supplementation holds immense potential for enhancing the lives of individuals and communities worldwide. We must continue to learn from successful community engagement models, thus adapting best practices, and fostering collaborative partnerships to enhance the communities' role at the forefront of vitamin D public health initiatives.

AI disclosure

During the preparation of this work, the authors used DeepL Write to seek improved options during academic writing and find any mistakes in some areas of this work. After using this tool/service, the authors reviewed and edited the content as needed and took full responsibility for the content of the publication.

References

Aggeletopoulou, I., Kalafateli, M., Geramoutsos, G., & Triantos, C. (2024). Recent advances in the use of vitamin D organic nanocarriers for drug delivery. *Biomolecules, 14*(9), 1090. https://doi.org/10.3390/biom14091090.

Allen, L., Dary, B., & Hurrell, R. (Eds.), (2006). Guidelines on food fortification with micronutrients..

Alnafisah, R. Y., Alragea, A. S., Alzamil, M. K., & Alqahtani, A. S. (2024). The Impact and Efficacy of Vitamin D Fortification. *Nutrients, 16*(24), 4322. https://doi.org/10.3390/nu16244322.

Amrein, K., Scherkl, M., Hoffmann, M., Neuwersch-Sommeregger, S., Köstenberger, M., Tmava Berisha, A., Martucci, G., Pilz, S., & Malle, O. (2020). Vitamin D deficiency 2.0: an update on the current status worldwide. *European Journal of Clinical Nutrition, 74*(11), 1498–1513. https://doi.org/10.1038/s41430-020-0558-y.

Anderson, E. L. (2014). Recommended solutions to the barriers to immunization in children and adults. *Missouri medicine, 111*(4), 344–348.

Armas, L. A., Dowell, S., Akhter, M., Duthuluru, S., Huerter, C., Hollis, B. W., Lund, R., & Heaney, R. P. (2007). Ultraviolet-B radiation increases serum 25-hydroxyvitamin D levels: the effect of UVB dose and skin color. *Journal of the American Academy of Dermatology, 57*(4), 588–593. https://doi.org/10.1016/j.jaad.2007.03.004.

Azizi, S., & Tariq, T. (2019). Vitamin D Deficiency Among Afghan Adolescents in Kabul. *Journal of College of Physicians and Surgeons Pakistan, 29*(11), 1072–1077. https://doi.org/10.29271/jcpsp.2019.11.1072.

Bailey, R. L. (2020). Current regulatory guidelines and resources to support research of dietary supplements in the United States. *Critical Reviews in Food Science and Nutrition, 60*(2), 298–309. https://doi.org/10.1080/10408398.2018.1524364.

Balachandar, R., Pullakhandam, R., Kulkarni, B., & Sachdev, H. S. (2021). Relative efficacy of vitamin D2 and vitamin D3 in improving vitamin D status: Systematic review and meta-analysis. *Nutrients, 13*(10), 3328. https://doi.org/10.3390/nu13103328.

Bansal, B., Bansal,, M., Bajpai, P., & Garewal, H. K. (2014). Hypocalcemic cardiomyopathy-different mechanisms in adult and pediatric cases. *The Journal of Clinical Endocrinology and Metabolism, 99*(8), 2627–2632. https://doi.org/10.1210/jc.2013-3352.

Basatemur, E., & Sutcliffe, A. (2015). Incidence of hypocalcemic seizures due to vitamin D deficiency in children in the United Kingdom and Ireland. *The Journal of Clinical Endocrinology and Metabolism, 100*(1), E91–E95. https://doi.org/10.1210/jc.2014-2773.

Benedik, E. (2022). Sources of vitamin D for humans. *International Journal for Vitamin and Nutrition Research, 92*(2), 118–125. https://doi.org/10.1024/0300-9831/a000733.

Bener, A., & Hoffmann, G. F. (2010). Nutritional Rickets among Children in a Sun Rich Country. *International Journal of Pediatric Endocrinology,* 1–7. https://doi.org/10.1155/2010/410502.

Berretta, M., Quagliariello, V., Bignucolo, A., Facchini, S., Maurea, N., Di Francia, R., Fiorica, F., Sharifi, S., Bressan, S., Richter, S. N., Camozzi, V., Rinaldi, L., Scaroni, C., & Montopoli, M. (2022). The multiple effects of vitamin D against chronic diseases: From reduction of lipid peroxidation to updated evidence from clinical studies. *Antioxidants, 11*(6), 1090. https://doi.org/10.3390/antiox11061090.

Brown, J., Nunez, S., Russell, M., & Spurney, C. (2009). Hypocalcemic rickets and dilated cardiomyopathy: case reports and review of literature. *Pediatric Cardiology, 30*(6), 818–823. https://doi.org/10.1007/s00246-009-9444-z.

Buttriss, J. L., Lanham-New, S. A., Steenson, S., Levy, L., Swan, G. E., Darling, A. L., Cashman, K. D., Allen, R.E., Durrant, L. R., Smith, C. P., Magee, P., Hill, T. R., Uday, S., Kiely, M., Delamare, G., Hoyland, A. E., Larsen, L., Street, L. N., Mathers, J. C., & Prentice, A. (2022). Implementation strategies for improving vitamin D status and increasing vitamin D intake in the UK: current controversies and future perspectives: proceedings of the 2nd Rank Prize Funds Forum on vitamin D. *The British Journal of Nutrition, 127*(10), 1567–1587. https://doi.org/10.1017/S0007114521002555.

Calvo, M. S., & Lamberg-Allardt, C. J. (2017). Vitamin D research and public health nutrition: A current perspective. *Public Health Nutrition, 20*(10), 1713–1717. https://doi.org/10.1017/S1368980017001835.

Carlberg, C. (2019). Nutrigenomics of vitamin D. *Nutrients, 11*(3), 676. https://doi.org/10.3390/nu11030676.

Carlberg, C., Raczyk, M., & Zawrotna, N. (2023). Vitamin D: A master example of nutrigenomics. *Redox Biology, 62*, 102695. https://doi.org/10.1016/j.redox.2023.102695.

Cashman, K. D., & O'Dea, R. (2019). Exploration of strategic food vehicles for vitamin D fortification in low/lower-middle income countries. *The Journal of Steroid Biochemistry and Molecular Biology, 195*, 105479. https://doi.org/10.1016/j.jsbmb.2019.105479.

Cashman, K. D. (2017). Vitamin D deficiency: A Public Health Issue in High- and Low-Income Countries or Just Hype? *World Review of Nutrition and Dietetics, 118*, 206–214. https://doi.org/10.1159/000484391.

Cashman, K. D. (2020). Vitamin D deficiency: Defining, prevalence, causes, and strategies of addressing. *Springer, Ireland Calcified Tissue International, 106*(1), 14–29. https://doi.org/10.1007/s00223-019-00559-4.

Cashman, K. D. (2022). Global differences in vitamin D status and dietary intake: A review of the data. *Endocrine Connections, 11*(1). https://doi.org/10.1530/EC-21-0282.

Cashman, K. D., Dowling, K. G., Škrabáková, Z., Gonzalez-Gross, M., Valtueña, J., De Henauw, S., Moreno, L., Damsgaard, C. T., Michaelsen, K. F., Mølgaard, C., Jorde, R., Grimnes, G., Moschonis, G., Mavrogianni, C., Manios, Y., Thamm, M., Mensink, G. B. M., Rabenberg, M., Busch, M. A., ... Kiely, M. (2016). Vitamin D deficiency in Europe: Pandemic? *American Journal of Clinical Nutrition, 103*(4), 1033–1044. https://doi.org/10.3945/ajcn.115.120873.

Cashman, K. D., & O'Neill, C. M. (2024). Strategic food vehicles for vitamin D fortification and effects on vitamin D status: A systematic review and meta-analysis of randomised controlled trials. *Journal of Steroid Biochemistry and Molecular Biology, 238*, 106448. https://doi.org/10.1016/j.jsbmb.2023.106448.

Chandaria, K., Daud, K. M., Syed, F., & Blair, M. (2011). What are the views of local people about vitamin D and its health effects: a community focus group study. *Archives of Disease in Childhood, 96*(Supplement 1), A11. https://doi.org/10.1136/adc.2011.212563.19.

Chien, M. C., Huang, C. Y., Wang, J. H., Shih, C. L., & Wu, P. (2024). Effects of vitamin D in pregnancy on maternal and offspring health-related outcomes: An umbrella review of systematic review and meta-analyses. *Nutrition & Diabetes, 14*(1), 35. https://doi.org/10.1038/s41387-024-00296-0.

Creo, A. L., Thacher, T. D., Pettifor, J. M., Strand, M. A., & Fischer, P. R. (2017). Nutritional rickets around the world: an update. *Paediatrics and International Child Health, 37*(2), 84–98. https://doi.org/10.1080/20469047.2016.1248170.

Cui, A., Zhang, T., Xiao, P., Fan, Z., Wang, H., & Zhuang, Y. (2023). Global and regional prevalence of vitamin D deficiency in population-based studies from 2000 to 2022: A pooled analysis of 7.9 million participants. *Frontiers in Nutrition, 10*. https://doi.org/10.3389/fnut.2023.1070808.

Daryabor, G., Gholijani, N., & Kahmini, F. R. (2023). A review of the critical role of vitamin D axis on the immune system. *Experimental and Molecular Pathology, 132-133*, 104866. https://doi.org/10.1016/j.yexmp.2023.104866.

Dawson-Hughes, B. (2024). Effect of vitamin D on risk of falls and fractures – The contribution of recent mega-trials. *Metabolism Open, 23*. https://doi.org/10.1016/j.metop.2024.100300.

Dunlop, E., Kiely, M. E., James, A. P., Singh, T., Pham, N. M., & Black, L. J. (2021). Vitamin D food fortification and biofortification increases serum 25-hydroxyvitamin D concentrations in adults and children: An updated and extended systematic review and meta-analysis of randomized controlled trials. *Journal of Nutrition, 151*(9), 2622–2635. https://doi.org/10.1093/jn/nxab180.

Ekbote, V. H., Khadilkar, A. V., Chiplonkar, S. A., Hanumante, N. M., Khadilkar, V. V., & Mughal, M. Z. (2011). A pilot randomized controlled trial of oral calcium and vitamin D supplementation using fortified laddoos in underprivileged Indian toddlers. *European Journal of Clinical Nutrition, 65*(4), 440–446. https://doi.org/10.1038/ejcn.2010.288.

Ekezie, W., Awwad, S., Krauchenberg, A., Karara, N., Dembiński, Ł., Grossman, Z., del Torso, S., Dornbusch, H. J., Neves, A., Copley, S., Mazur, A., Hadjipanayis, A., Grechukha, Y., Nohynek, H., Damnjanović, K., Lazić, M., Papaevangelou, V., Lapii, F., Stein-Zamir, C., Rath, B., & for the ImmuHubs Consortium (2022). Access to vaccination among disadvantaged, isolated and difficult-to-reach communities in the WHO European Region: A systematic review. *Vaccines, 10*(7), 1038. https://doi.org/10.3390/vaccines10071038.

EMA. (2024). *Good manufacturing practice*. European Medicines Agency. https://www.ema.europa.eu/en/human-regulatory-overview/research-development/compliance-research-development/good-manufacturing-practice.

FDA. (2024). Facts about the current good manufacturing practice (CGMP). *FDA*. https://www.fda.gov/drugs/pharmaceutical-quality-resources/facts-about-current-good-manufacturing-practice-cgmp.

Floreskul, V., Juma, F. Z., Daniel, A. B., Zamir, I., Rawdin, A., Stevenson, M., Mughal, Z., & Padidela, R. (2020). Cost-effectiveness of vitamin D supplementation in pregnant woman and young children in preventing rickets: A modeling study. *Frontiers in Public Health, 8*, 439. https://doi.org/10.3389/fpubh.2020.00439.

George, A. S., Mehra, V., Scott, K., Sriram, V., & Li, X. (2015). Community participation in health systems research: A systematic review assessing the state of research, the nature of interventions involved and the features of engagement with communities. *PLOS ONE, 10*(10), e0141091. https://doi.org/10.1371/journal.pone.0141091.

Giustina, A., Bouillon, R., Dawson-Hughes, B., Ebeling, P. R., Lazaretti-Castro, M., Lips, P., Marcocci, C., & Bilezikian, J. P. (2023). Vitamin D in the older population: A consensus statement. *Springer, Italy Endocrine, 79*(1), 31–44. https://doi.org/10.1007/s12020-022-03208-3.

Global Alliance for Improved Nutrition (GAIN) (n.d.). The malnutrition challenge Programmes/partnerships. GAIN. https://www.gainhealth.org/impact/countries/pakistan.

Goswami, R., Gupta, N., Goswami, D., Marwaha, R. K., Tandon, N., & Kochupillai, N. (2000). Prevalence and significance of low 25-hydroxyvitamin D concentrations in healthy subjects in Delhi. *The American Journal of Clinical Nutrition, 72*(2), 472–475. https://doi.org/10.1093/ajcn/72.2.472.

Guo, J., He, Q., & Li, Y. (2024). Machine learning-based prediction of vitamin D deficiency: NHANES 2001-2018. *Frontiers in Endocrinology, 15*. https://doi.org/10.3389/fendo.2024.1327058.

Gupta, N., Farooqui, K. J., Batra, C. M., Marwaha, R. K., & Mithal, A. (2017). Effect of oral versus intramuscular Vitamin D replacement in apparently healthy adults with Vitamin D deficiency. *Indian Journal of Endocrinology and Metabolism, 21*(1), 131–136. https://doi.org/10.4103/2230-8210.196007.

Gupta, R., Behera, C., Paudwal, G., Rawat, N., Baldi, A., & Gupta, P. N. (2018). Recent Advances in Formulation Strategies for Efficient Delivery of Vitamin D. *AAPS PharmSciTech, 20*(1), 11. https://doi.org/10.1208/s12249-018-1231-9.

Hassan Ali, H., M. Abdelrahman, R., H. A. Hemida, E., & Abdo Abd El-Haleem, S. (2021). Knowledge, practices and attitudes regarding vitamin D insufficiency among health care workers' women with COVID-19. *Egyptian Journal of Health Care, 12*(2), 1504–1525. https://doi.org/10.21608/ejhc.2021.191874.

Hatchell, K. E., Lu, Q., Mares, J. A., Michos, E. D., Wood, A. C., & Engelman, C. D. (2020). Multi-ethnic analysis shows genetic risk and environmental predictors interact to influence 25(OH)D concentration and optimal vitamin D intake. *Genetic Epidemiology, 44*(2), 208–217. https://doi.org/10.1002/gepi.22272.

Henn, M., Martin-Gorgojo, V., & Martin-Moreno, J. M. (2022). Vitamin D in cancer prevention: Gaps in current knowledge and room for hope. *Nutrients, 14*(21), 4512. https://doi.org/10.3390/nu14214512.

Heo, J. S., Ahn, Y. N., Kim, A. E., & Shin, S. M. (2022). Breastfeeding and vitamin D. *Clinical and Experimental Pediatrics, 65*(9), 418–429. https://doi.org/10.3345/cep.2021.00444.

Hilger, J., Friedel, A., Herr, R., Rausch, T., Roos, F., Wahl, D. A., Pierroz, D. D., Weber, P., & Hoffmann, K. (2014). A systematic review of vitamin D status in populations worldwide. *British Journal of Nutrition, 111*(1), 23–45. https://doi.org/10.1017/S0007114513001840.

Hoddinott, J., Gillespie, S., & Yosef, S. (2015). Public-private partnerships and the reduction of undernutrition in developing countries. *SSRN Electronic Journal*. https://doi.org/10.2139/ssrn.2741274.

Hoss, K. E., Salla, M., Khaled, S., Krayem, M., Hassan, H., & Khatib, S. E. (2023). Update on vitamin D deficiency and its impact on human health major challenges & technical approaches of food fortification. *Journal of Agriculture and Food Research, 12*, 100616. https://doi.org/10.1016/j.jafr.2023.100616.

Houston, D. K., Marsh, A. P., Neiberg, R. H., Demons, J. L., Campos, C. L., Kritchevsky, S. B., Delbono, O., & Tooze, J. A. (2023). Vitamin D Supplementation and Muscle Power, Strength and Physical Performance in Older Adults: A Randomized Controlled Trial. *The American journal of clinical nutrition, 117*(6), 1086–1095. https://doi.org/10.1016/j.ajcnut.2023.04.021.

Jabbour, J., Khalil, M., Ronzoni,, A. R., Mabry,, R., Al-Jawaldeh,, A., El-Adawy, M., & Sakr, H. (2023). Malnutrition and gender disparities in the Eastern Mediterranean Region: The need for action. *Frontiers in Nutrition, 10*. https://doi.org/10.3389/fnut.2023.1113662.

Jones, G. (2022). 100 years of vitamin D: Historical aspects of vitamin D. *Endocrine Connections, 11*(4). https://doi.org/10.1530/ec-21-0594.

Julies, P., Lynn, R. M., Pall, K., Leoni, M., Calder, A., Mughal, Z., Shaw, N., McDonnell, C., McDevitt, H., & Blair, M. (2020). Nutritional rickets under 16 years: UK surveillance results. *Archives of Disease in Childhood, 105*(6), 587–592. https://doi.org/10.1136/archdischild-2019-317934.

Jääskeläinen, T., Itkonen, S. T., Lundqvist, A., Erkkola, M., Koskela, T., Lakkala, K., Dowling, K. G., Hull, G. L., Kröger, H., Karppinen, J., Kyllönen, E., Härkänen, T., Cashman, K. D., Männistö, S., & Lamberg-Allardt, C. (2017). The positive impact of general vitamin D food fortification policy on vitamin D status in a representative adult Finnish population: evidence from an 11-y follow-up based on standardized 25-hydroxyvitamin D data. *The American Journal of Clinical Nutrition, 105*(6), 1512–1520. https://doi.org/10.3945/ajcn.116.151415.

Kalyani, R. R., Stein, B., Valiyil, R., Manno, R., Maynard, J. W., & Crews, D. C. (2010). Vitamin D treatment for the prevention of falls in older adults: systematic review and meta-analysis. *Journal of the American Geriatrics Society, 58*(7), 1299–1310. https://doi.org/10.1111/j.1532-5415.2010.02949.x.

Karim, F., Chowdhury, A. M., & Gani, M. S. (2003). Rapid assessment of the prevalence of lower limb clinical rickets in Bangladesh. *Public Health, 117*(2), 135–144. https://doi.org/10.1016/S0033-3506(02)00017-3.

Kaur, J, Khare, S, Sizar, O, & Givler, A (2025). *Vitamin D Deficiency*. StatPearls Publishing.

Khadgawat, R., Marwaha, R. K., Garg, M. K., Ramot, R., Oberoi, A. K., Sreenivas, V., Gahlot, M., Mehan, N., Mathur, P., & Gupta, N. (2013). Impact of vitamin D fortified milk supplementation on vitamin D status of healthy school children aged 10–14 years. *Osteoporosis International, 24*(8), 2335–2343. https://doi.org/10.1007/s00198-013-2306-9.

Khadilkar, A., Khadilkar, V., Chinnappa, J., Rathi, N., Khadgawat, R., Balasubramanian, S., Parekh, B., & Jog, P. (2017). Prevention and Treatment of Vitamin D and Calcium Deficiency in Children and Adolescents: Indian Academy of Pediatrics (IAP) Guidelines. *Indian Pediatrics, 54*(7), 567–573. https://doi.org/10.1007/s13312-017-1070-x.

Kiely, M., & Cashman, K. D. (2018). Summary outcomes of the ODIN project on food fortification for vitamin D deficiency prevention. *International Journal of Environmental Research and Public Health, 15*(11), 2342. https://doi.org/10.3390/ijerph15112342.

Kimball, S. M., Lee, J., & Vieth, R. (2017). Sunbeds with UVB radiation can produce physiological levels of serum 25-Hydroxyvitamin D in healthy volunteers. *Dermato-Endocrinology, 9*(1). https://doi.org/10.1080/19381980.2017.1375635.

Kupisz-Urbańska, M., Płudowski, P., & Marcinowska-Suchowierska, E. (2021). Vitamin D deficiency in older patients—Problems of sarcopenia, drug interactions, management in deficiency. *Nutrients, 13*(4), 1247. https://doi.org/10.3390/nu13041247.

Lavelli, V., D'Incecco, P., & Pellegrino, L. (2021). Vitamin D incorporation in foods: Formulation strategies, stability, and bioaccessibility as affected by the food matrix. *Foods, 10*(9), 1989. https://doi.org/10.3390/foods10091989.

Lee, C., Tanna, N., Blair, M., Yusuf, Y., Khalief, H., & Lakhanpaul, M. (2019). Getting underneath the skin: A community engagement event for optimal vitamin D status in an 'easily overlooked' group. *Health expectations : an international journal of public participation in health care and health policy, 22*(6), 1322–1330. https://doi.org/10.1111/hex.12978.

Libon, F., Courtois, J., Le Goff, C., Lukas, P., Fabregat-Cabello, N., Seidel, L., Cavalier, E., & Nikkels, A. F. (2017). Sunscreens block cutaneous vitamin D production with only a minimal effect on circulating 25-hydroxyvitamin D. *Archives of Osteoporosis, 12*(1). https://doi.org/10.1007/s11657-017-0361-0.

Lim, K., & Thadhani, R. (2020). Vitamin D toxicity. *Brazilian Journal of Nephrology, 42*(2), 238–244. https://doi.org/10.1590/2175-8239-jbn-2019-0192.

Lips, P. (2010). Worldwide status of vitamin D nutrition. *The Journal of Steroid Biochemistry and Molecular Biology, 121*(1), 297–300. https://doi.org/10.1016/j.jsbmb.2010.02.021.

Lips, P., Cashman, K. D., Lamberg-Allardt, C., Bischoff-Ferrari, H. A., Obermayer-Pietsch, B., Bianchi, M. L., Stepan, J., El-Hajj Fuleihan, G., & Bouillon, R. (2019). Current vitamin D status in European and Middle East countries and strategies to prevent vitamin D deficiency: a position statement of the European Calcified Tissue Society. *European Journal of Endocrinology, 180*(4), P23–P54. https://doi.org/10.1530/EJE-18-0736.

Lips, P., de Jongh, R. T., & van Schoor, N. M. (2021). Trends in Vitamin D Status Around the World. *JBMR Plus, 5*(12), e10585. https://doi.org/10.1002/jbm4.10585.

Long, J. (2024). FDA increases annual domestic, foreign dietary supplement inspections. *SupplySide Supplement Journal.* https://www.supplysidesj.com/supplement-regulations/fda-increases-annual-domestic-foreign-dietary-supplement-inspections.

Martin-Gorgojo, A., & Martin-Moreno, J. M. (2024). Insights into the Role of Vitamin D in the Prevention and Control of Cancer and Other Chronic Noncommunicable Diseases: Shedding Further Light on a Captivating Subject. *Nutrients, 16*(13), 2166. https://doi.org/10.3390/nu16132166.

Maryam, S., Saba, S., Haider, W., Afzal, M. S., Mukhtar, S., Durrance-Bagale, A., Arfeen, R. Z. U., Bangash, N., Shah, N. A., & Ahmed, H. (2022). Community-based social and demographic assessment of knowledge, attitudes, practices and medical conditions related to vitamin D deficiency in Gilgit Baltistan, Pakistan. *Journal of biosocial science, 54*(6), 1100–1124. https://doi.org/10.1017/S002193202100050X.

Mavar, M., Sorić, T., Bagarić, E., Sarić, A., & Matek Sarić, M. (2024). The power of vitamin D: Is the future in precision nutrition through personalized supplementation plans? *Nutrients, 16*(8), 1176. https://doi.org/10.3390/nu16081176.

McAree, T., Jacobs, B., Manickavasagar, T., Sivalokanathan, S., Brennan, L., Bassett, P., Rainbow, S., & Blair, M. (2013). Vitamin D deficiency in pregnancy – Still a public health issue. *Maternal & Child Nutrition, 9*(1), 23–30. https://doi.org/10.1111/mcn.12014.

Metreau, E, Young, K. E, & Eapen, S. G (2024). World Bank country classifications by income level for 2024-2025. https://blogs.worldbank.org/en/opendata/world-bank-country-classifications-by-income-level-for-2024-2025.

Mogire, R., Mutua, A., Kimita, W., Kamau, A., Bejon, P., Pettifor, J. M., Adeyemo, A., Williams, T. N., & Atkinson, S. H. (2020). Prevalence of vitamin D deficiency in Africa: a systematic review and meta-analysis. *The Lancet. Global health,* e134–e142. https://doi.org/10.1016/S2214-109X(19)30457-7.

Moon, R. J., Davies, J. H., Cooper, C., & Harvey, N. C. (2020). Vitamin D, and Maternal and Child Health. *Calcified Tissue International, 106*(1), 30–46. https://doi.org/10.1007/s00223-019-00560-x.

Munns, C., Simm, P., J, Rodda, C. P., Garnett, S. P., Zacharin, M. R., Ward, L. M., Geddes, J., Cherian, S., Zurynski, Y., & Cowell, C. T. APSU Vitamin D Study Group. (2012). Incidence of vitamin D deficiency rickets among Australian children: an Australian Paediatric Surveillance Unit study. *The Medical journal of Australia, 196*(7), 466–468. https://doi.org/10.5694/mja11.10662.

Naik, B., Kumar, V., Rizwanuddin, S., Mishra, S., Kumar, V., Saris, P. E. J., Khanduri, N., Kumar, A., Pandey, P., Gupta, A. K., Khan, J. M., & Rustagi, S. (2024). Biofortification as a solution for addressing nutrient deficiencies and malnutrition. *Heliyon, 10*(9), e30595. https://doi.org/10.1016/j.heliyon.2024.e30595.

Nair, R., & Maseeh, A. (2012). Vitamin D: The sunshine vitamin. *Journal of Pharmacology and Pharmacotherapeutics, 3*(2), 118–126. https://doi.org/10.4103/0976-500X.95506.

National Institutes of Health (2020). Dietary Supplements: What You Need to Know. https://ods.od.nih.gov/factsheets/WYNTK-Consumer/.

Nyakundi, P. N., Némethné Kontár, Z., Kovács, A., Járomi, L., Zand, A., & Lohner, S. (2023). Fortification of staple foods for household use with vitamin D: An overview of systematic reviews. *Nutrients, 15*(17), 3742. https://doi.org/10.3390/nu15173742.

Ofori, K. F., Antoniello, S., English, M. M., & Aryee, A. N. A. (2022). Improving nutrition through biofortification–A systematic review. *Frontiers in Nutrition, 9*, 1043655. https://doi.org/10.3389/fnut.2022.1043655.

Ogbu, D., Xia, E., & Sun, J. (2020). Gut instincts: Vitamin D/vitamin D receptor and microbiome in neurodevelopment disorders. *Open Biology, 10*(7). https://doi.org/10.1098/rsob.200063.

Oktaria, V., Graham, S. M., Triasih, R., Soenarto, Y., Bines, J. E., Ponsonby, L., Clarke, M. W., Dinari, R., Nirwati, H., & Danchin, M. (2020). The prevalence and determinants of vitamin D deficiency in Indonesian infants at birth and six months of age. *PLOS ONE, 15*(10). https://doi.org/10.1371/journal.pone.0239603.

Orriss, G. D. (1998). Food fortification: Safety and legislation. *Food and Nutrition Bulletin, 19*(2). https://journals. sagepub.com/doi/pdf/10.1177/156482659801900204.

Osendarp, S. J. M., Martinez, H., Garrett, G. S., Neufeld, L. M., De-Regil, L. M., Vossenaar, M., & Darnton-Hill, I. (2018). Large-Scale Food Fortification and Biofortification in Low- and Middle-Income Countries: A Review of Programs, Trends, Challenges, and Evidence Gaps. *Food and Nutrition Bulletin, 39*(2), 315–331. https://doi.org/10.1177/0379572118774229.

Oskarsson, V., Eliasson, M., Salomaa, V., Reinikainen, J., Männistö, S., Palmieri, L., Donfrancesco, C., Sans, S., Costanzo, S., de Gaetano, G., Iacoviello, L., Veronesi, G., Ferrario, M. M., Padro, T., Thorand, B., Huth, C., Zeller, T., Blankenberg, S., Anderson, A. S., Tunstall-Pedoe, H., … BiomarCaRE investigators (2022). Influence of geographical latitude on vitamin D status: cross-sectional results from the BiomarCaRE consortium. *The British journal of nutrition, 128*(11), 2208–2218. https://doi.org/10.1017/S0007114521005080.

Özdemir, A. A., Ercan Gündemir, Y., Küçük, M., Yıldıran Sarıcı, D., Elgörmüş, Y., Çağ, Y., & Bilek, G. (2018). Vitamin D deficiency in pregnant women and their infants. *Journal of Clinical Research in Pediatric Endocrinology, 10*(1), 44–50. https://doi.org/10.4274/jcrpe.4706.

Palacios, C., & Gonzalez, L. (2014). Is vitamin D deficiency a major global public health problem? *The Journal of Steroid Biochemistry and Molecular Biology, 144*, 138–145. https://doi.org/10.1016/j.jsbmb.2013.11.003.

Paul, S., Kaushik, R., Chawla, P., Upadhyay, S., Rawat, D., & Akhtar, A. (2024). Vitamin-D as a multifunctional molecule for overall well-being: An integrative review. *Clinical Nutrition ESPEN, 62*, 10–21. https://doi.org/ 10.1016/j.clnesp.2024.04.016.

De Paula, F. J. A., & Rosen, C. J. (2012). Vitamin D safety and requirements. *Archives of Biochemistry and Biophysics, 523*(1), 64–72. https://doi.org/10.1016/j.abb.2011.12.002.

Pilz, S., März, W., Cashman, K. D., Kiely, M. E., Whiting, S. J., Holick, M. F., Grant, W. B., Pludowski, P., Hiligsmann, M., Trummer, C., Schwetz, V., Lerchbaum, E., Pandis, M., Tomaschitz, A., Grübler, M. R., Gaksch, M., Verheyen, N., Hollis, B. W., Rejnmark, L., Karras, S. N., & Zittermann (2018). Rationale and Plan for Vitamin D Food Fortification: A Review and Guidance Paper. *Frontiers in Endocrinology, 9*, 373. https://doi.org/10.3389/fendo.2018.00373.

Płudowski, P., Kos-Kudła, B., Walczak, M., Fal, A., Zozulińska-Ziółkiewicz, D., Sieroszewski, P., Peregud-Pogorzelski, J., Lauterbach, R., Targowski, T., Lewiński, A., Spaczyński, R., Wielgoś, M., Pinkas, J., Jackowska, T., Helwich, E., Mazur, A., Ruchała, M., Zygmunt, A., Szalecki, M., Bossowski, A., … Misiorowski, W. (2023). Guidelines for Preventing and Treating Vitamin D Deficiency: A 2023 Update in Poland. *Nutrients, 15*(3), 695. https://doi.org/10.3390/nu15030695

Płudowski, P., Kos-Kudła, B., Walczak, M., Fal, A., Zozulińska-Ziółkiewicz, D., Sieroszewski, P., Peregud-Pogorzelski, J., Lauterbach, R., Targowski, T., Lewiński, A., Spaczyński, R., Wielgoś, M., Pinkas, J., Jackowska, T., Helwich, E., Mazur, A., Ruchała, M., Zygmunt, A., Szalecki, M., … Misiorowski, W. (2023). Guidelines for preventing and treating vitamin D deficiency: A 2023 update in Poland. *Nutrients, 15*(3), 695. https://doi.org/10.3390/nu15030695.

Polonowita, A. K., & Wimalawansa, S. J. (2023). Molecular quantum and logic process of consciousness—Vitamin D big-data in covid-19—A case for incorporating machine learning in medicine. *Journal of Parenteral and Pharmaceutical Sciences, 10*(12), 24–43. https://doi.org/10.5281/zenodo. 10435649.

Roth, D. E., Abrams, S. A., Aloia, J., Bergeron, G., Bourassa, M. W., Brown, K. H., Calvo, M. S., Cashman, K. D., Combs, G., De-Regil, L. M., Jefferds, M. E., Jones, K. S., Kapner, H., Martineau, A. R., Neufeld, L. M., Schleicher, R. L., Thacher, T. D., & Whiting, S. J. (2018). Global prevalence and disease burden of vitamin D deficiency: a roadmap for action in low- and middle-income countries. *Annals of the New York Academy of Sciences, 1430*(1), 44–79. https://doi.org/10.1111/nyas.13968.

Sablah, M., Klopp, J., Steinberg, D., & Baker, S. (2011). Private-public partnerships drive one solution to vitamin and mineral deficiencies:fortify west Africa. *SCN News, 39*, 40–44.

Sanlier, N., & Guney-Coskun, M. (2022). Vitamin D, the immune system, and its relationship with diseases. *Egyptian Pediatric Association Gazette, 70*(1). https://doi.org/10.1186/s43054-022-00135-w.

dos Santos Ribeiro, H. S.'A., Dagnino, D., & Schripsema, Jan (2021). Rapid and accurate verification of drug identity, purity and quality by 1H-NMR using similarity calculations and differential NMR. *Journal of Pharmaceutical and Biomedical Analysis, 199*, 114040. https://doi.org/10.1016/j.jpba.2021.114040.

Shraim, R., MacDonnchadha, C., Vrbanic, L., McManus, R., & Zgaga, L. (2022). Gene-environment interactions in vitamin D status and sun exposure: A systematic review with recommendations for future research. *Nutrients, 14*(13), 2735. https://doi.org/10.3390/nu14132735.

Shurson, J., & Urriola, P. (2019). Understanding the vitamin supply chain and relative risk of transmission of foreign animal diseases.

Shuck, J. Checking for Quality in Vitamin D Supplements. *News-Medical.* https://www.news-medical.net/whitepaper/20170301/Checking-for-Quality-in-Vitamin-D-Supplements.aspx.

Siddiqee, M. H., Bhattacharjee, B., Siddiqi, U. R., & MeshbahurRahman, M. (2021). High prevalence of vitamin D deficiency among the South Asian adults: a systematic review and meta-analysis. *BMC Public Health, 21*(1). https://doi.org/10.1186/s12889-021-11888-1.

Singleton, R. J., Day, G. M., Thomas, T. K., Klejka, J. A., Desnoyers, C. A., McIntyre, M. N. P., Compton, D. M., Thummel, K. E., Schroth, R. J., Ward, L. M., Lenaker, D. C., Lescher, R. K., & McLaughlin, J. B. (2022). Impact of a Prenatal Vitamin D Supplementation Program on Vitamin D Deficiency, Rickets and Early Childhood Caries in an Alaska Native Population. *Nutrients, 14*(19), 3935. https://doi.org/10.3390/nu14193935.

Strand, M. A., Perry, J., Jin, M., Tracer, D. P., Fischer, P. R., Zhang, P., Xi, W., & Li, S. (2007). Diagnosis of rickets and reassessment of prevalence among rural children in northern China. *Pediatrics International: Official Journal of the Japan Pediatric Society, 49*(2), 202–209. https://doi.org/10.1111/j.1442-200X.2007.02343.x.

Sultan, S., Taimuri, U., Basnan, S. A., Ai-Orabi, W. K., Awadallah, A., Almowald, F., & Hazazi, A. (2020). Low Vitamin D and Its Association with Cognitive Impairment and Dementia. *Journal of aging research, 2020*, 6097820. https://doi.org/10.1155/2020/6097820.

Tanna, N. K., Alexander, E. C., Lee, C., Lakhanpaul, M., Popat, R. M., Almeida-Meza, P., Tuck, A., Manikam, L., & Blair, M. (2021). Interventions to improve vitamin D status in at-risk ethnic groups during pregnancy and early childhood: A systematic review. *Public health nutrition, 24*(11), 3498–3519. https://doi.org/10.1017/S1368980021000756.

Temova Rakuša, Ž., Pišlar, M., Kristl, A., & Roškar, R. (2021). Comprehensive stability study of vitamin D3 in aqueous solutions and liquid commercial products. *Pharmaceutics, 13*(5), 617. https://doi.org/10.3390/pharmaceutics13050617.

Terock, J., Bonk, S., Frenzel, S., Wittfeld, K., Garvert, L., Hosten, N., Nauck, M., Völzke, H., Van der Auwera, S., & Grabe, H. J. (2022). Vitamin D deficit is associated with accelerated brain aging in the general population. *Psychiatry Research: Neuroimaging, 327*, 111558. https://doi.org/10.1016/j.pscychresns.2022.111558.

The World Bank (2024). *World Bank Country and Lending Groups.* The World Bank. https://datahelpdesk.worldbank.org/knowledgebase/articles/906519-world-bank-country-and-lending-groups.

Toffanello, E. D., Perissinotto, E., Sergi, G., Zambon, S., Musacchio, E., Maggi, S., Coin, A., Sartori, L., Corti, M. C., Baggio, G., Crepaldi, G., & Manzato, E. (2012). Vitamin D and physical performance in elderly subjects: the Pro.V.A study. *PloS One, 7*(4). https://doi.org/10.1371/journal.pone.0034950.

Trefilio, L. M., Bottino, L., de Carvalho Cardoso, R., Montes, G. C., & Fontes-Dantas, F. L. (2024). The impact of genetic variants related to vitamin D and autoimmunity: A systematic review. *Heliyon, 10*(7), e27700. https://doi.org/10.1016/j.heliyon.2024.e27700.

Trimarco, V., Manzi, M. V., Mancusi, C., Strisciuglio, T., Fucile, I., Fiordelisi, A., Pilato, E., Izzo, R., Barbato, E., Lembo, M., & Morisco, C. (2022). Insulin Resistance and Vitamin D Deficiency: A Link Beyond the Appearances. *Frontiers in cardiovascular medicine, 9*, 859793. https://doi.org/10.3389/fcvm.2022.859793.

Uauy, R., Hertrampf, E., & Reddy, M. (2002). Iron fortification of foods: Overcoming technical and practical barriers. *The Journal of Nutrition, 132*(4), 849S. https://doi.org/10.1093/jn/132.4.849S.

Unicef.org. (2018). *National Nutrition Survey 2018*. Islamabad: National Health Services, Regulations & Coordination Government of Pakistan. https://www.unicef.org/pakistan/media/2826/file/National%20Nutrition%20Survey%202018%20Volume%201.pdf.

van den Heuvel, E. G., Lips, P., Schoonmade, L. J., Lanham-New, S. A., & van Schoor, N. M. (2024). Comparison of the Effect of Daily Vitamin D2 and Vitamin D3 Supplementation on Serum 25-Hydroxyvitamin D Concentration (Total 25(OH)D, 25(OH)D2, and 25(OH)D3) and Importance of Body Mass Index: A Systematic Review and Meta-Analysis. *Advances in Nutrition (Bethesda, Md.), 15*(1), 100133. https://doi.org/10.1016/j.advnut.2023.09.016.

Voltan, G., Cannito, M., Ferrarese, M., Ceccato, F., & Camozzi, V. (2023). Vitamin D: An overview of gene regulation, ranging from metabolism to genomic effects. *Genes, 14*(9), 1691. https://doi.org/10.3390/genes14091691.

Wacker, M., & Holick, M. F. (2013). Sunlight and Vitamin D: A global perspective for health. *Dermato-endocrinology, 5*(1), 51–108. https://doi.org/10.4161/derm.24494.

Wang, H., Chen, W., Li, D., Yin, X., Zhang, X., Olsen, N., & Zheng, S. G. (2017). Vitamin D and Chronic Diseases. *Aging and disease, 8*(3), 346–353. https://doi.org/10.14336/AD.2016.1021.

World Health Organization (2020). Community engagement: a health promotion guide for universal health coverage in the hands of the people. https://www.who.int/publications/i/item/9789240010529.

World Health Organization (2024). Summary report on the Consultation on the development of regional guidelines on vitamin D supplementation for the WHO Eastern Mediterranean Region. In *WHO Regional Office for the Eastern Mediterranean* (pp. 1–14). https://applications.emro.who.int/docs/WHOEMNUT313E-eng.pdf.

Wyon, M. A., Wolman, R., Martin, C., & Galloway, S. (2021). The efficacy of different vitamin D supplementation delivery methods on serum 25(OH)D: A randomised double-blind placebo trial. *Clinical Nutrition, 40*(2), 388–393. https://doi.org/10.1016/j.clnu.2020.05.040.

Yang, J. (2023). Using nutrigenomics to guide personalized nutrition supplementation for bolstering immune system. *Health Information Science and Systems, 11*(1). https://doi.org/10.1007/s13755-022-00208-5.

Yoon, Y. S., Lee, H. I., & Oh, S. W. (2024). A life-stage approach to precision nutrition: A narrative review. *Cureus, 16*(8). https://doi.org/10.7759/cureus.66813.

Yu, C. K. H., Sykes, L., Sethi, M., Teoh, T. G., & Robinson, S. (2009). Vitamin D deficiency and supplementation during pregnancy. *Clinical Endocrinology, 70*(5), 685–690. https://doi.org/10.1111/j.1365-2265.2008.03403.x.

Yu, S. B., Lee, Y., Oh, A., Yoo, H. W., & Choi, J. H. (2020). Efficacy and safety of parenteral vitamin D therapy in infants and children with vitamin D deficiency caused by intestinal malabsorption. *Annals of pediatric endocrinology & metabolism, 25*(2), 112–117. https://doi.org/10.6065/apem.1938142.071.

Zareie, M., Abbasi, A., Faghih, S., & Aguayo, E. (2021). Influence of storage conditions on the stability of vitamin D3 and kinetic study of the vitamin degradation in fortified canola oil during the storage. *Journal of Food Quality, 2021*, 1–9. https://doi.org/10.1155/2021/5599140.

Zittermann, A. (2017). The biphasic effect of vitamin D on the musculoskeletal and cardiovascular system. *International Journal of Endocrinology, 2017*, 1–11. https://doi.org/10.1155/2017/3206240.

CHAPTER 32

Future directions in vitamin D research

Rehana Rehman[1], and Faiza Alam[2]

[1]*Department of Biological & Biomedical Sciences, Aga Khan University, Karachi, Pakistan* [2]*Pengiran-Anak-Puteri-Rashidah-Sa'adatul-Bolkiah Institute of Health Sciences, Universiti Brunei Darussalam, Bandar Seri Begawan, Brunei Darussalam*

32.1 Introduction

Vitamin D (VD) research can pave the way for improved healthcare strategies, precision medicine approaches, enhanced disease prevention and management, and opportunities for research and further exploration. The role of VD supplementation in therapeutic applications, exploration for research advancements, and devising strategic policy reforms for specific populations is addressed.

32.2 Emerging therapeutic roles of vitamin D

32.2.1 Supplementation strategies

It is recommended to have a daily intake of 400 International Units (IU) of VD, with some guidelines suggesting intakes of up to 800 IU/day to meet the target serum levels. For younger children, a "safe intake" of approximately 340–400 IU/day is suggested for ages 0– < 1 year and 400 IU/day for ages 1– < 4 years (Pilz et al., 2018). Future research from observational studies and well-designed RCTs should determine optimal doses, administration methods (oral, intramuscular, or fortified foods), and individualized requirements based on ethnicity, lifestyle, and comorbidities (Grant et al., 2025).

32.2.2 Vitamin D as an adjunct therapy

Ongoing trials should evaluate the potential of VD as an adjunct therapy in various medical conditions, including cancer treatment, infectious diseases, and reproductive health. Understanding synergistic effects with other therapies will improve its clinical applications (Švajger & Rožman, 2019).

32.2.3 Personalized medicine

Exploration of distinct variations involving VD metabolism and requirements may aid in the precision of nutrition and modified supplementation strategies for different health

The Impact of Vitamin D on Health and Disease. DOI: https://doi.org/10.1016/B978-0-443-34037-6.00005-4

conditions, including respiratory infections, mental health, autoimmune diseases, and cancers. Innovations in genomics and epigenetics studies can suggest VD supplementation based on genetic predispositions. Exploration of VD receptor (VDR) gene polymorphisms and metabolic pathways may polish personalized approaches to disease prevention and treatment, as current knowledge on the precise favourable effects of VD remains indecisive and necessitates further intervention (Krivosheev et al., 2023). VD treatment plans should emphasize supplementation strategies considering individual cardiovascular risk profiles, hypertension, and diabetes. Additionally, studies should be designed to identify high-risk subgroups that may have a potential benefit from personalized VD interventions, eventually enhancing cardiovascular health, highlighting the association between low VD levels and increased cardiovascular mortality (Mattioli et al., 2025).

32.2.4 Disease prevention

The role of VD has been explored in osteoporosis by controlling calcium deficiency and supporting overall bone health with a recommended daily dose of 800 IU in osteoporotic patients. Literature supports the prophylactic role of VD supplementation (2000 IU daily) for improvement in bone mineral density and reducing the incidence of fractures (Ahmad et al., 2024). In addition to that, it reduces the chances of falls, which contributes to fracture risk reduction in older adults (Yakabe et al., 2023). The findings emphasize the need for safe sunlight exposure and adequate dietary VD intake to improve maternal health outcomes (Huang et al., 2023).

Research highlights that prospects for VD research involve addressing the controversies surrounding its supplementation and the interpretation of scientific results. There is a need for well-designed randomized controlled trials to clarify its role beyond bone mineralization, as current studies often lack rigor. Additionally, exploring the impact of lifestyle factors on VD levels and supplementation will be crucial in developing evidence-based clinical practices and guidelines for its use in various health contexts. Further studies are essential to determine appropriate dosages and to clarify the role of VD in prevention and treatment strategies across different population groups (Mavar et al., 2024).

Future research prospects for VD should explore its role in the treatment of bone turnover and peripheral neuropathy. Interventional trials to determine the efficacy of VD supplementation in preventing and treating various chronic diseases, including cardiovascular, malignant, and autoimmune diseases, are required. The evolving themes in research, such as oxidative stress and Alzheimer's disease, also present opportunities for deeper exploration of VD's broader health impacts (Fig. 32.1).

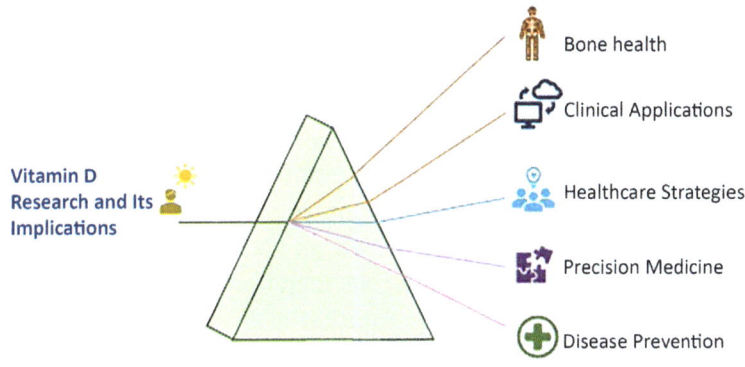

Figure 32.1
Unveiling the mulitfaceted impact of vitamin.

32.3 Advancing vitamin D research

Researchers may aim to clarify the molecular mechanisms by which VD applies its various health effects, including exploration of epigenetic alterations and genetic makeups influencing metabolic flexibility in the VD insufficiency milieu.

Future research is required to address unanswered questions about its broader health roles beyond musculoskeletal health, particularly in immune function and chronic diseases.

1. Assay variability and standardization issues: The lack of standardized methods for measuring serum 25-hydroxyVD [25(OH)D] levels leads to inconsistencies across studies, complicating data interpretation and the establishment of universal guidelines.

2. VD and multiomics integration: Integrative studies incorporating proteomics, metabolomics, and transcriptomics should be carried out to understand VD's role at the cellular and molecular levels and discover novel biomarkers for VD-related disorders and therapeutic targets.

3. Longitudinal studies on vitamin D and chronic diseases: There is a need for long-term, large-scale studies to establish causal relationships between VD status and chronic conditions like cardiovascular diseases, metabolic disorders, cancer, and autoimmune diseases. Investigating VD's impact on disease progression rather than correlation alone will be crucial. Additionally, exploring the long-term effects of VD supplementation on diverse populations, including nonobese individuals, and its interaction with factors such as ethnicity and body mass index (BMI) could provide valuable insights. Investigating the mechanisms by which VD influences glucose metabolism and diabetes progression is needed. Focusing on critically ill patients undergoing continuous renal replacement therapy (CRRT), as they experience significant losses of VD, can be another research domain. The upcoming VITDALIZE trial aims to investigate variations in VD plasma

levels during CRRT and the effects of high doses of cholecalciferol on mortality. Additionally, studies should consider pharmacokinetic variations and the need for tailored dosing strategies, such as loading doses, followed by monitoring blood concentrations to optimize treatment efficacy (Honore et al., 2020). Moreover, research may focus on understanding the genetic and epigenetic factors influencing VD's efficacy, as well as its potential to mitigate severe infections and improve health outcomes in populations with VD deficiency (Cashman, 2021).

4. Microbial transformation approaches: Recent literature links VD and gut microbiota, emphasizing their influence on immune function and metabolic health. Future studies need to probe the cross-talk between VD modulation and microbiome composition, further investigating the validity of targeted VD interventions to improve gut health.

5. Enzyme engineering: Further research may focus on VD synthesis, enhancing its physicochemical properties, and developing proficient delivery channels to diminish its side effects. Identification and engineering of fundamental enzymes and biosynthetic pathways, as well as utilization of microbial transformations to evolve novel VD products with enhanced absorption and function. This may tackle the health concerns related to vitamin deficiency and reduced metabolism, providing a potentially safe therapeutic approach (García-Domínguez et al., 2024).

6. Targeted vitamin D research for at-risk populations: Potential research prospects for VD should focus on specific risk groups rather than the general adult population, as current evidence does not support the efficacy of VD alone for significant health outcomes like fractures, cardiovascular disease, and cancer. Studies should adhere to the Heaney criteria for evaluating threshold nutrients and prioritize individuals with proven or likely VD deficiency.

7. Investigating the synergistic roles of vitamin D: The role of dietary calcium as a co-nutrient remains controversial and warrants further investigation (Sami & Abrahamsen, 2020). Other research projections for VD include designing randomized controlled trials (RCTs) that account for its unique metabolism and nutrient status. Adjustable VD supplementation based on interval serum 25-hydroxy cholecalciferol concentrations is suggested to achieve target levels indicated by observational studies. Additionally, incorporating Hill's criteria for causality and understanding the mechanisms by which VD affects various health outcomes will enhance study designs. This approach could inform medical and public health policies effectively (Grant et al., 2022).

8. VD and climate change: Air pollution, which is influenced by climate change, reduces sunlight exposure and, consequently, VD synthesis in the skin, leading to hypovitaminosis D. This deficiency is associated with obesity and various chronic diseases, suggesting that environmental factors, including pollution exacerbated by climate change, should be avoided to maintain optimal D status and overall health (Barrea et al., 2017). Studies highlight that climate change can reduce UV availability, which is crucial for VD synthesis in populations, particularly in higher latitudes. As ozone levels recover, UV

radiation may decrease, leading to potential VD deficiencies. Specifically, the study estimates reductions in VD-weighted UV daily doses of up to 30% in Antarctica by the century's end if anthropogenic emissions continue to rise, impacting public health due to insufficient VD levels (Correa et al., 2015).

9. Emerging fields: sports, mental health, and aging: Further research is desired to clarify VD's impact on muscle function, injury recovery, and athletic performance. Additionally, studies should investigate its role in mental health disorders, cognitive decline, and age-related diseases. Given the high prevalence of VD deficiency and its potential public health benefits, understanding the causal relationships between VD levels and these diseases is crucial. Additionally, exploring both genomic and nongenomic effects of VD on gene expression and cellular functions will enhance our understanding of its broader health implications (Pilz et al., 2010).

10. Application of advanced technologies: The use of novel large-scale technologies, such as nutrigenomics, nutrigenetics, and nutriepigenetics, will be pivotal in studying VD. These methods allow for comprehensive analyses involving transcriptomics, epigenomics, proteomics, and metabolomics to better understand nutritional pathways.

32.4 Public health initiatives and global policy development

With the prevalence of VD deficiency (levels < 20 ng/mL) in 25% of the United States and 60% of the Central European population, the need for public health initiatives and policy development is globally required to enhance public health (Grant 2025). Research in middle-income countries (LMICs) should emphasize effective public health policies, comprising fortification programs, supplementation policies, and education campaigns to diminish deficiency and related health risks. It is also important that data on the prevalence of deficiency should be carefully considered while planning for public health initiatives like dietary recommendations and supplementation programs (Cashman, 2024).

The strategies include promoting moderate sunlight exposure, encouraging fish consumption, fortifying foods with VD, and recommending VD supplements, particularly for at-risk groups like young children, pregnant women, and older adults. VD fortification in food, like milk and wheat flour, can significantly improve VD supply in populations (Cashman, 2021). Standardized fortification guidelines are held essential to ensure safety and efficacy in addressing VD deficiency by a combination of pharmaceutical interventions and coordinated public health efforts (Alnafisah et al., 2024). In addition to that, it is required to improve knowledge and awareness among the population to enhance supplement intake and address VD deficiency effectively (Saberi-Karimian et al., 2023).

These measures could form the basis for public health policies aimed at improving VD status globally (van Schoor et al., 2024). Nutrition Security: Addressing hidden hunger and ensuring nutrition security, particularly concerning VD intake, will be crucial in alleviating public health

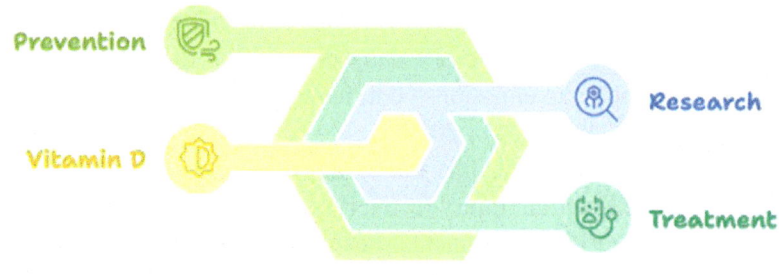

Future Directions of Vitamin D

Figure 32.2
Role of vitamin D in health future directions of vitamin D.

issues related to this micronutrient deficiency (Bendik et al., 2014). Therefore, the government and ministries of health should establish guidelines for the supplementation of VD and provide education and communication to encourage safe supplement use, especially in areas with limited exposure to sunlight (Whiting & Calvo, 2024). Accentuation of a holistic approach to well-being establishment and disease prevention will help in improving the guidelines (Wimalawansa et al., 2024). At the same time, the importance of ongoing evaluation and region-specific policies to optimize VD fortification strategies (Alnafisah et al., 2024) (Fig. 32.2).

AI disclosure

During the preparation of this work, the authors used Napkin to construct figures. After using this tool/service, the authors reviewed and edited the content as needed and took full responsibility for the content of the publication.

References

Ahmad, A., Khushal, A., Ali Shah, S. S., Islam, Z. U., Bashir, A., & Aziz, F. (2024). The role of vitamin D supplementation in preventing osteoporosis in postmenopausal women. *Innovative Research in Applied, Biological and Chemical Sciences, 2*(2), 223–227. https://doi.org/10.62497/irabcs.2024.63.

Alnafisah, R. Y., Alragea, A. S., Alzamil, M. K., & Alqahtani, A. S. (2024). The impact and efficacy of vitamin D fortification. *Multidisciplinary Digital Publishing Institute (MDPI), Saudi Arabia Nutrients, 16*(24). https://doi.org/10.3390/nu16244322, http://www.mdpi.com/journal/nutrients/.

Barrea, L., Savastano, S., Di Somma, C., Savanelli, M. C., Nappi, F., Albanese, L., Orio, F., & Colao, A. (2017). Low serum vitamin D-status, air pollution and obesity: A dangerous liaison. *Reviews in Endocrine and Metabolic Disorders, 18*(2), 207–214. https://doi.org/10.1007/s11154-016-9388-6.

Bendik, I., Friedel, A., Roos, F. F., Weber, P., & Eggersdorfer, M. (2014). Vitamin D: A critical and essential micronutrient for human health. *Frontiers Research Foundation, Switzerland Frontiers in Physiology, 5*. https://doi.org/10.3389/fphys.2014.00248, http://journal.frontiersin.org/Journal/10.3389/fphys.2014.00248/full.

Cashman, K. D. (2021). Global view of per capita daily vitamin D supply estimates as proxy measures for vitamin D intake data. *JBMR Plus, 5*(12). https://doi.org/10.1002/jbm4.10547, https://asbmr.onlinelibrary.wiley.com/journal/24734039.

Cashman, K. D. (2024). Vitamin D and other micronutrient deficiency prevention: The role of data in informing national, regional, and global policy. Cambridge University Press, Ireland. *Proceedings of the Nutrition Society.* https://doi.org/10.1017/S0029665124007626, http://journals.cambridge.org/PNS.

de Paula Correa, G. R., Godin-Beekmann, M., & Mahé, E. (2015). Climate change effects on the erythemal and vitamin D weighted UV daily doses in South America and Antartica: Impacts on the health of populations.

García-Domínguez, M., Gutiérrez-del-Río, I., Villar, C. J., Perez-Gomez, A., Sancho-Martinez, I., & Lombó, F. (2024). Structural diversification of vitamin D using microbial biotransformations. *SApplied Microbiology and Biotechnology, 108*(1). https://doi.org/10.1007/s00253-024-13244-w, https://www.springer.com/journal/253.

Grant, W. B., Boucher, B. J., Al Anouti, F., & Pilz, S. (2022). Comparing the evidence from observational studies and randomized controlled trials for nonskeletal health effects of vitamin D. *MDPI, United States Nutrients, 14*(18). https://doi.org/10.3390/nu14183811, http://www.mdpi.com/journal/nutrients/.

Grant, W. B., Wimalawansa, S. J., Pludowski, P., & Cheng, R. Z. (2025). Vitamin D: Evidence-based health benefits and recommendations for population guidelines. *Nutrients, 17*(2). https://doi.org/10.3390/nu17020277, http://www.mdpi.com/journal/nutrients/.

Honore, P. M., Mugisha, A., Kugener, L., Redant, S., Attou, R., Gallerani, A., & De Bels, D. (2020). Who may benefit most from future vitamin D intervention trials: Do not forget patients on continuous renal replacement therapy. *Critical Care, 24*(1). https://doi.org/10.1186/s13054-020-02910-w, http://ccforum.com/content/17.

Huang, Y. L., Pham, T. T. M., Chen, Y. C., Chang, J. S., Chao, J. C. J., & Bai, C. H. (2023). Effects of climate, sun exposure, and dietary intake on vitamin D concentrations in pregnant women: A population-based study. *MDPI, Taiwan Nutrients, 15*(5). https://doi.org/10.3390/nu15051182, http://www.mdpi.com/journal/nutrients/.

Krivosheev, V. V., Kozlovsky, I. V., Nikitina, L. U., & Fedorov, A. V. (2023). International experience of drug correction of vitamin D level depending on its initial level in blood serum and the age of the patient (review and mathematical analysis). *Sanitarnyj vrač (Sanitary Doctor)*, (8), 521–534. https://doi.org/10.33920/med-08-2308-05.

Mattioli, A. V., Coppi, F., Severino, P., Penna, C., Pagliaro, P., Dei Cas, A., Bucciarelli, V., Madonna, R., Tarperi, C., Schena, F., Cetrullo, S., Angelone, T., Rocca, C., Parenti, A., Palazzuoli, A., Margonato, A., Paolillo, S., Perrone Filardi, P., Barillà, F., ... Fedele, F. (2025). A personalized approach to vitamin D supplementation in cardiovascular health beyond the bone: An expert consensus by the Italian National Institute for Cardiovascular Research. *Multidisciplinary Digital Publishing Institute (MDPI), Italy Nutrients, 17*(1). https://doi.org/10.3390/nu17010115, http://www.mdpi.com/journal/nutrients/.

Mavar, M., Sorić, T., Bagarić, E., Sarić, A., & Matek Sarić, M. (2024). The power of vitamin D: Is the future in precision nutrition through personalized supplementation plans? *Nutrients, 16*(8), 1176. https://doi.org/10.3390/nu16081176.

Pilz, S., Trummer, C., Pandis, M., Schwetz, V., Aberer, F., Grübler, M., Verheyen, N., Tomaschitz, A., & März, W. (2018). Vitamin D: Current guidelines and future outlook. *Anticancer Research, 38*(2), 1145–1151. https://doi.org/10.21873/anticanres.12333, http://ar.iiarjournals.org/content/38/2/1145.full.pdf.

Pilz, S., Fahrleitner-Pammer, A., Polt, G., Grammer, T., Dobnig, H., & März, W. (2010). Vitamin-D-Mangel – Ein Risikofaktor für kardiovaskuläre Erkrankungen und mehr. *Der Klinikarzt, 39*(03), 120–128. https://doi.org/10.1055/s-0030-1253320.

Saberi-Karimian, M., Ghazizadeh, H., Zanganeh Baygi, M., Minaie, M., Sadeghi, F., Pouraram, H., Elmadfa, I., Esmaily, H., Khadem Rezaian, M., Tavallaei, S., Mohammadi Bajgiran, M., Zare Feyz-abadi, R., Timar, A., Sharifan, P., Bahrami Taghanaki, H. R., Gholian, M., Farahmand, S. K., Abasalti, Z., Farkhani, E. M., ... Ghayour-Mobarhan, M. (2023). The national health program for vitamin D supplementation in a developing country. *Clinical Nutrition ESPEN, 54*, 52–59. https://doi.org/10.1016/j.clnesp.2023.01.012, http://www.journals.elsevier.com/clinical-nutrition-espen.

Sami, A., & Abrahamsen, B. (2020). The latest evidence from vitamin D intervention trials for skeletal and nonskeletal outcomes. *Calcified Tissue International, 106*(1), 88–93. https://doi.org/10.1007/s00223-019-00616-y, http://link.springer.de/link/service/journals/00223/index.htm.

Švajger, U., & Rožman, P. J. (2019). Synergistic effects of interferon-γ and vitamin D3 signaling in induction of ILT-3highPDL-1high tolerogenic dendritic cells. *Frontiers Media S.A., Slovenia Frontiers in Immunology, 10*. https://doi.org/10.3389/fimmu.2019.02627, https://www.frontiersin.org/journals/immunology#.

van Schoor, N., de Jongh, R., & Lips, P. (2024). *Worldwide vitamin D status*. Elsevier BV, 47–75. http://doi.org/10.1016/b978-0-323-91338-6.00004-5.

Whiting, S. J., & Calvo, M. S. (2024). *Vitamin D supplement use as a public health strategy to augment diet and sustain population adequacy*. Elsevier BV, 115–133. http://doi.org/10.1016/b978-0-323-91338-6.00007-0.

Yakabe, M., Hosoi, T., Matsumoto, S., Fujimori, K., Tamaki, J., Nakatoh, S., Ishii, S., Okimoto, N., Kamiya, K., Akishita, M., Iki, M., & Ogawa, S. (2023). Prescription of vitamin D was associated with a lower incidence of hip fractures. *Scientific Reports, 13*(1). https://doi.org/10.1038/s41598-023-40259-6.

Index

Note: Page numbers followed by "*f*" and "*t*" refer to figures and tables, respectively.

Printed and bound by CPI Group (UK) Ltd, Croydon, CR0 4YY

18/12/2025

02021940-0006